WHAT IS A CALORIE?

Americans, on average, consume 2,095 calories a day: men eat more at 2,478 calories per day, while women eat less, roughly 1,732 calories per day. The number of calories in a food is determined by burning the food. The amount of heat produced by the burning food is measured and converted into calories. The same thing happens when food is used, or "burned," in your body—it gives off heat. By measuring the amount of heat given off by the body, the calorie cost of keeping you going can be measured. That's also how the number of calories used in jogging, bicycling, cleaning house, and other activities is determined. Your daily level of activity must burn as many calories as you consume, or you gain weight!

ANNETTE B. NATOW, Ph.D., R.D., and JO-ANN HESLIN, M.A., R.D., are the authors of twenty-one books on nutrition. Both are former faculty members of Adelphi University and the State University of New York, Downstate Medical Center. They are editors of the *Journal of Nutrition for the Elderly,* serve as editorial board members for the *Environmental Nutrition Newsletter,* and are frequent conbributors to magazines and journals.

Books by Annette B. Natow and Jo-Ann Heslin

The Antioxidant Vitamin Counter
The Calorie Counter
The Cholesterol Counter (Fourth Edition)
The Diabetes Carbohydrate and Calorie Counter
The Fast Food Nutrition Counter
The Fat Attack Plan
The Fat Counter (Fourth Edition)
The Iron Counter
Megadoses
No-Nonsense Nutrition for Kids
The Pocket Encyclopedia of Nutrition
The Pocket Fat Counter
The Pocket Protein Counter
The Pregnancy Nutrition Counter
The Protein Counter
The Sodium Counter
The Supermarket Nutrition Counter (Second Edition)

Published by POCKET BOOKS

THE
CALORIE
COUNTER

**Annette B. Natow, Ph.D., R.D.
and Jo-Ann Heslin, M.A., R.D.**

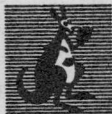

POCKET BOOKS

New York   London   Toronto   Sydney   Tokyo   Singapore

An *Original* Publication of POCKET BOOKS

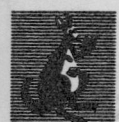

POCKET BOOKS, a division of Simon & Schuster Inc.
1230 Avenue of the Americas, New York, NY 10020

Copyright © 1997 by Jo-Ann Heslin and Annette Natow

ISBN: 0-671-89474-9

First Pocket Books printing September 1997

10 9 8 7 6 5 4 3 2 1

POCKET and colophon are registered trademarks of Simon & Schuster Inc.

Cover design by Kevin McKeveny

Printed in the U.S.A.

To our families, who support us through every project:
Harry, Allen, Irene, Sarah, Meryl, Laura, Marty, George,
Emily, Steven, Joe, Kristen and Karen

ACKNOWLEDGMENTS

Without the tireless cooperation of Steven and Stephen, *The Calorie Counter* would never have been completed. Our thanks to all the food manufacturers and processors who shared product information. A special thanks to our editor, Gary Goldstein, and our agent, Nancy Trichter.

"Man is to be compared to a clock, going all the time, rather than to an automobile engine, working only at intervals. . . . In order to have energy to spend . . . we must first acquire it . . . protein, fat and carbohydrate . . . are the fuels which supply energy for the human machine."

MARY SWARTZ ROSE, Ph.D.
Feeding the Family
The Macmillan Company, 1919

SOURCES OF DATA

———◇———

Values in this counter have been obtained from the Composition of Foods, United States Department of Agriculture, Agricultural Handbooks: No. 8-1, Dairy and Egg Products; No. 8-2, Spices and Herbs; No. 8-3, Baby Foods; No. 8-4, Fats and Oils; No. 8-5, Poultry Products; No. 8-6, Soups, Sauces and Gravies; No. 8-7, Sausages and Luncheon Meats; No. 8-8, Breakfast Cereals; No. 8-9, Fruit and Fruit Juices; No. 8-10, Pork Products; No. 8-11, Vegetables and Vegetable Products; No. 8-12, Nut and Seed Products; No. 8-13, Beef Products; No. 8-14, Beverages; No. 8-15, Finfish and Shellfish Products; No. 8-16, Legumes and Legume Products; No. 8-17, Lamb, Veal and Game Products; No. 8-18, Baked Products; No. 8-19, Snacks and Sweets; No. 8-20, Cereal Grains and Pasta; No. 8-21, Fast Foods; Supplements 1989, 1990, 1991, 1992.

"Nutritive Value of Foods." United States Department of Agriculture, Home and Garden Bulletin No. 72.

J. Davies and J. Dickerson, *Nutrient Content of Food Portions*. Cambridge, UK: The Royal Society of Chemistry, 1991.

G. A. Leveille, M. E. Zabik, and K. J. Morgan, *Nutrients in Foods*. Cambridge, MA: The Nutrition Guild, 1983.

A. Moller, E. Saxholt, and B. E. Mikkelsen, *Food Composition Tables: Amino-acids, Carbohydrates and Fatty Acids in Danish Foods*. 1991.

Souci, Fachman, and Kraut, *Food Composition and Nutrition Tables*. Stuttgart: Wissenschaftliche Verlagsgesellschaft MbH, 1989.

Information from food labels, manufacturers and processors. The values are based on research conducted prior to 1997. Manufacturers' ingredients are subject to change, so current values may vary from those listed in the book. If the serving size on the package label is different from that listed in this counter, use the nutrition information provided as a guide. If the nutrition information listed in the Nutrition Facts panel is different from the information in this counter, assume that the product has been recently reformulated.

INTRODUCTION

—◇—

Regardless of what you heard from experts or read in the newspaper CALORIES STILL COUNT.

The correct message is simple: EXCESS CALORIES PUT ON POUNDS. Every 3500 calories you eat that you don't use to keep your body going winds up being stored as one pound of fat. This message got muddied lately as a lot of emphasis was put on reducing fat. The implication was that if you were careful about how much fat you ate, you could forget about calories. That simply is not true. Calories count. Over the last ten years fat consumption has been going down steadily and at the same time weight keeps going up. One third of Americans are over-weight—8 percent more than a decade ago. A study from the National Institutes of Health shows that Americans aged 25 to 30 now weigh an average of 171 pounds up from 161 pounds in 1986.

While reducing the amount of fat you eat is good advice to keep you healthy, you cannot disregard the total number of calories you eat if you want to maintain or get to your best weight. Some lowfat foods, and even foods labeled reduced fat, still contain lots of calories. Eating too much of them will sabotage your efforts to stay at your best weight. This is where *The Calorie Counter* will help. In it you'll find calorie counts for more than 22,000 foods, so you can easily find out how many calories are in the foods you eat.

CALORIES—CAUTION: Americans are eating 230 calories more each day than they did in 1978. These calories add up!

Eating too many calories can make you fat and that can increase your risk for:

heart attack
stroke
high blood pressure
high blood cholesterol and triglyceride levels
diabetes
some cancers
gall bladder disease
gout
hiatus hernia
indigestion
osteoarthritis
foot problems
surgery complications
short periods of not breathing while sleeping (sleep apnea)

WHAT IS A CALORIE?

The number of calories in a food is determined by burning the food. The amount of heat produced by the burning food is measured and converted into calories. The same thing happens when food is used or "burned" in your body—it gives off heat. By measuring the amount of heat given off, the calorie cost of keeping the body going can be measured. That's also how the number of calories used up in jogging, bicycling, cleaning house and other activities is measured. Americans, on average, consume 2,095 calories a day. Men eat more—2,478 calories, women less—1,732 calories.

CALORIES IN FOOD

Practically everything you eat and drink contains calories, except for water. The carbohydrate, protein and fat in foods supply the calories. Carbohydrate and protein each contain 4 calories in a gram (about ¼ of a teaspoon) while fat has more than double that amount, 9 calories in a gram.

For example, a teaspoon of sugar, all carbohydrate, or unsweetened gelatin, all protein, has 16 calories, while a teaspoon of oil, all fat, has 40 calories.

It follows that foods that are high in fat contain more calories than foods that are high in carbohydrate or protein. On the other hand, foods that are high in water and indigestible fiber, like vegetables and fruits, have fewer calories. It gets complicated because most foods and drinks are combinations of carbohydrate, protein, fat, water and, often, fiber, so the best way for you to find out how many calories are in a specific food is to look it up in *The Calorie Counter.*

How Many Calories Do You Need?

It depends on your best weight.

1. How to find your best weight

You can always look at one of those height/weight charts. But which one? There are several, and experts don't agree on which one to use. One simple approach is to use your weight in your early twenties as a benchmark. If your weight was normal then, that's a good weight to maintain for the rest of your life, if you can. Still another easy and reliable way to estimate your best weight is to use the following simple formulas.

BMI—BODY MASS INDEX

BMI is often used to determine if a person is overweight. Weight and height are calculated together to estimate body fat.

To figure your BMI:

1. Multiply your weight in pounds by 700.
2. Divide that number by height in inches.
3. Then divide that result by height in inches again.

Desirable body fat levels increase as people age. An easy rule of thumb you can use as a guide is: a person is overweight with a BMI of 25 to 30, while a BMI of more than 30 indicates obesity.

Women: Give yourself 100 pounds for the first 5 feet of your height and add 5 pounds for each additional inch over 5 feet (or subtract 5 pounds for each inch under 5 feet). For example, if you're 5 feet, 4 inches tall:

   100 pounds (for first 5 feet)
   <u>+ 20 pounds</u> (4 additional inches times 5 pounds each)
   120 pounds is a good weight

Men: Give yourself 106 pounds for the first 5 feet of your height and add 6 pounds for each additional inch over 5 feet (or subtract 6 pounds for each inch under 5 feet). For example, if you're 5 feet, 9 inches tall:

   106 pounds (for the first 5 feet)
   <u>+ 54 pounds</u> (9 additional inches times 6 pounds each)
   160 pounds is a good weight

2. How many calories do you need to maintain or to reach your best weight?

You can make a pretty good estimate of the number of calories you need each day once you have figured out your best weight. The more active you are, the more calories you need:

13 calories a pound if you are not very active
15 calories a pound if you are moderately active
17 calories a pound if you are very active
20 calories a pound if you are extremely active

For example, if you are moderately active and your best weight is 145 pounds, you need 2175 calories a day to maintain your weight (145 X 15 calories = 2175 calories).

You can see that calories and activity go hand in hand. The more active you are, the more calories you use up. And you don't have to run in a marathon to make this work for you. Besides using up calories, new research points to the value of moderate activity in improving health and fitness. A paper published by a group of 20 health and fitness experts in the *Journal of the American Medical Association* recommends that every American adult accumulate 30 minutes or more of moderate intensity physical activity every day. This includes walking, climbing stairs, gardening or even cleaning house. And the thirty minutes do not have to be done all at once. Activity throughout the day adds up. In the words of former United States Surgeon General C. Everett Koop, "Just get off your seat and on your feet."

Keep moving—it adds up:
Take the stairs, instead of an elevator
Park your car at the far end of the parking lot
For short errands, walk instead of taking the car
When you have just a few dishes, wash them by hand
Use hand power instead of electric appliances when beating, mixing, slicing food or opening cans

Using Your Calorie Counter

This book lists the calorie content of more than 22,000 foods. Now you can compare the calorie values in your favorite foods and choose substitutes for them before you go out to grocery shop or to eat. This will help you save time while making choices when you are deciding what to buy or eat.

The Calorie Counter has foods listed alphabetically. For each category, you will find nonbranded (generic) foods listed first, in alphabetical order, followed by an alphabetical listing of brand-name foods. The nonbranded listing will help you determine fat values for foods when you do not find your favorite brand listed. They also help you to evaluate generic and store brands. Large categories are divided into subcategories such as canned, fresh, frozen, and refrigerated to make it easier to find what you are looking for. Many categories have take-out and home-recipe subcategories. Look there for foods you take-out or order in a store or restaurant because these foods are not nutrition labeled.

Most foods are listed alphabetically. But in some cases, foods are grouped by category. For example, a tuna salad sandwich and tuna salad are found under the category TUNA DISHES. Other group categories include:

DEFINITIONS

———◇———

as prep (as prepared): refers to food that has been prepared according to package directions

home recipe: describes homemade dishes; those included can be used as a guide to the fat values of similar products you may prepare or take-out food you buy ready-to-eat

lean and fat: describes meat with some fat on its edges that is not cut away before cooking or poultry prepared with skin and fat as purchased

lean only: lean portion, trimmed of all visible fat

shelf stable: refers to prepared products found on the supermarket shelf that are ready to eat or be heated and do not require refrigeration

take-out: describes prepared dishes that you purchase ready-to-eat; those included serve as a guide to the fat values of similar products you may purchase

ABBREVIATIONS

———◇———

avg	=	average
diam	=	diameter
fl	=	fluid
frzn	=	frozen
g	=	gram
in	=	inch
lb	=	pound
lg	=	large
med	=	medium
mg	=	milligram
oz	=	ounce
pkg	=	package
pt	=	pint
prep	=	prepared
qt	=	quart
reg	=	regular
serv	=	serving
sm	=	small
sq	=	square
tbsp	=	tablespoon
tr	=	trace
tsp	=	teaspoon
w/	=	with
w/o	=	without
<	=	less than

EQUIVALENT MEASURES

———◇———

3 teaspoons	=	1 tablespoon
4 tablespoons	=	¼ cup
8 tablespoons	=	½ cup
12 tablespoons	=	¾ cup
16 tablespoons	=	1 cup
1000 milligrams	=	1 gram
28 grams	=	1 ounce

Liquid Measurements

2 tablespoons	=	1 ounce
2 ounces	=	¼ cup
4 ounces	=	½ cup
6 ounces	=	¾ cup
8 ounces	=	1 cup
2 cups	=	1 pint
4 cups	=	1 quart

Dry Measurements

4 ounces	=	¼ pound
8 ounces	=	½ pound
12 ounces	=	¾ pound
16 ounces	=	1 pound

NOTES

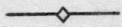

Discrepancies in figures are due to rounding, product reformulation and reevaluation. Labeling law allows rounding of values. Because most of the data is analysis data, obtained directly from manufacturers and not from labels, in some cases our values may not be exactly the same as label information, because they have not been rounded.

NOTES

Discrepancies in figures are due to rounding, product reformulation and reevaluation. Labeling law allows rounding of values. Because most of the data is analysis data, obtained directly from manufacturers and not from labels, in some cases our values may not be exactly the same as label information, because they have not been rounded.

BRAND-NAME,

GENERIC,

AND

TAKE-OUT FOODS

PART · ONE

BRAND-NAME,

GENERIC,

AND

TAKE-OUT FOODS

FOOD	PORTION	CALS.
ABALONE		
fresh fried	3 oz	161
raw	3 oz	89
ACEROLA		
fresh	1	2
ACEROLA JUICE		
juice	1 cup	51
ADZUKI BEANS		
CANNED		
sweetened	1 cup	702
Eden		
Organic	½ cup (4.1 oz)	100
DRIED		
cooked	1 cup	294
READY-TO-USE		
yokan sliced	3¼ in slices	112
AKEE		
fresh	3½ oz	223
ALE		
(see BEER AND ALE, MALT)		
ALFALFA		
sprouts	1 tbsp	1
sprouts	1 cup	40
ALLIGATOR		
tail cooked	3½ oz	143
ALLSPICE		
ground	1 tsp	5
ALMONDS		
almond butter honey & cinnamon	1 tbsp	96
almond butter w/ salt	1 tbsp	101
almond butter w/o salt	1 tbsp	101
almond meal	1 oz	116
almond paste	1 oz	127
dried blanched	1 oz	166
dried unblanched	1 oz	167
dry roasted unblanched	1 oz	167
dry roasted unblanched salted	1 oz	167
oil roasted blanched	1 oz	174
oil roasted blanched salted	1 oz	174

FOOD	PORTION	CALS.
oil roasted unblanched	1 oz	176
toasted unblanched	1 oz	167
Beer Nuts		
Almonds	1 pkg (1 oz)	180
Dole		
Blanched Slivered	1 oz	170
Blanched Whole	1 oz	170
Chopped Natural	1 oz	170
Sliced Natural	1 oz	170
Whole Natural	1 oz	170
Erewhon		
Almond Butter	1 tbsp (16 g)	90
Hain		
Almond Butter Natural Raw	2 tbsp	190
Almond Butter Toasted	2 tbsp	220
Lance		
Smoked	1 pkg (0.7 oz)	120
Nutella		
Spread	1 tbsp (0.5 oz)	85
Planters		
Almonds	1 oz	170
Gold Measure Slivered	1 pkg (2 oz)	340
Honey Roasted	1 oz	160

AMARANTH
(*see also* CEREAL, COOKIES)

cooked	½ cup	59
uncooked	½ cup	366
Arrowhead		
Seeds	¼ cup (1.6 oz)	170
Health Valley		
Amaranth Cereal With Bananas	½ cup (1 oz)	110
Amaranth Crunch With Raisins	¼ cup (1 oz)	110
Amaranth Flakes 100% Organic	½ cup (1 oz)	90
Fast Menu Amaranth With Garden Vegetables	7½ oz	140

ANASAZI BEANS
DRIED

Arrowhead		
Dried	¼ cup (1.5 oz)	150
Bean Cuisine		
Dried	½ cup	115

FOOD	PORTION	CALS.
ANCHOVY		
CANNED		
in oil	5	42
in oil	1 can (1.6 oz)	95
FRESH		
fillets	3 (0.4 oz)	21
raw	3 oz	62
ANGLERFISH		
raw	3½ oz	72
ANISE		
seed	1 tsp	7
ANTELOPE		
roasted	3 oz	127
APPLE		
CANNED		
sliced sweetened	1 cup	136
Luck's		
Fried Apples	8 oz	190
White House		
Escalloped Apples	4 oz	120
Sliced	4 oz	55
Spiced Apple Rings	1 ring	25
DRIED		
cooked w/ sugar	½ cup	116
cooked w/o sugar	½ cup	172
rings	10	155
Del Monte		
Sliced	⅓ cup (1.4 oz)	80
Mariani		
Apples	¼ cup	150
Sonoma		
Pieces	10-12 pieces (1.4 oz)	110
FRESH		
apple	1	81
w/o skin sliced	1 cup	62
w/o skin sliced & cooked	1 cup	91
w/o skin sliced & microwaved	1 cup	96
Dole		
Apple	1	80
Tastee		
Candy Apple	1 (3 oz)	160
Caramel Apple	1 (3 oz)	160

FOOD	PORTION	CALS.
FROZEN		
sliced w/o sugar	½ cup	41
Mrs. Paul's		
Apple Fritters	2	270
Stouffer's		
Escalloped	1 cup (6 oz)	180
APPLE JUICE		
frzn as prep	1 cup	111
frzn not prep	6 oz	349
juice	1 cup	116
After The Fall		
Organic	1 bottle (10 oz)	110
Vermont Apple	1 bottle (8 oz)	90
Vermont Apple	1 bottle (10 oz)	110
Vermont Harvest Moon Sparkling Apple Cider	8 fl oz	110
Apple & Eve		
Cider	6 fl oz	80
Juice	6 fl oz	80
Nothin' But Juice	6 fl oz	78
Bruce		
Lite	½ cup	88
Hi-C		
Jammin' Apple	8 fl oz	130
Hood		
Select Cider	1 cup (8 oz)	120
Juice Works	6 oz	100
Minute Maid		
Box	8.45 fl oz	120
Juices To Go	1 can (11.5 fl oz)	160
Juices To Go	1 bottle (10 fl oz)	140
Naturals	8 fl oz	110
Mott's		
From Concentrate as prep	8 fl oz	120
Fruit Basket Cocktail as prep	8 fl oz	120
Natural	8 fl oz	120
Ocean Spray		
Juice	8 fl oz	110
Odwalla		
Live Apple	8 fl oz	140
Red Cheek		
From Concentrate	8 fl oz	120
Natural	8 fl oz	120

FOOD	PORTION	CALS.
S&W		
100% Unsweetened	6 oz	85
Seneca		
Clarified frzn, as prep	8 fl oz	120
Granny Smith frzn as prep	8 fl oz	120
Natural frzn as prep	8 fl oz	120
Sippin' Pak		
100% Pure	8.45 fl oz	110
Sipps		
Juice	8.45 oz	130
Snapple		
Apple Crisp	10 fl oz	140
Tree Of Life		
East Coast Apple	8 fl oz	120
Tree Top		
Cider	6 oz	90
Cider frzn as prep	6 oz	90
Frzn, as prep	6 oz	90
Juice	6 oz	90
Sparkling Juice	6 oz	90
Unfiltered	6 oz	90
Unfiltered frzn as prep	6 oz	90
w/ Vitamin C	6 oz	90
Tropicana		
Season's Best	8 fl oz	110
Season's Best	1 bottle (10 fl oz)	140
Season's Best	1 container (6 fl oz)	80
Season's Best	1 container (8 fl oz)	110
Season's Best	1 container (10 fl oz)	140
Season's Best	1 bottle (7 fl oz)	100
Season's Best	1 can (11.5 fl oz)	160
Veryfine		
100%	8 oz	107
White House		
Juice	6 oz	90
APPLESAUCE		
sweetened	½ cup	97
unsweetened	½ cup	53
Eden		
Applesauce	½ cup (4.3 oz)	50
Mott's		
Chunky	5 oz	110
Cinnamon	5 oz	120

FOOD	PORTION	CALS.
Mott's (CONT.)		
Fruit Snacks Apple Spice	4 oz	70
Fruit Snacks Cinnamon	4 oz	90
Fruit Snacks Strawberry	4 oz	80
Fruit Snacks Sweetened	4 oz	90
Sweetened	5 oz	110
S&W		
Diet	½ cup	55
Gravenstein Sweetened	½ cup	90
Gravenstein Unsweetened	½ cup	55
Sweetened	½ cup	55
Unsweetened	½ cup	25
Seneca		
Cinnamon	½ cup	100
Golden Delicious	½ cup	100
McIntosh	½ cup	100
Natural	½ cup	60
Regular	½ cup	100
Tree Of Life		
Applesauce	½ cup (4.3 oz)	50
Tree Top		
Cinnamon	½ cup	80
Natural	½ cup	60
Original	½ cup	80
White House		
Chunky	4 oz	80
Cinnamon	4 oz	100
Natural Packed w/ Apple Juice	4 oz	60
Regular	4 oz	80
Unsweetened	4 oz	50

APRICOT JUICE

FOOD	PORTION	CALS.
nectar	1 cup	141
Del Monte		
Nectar	8 fl oz	140
Kern's		
Nectar	6 fl oz	110
Libby		
Nectar	1 can (11.5 fl oz)	220
S&W		
Nectar	6 oz	35

APRICOTS
CANNED

FOOD	PORTION	CALS.
halves heavy syrup pack w/ skin	1 cup (9.1 oz)	214

FOOD	PORTION	CALS.
halves water pack w/ skin	1 cup (8.5 oz)	65
halves water pack w/o skin	1 cup (8 oz)	51
heavy sirup w/ skin	3 halves	70
juice pack w/ skin	3 halves	40
light sirup w/ skin	3 halves	54
puree from heavy syrup pack w/ skin	¾ cup (9.1 oz)	214
puree from light pack w/ skin	¾ cup (8.9 oz)	160
puree from water pack w/ skin	¾ cup (8.5 oz)	65
water pack w/ skin	3 halves	22
water pack w/o skin	4 halves	20
Del Monte		
Halves Unpeeled In Heavy Syrup	½ cup (4.5 oz)	100
Halves Unpeeled Lite	½ cup (4.3 oz)	60
Libby		
Halves Unpeeled Lite	½ cup (4.4 oz)	60
S&W		
Halves Diet	½ cup	35
Halves Unpeeled In Heavy Syrup	½ cup	110
Halves Unsweetened	½ cup	35
Whole Peeled Diet	½ cup	28
Whole Peeled In Heavy Syrup	½ cup	100
DRIED		
halves	10	83
halves cooked w/o sugar	½ cup	106
Del Monte		
Sun Dried	⅓ cup (1.4 oz)	80
Mariani		
Apricots	¼ cup	140
Sonoma		
Dried	10 pieces (1.4 oz)	120
FRESH		
apricots	3	51
FROZEN		
sweetened	½ cup	119

ARROWHEAD
fresh boiled	1 med (⅓ oz)	9

ARROWROOT
flour	1 cup	457

ARTICHOKE
CANNED
Progresso
Hearts	2 pieces (2.9 oz)	35

FOOD	PORTION	CALS.
Progresso (CONT.)		
Hearts Marinated	⅓ cup (3 oz)	160
S&W		
Hearts Marinated	½ cup	225
FRESH		
boiled	1 med (4 oz)	60
hearts cooked	½ cup	42
sunchoke raw sliced	½ cup	57
Dole		
Large	1	23
FROZEN		
cooked	1 pkg (9 oz)	108
Birds Eye		
Hearts Deluxe	½ cup	30
ARUGULA		
raw	½ cup	2
ASPARAGUS		
CANNED		
spears	½ cup	24
Del Monte		
Salad Tips Tender Green	½ cup (4.4 oz)	20
Spears Cut Tender Green	½ cup (4.4 oz)	20
Spears Extra Long Tender Green	½ cup (4.4 oz)	20
Spears Tender Green	½ cup (4.4 oz)	20
Tips Tender Green	½ cup (4.4 oz)	20
Owatonna		
Spears Cut	½ cup	20
S&W		
Points Water Pack	½ cup	17
Spears Colossal Fancy	½ cup	20
Spears Fancy	½ cup	18
Seneca		
Asparagus	½ cup	20
FRESH		
cooked	4 spears	14
cooked	½ cup	22
raw	½ cup	16
raw	4 spears	14
Dole		
Spears	5	18
FROZEN		
cooked	4 spears	17
cooked	1 pkg (10 oz)	82

FOOD	PORTION	CALS.
Big Valley		
Spears	5-6 (3 oz)	20
Birds Eye		
Cut	½ cup	23
Spears	½ cup	25
Green Giant		
Harvest Fresh Cuts	½ cup	25

AVOCADO
FRESH

California Avocado	½	153
California Avocado, mashed	1 cup	407
avocado	1	324
puree	1 cup	370

BABY FOOD
Nutritional guidelines for infants are different from those recommended for older children and adults. Check with a pediatrician for advice on feeding children under the age of 2.

BAKED SELECTIONS

Gerber		
Chunky Animal Cookies	2 (0.5 oz)	60
Chunky Biter Biscuits	1 (0.4 oz)	50
Chunky Zwieback Toast	2 (0.5 oz)	70
Graduates Animal Crackers Cinnamon	2 (0.2 oz)	30
Graduates Arrowroot Cookies	2 (0.4 oz)	50
Graduates Pretzels	2 (0.4 oz)	45

CEREAL

Beech-Nut		
Stage 1 Barley	½ oz	60
Stage 1 Oatmeal	½ oz	60
Stage 1 Oatmeal & Apples	1 jar (4 oz)	70
Stage 1 Rice	½ oz	60
Stage 2 Mixed	½ oz	50
Stage 2 Mixed & Apples	1 jar (4 oz)	70
Stage 2 Oatmeal & Chiquita Bananas	½ oz	60
Stage 2 Rice & Apples	1 jar (4 oz)	70
Stage 2 Rice & Chiquita Bananas	½ oz	60
Stage 2 Rice & Golden Delicious Apples	½ oz	60
Earth's Best		
Brown Rice	5 tbsp (0.5 oz)	60
Mixed Grain	5 tbsp (0.5 oz)	60
Peach Oatmeal Banana	1 jar (4.5 fl oz)	60
Prunes & Oatmeal	1 jar (4.5 fl oz)	100

FOOD	PORTION	CALS.
Gerber		
1st Foods Barley	4 tbsp (0.5 oz)	60
1st Foods Oatmeal	4 tbsp (0.5 oz)	50
1st Foods Rice	4 tbsp (0.5 oz)	60
2nd Foods High Protein	4 tbsp (0.5 oz)	50
2nd Foods Mixed	4 tbsp (0.5 oz)	60
2nd Foods Mixed With Applesauce & Bananas	1 jar (4 oz)	90
2nd Foods Mixed With Banana	4 tbsp (0.5 oz)	60
2nd Foods Oatmeal With Applesauce & Bananas	1 jar (4 oz)	90
2nd Foods Oatmeal With Bananas	4 tbsp (0.5 oz)	60
2nd Foods Rice With Applesauce & Bananas	1 jar (4 oz)	90
2nd Foods Rice With Bananas	4 tbsp (0.5 oz)	60
3rd Foods Mixed With Applesauce & Bananas	1 jar (6 oz)	140
3rd Foods Oatmeal With Applesauce & Bananas	1 jar (6 oz)	140
3rd Foods Rice With Mixed Fruit	1 jar (6 oz)	130
Tropical Foods Corn Cereal	4 tbsp (0.5 oz)	60
Tropical Foods Rice With Mango	4 tbsp (0.5 oz)	50
Health Valley		
Brown Rice 100% Organic	1 tbsp (0.5 oz)	60
Sprouted Baby Cereal 100% Organic	1 tbsp (0.5 oz)	60
DESSERT		
Beech-Nut		
Stage 2 Apple & Strawberry Dessert	1 jar (4 oz)	100
Stage 2 Apple Peach & Strawberry Dessert	1 jar (4 oz)	100
Stage 2 Apple Yogurt Dessert	1 jar (4 oz)	100
Stage 2 Banana Pineapple Dessert	1 jar (4 oz)	100
Stage 2 Banana Pudding (Spanish Label)	1 jar (4 oz)	110
Stage 2 Banana Yogurt Dessert	1 jar (4 oz)	120
Stage 2 Cottage Cheese With Pears Dessert	1 jar (4 oz)	120
Stage 2 Dutch Apple Dessert	1 jar (4 oz)	100
Stage 2 Flan De Vanilla	1 jar (4 oz)	120
Stage 2 Fruit Dessert	1 jar (4 oz)	80
Stage 2 Frutas Islenas Dessert	1 jar (4 oz)	100
Stage 2 Guava Tropical Fruit Dessert	1 jar (4 oz)	90
Stage 2 Mango Tropical Fruit Dessert	1 jar (4 oz)	110
Stage 2 Mixed Fruit Yogurt Dessert	1 jar (4 oz)	100
Stage 2 Papaya Tropical Fruit Dessert	1 jar (4 oz)	100
Stage 2 Vanilla Custard Pudding	1 jar (4 oz)	120

FOOD	PORTION	CALS.
Beech-Nut (CONT.)		
Stage 3 Cottage Cheese With Pears	1 jar (6 oz)	180
Stage 3 Fruit Dessert	1 jar (6 oz)	120
Stage 3 Mixed Fruit Yogurt Dessert	1 jar (6 oz)	170
Stage 3 Vanilla Custard Pudding	1 jar (6 oz)	190
Gerber		
2nd Foods Banana Apple Dessert	1 jar (4 oz)	80
2nd Foods Banana Yogurt Dessert	1 jar (4 oz)	90
2nd Foods Cherry Vanilla Pudding	1 jar (4 oz)	80
2nd Foods Dutch Apple	1 jar (4 oz)	100
2nd Foods Fruit Dessert	1 jar (4 oz)	100
2nd Foods Hawaiian Delight	1 jar (4 oz)	90
2nd Foods Mixed Fruit Yogurt Dessert	1 jar (4 oz)	90
2nd Foods Peach Cobbler	1 jar (4 oz)	90
2nd Foods Peach Yogurt Dessert	1 jar (4 oz)	90
2nd Foods Vanilla Custard Pudding	1 jar (4 oz)	100
3rd Foods Dutch Apple	1 jar (6 oz)	130
3rd Foods Fruit Dessert	1 jar (6 oz)	120
3rd Foods Hawaiian Delight	1 jar (6 oz)	150
3rd Foods Peach Cobbler	1 jar (6 oz)	130
3rd Foods Vanilla Custard Pudding	1 jar (6 oz)	150
Tropical Foods Banana Vanilla Dessert	1 jar (4 oz)	100
Tropical Foods Guava With Tapioca	1 jar (4 oz)	80
Tropical Foods Mango Banana Passion Fruit	1 jar (4 oz)	80
Tropical Foods Mango With Tapioca	1 jar (4 oz)	80
Tropical Foods Papaya Pineapple Dessert	1 jar (4 oz)	90
Tropical Foods Papaya With Tapioca	1 jar (4 oz)	70
Tropical Foods Peaches Mango	1 jar (4 oz)	80
DINNER		
Beech-Nut		
Stage 2 Beef & Egg Noodle	1 jar (4 oz)	100
Stage 2 Beef Supreme	1 jar (4 oz)	130
Stage 2 Chicken & Rice	1 jar (4 oz)	80
Stage 2 Chicken Noodle	1 jar (4 oz)	70
Stage 2 Chicken Soup	1 jar (4 oz)	90
Stage 2 Turkey Supreme	1 jar (4 oz)	90
Stage 2 Vegetable Chicken	1 jar (4 oz)	80
Stage 2 Vegetable Ham	1 jar (4 oz)	80
Stage 2 Vegetable Lamb	1 jar (4 oz)	80
Stage 2 Vegetables Turkay Rice	1 jar (4 oz)	70
Stage 3 Beef & Egg Noodle	1 jar (6 oz)	130
Stage 3 Chicken Noodle	1 jar (6 oz)	110
Stage 3 Macaroni & Beef	1 jar (6 oz)	130

FOOD	PORTION	CALS.
Beech-Nut (CONT.)		
Stage 3 Spaghetti & Beef	1 jar (6 oz)	130
Stage 3 Turkey Rice	1 jar (6 oz)	100
Stage 3 Vegetable Chicken	1 jar (6 oz)	110
Table Time Chicken & Stars	1 bowl (6 oz)	150
Table Time Macaroni & Cheese	1 bowl (6 oz)	200
Table Time Seashells In Tomato Sauce	1 bowl (6 oz)	150
Table Time Spaghetti Rings In Meat Sauce	1 bowl (6 oz)	160
Table Time Turkey Stew With Rice	1 bowl (6 oz)	150
Table Time Vegetable Stew With Beef	1 bowl (6 oz)	110
Earth's Best		
Corn Rice & Cheese Dinner	1 jar (4.5 fl oz)	120
Macaroni & Cheese	1 jar (4.5 oz)	100
Pasta Dinner	1 jar (4.5 fl oz)	90
Potato & Green Bean Dinner	1 jar (4.5 fl oz)	100
Rice & Lentil Dinner	1 jar (4.5 fl oz)	80
Summer Vegetable Dinner	1 jar (4.5 oz)	90
Gerber		
2nd Foods Apples & Chicken	1 jar (4 oz)	70
2nd Foods Apples & Ham	1 jar (4 oz)	70
2nd Foods Apples & Turkey	1 jar (4 oz)	80
2nd Foods Beef Egg Noodle	1 jar (4 oz)	80
2nd Foods Broccoli & Chicken	1 jar (4 oz)	50
2nd Foods Carrots & Beef	1 jar (4 oz)	70
2nd Foods Chicken Noodle	1 jar (4 oz)	70
2nd Foods Green Beans & Turkey	1 jar (4 oz)	70
2nd Foods Macaroni Cheese	1 jar (4 oz)	80
2nd Foods Macaroni Tomato Beef	1 jar (4 oz)	70
2nd Foods Turkey Rice	1 jar (4 oz)	70
2nd Foods Vegetable Bacon	1 jar (4 oz)	90
2nd Foods Vegetable Beef	1 jar (4 oz)	70
2nd Foods Vegetable Chicken	1 jar (4 oz)	70
2nd Foods Vegetable Ham	1 jar (4 oz)	70
2nd Foods Vegetable Turkey	1 jar (4 oz)	60
3rd Foods Beef Egg Noodle	1 jar (6 oz)	110
3rd Foods Chicken Noodle	1 jar (6 oz)	100
3rd Foods Macaroni Tomato Beef	1 jar (6 oz)	110
3rd Foods Spaghetti Tomato Sauce Beef	1 jar (6 oz)	120
3rd Foods Turkey Rice	1 jar (6 oz)	100
3rd Foods Vegetable Beef	1 jar (6 oz)	120
3rd Foods Vegetable Chicken	1 jar (6 oz)	100
3rd Foods Vegetable Ham	1 jar (6 oz)	110
3rd Foods Vegetable Turkey	1 jar (6 oz)	100
Chunky Homestyle Noodles & Beef	1 jar (6 oz)	150

FOOD	PORTION	CALS.
Gerber (CONT.)		
Chunky Macaroni Alphabets With Beef & Sauce	1 jar (6.3 oz)	140
Chunky Noodles & Chicken With Carrots & Peas	1 jar (6 oz)	110
Chunky Rice With Beef & Tomato Sauce	1 jar (6.3 oz)	140
Chunky Saucy Rice With Chicken	1 jar (6 oz)	120
Chunky Spaghetti Tomato Sauce Beef	1 jar (6.3 oz)	150
Chunky Vegetables & Beef	1 jar (6.3 oz)	130
Chunky Vegetables & Chicken	1 jar (6.3 oz)	140
Chunky Vegetables & Ham	1 jar (6.3 oz)	130
Chunky Vegetables & Turkey	1 jar (6.3 oz)	110
Graduates Chicken Stew With Noodles	1 bowl (6 oz)	120
Graduates Macaroni And Beef in Sauce	1 bowl (6 oz)	150
Graduates Spaghetti With Mini Meatballs & Sauce	1 bowl (6 oz)	160
Graduates Tomato Sauce With Beef Ravioli	1 bowl (6 oz)	170
Graduates Tomato Sauce With Cheese Ravioli	1 bowl (6 oz)	170
Graduates Turkey Stew With Rice	1 bowl (6 oz)	100
Graduates Vegetable Stew With Beef	1 bowl (6 oz)	130
Tropical Foods Beans & Rice	1 jar (4 oz)	60
FRUIT		
Beech-Nut		
Stage 1 Applesauce Golden Delicious	1 jar (2.5 oz)	50
Stage 1 Applesauce Golden Delicious	1 jar (4 oz)	70
Stage 1 Bananas Chiquita	1 jar (2.5 oz)	70
Stage 1 Bananas Chiquita	1 jar (4 oz)	110
Stage 1 Chiquita Bananas With Pears & Apples	1 jar (4 oz)	90
Stage 1 Peaches Yellow Cling	1 jar (2.5 oz)	45
Stage 1 Peaches Yellow Cling	1 jar (4 oz)	70
Stage 1 Pears Bartlett	1 jar (2.5 oz)	50
Stage 1 Pears Bartlett	1 jar (4 oz)	70
Stage 2 Apples & Apricots	1 jar (4 oz)	70
Stage 2 Apples & Bananas	1 jar (4 oz)	60
Stage 2 Apples & Blueberries	1 jar (4 oz)	70
Stage 2 Apples & Cherries	1 jar (4 oz)	80
Stage 2 Apples & Pears	1 jar (4 oz)	80
Stage 2 Apples Pears & Bananas	1 jar (4 oz)	90
Stage 2 Apricots With Pears & Apples	1 jar (4 oz)	90
Stage 2 Bartlett Pears & Pineapple	1 jar (4 oz)	70
Stage 2 Peaches & Bananas	1 jar (4 oz)	70
Stage 2 Plums With Apples & Rice	1 jar (4 oz)	90

FOOD	PORTION	CALS.
Beech-Nut (CONT.)		
Stage 2 Prunes With Pears	1 jar (4 oz)	110
Stage 3 Apples & Bananas	1 jar (6 oz)	90
Stage 3 Apples & Cherries	1 jar (6 oz)	110
Stage 3 Applesauce	1 jar (6 oz)	100
Stage 3 Apricots With Pears & Apples	1 jar (6 oz)	130
Stage 3 Bananas Chiquita	1 jar (6 oz)	160
Stage 3 Peaches	1 jar (6 oz)	100
Stage 3 Pears Bartlett	1 jar (6 oz)	110
Earth's Best		
Apples	1 jar (4.5 oz)	70
Apples & Apricots	1 jar (4.5 fl oz)	70
Apples & Blueberries	1 jar (4.5 fl oz)	70
Apples & Plums	1 jar (4.5 fl oz)	70
Bananas	1 jar (4.5 oz)	90
Pear	1 jar (4.5 fl oz)	60
Plums Bananas & Rice	1 jar (4.5 fl oz)	90
Gerber		
1st Foods Applesauce	1 jar (2.5 oz)	25
1st Foods Bananas	1 jar (2.5 oz)	70
1st Foods Peaches	1 jar (2.5 oz)	30
1st Foods Pears	1 jar (2.5 oz)	40
1st Foods Prunes	1 jar (2.5 oz)	70
2nd Foods Apple Blueberry	1 jar (4 oz)	50
2nd Foods Applesauce	1 jar (4 oz)	60
2nd Foods Applesauce Apricot	1 jar (4 oz)	60
2nd Foods Apricots With Tapioca	1 jar (4 oz)	80
2nd Foods Banana With Pineapple & Tapioca	1 jar (4 oz)	60
2nd Foods Banana With Tapioca	1 jar (4 oz)	90
2nd Foods Peaches	1 jar (4 oz)	70
2nd Foods Pear Pineapple	1 jar (4 oz)	60
2nd Foods Pears	1 jar (4 oz)	60
2nd Foods Plums With Tapioca	1 jar (4 oz)	80
2nd Foods Prunes With Tapioca	1 jar (4 oz)	90
JUICE		
Beech-Nut		
Stage 1 Apple	4 fl oz	60
Stage 1 Pear	4 fl oz	60
Stage 1 White Grape	4 fl oz	100
Stage 2 Apple Banana	4 fl oz	70
Stage 2 Apple Cherry	4 fl oz	70
Stage 2 Apple Cranberry	4 fl oz	60
Stage 2 Apple Grape	4 fl oz	70

FOOD	PORTION	CALS.
Beech-Nut (CONT.)		
Stage 2 Juice Plus Grape	4 fl oz	100
Stage 2 Mango Nectar (Spanish Label)	4 fl oz	80
Stage 2 Mixed Fruit	4 fl oz	70
Stage 2 Papaya Nectar (Spanish Label)	4 fl oz	80
Stage 2 Tropical Blend	4 fl oz	90
Stage 2 Tropical Blend Nectar (Spanish Label)	4 fl oz	90
Stage 3 Orange	4 fl oz	60
Earth's Best		
Apple	1 bottle (4.2 fl oz)	60
Apple Banana	1 bottle (4.2 fl oz)	60
Apple Grape	1 bottle (4.2 fl oz)	60
Apples & Bananas	1 jar (4.5 fl oz)	80
Pear	1 bottle (4.2 fl oz)	60
Gerber		
1st Foods Apple	4 fl oz	60
1st Foods Pear	4 fl oz	60
1st Foods Red Grape	4 fl oz	80
1st Foods White Grape	4 fl oz	80
2nd Foods Apple Banana	4 fl oz	60
2nd Foods Apple Cherry	4 fl oz	60
2nd Foods Apple Grape	4 fl oz	60
2nd Foods Apple Peach	4 fl oz	60
2nd Foods Apple Plum	4 fl oz	60
2nd Foods Apple Prune	4 fl oz	60
2nd Foods Apple With Yogurt	4 fl oz	100
2nd Foods Mixed Fruit	4 fl oz	60
2nd Foods Mixed Fruit with Yogurt	4 fl oz	100
2nd Foods Orange	4 fl oz	60
2nd Foods Pear Peach With Yogurt	4 fl oz	90
3rd Foods Apple Carrot	4 fl oz	50
3rd Foods Apple Sweet Potato	4 fl oz	60
3rd Foods Orange Carrot	4 fl oz	50
3rd Foods Pineapple Carrot	4 fl oz	60
Graduates Apple	4 fl oz	80
Graduates Apple Banana	4 fl oz	90
Graduates Apple Cherry	4 fl oz	80
Graduates Apple Grape	4 fl oz	90
Tropical Foods Guava With Mixed Fruit	4 fl oz	70
Tropical Foods Mango With Mixed Fruit	4 fl oz	70
Tropical Foods Papaya With Mixed Fruit	4 fl oz	70
MEAT		
Beech-Nut		
Stage 1 Beef & Broth	1 jar (2.5 oz)	90

FOOD	PORTION	CALS.
Beech-Nut (CONT.)		
Stage 1 Chicken & Broth	1 jar (2.5 oz)	70
Stage 1 Lamb & Broth	1 jar (2.5 oz)	60
Stage 1 Turkey & Broth	1 jar (2.5 oz)	90
Stage 1 Veal & Broth	1 jar (2.5 oz)	60
Gerber		
2nd Foods Beef	1 jar (2.5 oz)	80
2nd Foods Chicken	1 jar (2.5 oz)	90
2nd Foods Egg Yolks	1 jar (2.5 oz)	130
2nd Foods Ham	1 jar (2.5 oz)	90
2nd Foods Lamb	1 jar (2.5 oz)	80
2nd Foods Turkey	1 jar (2.5 oz)	80
2nd Foods Veal	1 jar (2.5 oz)	70
3rd Foods Beef	1 jar (2.5 oz)	80
3rd Foods Chicken	1 jar (2.5 oz)	90
3rd Foods Ham	1 jar (2.5 oz)	90
3rd Foods Turkey	1 jar (2.5 oz)	90
3rd Foods Veal	1 jar (2.5 oz)	80
Graduates Chicken Sticks	1 jar (2.5 oz)	110
Graduates Meat Sticks	1 jar (2.5 oz)	110
Graduates Turkey Sticks	1 jar (2.5 oz)	120
VEGETABLE		
Beech-Nut		
Stage 1 Butternut Squash	1 jar (2.5 oz)	30
Stage 1 Butternut Squash	1 jar (4 oz)	50
Stage 1 Carrots Sweet Tender	1 jar (4 oz)	50
Stage 1 Carrots Tender Sweet	1 jar (2.5 oz)	30
Stage 1 Green Beans (Spanish Label)	1 jar (2.5 oz)	20
Stage 1 Green Beans Tender Young	1 jar (4 oz)	35
Stage 1 Peas Tender Sweet	1 jar (4 oz)	60
Stage 1 Peas Tender Sweet	1 jar (2.5 oz)	40
Stage 1 Sweet Potatoes Tender Golden	1 jar (2.5 oz)	50
Stage 1 Sweet Potatoes Tender Golden	1 jar (4 oz)	80
Stage 2 Carrots & Peas	1 jar (4 oz)	50
Stage 2 Creamed Corn	1 jar (4 oz)	90
Stage 2 Garden Vegetables	1 jar (4 oz)	50
Stage 2 Mixed Vegetables	1 jar (4 oz)	45
Stage 3 Carrots	1 jar (6 oz)	70
Stage 3 Green Beans	1 jar (6 oz)	50
Stage 3 Sweet Potatoes	1 jar (6 oz)	110
Earth's Best		
Carrots	1 jar (4.5 fl oz)	40
Carrots & Parsnips	1 jar (4.5 fl oz)	60
Corn & Butternut Squash	1 jar (4.5 fl oz)	90

FOOD	PORTION	CALS.
Earth's Best (CONT.)		
Garden Vegetables	1 jar (4.5 fl oz)	70
Green Beans & Rice	1 jar (4.5 fl oz)	40
Peas & Brown Rice	1 jar (4.5 fl oz)	80
Spinach & Potatoes	1 jar (4.5 fl oz)	60
Sweet Potatoes	1 jar (4.5 fl oz)	60
Winter Squash	1 jar (4.5 fl oz)	50
Gerber		
1st Foods Carrots	1 jar (2.5 oz)	25
1st Foods Green Beans	1 jar (2.5 oz)	25
1st Foods Peas	1 jar (2.5 oz)	30
1st Foods Squash	1 jar (2.5 oz)	25
1st Foods Sweet Potatoes	1 jar (2.5 oz)	45
2nd Foods Beets	1 jar (4 oz)	45
2nd Foods Carrots	1 jar (4 oz)	30
2nd Foods Creamed Corn	1 jar (4 oz)	80
2nd Foods Creamed Spinach	1 jar (4 oz)	50
2nd Foods Garden Vegetables	1 jar (4 oz)	45
2nd Foods Green Beans	1 jar (4 oz)	35
2nd Foods Mixed Vegetables	1 jar (4 oz)	50
2nd Foods Peas	1 jar (4 oz)	60
2nd Foods Squash	1 jar (4 oz)	35
2nd Foods Sweet Potatoes	1 jar (4 oz)	70
3rd Foods Broccoli Carrots Cheese	1 jar (6 oz)	80
3rd Foods Carrots	1 jar (6 oz)	50
3rd Foods Creamed Green Beans	1 jar (6 oz)	80
3rd Foods Mixed Vegetables	1 jar (6 oz)	70
3rd Foods Peas	1 jar (6 oz)	80
3rd Foods Squash	1 jar (6 oz)	60
3rd Foods Sweet Potatoes	1 jar (6 oz)	100
Graduates Carrots	1 jar (4.5 oz)	30
Graduates Green Beans	1 jar (4.5 oz)	30
Graduates Peas	1 jar (4.5 oz)	60
Graduates Potatoes	1 jar (4.5 oz)	50
BACON		
(*see also* BACON SUBSTITUTES)		
breakfast strips cooked	3 strips (34 g)	156
breakfast strips beef cooked	3 strips (34 g)	153
cooked	3 strips	109
gammon lean & fat grilled	4.2 oz	274
grilled	2 slices (1.7 oz)	86
Armour		
Lower Salt cooked	1 strip	38

FOOD	PORTION	CALS.
Armour (CONT.)		
Star cooked	1 strip	38
Black Label		
Center Cut cooked	3 slices (0.5 oz)	70
Cooked	2 slices (0.5 oz)	80
Low Salt cooked	2 slices (0.5 oz)	80
Hillshire		
Bacon	1 slice	120
Hormel		
Bacon Bits	1 tsp (7 g)	30
Bacon Pieces	1 tsp (7 g)	25
Microwave cooked	2 slices (0.5 oz)	70
Jones		
Sliced	1 slice	130
Nathan's		
Beef cooked	3 slices	100
Old Smokehouse		
Cooked	2 slices (0.5 oz)	80
Oscar Mayer		
Bacon Bits	1 tbsp (7 g)	25
Center Cut cooked	3 slices (0.5 oz)	70
Cooked	2 slices (0.4 oz)	60
Lower Sodium cooked	2 slices (0.5 oz)	60
Thick Cut cooked	1 slice (0.4 oz)	50
Range Brand		
Cooked	2 slices (0.7 oz)	100
Red Label		
Cooked	2 slices (0.5 oz)	80
Shannon		
Irish	1 oz	70
BACON SUBSTITUTES		
bacon substitute	1 strip	25
Bac-Os		
Pieces	2 tsp (5 g)	25
Harvest Direct		
Bacon Bits	3.5 oz	320
Lightlife		
Fakin' Bacon	3 strips (2 oz)	79
Louis Rich		
Turkey Bacon	1 slice (0.5 oz)	30
McCormick		
Bac'n Pieces	2 tsp	20
Morningstar Farms		
Breakfast Strips	3 (25 g)	80

FOOD	PORTION	CALS.
Mr. Turkey		
Slice	1	25
Worthington		
Stripples	4 strips (33 g)	120
BAGEL		
FRESH		
cinnamon raisin	1 (3½ in)	194
cinnamon raisin toasted	1 (3½ in)	194
egg	1 (3½ in)	197
egg toasted	1 (3½ in)	197
oat bran	1 (3½ in)	181
oat bran toasted	1 (3½ in)	181
onion	1 (3½ in)	195
plain	1 (3½ in)	195
plain toasted	1 (3½ in)	195
poppy seed	1 (3½ in)	195
Alvarado St. Bakery		
Sprouted Wheat	1 (3.3 oz)	260
Sprouted Wheat Cinnamon/Raisin	1 (3.3 oz)	280
Sprouted Wheat Onion/Poppyseed	1 (3.3 oz)	320
Sprouted Wheat Sesame	1 (3.3 oz)	320
FROZEN		
Great Starts		
Ham & Cheese On A Bagel	3 oz	240
Lender's		
Cinnamon'N Raisin	1 (2.5 oz)	200
Egg	1 (2 oz)	150
Onion	1 (2 oz)	160
Plain	1 (2 oz)	150
Sara Lee		
Cinnamon & Raisin	1 (3 oz)	240
Cinnamon Raisin	1 (2.5 oz)	200
Egg	1 (2.5 oz)	200
Egg	1 (3 oz)	250
Oat Bran	1 (2.5 oz)	180
Oat Bran	1 (3 oz)	220
Onion	1 (3 oz)	230
Onion	1 (2.5 oz)	190
Plain	1 (3 oz)	230
Plain	1 (2.5 oz)	190
Poppy Seed	1 (3 oz)	230
Poppy Seed	1 (2.5 oz)	190
Sesame Seed	1 (3 oz)	240

FOOD	PORTION	CALS.
Sara Lee (CONT.)		
Sesame Seed	1 (2.5 oz)	190
Tree Of Life		
Onion	1 (3 oz)	210
Plain	1 (3 oz)	210
Poppy	1 (3 oz)	210
Raisin	1 (3 oz)	210
Sesame	1 (3 oz)	210
Weight Watchers		
Sandwich Ham And Cheese	1 (3 oz)	200

BAKING POWDER

FOOD	PORTION	CALS.
baking powder	1 tsp	2
low sodium	1 tsp	5
Calumet		
Baking Powder	1 tsp	3
Clabber Girl		
Baking Powder	1 tsp	0
Davis		
Baking Powder	1 tsp	6
Watkins		
Baking Powder	¼ tsp (1 g)	0

BAKING SODA

FOOD	PORTION	CALS.
baking soda	1 tsp	0
Arm & Hammer		
Baking Soda	1 tsp	0

BALSAM PEAR

FOOD	PORTION	CALS.
leafy tips cooked	½ cup	10
leafy tips raw	½ cup	7
pods cooked	½ cup	12

BAMBOO SHOOTS

FOOD	PORTION	CALS.
CANNED		
sliced	1 cup	25
Empress		
Sliced	2 oz	14
Ka-Me		
Sliced	½ cup (4.5 oz)	15
La Choy		
Sliced	¼ cup	6
FRESH		
cooked	½ cup	15
raw	½ cup	21

FOOD	PORTION	CALS.
BANANA		
banana chips	1 oz	147
DRIED		
powder	1 tbsp	21
FRESH		
banana	1	105
mashed	1 cup	207
Chiquita		
Fresh	1 (3½ oz)	110
Dole		
Banana	1	120
BANANA JUICE		
Libby		
Nectar	1 can (11.5 fl oz)	190
BARBECUE SAUCE		
(*see also* SAUCE)		
barbecue	1 cup	188
Bull's Eye		
Original	2 tbsp	50
Hain		
Honey	1 tbsp	14
Healthy Choice		
Hickory	2 tbsp (1.1 oz)	26
Hot & Spicy	2 tbsp (1.1 oz)	25
Original	2 tbsp (1.1 oz)	25
Heinz		
Select	1 oz	40
Select Hickory	1 oz	35
Thick & Rich Cajun Style	1 oz	35
Thick & Rich Chunky	1 oz	30
Thick & Rich Hawaiian Style	1 oz	40
Thick & Rich Hickory Smoke	1 oz	35
Thick & Rich Mesquite Smoke	1 oz	30
Thick & Rich Mushroom	1 oz	30
Thick & Rich Old Fashioned	1 oz	35
Thick & Rich Onion	1 oz	30
Thick & Rich Original	1 oz	35
Thick & Rich Texas Hot	1 oz	30
House Of Tsang		
Hong Kong	1 tbsp (0.6 oz)	10
Hunt's		
Hickory	2 tbsp (1.2 oz)	38
Homestyle	1 tbsp	20

FOOD	PORTION	CALS.
Hunt's (CONT.)		
Honey Mustard	1 tbsp (1.2 oz)	50
Light	2 tbsp (1.2 oz)	23
Mesquite Barbecue	2 tbsp (1.2 oz)	40
Mild	2 tbsp (1.2 oz)	41
Mild Dijon	2 tbsp (1.2 oz)	39
Original	2 tbsp (1.2 oz)	39
Texas Style	1 tbsp	25
Kraft		
Char-Grill	2 tbsp (1.2 oz)	60
Extra Rich Original	2 tbsp (1.2 oz)	50
Garlic	2 tbsp (1.2 oz)	40
Hickory Smoke	2 tbsp (1.2 oz)	40
Hickory Smoke Onion Bits	2 tbsp (1.2 oz)	50
Honey	2 tbsp (1.2 oz)	50
Hot	2 tbsp (1.2 oz)	40
Hot Hickory Smoke	2 tbsp (1.2 oz)	40
Italian Seasonings	2 tbsp (1.2 oz)	45
Kansas City Style	2 tbsp (1.2 oz)	45
Mesquite Smoke	2 tbsp (1.2 oz)	40
Onion Bits	2 tbsp (1.2 oz)	50
Original	2 tbsp (1.2 oz)	40
Teriyaki	2 tbsp (1.2 oz)	60
Thick'N Spicy Hickory Smoke	2 tbsp (1.2 oz)	50
Thick'N Spicy Honey	2 tbsp (1.2 oz)	60
Thick'N Spicy Kansas City Style	2 tbsp (1.2 oz)	60
Thick'N Spicy Mesquite Smoke	2 tbsp (1.2 oz)	50
Thick'N Spicy Original	2 tbsp (1.2 oz)	50
Lawry's		
Dijon Honey	¼ cup	203
Maull's		
Beer Non-Alcholic	3.5 oz	128
Regular	3.5 oz	123
Smoky	3.5 oz	124
Sweet-N-Mild	3.5 oz	167
Sweet-N-Smoky	3.5 oz	160
With Onion Bits	3.5 oz	126
Red Wing		
"K" Sauce	2 tbsp (1.2 oz)	45
Watkins		
Bold	2 tsp (0.4 oz)	25
Honey	2 tsp (0.4 oz)	25
Mesquite	2 tsp (0.4 oz)	25
Original	2 tsp (0.4 oz)	25

FOOD	PORTION	CALS.
Watkins (CONT.)		
Smokehouse	2 tsp (0.4 oz)	25
BARLEY		
pearled cooked	½ cup	97
pearled uncooked	½ cup	352
Arrowhead		
Barley	¼ cup (1.7 oz)	170
Hulless	¼ cup (1.6 oz)	140
Quaker		
Medium Pearled	¼ cup	172
Quick Pearled	¼ cup	172
Scotch		
Medium Pearled	¼ cup	172
Quick Pearled	¼ cup	172
BASIL		
fresh chopped	2 tbsp	1
ground	1 tsp	4
leaves fresh	5	1
Watkins		
Liquid Spice	1 tbsp (0.5 oz)	120
BASS		
freshwater raw	3 oz	97
sea cooked	3 oz	105
sea raw	3 oz	82
striped baked	3 oz	105
BAY LEAF		
crumbled	1 tsp	2
Watkins		
Bay Leaves	¼ tsp (0.5 g)	0
BEAN SPROUTS		
(see also individual bean names)		
CANNED		
La Choy	⅔ cup	8
BEANS		
(see also individual names)		
CANNED		
baked beans plain	½ cup	118
baked beans vegetarian	½ cup	118
baked beans w/ beef	½ cup	161
baked beans w/ franks	½ cup	182
baked beans w/ pork	½ cup	133

FOOD	PORTION	CALS.
baked beans w/ pork & sweet sauce	½ cup	140
baked beans w/ pork & tomato sauce	½ cup	123
refried beans	½ cup	134
Allen		
Baked	½ cup (4.5 oz)	150
B&M		
99% Fat Free Baked Beans	½ cup (4.6 oz)	160
Baked With Honey	½ cup (4.7 oz)	170
Barbeque Baked Beans	½ cup (4.7 oz)	170
Brick Oven Baked	½ cup (4.6 oz)	180
Extra Hearty Baked	½ cup (4.6 oz)	190
Brick Oven		
Baked Beans	½ cup	160
Brown Beauty		
Mexican Beans With Jalapeno	½ cup (4.5 oz)	120
Bush's		
Baked	½ cup (4.6 oz)	150
Baked With Onions	½ cup (4.6 oz)	150
Homestyle Baked	½ cup (4.6 oz)	160
Vegetarian	½ cup (4.6 oz)	140
Campbell		
Barbecue Beans	½ can (7⅞ oz)	210
Home Style Beans	½ can (8 oz)	220
Hot Chili Beans	½ can (7¾ oz)	180
Old Fashioned Beans In Molasses & Brown Sugar Sauce	½ can (8 oz)	230
Pork & Beans In Tomato Sauce	½ can (8 oz)	200
Vegetarian	½ can (7¾ oz)	170
Casa Fiesta		
Refried	3.5 oz	110
Chi-Chi's		
Ranchero Beans	½ cup (4.3 oz)	100
Refried	½ cup (4.2 oz)	130
Crest Top		
Pork And Beans	½ cup (4.5 oz)	130
Friend's		
Maple Baked	8 oz	240
Original Baked	½ cup (4.6 oz)	170
Gebhardt		
Chili	4 oz	115
Refried	4 oz	100
Refried Jalapeno	4 oz	115

FOOD	PORTION	CALS.
Green Giant		
Pork And Beans In Tomato Sauce	½ cup	90
Three Bean Salad	½ cup	70
Hanover		
Four Bean Salad	½ cup	80
Health Valley		
Boston Baked	7½ oz	190
Boston Baked No Salt Added	7.5 oz	190
Fast Menu Honey Baked Organic Beans With Tofu Weiner	7½ oz	150
Vegetarian With Miso	7½ oz	180
Heartland		
Iron Kettle Baked	½ cup (4.6 oz)	150
Hormel		
Beans & Wieners	1 can (7.5 oz)	290
Hunt's		
Big John's Beans 'n Fixin's	4 oz	170
Pork And Beans	4 oz	135
Kid's Kitchen		
Beans & Wieners	1 cup (7.5 oz)	310
Little Pancho		
Refried & Green Chili	½ cup	80
Luck's		
Cut Green & Shelled Beans Seasoned w/ Pork	7.25 oz	200
Mixed Beans Seasoned w/ Pork	7.25 oz	200
McIlhenny		
Spicy	1 oz	7
Old El Paso		
Mexe-Beans	½ cup (4.6 oz)	110
Refried	½ cup (4.2 oz)	110
Refried Fat Free	½ cup (4.4 oz)	110
Refried Spicy	½ cup (4.3 oz)	140
Refried Vegetarian	½ cup (4.1 oz)	100
Refried With Cheese	½ cup (4.2 oz)	130
Refried With Green Chilies	½ cup (4.3 oz)	110
Refried With Sausage	½ cup (4.1 oz)	200
Rosarita		
Refried	4 oz	100
Refried Spicy	4 oz	100
Refried Vegetarian	4 oz	100
Refried With Bacon	4 oz	110
Refried With Green Chilies	4 oz	90
Refried With Nacho Cheese	4 oz	110

FOOD	PORTION	CALS.
Rosarita (CONT.)		
Refried With Onions	4 oz	110
S&W		
Barbecue Beans Texas Style	½ cup	135
Maple Sugar Beans	½ cup	150
Mixed Bean Salad Marinated	½ cup	90
Pork 'N Beans	½ cup	130
Smokey Ranch	½ cup	130
Trappey		
Mexi-Beans With Jalapeno	½ cup (4.5 oz)	130
Pork And Beans	½ cup (4.5 oz)	110
Pork And Beans With Jalapeno	½ cup (4.5 oz)	130
Van Camp's		
Baked Beans Fat Free	½ cup (4.6 oz)	130
Baked Beans Premium	½ cup (4.6 oz)	140
Beanee Weenee	1 cup (9 oz)	320
Beanee Weenee Baked Flavor	1 cup (9 oz)	410
Beanee Weenee Barbeque	1 cup (9 oz)	340
Brown Sugar Beans	½ cup (4.6 oz)	170
Mexican Style Chili Beans	½ cup (4.6 oz)	110
Pork And Beans	½ cup (4.6 oz)	110
Vegetarian In Tomato Sauce	½ cup (4.6 oz)	110
Wagon Master		
Pork And Beans	½ cup (4.5 oz)	110
FROZEN		
Hanover		
Romano Bean Medley	½ cup	25
MIX		
Bean Cuisine		
Florentine Beans With Bow Ties	½ cup	199
Pasta & Beans Country French With Gemelli	½ cup	214
TAKE-OUT		
baked beans	½ cup	190
barbecue beans	3.5 oz	120
four bean salad	3.5 oz	100
refried beans	½ cup	43
three bean salad	¾ cup	230

BEAR

simmered	3 oz	220

BEAVER

roasted	3 oz	140
simmered	3 oz	141

FOOD	PORTION	CALS.

BEECHNUTS
dried · 1 oz · 164

BEEF
(see also BEEF DISHES, VEAL)

Beef is graded according to its marbling, the little flecks of fat in the muscle. Beef graded "Prime" has the highest percentage of fat, followed by "Choice" with less fat and "Select" with the least fat.

CANNED

corned beef	1 oz	71
corned beef	3 oz	85

Armour

Chopped Beef	2 oz	170
Corned Beef	2 oz	120
Potted Meat	¼ cup (2.2 oz)	90
Potted Meat	1 can (3 oz)	120
Tripe	3 oz	90

Hormel

Corned Beef	2 oz	120
Potted Meat	4 tbsp (2 oz)	60

Treet

50% Less Fat	2 oz	120
Beef	2 oz	150

Underwood

Roast Beef	2.08 oz	140
Roast Beef Mesquite Smoked	2.08 oz	126
Roast Beef Light	2.08 oz	90

DRIED

Hormel

Pillow Pack	10 slices (1 oz)	45
Sliced	10 slices (1 oz)	50

FRESH

Note that the values for cooked beef may differ slightly from values for raw beef. When meat is cooked some moisture and fat is lost changing the nutrition value slightly. As a rule of thumb it can be assumed that a 4 oz raw portion will equal a 3 oz cooked portion of meat.

bottom round lean & fat trim 0 in Choice roasted	3 oz	172
bottom round lean & fat trim 0 in Select braised	3 oz	171
bottom round lean & fat trim 0 in Select roasted	3 oz	150

FOOD	PORTION	CALS.
bottom round lean & fat trim 0 in braised	3 oz	193
bottom round lean & fat trim ¼ in Choice braised	3 oz	241
bottom round lean & fat trim ¼ in Choice roasted	3 oz	221
bottom round lean & fat trim ¼ in Select braised	3 oz	220
bottom round lean & fat trim ¼ in Select roasted	3 oz	199
brisket flat half lean & fat trim 0 in braised	3 oz	183
brisket flat half lean & fat trim ¼ in braised	3 oz	309
brisket point half lean & fat trim 0 in braised	3 oz	304
brisket point half lean & fat trim ¼ in braised	3 oz	343
brisket whole lean & fat trim 0 in braised	3 oz	247
brisket whole lean & fat trim ¼ in braised	3 oz	327
chuck arm pot roast lean & fat trim 0 in braised	3 oz	238
chuck arm pot roast lean & fat trim ¼ in braised	3 oz	282
chuck blade roast lean & fat trim 0 in braised	3 oz	284
chuck blade roast lean & fat trim ¼ in braised	3 oz	293
corned beef brisket cooked	3 oz	213
eye of round lean & fat trim 0 in Choice roasted	3 oz	153
eye of round lean & fat trim 0 in Select roasted	3 oz	137
eye of round lean & fat trime ¼ in Select roasted	3 oz	184
flank lean & fat trim 0 in braised	3 oz	224
flank lean & fat trim 0 in broiled	3 oz	192
ground extra lean broiled medium	3 oz	217
ground extra lean broiled well done	3 oz	225
ground extra lean fried medium	3 oz	216
ground extra lean fried well done	3 oz	224
ground extra lean raw	4 oz	265
ground lean broiled medium	3 oz	231
ground lean broiled well done	3 oz	238
ground regular broiled medium	3 oz	246
ground regular broiled well done	3 oz	248
ground low-fat w/ carrageenan raw	4 oz	160
porterhouse steak lean & fat trim ¼ in Choice broiled	3 oz	260
porterhouse steak lean only trim ¼ in Prime broiled	3 oz	185

FOOD	PORTION	CALS.
rib eye small end lean & fat trim 0 in Choice broiled	3 oz	261
rib large end lean & fat trim 0 in roasted	3 oz	300
rib large end lean & fat trim ¼ in broiled	3 oz	295
rib large end lean & fat trim ¼ in roasted	3 oz	310
rib small end lean & fat trim 0 in broiled	3 oz	252
rib small end lean & fat trim ¼ in broiled	3 oz	285
rib small end lean & fat trim ¼ in roasted	3 oz	295
rib whole lean & fat trim ¼ in Choice broiled	3 oz	306
rib whole lean & fat trim ¼ in Choice roasted	3 oz	320
rib whole lean & fat trim ¼ in Prime roasted	3 oz	348
rib whole lean & fat trim ¼ in Select broiled	3 oz	274
rib whole lean & fat trim ¼ in Select roasted	3 oz	286
shank crosscut lean & fat trim ¼ in Choice simmered	3 oz	224
short loin top loin lean & fat trim 0 in Choice broiled	1 steak (5.4 oz)	353
short loin top loin lean & fat trim 0 in Choice broiled	3 oz	193
short loin top loin lean & fat trim 0 in Select broiled	1 steak (5.4 oz)	309
short loin top loin lean & fat trim ¼ in Choice braised	3 oz	253
short loin top loin lean & fat trim ¼ in Choice broiled	1 steak (6.3 oz)	536
short loin top loin lean & fat trim ¼ in Prime broiled	1 steak (6.3 oz)	582
short loin top loin lean & fat trim ¼ in Select broiled	1 steak (6.3 oz)	473
short loin top loin lean only trim 0 in Choice broiled	1 steak (5.2 oz)	311
short loin top loin lean only trim ¼ in Choice broiled	1 steak (5.2 oz)	314
shortribs lean & fat Choice braised	3 oz	400
t-bone steak lean & fat trim ¼ in Choice	3 oz	253
t-bone steak lean only trim ¼ in Choice broiled	3 oz	182
tenderloin lean & fat trim 0 in Select broiled	3 oz	194
tenderloin lean & fat trim ¼ in Choice broiled	3 oz	259
tenderloin lean & fat trim ¼ in Choice roasted	3 oz	288
tenderloin lean & fat trim ¼ in Choice broiled	3 oz	208
tenderloin lean & fat trim ¼ in Prime broiled	3 oz	270

FOOD	PORTION	CALS.
tenderloin lean & fat trim ¼ in Select roasted	3 oz	275
tenderloin lean only trim 0 in Select broiled	3 oz	170
tenderloin lean only trim ¼ in Choice broiled	3 oz	188
tenderloin lean only trim ¼ in Select broiled	3 oz	169
tip round lean & fat trim 0 in Choice roasted	3 oz	170
tip round lean & fat trim 0 in Select roasted	3 oz	158
tip round lean & fat trim ¼ in Choice roasted	3 oz	210
tip round lean & fat trim ¼ in Prime roasted	3 oz	233
tip round lean & fat trim ¼ in Select roasted	3 oz	191
top round lean & fat trim 0 in Choice braised	3 oz	184
top round lean & fat trim 0 in Select braised	3 oz	170
top round lean & fat trim ¼ in Choice braised	3 oz	221
top round lean & fat trim ¼ in Choice broiled	3 oz	190
top round lean & fat trim ¼ in Choice fried	3 oz	235
top round lean & fat trim ¼ in Prime broiled	3 oz	195
top round lean & fat trim ¼ in Select braised	3 oz	175
top round lean & fat trim ¼ in Select braised	3 oz	199
top sirloin lean & fat trim 0 in Choice broiled	3 oz	194
top sirloin lean & fat trim 0 in Select broiled	3 oz	166
top sirloin lean & fat trim ¼ in Choice broiled	3 oz	228
top sirloin lean & fat trim ¼ in Choice fried	3 oz	277
top sirloin lean & fat trim ¼ in Select broiled	3 oz	208
tripe raw	4 oz	111
Dakota Lean		
Chuck Roast raw	3 oz	80
Eye Round raw	3 oz	80
Flank Steak raw	3 oz	80
Ground raw	3 oz	88
Outside Round raw	3 oz	80
Ribeye raw	3 oz	90
Sirloin Tip raw	3 oz	90
Strip Loin raw	3 oz	90
Tenderloin raw	3 oz	70
Top Round raw	3 oz	80
Double J		
Filet	3.5 oz	130
NY Strip	3.5 oz	133
Rib Eye	3.5 oz	134
Top Butt	3.5 oz	136
Healthy Choice		
Ground Extra Lean	4 oz	130
Laura's Lean		
Eye Of Round	4 oz	150
Flank Steak	4 oz	160

FOOD	PORTION	CALS.
Laura's Lean (CONT.)		
Ground	4 oz	180
Ground Round	4 oz	160
Ribeye Steak	4 oz	150
Sirloin Tip Round	4 oz	140
Sirloin Top Butt	4 oz	140
Strip Steak	4 oz	150
Tenderloins	4 oz	150
Top Round	4 oz	140
FROZEN		
patties broiled medium	3 oz	240
READY-TO-USE		
Healthy Choice		
Deli-Thin Roast Beef	6 slices (2 oz)	60
Fresh-Trak Roast Beef	1 slice (1 oz)	30
Oscar Mayer		
Deli-Thin Roast Beef	4 slices (1.8 oz)	60
Weight Watchers		
Deli Thin Oven Roasted Cured	5 slices (⅓ oz)	10
TAKE-OUT		
roast beef medium	2 oz	70
roast beef rare	2 oz	70
BEEF DISHES		
CANNED		
corned beef hash	3 oz	155
Armour		
Corned Beef Hash	1 cup (8.3 oz)	440
Roast Beef Hash	1 cup (8.4 oz)	400
Roast Beef In Gravy	½ cup (4.6 oz)	150
Stew	1 cup (8.6 oz)	220
Dinty Moore		
American Classics Roast Beef With Mashed Potatoes	1 bowl (10 oz)	240
Beef Stew	1 can (7.5 oz)	190
Beef Stew	1 cup (8.3 oz)	230
Meatball Stew	1 cup (8.4 oz)	260
Sliced Potatoes & Beef	1 can (7.5 oz)	230
Hormel		
Beef Goulash	1 can (7.5 oz)	230
Corned Beef Hash	1 cup (8.3 oz)	390
Roast Beef Hash	1 cup (8.3 oz)	390
Roast Beef With Gravy	2 oz	60
Mary Kitchen		
Corned Beef Hash	1 can (7.5 oz)	350

FOOD	PORTION	CALS.
Mary Kitchen (CONT.)		
Roast Beef Hash	1 can (7.5 oz)	348
Wolf Brand		
Beef Stew	1 cup	179
FROZEN		
Chefwich		
Beef w/ Barbecue Sauce	1	340
Hot Pocket		
Stuffed Sandwich Barbecue	1 (4.5 oz)	340
Stuffed Sandwich Beef & Cheddar	1 (4.5 oz)	360
Stuffed Sandwich Beef Fajita	1 (4.5 oz)	360
Lean Pockets		
Stuffed Sandwich Beef & Broccoli	1 (4.5 oz)	250
Luigino's		
Creamed Sauce Shaved Cured Beef With Croutons	1 pkg (8 oz)	360
Egg Noodles Rich Gravy Swedish Meatballs	1 cup (7.5 oz)	280
Egg Noodles Rich Gravy Swedish Meatballs	1 pkg (9 oz)	340
Ovenstuffs		
Beef/Cheddar Deli Melt	1 (4.75 oz)	390
Tyson		
Microwave BBQ Sandwich	1 sandwich	200
Weight Watchers		
Reuben Pocket Sandwich	1 (5 oz)	250
MIX		
Casbah		
Gyro as prep	1 patty (2 oz)	145
Hamburger Helper		
Beef Noodle as prep	1 cup	330
Beef Romanoff as prep	1 cup	350
Beef Taco as prep	1 cup	330
Cheddar 'n Bacon as prep	1 cup	380
Cheeseburger Macaroni as prep	1 cup	370
Cheesy Italian as prep	1 cup	370
Chili Macaroni as prep	1 cup	330
Hamburger Hash as prep	1 cup	320
Hamburger Stew as prep	1 cup	300
Lasagne as prep	1 cup	340
Meat Loaf as prep	5 oz	360
Nacho Cheese as prep	1 cup	360
Pizza Dish as prep	1 cup	360
Pizzabake as prep	⅙ pkg (4.5 oz)	320

FOOD	PORTION	CALS.
Hamburger Helper (CONT.)		
Potatoes Stroganoff as prep	1 cup	330
Rice Oriental as prep	1 cup	340
Sloppy Joe Bake as prep	5 oz	340
Spaghetti as prep	1 cup	340
Stroganoff as prep	1 cup	390
Tacobake as prep	⅙ pkg (5.75 oz)	320
Zesty Italian as prep	1 cup	340
SHELF-STABLE		
Dinty Moore		
American Classics Beef Stew	1 bowl (10 oz)	260
American Classics Meatloaf With Mashed Potatoes	1 bowl (10 oz)	300
American Classics Salisbury Steak	1 bowl (10 oz)	310
Microwave Cup Beef Stew	1 cup (7.5 oz)	190
Microwave Cup Corned Beef Hash	1 cup (7.5 oz)	350
Microwave Cup Hearty Burger Stew	1 cup (7.5 oz)	240
Microwave Cup Meatball Stew	1 cup (7.5 oz)	240
Lunch Bucket		
Beef Stew	1 pkg (7.5 oz)	180
Micro Cup Meals		
Beef Stew	1 cup (7.5 oz)	180
TAKE-OUT		
bubble & squeak	5 oz	186
cornish pasty	1 (8 oz)	847
irish stew	1 cup (7 oz)	280
kebab indian	1 (5.4 oz)	553
kheena	6.7 oz	781
koftas	5	280
roast beef sandwich plain	1	346
roast beef sandwich w/ cheese	1	402
roast beef submarine sandwich w/ tomato lettuce & mayonnaise	1	411
samosa	2 (4 oz)	652
shepherds pie	6 oz	196
steak & kidney pie w/ top crust	1 slice (5 oz)	400
steak sandwich w/ tomato lettuce salt & mayonnaise	1	459
stew	6 oz	208
stew w/ vegetables	1 cup	220
stroganoff	¾ cup	260
swiss steak	4.6 oz	214
toad in the hole	1 (4.7 oz)	383

FOOD	PORTION	CALS.
BEEFALO		
roasted	3 oz	160
BEER AND ALE		
ale brown	10 oz	77
ale pale	10 oz	88
beer light	12 oz can	100
beer regular	12 oz can	146
lager	10 oz	80
pilsener lager beer	7 fl oz	85
stout	10 oz	102
Amstel		
Light	12 oz	95
Anheuser Busch		
Natural Light	12 oz	110
Bud		
Light	12 oz	108
Coors		
Beer	12 oz	132
Extra Gold	12 oz	147
Light	12 oz	101
Hamm's		
Beer	12 oz	137
Nonalcoholic	12 oz	55
Killian's		
Beer	12 oz	212
Kingsbury		
Nonalcoholic	12 fl oz	60
Michelob		
Light	12 oz	134
Miller		
Lite	12 oz	96
Molson		
Light	12 oz	109
Old Milwaukee		
Beer	12 oz	145
Light	12 oz	122
Olympia		
Beer	12 oz	143
Pabst		
Beer	12 oz	143
Nonalcoholic	12 oz	55
Piels		
Light	12 oz	136

FOOD	PORTION	CALS.
Schaefer		
Beer	12 oz	138
Light	12 oz	111
Schlitz		
Beer	12 oz	145
Light	12 oz	99
Schmidts		
Light	12 oz	96
Signature		
Beer	12 oz	150
Spirit		
Nonalcoholic	12 oz	80
Stroh		
Beer	12 oz	142
Light	12 oz	115
Winterfest		
Beer	12 oz	167
NONALCOHOLIC		
alcohol free beer	7 fl oz	50
Guiness		
Kaliber	12 oz	43

BEET JUICE
juice	3½ oz	36

BEETS
CANNED		
harvard	½ cup	89
pickled	½ cup	75
sliced	½ cup	27
Del Monte		
Pickled Crinkle Style Sliced	½ cup (4.5 oz)	80
Sliced	½ cup (4.3 oz)	35
Whole	½ cup (4.3 oz)	35
Whole Tiny	½ cup (4.3 oz)	35
S&W		
Diced Tender	½ cup	40
Julienne French Style	½ cup	40
Pickled Whole Extra Small	½ cup	70
Pickled w/ Red Wine Vinegar Sliced	½ cup	70
Sliced Small Premium	½ cup	40
Sliced Water Pack	½ cup	35
Whole Small	½ cup	40
Seneca		
Cut	½ cup	35

FOOD	PORTION	CALS.
Seneca (CONT.)		
Diced	½ cup	35
Harvard	½ cup	90
Pickled	2 tbsp	20
Pickled With Onions	2 tbsp	20
Sliced	½ cup	35
Whole	½ cup	35
FRESH		
greens cooked	½ cup	20
greens raw	½ cup	4
greens raw chopped	½ cup	4
raw sliced	½ cup (2.4 oz)	29
sliced cooked	½ cup (3 oz)	38
whole cooked	2 (3.5 oz)	44
whole raw	2 (5.7 oz)	70

BEVERAGES

(*see* BEER AND ALE, CHAMPAGNE, COFFEE, DRINK MIXERS, FRUIT DRINKS, ICE TEA, MALT, MINERAL WATER/BOTTLED WATER, LIQUOR/LIQUEUR, SODA, TEA/HERBAL TEA, WINE, WINE COOLER)

BISCUIT
FROZEN
Great Starts

FOOD	PORTION	CALS.
Egg Canadian Bacon & Cheese	5.2 oz	420
Sausage	4.7 oz	410
Jimmy Dean		
Chicken Twin	2 (3.2 oz)	280
Sausage Twin	2 (3.4 oz)	330
Steak Twin	2 (3.2 oz)	270
Rudy's Farm		
Ham Twin	2 (3 oz)	160
Sausage & Cheese Twin	2 (3 oz)	290
Sausage Twin	2 (2.7 oz)	296
Weight Watchers		
Sausage Biscuit	1 (3 oz)	230
HOME RECIPE		
buttermilk	1 (2 oz)	212
oatcakes	2 (4 oz)	115
plain	1 (2 oz)	212
MIX		
buttermilk	1 (2 oz)	191
plain	1 (2 oz)	191
Arrowhead		
Biscuit Mix	¼ cup (1.2 oz)	120

FOOD	PORTION	CALS.
Bisquick		
Mix	½ cup (2 oz)	240
Reduced Fat	½ cup (2 oz)	210
Health Valley		
Buttermilk Biscuit Mix not prep	1 oz	100
Jiffy		
As prep	1	150
Biscuit	¼ cup (1.1 oz)	130
Buttermilk as prep	1	170
READY-TO-EAT		
Arnold		
Old Fashioned	1	60
REFRIGERATED		
buttermilk	1 (1 oz)	98
plain	1 (1 oz)	98
1869 Brand		
Baking Powder	1	100
Butter Tastin'	1	100
Buttermilk	1	100
Ballard		
Ovenready	1	50
Ovenready Buttermilk	1	50
Big Country		
Southern Style	1	100
Hungry Jack		
Butter Tastin' Flaky	1	90
Buttermilk Flaky	1	90
Buttermilk Fluffy	1	90
Extra Rich Buttermilk	1	50
Flaky	1	80
Honey Tastin' Flaky	1	90
Pillsbury		
Big Country Butter Tastin'	1	100
Big Country Buttermilk	1	100
Butter	1	50
Buttermilk	1	50
Country	1	50
Deluxe Heat N' Eat Buttermilk	2	170
Good'N Buttery Fluffy	1	90
Hearty Grains Multi-Grain	1	80
Hearty Grains Oatmeal Raisin	1	90
Heat N' Eat Big Premium	2	280
Tender Layer Buttermilk	1	50

FOOD	PORTION	CALS.
Roman Meal		
Biscuit	2 (2.4 oz)	180
Honey Nut Oat Bran	1 (1.5 oz)	131
TAKE-OUT		
buttermilk	1	127
plain	1 (35 g)	276
w/ egg	1	315
w/ egg & bacon	1	457
w/ egg & sausage	1	582
w/ egg & steak	1	474
w/ egg cheese & bacon	1	477
w/ ham	1	387
w/ sausage	1	485
w/ steak	1	456

BISON
roasted	3 oz	122

BLACK BEANS
CANNED

Allen		
Seasoned	½ cup (4.5 oz)	120
Eden		
Organic	½ cup (4.3 oz)	100
Health Valley		
Fast Menu Organic Black Beans With Tofu Weiners	7½ oz	150
Fast Menu Western Black Beans With Garden Vegetable	7½ oz	160
Old El Paso		
Black Beans	½ cup (4.6 oz)	100
Refried	½ cup (4.2 oz)	120
Progresso		
Black Beans	½ cup (4.6 oz)	100
Trappey		
Seasoned	½ cup (4.5 oz)	120
DRIED		
cooked	1 cup	227
MIX		
Bean Cuisine		
Black Turtle	½ cup	115
Pasta & Beans Black Beans With Fusilli	½ cup	174
Mahatma		
Black Beans & Rice	1 cup	200

BLACKBERRIES
CANNED

in heavy syrup	½ cup	118

FOOD	PORTION	CALS.
Allen-Wolco		
Blackberries	½ cup (5.3 oz)	60
FRESH		
blackberries	½ cup	37
FROZEN		
unsweetened	1 cup	97
Big Valley		
Blackberries	⅔ cup (4.9 oz)	70

BLACKEYE PEAS
CANNED		
w/pork	½ cup	199
Allen		
Blackeye Peas	½ cup (4.5 oz)	110
Fresh Shell	½ cup (4.4 oz)	120
With Bacon	½ cup (4.5 oz)	105
With Snaps	½ cup (4.4 oz)	120
Dorman		
Fresh Shell	½ cup (4.4 oz)	120
East Texas Fair		
Blackeye Peas	½ cup (4.5 oz)	110
Fresh Shell	½ cup (4.4 oz)	120
With Snaps	½ cup (4.4 oz)	120
Homefolks		
Fresh Shell	½ cup (4.4 oz)	120
With Jalapeno	½ cup (4.4 oz)	120
With Snaps	½ cup (4.4 oz)	120
Luck's		
Seasoned w/ Pork	7.25 oz	200
Sunshine		
With Bacon	½ cup (4.5 oz)	105
Trappey		
With Bacon	½ cup (4.5 oz)	120
With Bacon & Jalapeno	½ cup (4.4 oz)	110
DRIED		
cooked	1 cup	198
FROZEN		
Fresh Like	3.5 oz	138

BLINTZE
Empire		
Apple	2 (4.4 oz)	220
Blueberry	2 (4.4 oz)	190
Cheese	2 (4.4 oz)	200
Cherry	2 (4.4 oz)	200

FOOD	PORTION	CALS.
Empire (CONT.)		
Potato	2 (4.4 oz)	190
Golden		
Apple Raisin	1 (2.25 oz)	80
Blueberry	1 (2.25 oz)	90
Cheese	1 (2.25 oz)	80
Cherry	1 (2.25 oz)	95
Potato	1 (2.25 oz)	90
TAKE-OUT		
cheese	2	186

BLUEBERRIES
CANNED		
in heavy sirup	1 cup	225
S&W		
In Heavy Syrup	½ cup	111
DRIED		
Sonoma		
Dried	¼ cup (1.3 oz)	140
FRESH		
blueberries	1 cup	82
FROZEN		
unsweetened	1 cup	78
Big Valley		
Blueberries	¾ cup (4.9 oz)	70

BLUEBERRY JUICE
After The Fall		
Maine Coast	1 cup (8 oz)	90

BLUEFIN
fillet baked	4.1 oz	186

BLUEFISH
fresh baked	3 oz	135

BOAR
wild roasted	3 oz	136

BOK CHOY
Dole		
Shredded	½ cup	5

BORAGE
fresh chopped cooked	3½ oz	25
raw chopped	½ cup	9

BOYSENBERRIES
in heavy sirup	1 cup	226
unsweetened frzn	1 cup	66

FOOD	PORTION	CALS.
BOYSENBERRY JUICE		
Smucker's		
Juice	8 oz	120
Juice Sparkler	10 oz	130
BRAINS		
beef pan-fried	3 oz	167
beef simmered	3 oz	136
lamb braised	3 oz	124
lamb fried	3 oz	232
pork, braised	3 oz	117
veal braised	3 oz	115
veal fried	3 oz	181
Armour		
Pork Brains In Milk Gravy	⅔ cup (5.5 oz)	150
BRAN		
corn	⅓ cup	56
oat cooked	½ cup	44
oat dry	½ cup	116
rice dry	⅓ cup	88
wheat dry	½ cup	65
Arrowhead		
Oat Bran	⅓ cup (1.4 oz)	150
Wheat Bran	¼ cup (0.6 oz)	30
Good Shepherd		
Wheat Bran	1 oz	80
H-O		
Super Bran	⅓ cup	110
Health Valley		
Fast Menu Oat Bran Pilaf With Garden Vegetables	7½ oz	210
Hodgson Mill		
Oat	¼ cup (1.3 oz)	120
Wheat	¼ cup (0.5 oz)	30
Kretschmer		
Toasted Wheat Bran	⅓ cup	57
Mother's		
Oat Bran	½ cup	150
Quaker		
Oat Bran	½ cup	150
Unprocessed	2 tbsp	8
Roman Meal		
Oat	1 oz	94

FOOD	PORTION	CALS.
Stone-Buhr		
Oat	⅓ cup (1 oz)	90

BRAZIL NUTS
dried unblanched | 1 oz | 186

BREAD
(*see also* BAGEL, BISCUIT, BREADSTICK, CROISSANT, ENGLISH MUFFIN, MUFFIN, ROLL, SCONE)

FOOD	PORTION	CALS.
CANNED		
boston brown	1 slice (1.6 oz)	88
B&M		
Brown Bread	½ in slice (2 oz)	130
Brown Bread Raisins	½ in slice (2 oz)	130
S&W		
Brown Bread New England Recipe	2 slices	76
FROZEN		
Kineret		
Challah	⅛ loaf (2 oz)	150
HOME RECIPE		
banana	1 slice (2 oz)	195
cornbread as prep w/ 2% milk	1 piece (2.3 oz)	173
cornbread as prep w/ whole milk	1 piece (2.3 oz)	176
datenut	½ in slice	92
irish soda bread	1 slice (2 oz)	174
pita whole wheat	1-6 in	247
pumpkin	1 slice (1 oz)	94
white as prep w/ nonfat dry milk	1 slice	78
white as prep w/ 2% milk	1 slice	81
white as prep w/ whole milk	1 slice	82
whole wheat	1 slice	79
MIX		
cornbread	1 piece (2 oz)	189
Aunt Jemima		
Corn Bread Easy Mix	⅓ cup (1.3 oz)	150
Ballard		
Corn Bread	⅛ bread	140
Dromedary		
Corn Bread	1 piece (2 in x 2 in)	130
Natural Ovens		
Cracked Wheat	2 slices (2.4 oz)	140
English Muffin Bread	2 slices (2.4 oz)	140
Executive Fitness Sunny Millet	2 slices (2.6 oz)	160
Garden Bread	1 oz	50
Glorious Cinnamon & Raisin Fat Free	2 slices (2.1 oz)	110

FOOD	PORTION	CALS.
Natural Ovens (CONT.)		
Honey 'N Flax	2 slices (2.5 oz)	140
Hunger Filler Bread	2 slices (2.1 oz)	110
Light Wheat	2 slices (2.2 oz)	84
Nutty Natural Wheat Bread	2 slices (2.5 oz)	140
Seven Grain Herb	2 slices (2.5 oz)	140
Soft Hearth Whole Wheat	2 slices (2 oz)	100
Soft Sandwich Very Low Fat	2 slices (2.3 oz)	110
Stay Slim	2 slices (2 oz)	100
Zia Foods		
Cornbread Blue Cornmeal	1 piece (1.2 oz)	110
READY-TO-EAT		
cracked wheat	1 slice	65
egg	1 slice (1.4 oz)	115
french	1 loaf (1 lb)	1270
french	1 slice (1 oz)	78
gluten	1 slice	47
italian	1 loaf (1 lb)	1255
italian	1 slice (1 oz)	81
navajo fry	1 (5 in diam)	296
navajo fry	1 (10.5 in diam)	527
oat bran	1 slice	71
oat bran reduced calorie	1 slice	46
oatmeal	1 slice	73
oatmeal reduced calorie	1 slice	48
pita	1 reg (2 oz)	165
pita	1 sm (1 oz)	78
pita whole wheat	1 reg (2 oz)	170
pita whole wheat	1 sm (1 oz)	76
protein	1 slice	47
pumpernickel	1 slice	80
raisin	1 slice	71
rice bran	1 slice	66
rye	1 slice	83
rye reduced calorie	1 slice	47
seven grain	1 slice	65
sourdough	1 slice (1 oz)	78
vienna	1 slice (1 oz)	78
wheat reduced calorie	1 slice	46
wheat berry	1 slice	65
wheat bran	1 slice	89
wheat germ	1 slice	74
white	1 slice	67
white reduced calorie	1 slice	48

FOOD	PORTION	CALS.
white toasted	1 slice	67
white cubed	1 cup	80
whole wheat	1 slice	70
Alvarado St. Bakery		
Barley	1 slice (1.2 oz)	70
California Style	1 slice (1.2 oz)	60
French	1 slice (1.2 oz)	80
Multi-Grain	1 slice (1.2 oz)	60
Multi-Grain No-Salt	1 slice (1.2 oz)	60
Oat Berry	1 slice (1.2 oz)	70
Raisin	1 slice (1.1 oz)	80
Rye Seed	1 slice (1.2 oz)	60
Sourdough	1 slice (1.2 oz)	80
Wheat	1 slice (1.3 oz)	90
America's Own		
Wheat Cottage	1 slice	70
White Cottage	1 slice	70
Arnold		
12 Grain Natural	1 slice (0.8 oz)	60
Augusto Pan De Aqua	1 oz	80
Bran'nola Country Oat	1 slice (1.3 oz)	90
Bran'nola Dark Wheat	1 slice (1.3 oz)	90
Bran'nola Hearty Wheat	1 slice (1.3 oz)	100
Bran'nola Nutty Grains	1 slice (1.3 oz)	90
Bran'nola Original	1 slice (1.3 oz)	90
Cinnamon Chip	1 slice	80
Cinnamon Raisin	1 slice (0.9 oz)	70
Country Bran Bakery Light	1 slice (0.8 oz)	40
Cranberry	1 slice (0.9 oz)	70
French Stick Francisco	1 slice (1 oz)	70
French Stick Savoni	1 oz	80
Italian Bakery Light	1 slice (0.7 oz)	40
Italian Francisco	1 slice (1 oz)	70
Italian Stick Francisco	1 oz	90
Oatmeal Bakery	1 slice	60
Oatmeal Bakery Light	1 slice	40
Oatmeal Raisin	1 slice (0.9 oz)	60
Pita Wheat	½ pocket (1 oz)	71
Pita White	½ pocket (0.5 oz)	71
Pumpernickel	1 slice (1.1 oz)	70
Rye Bakery Soft Light	1 slice (1.1 oz)	40
Rye Bakery Soft Seeded	1 slice (1.1 oz)	70
Rye Bakery Soft Unseeded	1 slice (1.1 oz)	70
Rye Dill	1 slice (1.1 oz)	60

FOOD	PORTION	CALS.
Arnold (CONT.)		
Rye Real Jewish Dijon	1 slice	70
Rye Real Jewish Melba Thin	1 slice (0.7 oz)	40
Rye Real Jewish Unseeded	1 slice	80
Rye Real Jewish With Caraway	1 slice	70
Rye Real Jewish Without Seeds	1 slice (1.1 oz)	70
Sourdough Francisco	1 slice	90
Wheat Brick Oven	1 slice (0.8 oz)	60
Wheat Golden Light	1 slice (0.8 oz)	40
Wheat Natural	1 slice (1.3 oz)	80
Wheat Berry Honey	1 slice (1.1 oz)	80
White Brick Oven	1 slice (0.8 oz)	60
White Country	1 slice (1.3 oz)	100
White Extra Fiber Brick Oven	1 slice (0.9 oz)	50
White Light Brick Oven	1 slice (0.8 oz)	40
White Premium Light	1 slice	40
White Thin Sliced Brick Oven	1 slice	40
Whole Wheat 100% Light Brick Oven	1 slice (0.8 oz)	40
Whole Wheat 100% Stoneground	1 slice (0.8 oz)	50
August Bros.		
Pumpernickel	1 slice	80
Rye Onion	1 slice	80
Rye Thin Unseeded	1 slice	40
Rye With Seeds	1 slice (1 lb loaf)	80
Rye Without Seeds	1 slice	80
Rye N' Pump	1 slice	90
Beefsteak		
Pumpernickel	1 slice (1 oz)	70
Rye Hearty	1 slice (1 oz)	70
Rye Light	2 slices (1.6 oz)	70
Rye Mild	2 slices (1.4 oz)	90
Rye Soft	1 slice (1 oz)	70
Wheat Hearty	1 slice (1 oz)	70
Wheat Soft	1 slice (1 oz)	70
White Robust	1 slice (1 oz)	70
Bread Du Jour		
Austrian Wheat	3 in slice (1 oz)	130
French	3 in slice (1 oz)	130
Brownberry		
Bran'nola Country Oat	1 slice	90
Bran'nola Hearty Wheat	1 slice	88
Bran'nola Nutty Grains	1 slice	85
Bran'nola Original	1 slice	85
Health Nut	1 slice	71

FOOD	PORTION	CALS.
Brownberry (CONT.)		
Oatmeal Natural	1 slice	63
Oatmeal Soft	1 slice	48
Raisin Bran	1 slice	61
Raisin Cinnamon	1 slice	66
Raisin Walnut	1 slice	68
Wheat Apple Honey	1 slice	69
Wheat Soft	1 slice	74
Cedar's		
Mountain Bread Six Grain	1 piece (2.4 oz)	200
Damascus Bakeries		
Mountain Shepard Lahvash	⅓ loaf (2 oz)	135
Dicarlo's		
Foccaccia	⅛ bread (2 oz)	130
French Parisian	2 slices (1 oz)	70
Freihofer's		
Country Potato	1 slice (1.3 oz)	100
Country White	1 slice (1.3 oz)	100
Wheat	1½ slices	70
Wheat Light	1 slice (1.6 oz)	80
White Light	2 slices (1.6 oz)	80
Whole Wheat 100%	1 slice (1.3 oz)	90
Home Pride		
Hearty Buttermilk & Biscuit White	1 slice (1.3 oz)	100
Hearty Deli Rye	1 slice (2 oz)	140
Hearty Golden Honey Wheat	1 slice (1.3 oz)	90
Hearty Honey Oats & Cracked Wheat	1 slice (1.4 oz)	100
Hearty Seven Grain Multi Grain	1 slice (1.3 oz)	100
Honey Wheat	1 slice (1 oz)	70
Seven Grain	1 slice (0.9 oz)	60
Wheat	1 slice (0.9 oz)	70
Wheat Light	3 slices (2.1 oz)	110
White	1 slice (0.9 oz)	70
White Light	3 slices (0.9 oz)	110
Whole Wheat Hearty 100% Stoneground	1 slice (1.4 oz)	90
Malsovit		
Bread	1 slice	66
Raisin	1 slice	77
Matthew's		
9 Grain & Nut	1 slice	80
Cinnamon	1 slice	70
Golden	1 slice	70
Oat Bran	1 slice	65
Pita Whole Wheat	1	210

FOOD	PORTION	CALS.
Matthew's (CONT.)		
Sodium Free	1 slice	70
Whole Wheat	1 slice	70
Meditarranean Magic		
Focaccia	⅕ loaf (1.8 oz)	140
Monks' Bread		
Hi-Fibre	1 slice	50
Raisin	1 slice	70
Sunflower & Bran	1 slice	70
White	1 slice	60
Whole Wheat 100% Stoneground	1 slice	70
Parisian		
French Stick Extra Sour	2 oz	150
French Stick Sweet	2 oz	154
Pepperidge Farm		
7 Grain Hearty Slice	2 slices	180
Cinnamon	1 slice	90
Cracked Wheat	1 slice	70
Crunchy Oat 1½ lb Loaf	2 slices	190
Date Walnut	1 slice	90
French Fully Baked	2 oz	150
French Twin	1 oz	80
Honey Bran	1 slice	90
Italian Brown & Serve	1 oz	80
Italian Sliced	1 slice	70
Oatmeal	1 slice	70
Oatmeal 1½ lb Loaf	1 slice	90
Oatmeal Light	1 slice	45
Oatmeal Very Thin Sliced	1 slice	40
Pumpernickel Family	1 slice	80
Pumpernickel Party	4 slices	60
Raisin With Cinnamon	1 slice	90
Rye Dijon	1 slice	50
Rye Dijon Thick Sliced	1 slice	70
Rye Family	1 slice (32 g)	80
Rye Party	4 slices	60
Rye Seedless Family	1 slice	80
Rye Soft	1 slice	70
Sesame Wheat	2 slices	190
Sprouted Wheat	1 slice	70
Vienna Light	1 slice	45
Vienna Thick Sliced	1 slice	70
Wheat 1½ lb Loaf	1 slice	90
Wheat Family	1 slice	70

FOOD	PORTION	CALS.
Pepperidge Farm (CONT.)		
Wheat Light	1 slice	45
Wheat Very Thin Sliced	1 slice	35
White Country	2 slices	190
White Large Family Thin Slice	1 slice	70
White Sandwich	2 slices	130
White Thin Slice	1 slice	80
White Toasting	1 slice	90
White Very Thin Sliced	1 slice	40
Whole Wheat Thin Slice	1 slice	60
Roman Meal		
Brown & Serve Mini Loaf	½ loaf (2 oz)	136
Cracked Wheat	1 slice (1.4 oz)	92
Hearty Wheat Light	1 slice (0.8 oz)	42
Honey Nut Oat Bran	1 slice (1 oz)	72
Honey Oat Bran	1 slice (1 oz)	70
Oat	1 slice (1 oz)	69
Oat Bran	1 slice (1 oz)	68
Oat Bran Light	1 slice (0.8 oz)	42
Round Top	1 slice (1 oz)	67
Sandwich	1 slice (0.8 oz)	55
Seven Grain	1 slice (1 oz)	67
Seven Grain Light	1 slice (0.8 oz)	42
Sourdough Light	1 slice (0.8 oz)	41
Sourdough Whole Grain Light	1 slice (0.8 oz)	40
Sun Grain	1 slice (1 oz)	70
Twelve Grain	1 slice (1 oz)	70
Twelve Grain Light	1 slice (0.8 oz)	42
Wheat Light	1 slice (0.8 oz)	41
Wheatberry Honey	1 slice (1 oz)	67
Wheatberry Light	1 slice (0.8 oz)	42
White Light	1 slice (0.8 oz)	41
Whole Grain 100%	1 slice (1.4 oz)	91
Whole Grain Sourdough	1 slice (1 oz)	66
Whole Wheat 100%	1 slice (1 oz)	64
Whole Wheat 100% Light	1 slice (0.8 oz)	42
Sahara		
Pita Oat Bran	½ pocket (1 oz)	66
Pita White	½ pocket	78
Stroehmann		
White Whole Special Recipe	1 slice	70
White Whole Special Recipe Kids	1 slice	60
Sunmaid		
Raisin	1 slice	70

FOOD	PORTION	CALS.
Tree Of Life		
100% Spelt	1 slice (1.8 oz)	130
Millet	1 slice (1.8 oz)	130
Rye Sour Dough	1 slice (1.8 oz)	110
Sprouted Seven Grain	1 slice (1.8 oz)	110
Wonder		
Calcium Enriched	1 slice (1 oz)	70
Cinnamon Raisin	1 slice (1 oz)	70
Cracked Wheat	1 slice (1 oz)	70
French	1 slice (1 oz)	80
French Light	2 slices (1.6 oz)	80
Granola	1 slice (1.5 oz)	100
Honey Bran Light	2 slices (1.6 oz)	80
Italian	1 slice (1.1 oz)	80
Italian Family	1 slice (1 oz)	70
Italian Light	2 slices (1.6 oz)	80
Kid	1 slice (0.9 oz)	70
Light Calcium Enriched	2 slices (1.6 oz)	80
Nine Grain Light	2 slices (1.6 oz)	80
Oatmeal Light	2 slices (1.6 oz)	90
Rye	1 slice (1 oz)	70
Rye Light	2 slices (1.6 oz)	70
Sourdough	1 slice (1.2 oz)	90
Sourdough Light	2 slices (1.6 oz)	80
Texas Toast	1 slice (1.4 oz)	100
Vienna	1 slice (1 oz)	70
Wheat Calcium Light	2 slices (1.6 oz)	80
Wheat Family	1 slice (0.9 oz)	70
Wheat Golden Country Style	2 slices (1.4 oz)	100
Wheat Light	2 slices (1.6 oz)	80
White	1 slice (0.9 oz)	70
White Calcium	2 slices (1.6 oz)	100
White Calcium Light	2 slices (1.6 oz)	80
White Light	2 slices (1.6 oz)	80
White With Buttermilk	1 slice (1 oz)	80
Whole Wheat 100%	1 slice (1 oz)	70
Whole Wheat 100% Soft	2 slices (1.6 oz)	110
Whole Wheat 100% Stoneground	1 slice (1.2 oz)	80
REFRIGERATED		
Pillsbury		
Crusty French Loaf	1 in slice	60
Hearty Grains Country Oatmeal Twists	1	80
Hearty Grains Cracked Wheat Twists	1	80
Pipin'Hot Wheat Loaf	1 in slice	70

FOOD	PORTION	CALS.
Pillsbury (CONT.)		
Pipin'Hot White Loaf	1 in slice	70
Roman Meal		
Loaf	1 slice (1 oz)	85
Stefano's		
Stuffed Bread Broccoli & Cheese	½ bread (6 oz)	450
TAKE-OUT		
chapatis as prep w/ fat	1 (2½ oz)	230
chapatis as prep w/o fat	1 (2½ oz)	141
cornbread	2 in x 2 in (1.4 oz)	107
cornstick	1 (1.3 oz)	101
focaccia onion	1 piece (4.6 oz)	282
focaccia rosemary	1 piece (3.5 oz)	251
focaccia tomato olive	1 piece (4.7 oz)	270
naan	1 (6 oz)	571
papadums fried	2 (1.5 oz)	81
paratha	1 (4.4 oz)	403

BREAD COATING

FOOD	PORTION	CALS.
Don's Chuck Wagon		
All Purpose Mix	¼ cup (1 oz)	100
Fish & Chips Mix	¼ cup (1 oz)	100
Fish Mix	¼ cup (1 oz)	95
Frying Mix Chicken	¼ cup (1 oz)	95
Frying Mix Seafood Seasoned	¼ cup (1 oz)	95
Mushroom Mix	¼ cup (1 oz)	95
Onion Ring Mix	¼ cup (1 oz)	100
Golden Dipt		
Breading Frying Mix	1 oz	90
Chicken Frying Mix	1 oz	90
Onion Ring Mix	1 oz	100
Ka-Me		
Tempura Batter Mix	1 oz	100
Little Crow		
Fryin' Magic	0.5 oz	43
Mrs. Dash		
Crispy Coating	0.5 oz	63
Oven Fry		
Homestyle Flour Recipe For Chicken	¼ pkg	85
Shake 'N Bake		
Extra Crispy Oven Fry For Pork	¼ pkg (1 oz)	120
Italian Herb Recipe	¼ pkg (½ oz)	77
Original Barbecue For Chicken	¼ pkg (½ oz)	93
Original Barbecue For Pork	¼ pkg (½ oz)	38

FOOD	PORTION	CALS.
Shake 'N Bake (CONT.)		
Original Country Mild	¼ pkg (½ oz)	76
Original For Chicken	¼ pkg (½ oz)	75
Original For Fish	¼ pkg (½ oz)	73
Original For Pork	¼ pkg (½ oz)	41

BREAD MACHINE MIX

FOOD	PORTION	CALS.
Dromedary		
Country White	½ in slice (2 oz)	140
Italian Herb	½ in slice (1.8 oz)	140
Stoneground Wheat	½ in slice (1.8 oz)	140
Pillsbury		
Cracked Wheat	1/12 pkg (1.3 oz)	130
Sassafras		
Apricot Oatmeal	1 slice (1.4 oz)	140
Wanda's		
Dried Tomato Cheddar	¼ cup mix per serv (1.2 oz)	140
European White	¼ cup mix per serv (1.2 oz)	130
Oatmeal	¼ cup mix per serv (1.2 oz)	120
Oatmeal Cinnamon	¼ cup mix per serv (1.2 oz)	120
Old World Rye	¼ cup mix per serv (1.9 oz)	90
Onion	¼ cup mix per serv (1.2 oz)	120
Orange Cinnamon	¼ cup mix per serv (1.3 oz)	130
Oregano Garlic	¼ cup mix per serv (1.2 oz)	130
Rosemary Basil	¼ cup mix per serv (1.2 oz)	130
Rye	¼ cup mix per serv (1.2 oz)	120
Rye Caraway	¼ cup mix per serv (1.2 oz)	120
Sourdough	¼ cup mix per serv (1.2 oz)	120
Sunflower Sesame Poppyseed	¼ cup mix per serv (1.2 oz)	120
Ten Grain	¼ cup mix per serv (1.4 oz)	140

FOOD	PORTION	CALS.
Wanda's (CONT.)		
Wheat	¼ cup mix per serv (1.2 oz)	130
White	¼ cup mix per serv (1.2 oz)	130
Whole Wheat	¼ cup mix per serv (1.3 oz)	130

BREADCRUMBS

FOOD	PORTION	CALS.
dry	1 cup	426
dry seasonsed	1 cup (4 oz)	441
fresh	⅔ cup	76
4C		
Salt Free	1 tbsp (0.5 oz)	50
Seasoned	1 tbsp (.5 oz)	50
Toasted	1 tbsp (0.5 oz)	50
Toasted Salt Free	1 tbsp (0.5 oz)	50
Arnold		
Italian	½ oz	50
Plain	½ oz	50
Contadina		
Plain	⅓ cup	100
Devonsheer		
Italian Style	1 oz	104
Plain	1 oz	108
Friday's		
Seasoned	1 oz	56
Jaclyn's		
Organic Whole Wheat Italian Style	½ oz	28
Progresso		
Italian Style	¼ cup (1 oz)	110
Lemon Herb	¼ cup (0.9 oz)	100
Plain	¼ cup (1 oz)	100
Tomato Basil	¼ cup (1.1 oz)	120

BREADFRUIT

FOOD	PORTION	CALS.
breadfruit	3.5 oz	109
fresh	¼ small	99
seeds cooked	1 oz	48
seeds raw	1 oz	54
seeds roasted	1 oz	59

BREADNUTTREE SEEDS

FOOD	PORTION	CALS.
dried	1 oz	104

BREADSTICKS

FOOD	PORTION	CALS.
onion poppyseed home recipe	1	64

FOOD	PORTION	CALS.
plain	1	41
plain	1 sm	25
Angonoa		
Cheese	5 (1 oz)	120
Cheese Mini	16 (1 oz)	120
Garlic	6 (1 oz)	120
Italian Style Plain	5 (1 oz)	120
Low Sodium With Sesame Seed	6 (1 oz)	130
Onion	6 (1 oz)	120
Pizza Mini	26 (1 oz)	120
Sesame Mini	16 (1 oz)	130
Sesame Royale	6 (1 oz)	130
Whole Wheat Mini	14 (1 oz)	130
Bread Du Jour		
Italian	1 (1.9 oz)	130
Sourdough	1 (1.9 oz)	130
J.J. Cassone		
Garlic	1 (1.6 oz)	150
Keebler		
Garlic	2	30
Onion	2	30
Plain	2	30
Sesame	2	30
Lance		
Cheese	2	20
Garlic	2	30
Plain	2	30
Sesame	2	30
Pillsbury		
Soft Bread Sticks	1	100
Roman Meal		
Brown & Serve Soft	1 (2.7 oz)	181
Refrigerated	1 (1.4 oz)	117
Stella D'Oro		
Deli Garlic Fat Free	5	60
Deli Original Fat Free	5	60
Garlic	1	35
Grissini Garlic Fat Free	3	60
Grissini Original Fat Free	3	60
Onion	1	40
Regular	1	40
Regular Sodium Free	2	80
Sesame Low Fat	2	70
Sesame Sodium Free	1	50

FOOD	PORTION	CALS.
Stella D'Oro (CONT.)		
Traditional Garlic Fat Free	2	70
Traditional Original Fat Free	2	70
Wheat	1	40

BREAKFAST BAR

(*see also* BREAKFAST DRINKS, NUTRITIONAL SUPPLEMENTS)

Carnation		
Chewy Chocolate Chip	1 (1.26 oz)	150
Chewy Peanut Butter Chocolate Chip	1 (1.26 oz)	140
Glenny's		
Sunrise Bee Pollen	1 (1.5 oz)	190
Sunrise Ginseng	1 (1.5 oz)	160
Sunrise Spirulina	1 (1.5 oz)	140
Nutri-Grain		
Apple Cinnamon	1 (1.3 oz)	140
Blueberry	1 (1.3 oz)	140
Peach	1 (1.3 oz)	140
Raspberry	1 (1.3 oz)	140
Strawberry	1 (1.3 oz)	140

BREAKFAST DRINKS

(*see also* BREAKFAST BAR, NUTRITIONAL SUPPLEMENTS)

orange drink powder	3 rounded tsp	93
orange drink powder as prep w/water	6 oz	86
Carnation		
Instant Breakfast Cafe Mocha	1 pkg + skim milk (9 fl oz)	220
Instant Breakfast Cafe Mocha	1 pkg	130
Instant Breakfast Cafe Mocha	1 can (10 fl oz)	220
Instant Breakfast Classic Chocolate Malt	1 pkg + skim milk (9 fl oz)	220
Instant Breakfast Classic Chocolate Malt	1 pkg	130
Instant Breakfast Creamy Milk Chocolate	1 pkg + skim milk (9 fl oz)	220
Instant Breakfast Creamy Milk Chocolate	1 pkg	130
Instant Breakfast Creamy Milk Chocolate	8 fl oz	220
Instant Breakfast Creamy Milk Chocolate	1 can (10 fl oz)	220
Instant Breakfast French Vanilla	1 pkg	130
Instant Breakfast French Vanilla	1 pkg + skim milk	220
Instant Breakfast No Sugar Added Classic Chocolate	1 pkg	70
Instant Breakfast No Sugar Added Classic Chocolate	1 pkg + skim milk (9 fl oz)	160
Instant Breakfast No Sugar Added Creamy Milk Chocolate	1 pkg	70

FOOD	PORTION	CALS.
Carnation (CONT.)		
Instant Breakfast No Sugar Added Creamy Milk Chocolate	1 pkg + skim milk (9 fl oz)	160
Instant Breakfast No Sugar Added French Vanilla	1 pkg + skim milk (9 fl oz)	150
Instant Breakfast No Sugar Added French Vanilla	1 pkg	70
Instant Breakfast No Sugar Added Strawberry Creme	1 pkg + skim milk (9 fl oz)	150
Instant Breakfast No Sugar Added Strawberry Creme	1 pkg	70
Instant Breakfast Strawberry Creme	1 pkg + skim milk	220
Instant Breakfast Strawberry Creme	1 pkg	130
Pillsbury		
Instant Breakfast Chocolate Malt as prep w/ milk	1 serving	290
Instant Breakfast Chocolate as prep w/ milk	1 serving	290
Instant Breakfast Strawberry as prep w/ milk	1 serving	290
Instant Breakfast Vanilla as prep w/ whole milk	1 serving	300

BROAD BEANS

canned	1 cup	183
dried cooked	1 cup	186
fresh cooked	3½ oz	56

BROCCOLI

FRESH		
chopped cooked	½ cup	22
raw chopped	½ cup	12
Dole		
Spear	1 med	40
FROZEN		
chopped cooked	½ cup	25
spears cooked	½ cup	25
spears cooked	10 oz pkg	69
Big Valley		
Chopped	¾ cup (3 oz)	25
Cuts	¾ cup (3 oz)	25
Birds Eye		
Baby Spears Deluxe	⅔ cup	30
Chopped	⅔ cup	25
Farm Fresh Spears	¾ cup	30

FOOD	PORTION	CALS.
Birds Eye (CONT.)		
Florets Deluxe	½ cup	25
Polybag Cuts	½ cup	25
Polybag Deluxe Florets	⅔ cup	25
Spears	⅔ cup	25
With Cheese Sauce	½ pkg	110
Fresh Like		
Spear	3.5 oz	26
Green Giant		
Cut	½ cup	16
Cuts	½ cup	12
Harvest Fresh Spears	½ cup	20
In Butter Sauce	½ cup	40
In Cheese Sauce	½ cup	60
Mini Spears Select	4-5 spears	18
One Serve Cuts In Butter Sauce	1 pkg	45
Valley Combinations Broccoli Fanfare	½ cup	80
Hanover		
Cut	½ cup	25
Florets	½ cup	30
Pepperidge Farm		
Broccoli With Cheese In Pastry	1	230
Tree Of Life		
Broccoli	1 cup (3.1 oz)	25

BROWNIE
FROZEN
Pepperidge Farm

Monterey Hot Fudge Chocolate Chunk Brownie	1	480
Newport Hot Fudge Brownie	1	400
Weight Watchers		
Brownie A La Mode	1 (6.42 oz)	190
Chocolate Frosted Brownie	1 (1.25 oz)	100
Deluxe Fudge Brownie Parfait	1 (5.3 oz)	190
Peanut Butter Double Fudge	1 (1.23 oz)	110
HOME RECIPE		
plain	1 (0.8 oz)	112
w/nuts	1 (0.8 oz)	95
MIX		
plain	1 (1.2 oz)	139
plain low calorie	1 (0.8 oz)	84
Betty Crocker		
Brownie With Hot Fudge MicroRave Single	1	350

FOOD	PORTION	CALS.
Betty Crocker (CONT.)		
Frosted MicroRave	1	180
Fudge Family Size	1	150
Fudge Light	1	100
Fudge MicroRave	1	150
Fudge Regular Size	1	150
Supreme Caramel	1	120
Supreme Frosted	1	160
Supreme German Chocolate	1	160
Supreme Original	1	140
Supreme Party	1	160
Supreme Walnut	1	140
Walnut MicroRave	1	160
Estee		
Lite	2	100
Jiffy		
Fudge as prep	1	160
Pillsbury		
Deluxe Family- Size Fudge Brownie	2 in sq	150
Deluxe Fudge Brownie	2 in sq	150
Deluxe Fudge Brownie With Walnuts	2 in sq	150
Fudge Microwave	1	190
The Ultimate Carmel Fudge Chunk Brownie	2 in sq	170
The Ultimate Chunky Triple Fudge Brownie	2 in sq	170
The Ultimate Double Fudge Brownie	2 in sq	160
The Ultimate Rockey Road Fudge Brownie	2 in sq	170
READY-TO-EAT		
plain	1 lg (2 oz)	227
plain	1 sm (1 oz)	115
w/ nuts	1 (1 oz)	100
w/o nuts	1 (2 oz)	243
Frito Lay		
Fudge Nut	3 oz	360
Greenfield		
Brownie HomeStyle	1 (1.4 oz)	120
Hostess		
Brownie Bites	5 (2 oz)	260
Brownie Bites Walnut	5 (2 oz)	270
Lance		
Brownie	1 pkg (78 g)	320
Little Debbie		
Fudge	1 pkg (2.1 oz)	270
Fudge	1 pkg (3.6 oz)	450

FOOD	PORTION	CALS.
Little Debbie (CONT.)		
Fudge	1 pkg (2.9 oz)	360
Fudge	1 pkg (2.5 oz)	310
Pepperidge Farm		
Charlotte Fudgey Brownie	1	220
Tahoe Milk Chocolate Pecan	1	210
Westport Fudgey Brownies w/ Walnuts	1	220
Sweet Rewards		
Double Fudge	1 (1.1 oz)	110
Fat Free Brownie	1 bar (1 oz)	90
Tastykake		
Brownie	1 (85 g)	340

BRUSSELS SPROUTS
FRESH

cooked	½ cup	30
cooked	1 sprout	8
raw	1 sprout	8
raw	½ cup	19
Dole		
Sprouts	½ cup	19
FROZEN		
cooked	½ cup	33
Big Valley		
Whole	5-8 pieces (3 oz)	35
Birds Eye		
Brussels Sprouts	½ cup	35
Fresh Like		
Sprouts	3.5 oz	37
Green Giant		
In Butter Sauce	½ cup	40
Sprouts	½ cup	25
Hanover		
Brussels Sprouts	½ cup	40

BUCKWHEAT

flour whole groat	1 cup	402
groats roasted cooked	½ cup	91
groats roasted uncooked	½ cup	283
Wolff's		
Brown Groats Roasted	1 cup (8 oz)	900
Flour	1 cup (8 oz)	860
Kasha Coarse cooked	¼ cup (1.6 oz)	170
Kasha Fine cooked	¼ cup (1.6 oz)	170
Kasha Medium cooked	¼ cup (1.6 oz)	170

FOOD	PORTION	CALS.
Wolff's (CONT.)		
Kasha Whole cooked	¼ cup (1.6 oz)	170
White Grits	1 cup (8 oz)	840
BUFFALO		
water roasted	3 oz	111
BULGUR		
cooked	½ cup	76
uncooked	½ cup	239
Casbah		
Pilaf Mix as prep	1 cup	200
Salad Mix as prep	⅔ cup	90
Good Shepherd		
Bulgur	¼ cup (43 g)	150
Hodgson Mill		
Bulgur	¼ cup (1.4 oz)	120
BURBOT (FISH)		
fresh baked	3 oz	98
BURDOCK ROOT		
cooked	1 cup	110
raw	1 cup	85
BUTTER		
(*see also* BUTTER BLENDS, BUTTER SUBSTITUTES, MARGARINE)		
clarified butter	3½ oz	876
stick	1 pat	36
stick	1 stick (4 oz)	813
whipped	4 oz	542
whipped	1 pat	27
Cabot		
Stick	1 tsp	35
Unsalted Stick	1 tsp	35
Crystal		
Salted Stick	1 tbsp (0.5 oz)	102
Unsalted Stick	1 tbsp (0.5 oz)	102
Hotel Bar		
Stick	1 tsp	35
Keller's		
Stick	1 tsp	35
Land O'Lakes		
Light Stick	1 tbsp	50
Light Unsalted Stick	1 tbsp	50
Stick	1 tbsp (0.5 oz)	100

FOOD	PORTION	CALS.
Land O'Lakes (CONT.)		
Unsalted Stick	1 tbsp (0.5 oz)	100
Unsalted Tub	1 tbsp	60
Whipped	1 tbsp (0.3 oz)	70

BUTTER BEANS
CANNED
Allen

Baby	½ cup (4.5 oz)	120
Large	½ cup (4.5 oz)	120
Hanover		
Butter Beans	½ cup	80
In Sauce	½ cup	100
Luck's		
Speckled Seasoned w/ Pork	7.5 oz	230
S&W		
Tender Cooked	½ cup	100
Sunshine		
Butter Beans	½ cup (4.5 oz)	120
Trappey		
Baby White With Bacon	½ cup (4.5 oz)	130
Large White With Bacon	½ cup (4.5 oz)	110
Van Camp's		
Butter Beans	½ cup	110

BUTTER BLENDS
(*see also* BUTTER, BUTTER SUBSTITUTES, MARGARINE)

stick	1 stick	811
Blue Bonnet		
Better Blend Stick	1 tbsp	90
Better Blend Tub	1 tbsp	90
Better Blend Unsalted Stick	1 tbsp	90
Country Morning		
Blend Light Stick	1 tbsp (0.5 oz)	50
Blend Light Tub	1 tbsp (0.5 oz)	50
Blend Stick	1 tbsp	100
Blend Tub	1 tbsp	100
Blend Unsalted Stick	1 tbsp	100
Downey's		
Cinnamon Honey-Butter Tub	1 tbsp	52
Original Honey-Butter Tub	1 tbsp	52
Le Slim Cow		
Tub	1 tbsp	40

FOOD	PORTION	CALS.

Touch Of Butter
| Tub | 1 tbsp (0.5 oz) | 60 |

BUTTER SUBSTITUTES
(see also BUTTER BLENDS, MARGARINE)

Butter Buds
| Mix | 1 tsp (2 g) | 5 |
| Sprinkles | 1 tsp (2 g) | 5 |

Molly McButter
w/ Bacon	½ tsp (1 g)	4
w/ Cheese	½ tsp (0.9 g)	4
w/ Sour Cream	½ tsp (1.1 g)	4

Mrs. Bateman's
| Baking Butter | 1 tbsp (0.5 oz) | 40 |

Watkins
| Butter Sprinkles | 1 tsp (2 g) | 5 |
| Imitation Butter Flavored Mist | 1 tbsp (0.5 oz) | 120 |

BUTTERBUR
| canned fuki chopped | 1 cup | 3 |
| fresh fuki raw | 1 cup | 13 |

BUTTERFISH
| baked | 3 oz | 159 |
| fillet baked | 1 oz | 47 |

BUTTERNUTS
| dried | 1 oz | 174 |

BUTTERSCOTCH
(see also CANDY)

Nestle
| Morsels Butterscotch | 1 tbsp | 80 |

CABBAGE
FRESH
chinese pak-choi raw shredded	½ cup	5
chinese pak-choi shredded cooked	½ cup	10
chinese pe-tsai raw shredded	1 cup	12
chinese pe-tsai shredded cooked	1 cup	16
danish raw	1 head (2 lbs)	228
danish raw shredded	½ cup (1.2 oz)	9
danish shredded cooked	½ cup (2.6 oz)	17
green raw	1 head (2 lbs)	228
green raw shredded	½ cup (1.2 oz)	9
green shredded cooked	½ cup (2.6 oz)	17
red raw shredded	½ cup	10

FOOD	PORTION	CALS.
red shredded cooked	½ cup	16
savoy raw shredded	½ cup	10
savoy shredded cooked	½ cup	18
Dole		
Cabbage	1/12 med head	18
Napa shredded	½ cup	6
Fresh Express		
Cole Slaw	1½ cups (3 oz)	25
HOME RECIPE		
coleslaw w/ dressing	¾ cup	147
TAKE-OUT		
coleslaw w/ dressing	½ cup	42
stuffed cabbage	1 (6 oz)	373
sweet & sour red cabbage	4 oz	61
vinegar & oil coleslaw	3.5 oz	150

CAKE

(*see also* BROWNIE, COOKIE, DANISH PASTRY, DOUGHNUT, PIE)

FROSTING/ICING

FOOD	PORTION	CALS.
chocolate as prep w/ butter	1/12 box (1.5 oz)	161
chocolate as prep w/ butter	1 box (13.7 oz)	1908
chocolate as prep w/ butter home recipe	1/12 recipe (1.8 oz)	200
chocolate as prep w/ butter home recipe	1 recipe (21.1 oz)	2409
chocolate as prep w/ margarine	1/12 box (1.5 oz)	161
chocolate as prep w/ margarine	1 box (13.7 oz)	1909
chocolate as prep w/ margarine home recipe	1 recipe (21.1 oz)	2411
chocolate as prep w/ margarine home recipe	1/12 recipe (1.8 oz)	200
chocolate ready-to-use	1/12 pkg (1.3 oz)	151
chocolate ready-to-use	1 pkg (16 oz)	1834
coconut ready-to-use	1 pkg (16 oz)	1903
coconut ready-to-use	1/12 pkg (1.3 oz)	157
cream cheese ready-to-use	1/12 pkg (1.3 oz)	157
cream cheese ready-to-use	1 pkg (16 oz)	1906
glaze home recipe	1 recipe (11.5 oz)	1173
glaze home recipe	1/12 recipe (1 oz)	97
seven minute home recipe	1/12 recipe (1.1 oz)	102
seven minute home recipe	1 recipe (13.6 oz)	1231
sour cream ready-to-use	1/12 pkg (1.3 oz)	157
sour cream ready-to-use	1 pkg (16 oz)	1904
vanilla as prep w/ butter	1/12 pkg (1.5 oz)	182
vanilla as prep w/ butter	1 pkg (14.5 oz)	2188
vanilla as prep w/ butter home recipe	1 recipe (20.1 oz)	1972
vanilla as prep w/ butter home recipe	1/12 recipe (1.7 oz)	165
vanilla as prep w/ margarine	1/12 pkg (1.5 oz)	182

FOOD	PORTION	CALS.
vanilla as prep w/ margarine	1 pkg (14.5 oz)	2190
vanilla as prep w/ margarine home recipe	1 recipe (20.1 oz)	2326
vanilla as prep w/ margarine home recipe	1/12 recipe (1.7 oz)	195
vanilla ready-to-use	1/12 pkg (1.3 oz)	159
vanilla ready-to-use	1 pkg (16 oz)	1936
white as prep w/ water	1/12 pkg (0.9 oz)	64
white as prep w/ water	1 pkg (11.1 oz)	770
Betty Crocker		
Butter Pecan Ready-to-Spread	1/12 tub	170
Cherry Ready-to-Spread	1/12 tub	160
Chocolate Ready-to-Spread	1/12 tub	160
Chocolate Chip Ready-to-Spread	1/12 tub	170
Chocolate Fudge as prep	1/12 mix	180
Chocolate Light Ready-to-Spread	1/12 tub	130
Chocolate With Candy Coated Chocolate Chips Ready-to-Spread	1/12 tub	160
Chocolate With Dinosaurs Ready-to-Spread	1/12 tub	160
Chocolate With Turbo Racers Ready-to-Spread	1/12 tub	160
Coconut Pecan Ready-to-Spread	1/12 tub	160
Coconut Pecan as prep	1/12 mix	180
Cream Cheese Ready-to-Spread	1/12 tub	170
Creamy Milk Chocolate as prep	1/12 mix	170
Creamy Vanilla as prep	1/12 mix	170
Dark Dutch Fudge Ready-to-Spread	1/12 tub	160
Lemon Ready-to-Spread	1/12 tub	170
Milk Chocolate Light Ready-to-Spread	1/12 tub	140
Milk Chocolate Ready-to-Spread	1/12 tub	160
Rainbow Chip Ready-to-Spread	1/12 tub	170
Sour Cream Chocolate Ready-to-Spread	1/12 tub	160
Sour Cream White Ready-to-Spread	1/12 tub	160
Vanilla Ready-to-Spread	1/12 tub	160
Vanilla Light Ready-to-Spread	1/12 tub	140
Vanilla With Teddy Bears Ready-to-Spread	1/12 tub	160
White Fluffy as prep	1/12 mix	70
Duncan Hines		
Chocolate Creamy Homestyle	1 oz	130
Milk Chocolate Creamy Homestyle	1 oz	130
Vanilla Creamy Homestyle	1 oz	140
Estee		
Lite Frosting as prep	3 tbsp (0.7 oz)	100
Jiffy		
Fudge	1/4 cup (1.2 oz)	150

FOOD	PORTION	CALS.
Jiffy (CONT.)		
White	¼ cup (1.2 oz)	150
Pillsbury		
Cake & Cookie Decorator Chocolate	1 tbsp	60
Cake & Cookie Decorator all colors except chocolate	1 tbsp	70
Chocolate Fudge	for ⅛ cake	110
Coconut Almond Frosting Mix	for ¹⁄₁₂ cake	160
Coconut Pecan Frosting Mix	for ¹⁄₁₂ cake	150
Fluffy White Frosting Mix	for ¹⁄₁₂ cake	60
Frost It Hot Chocolate	for ⅛ cake	50
Frost It Hot Fluffy White	for ⅛ cake	50
Frosting Supreme Caramel Pecan	for ¹⁄₁₂ cake	160
Frosting Supreme Chocolate Chip	for ¹⁄₁₂ cake	150
Frosting Supreme Chocolate Fudge	for ¹⁄₁₂ cake	150
Frosting Supreme Chocolate Mint	for ¹⁄₁₂ cake	150
Frosting Supreme Coconut Almond	for ¹⁄₁₂ cake	150
Frosting Supreme Coconut Pecan	for ¹⁄₁₂ cake	160
Frosting Supreme Cream Cheese	for ¹⁄₁₂ cake	160
Frosting Supreme Double Dutch	for ¹⁄₁₂ cake	140
Frosting Supreme Lemon	for ¹⁄₁₂ cake	160
Frosting Supreme Milk Chocolate	for ¹⁄₁₂ cake	150
Frosting Supreme Mocha	for ¹⁄₁₂ cake	150
Frosting Supreme Sour Cream Vanilla	for ¹⁄₁₂ cake	160
Frosting Supreme Strawberry	for ¹⁄₁₂ cake	160
Frosting Supreme Vanilla	for ¹⁄₁₂ cake	160
Funetti Chocolate Fudge	¹⁄₁₂ can	140
Funfetti Vanilla Pink	¹⁄₁₂ can	150
Funfetti Vanilla White	¹⁄₁₂ can	150
Vanilla	for ⅛ cake	120
FROZEN		
boston cream pie	⅙ cake (3.2 oz)	232
eclair w/ chocolate icing & custard filling	1	205
Pepperidge Farm		
Amhurst Apple Crumb Coffee Cake	1	220
Apple 'N Spice Bake Dessert Lights	1 piece (4¼ oz)	170
Apple Turnover	1	300
Berkshire Apple Crisp	1	250
Blueberry Turnovers	1	310
Boston Cream Supreme	1 piece (2⅞ oz)	290
Butter Pound	1 slice (1 oz)	130
Carrot Classic	1 cake	260
Carrot w/ Cream Cheese Icing	1 slice (1½ oz)	150
Charleston Peach Melba Shortcake	1	220

FOOD	PORTION	CALS.

Pepperidge Farm (CONT.)

FOOD	PORTION	CALS.
Cherries Supreme Dessert Lights	1 piece (3¼ oz)	170
Cherry Turnover	1	310
Chocolate Supreme	1 piece (2⅞ oz)	300
Chocolate Fudge Large Layer	1 slice (1⅝ oz)	180
Chocolate Fudge Strip Large Layer	1 piece (1⅝ oz)	170
Chocolate Mousse Cake Dessert Lights	1 piece (2½ oz)	190
Cholesterol Free Pound	1 slice (1 oz)	110
Coconut Classic	1 cake	230
Coconut Large Layer	1 slice (1⅝ oz)	180
Devil's Food Large Layer	1 slice (1⅝ oz)	180
Double Chocolate Classic	1 cake	250
Fruit Squares Apple	1	220
Fruit Squares Cherry	1	230
Fudge Golden Classic	1 cake	260
German Chocolate Classic	1 cake	250
German Chocolate Large Layer	1 slice (1⅝ oz)	180
Golden Large Layer	1 slice (1⅝ oz)	180
Lemon Cake Supreme Dessert Lights	1 piece (2¾ oz)	170
Lemon Coconut Classic Cake	3 oz	280
Lemon Coconut Supreme	1 piece (3 oz)	280
Lemon Cream Supreme	1 piece (1⅝ oz)	170
Manhattan Strawberry Cheesecake	1	300
Peach Melba Supreme	1 (3⅛ oz)	270
Peach Parfait Dessert Lights	1 piece (4¼ oz)	150
Peach Turnover	1	310
Pineapple Cream Supreme	1 piece (2 oz)	190
Raspberry Turnovers	1	310
Raspberry Vanilla Swirl Dessert Lights	1 piece (3¼ oz)	160
Strawberry Shortcake Dessert Lights	1 piece (3 oz)	170
Strawberry Cream Supreme	1 piece (2 oz)	190
Strawberry Strip Large Layer	1 piece (1½ oz)	160
Vanilla Fudge Swirl Classic	1 cake	250
Vanilla Large Layer	1 slice (1⅝ oz)	190

Pet-Ritz

FOOD	PORTION	CALS.
Cobbler Apple	⅙ cake (4.33 oz)	290
Cobbler Blackberry	⅙ cake (4.33 oz)	250
Cobbler Blueberry	⅙ cake (4.33 oz)	270
Cobbler Cherry	⅙ cake (4.33 oz)	280
Cobbler Peach	⅙ cake (4.33 oz)	260
Cobbler Strawberry	⅙ cake (4.33 oz)	290

Sara Lee

FOOD	PORTION	CALS.
Apple Crisp Light	1 (3 oz)	150
Banana Single Layer Iced	1 slice (1.7 oz)	170

FOOD	PORTION	CALS.
Sara Lee (CONT.)		
Black Forest Light	1 (3.6 oz)	170
Black Forest Two Layer	1 slice (2.5 oz)	190
Carrot Light	1 (2.5 oz)	170
Carrot Single Layer Iced	1 slice (2.4 oz)	250
Cheesecake Original Strawberry	1 slice (3.2 oz)	222
Cheesecake Original Cherry	1 slice (3.2 oz)	243
Cheesecake Original Plain	1 slice (2.8 oz)	230
Chocolate Free & Light	1 slice (1.7 oz)	110
Coffee Cake All Butter Butter Streusel	1 slice (1.4 oz)	160
Coffee Cake All Butter Cheese	1 slice (2 oz)	210
Coffee Cake All Butter Pecan	1 slice (1.4 oz)	160
Double Chocolate Light	1 (2.5 oz)	150
Double Chocolate Three Layer	1 slice (2.2 oz)	220
French Cheesecake Light	1 (3.2 oz)	150
French Cheese	1 slice (2.9 oz)	250
Lemon Cream Light	1 (3.2 oz)	180
Pound Free & Light	1 slice (1 oz)	70
Pound All Butter Family Size	1 slice (1 oz)	130
Pound All Butter Original	1 slice (1 oz)	130
Strawberry French Cheesecake Light	1 (3.5 oz)	150
Strawberry Shortcake Two Layer	1 slice (2.5 oz)	190
Strawberry Yogurt Dessert Free & Light	1 slice (2.2 oz)	120
Weight Watchers		
Brownie Cheesecake	1 cake (3.5 oz)	200
Caramel Fudge A La Mode	1 cake (6.07 oz)	180
Chocolate Eclair	1 (2.1 oz)	150
Coffee Cake Cinnamon Streusel	1 (2.25 oz)	190
Double Fudge	1 piece (2.75 oz)	190
Strawberry Cheesecake	1 (3.9 oz)	190
Strawberry Shortcake A La Mode	1 (6.49 oz)	180
Toasted Almond Amaretto Cheesecake	1 (3 oz)	170
Triple Chocolate Cheesecake	1 (3.15 oz)	200
HOME RECIPE		
angelfood	1/12 cake (1.9 oz)	142
apple crisp	1 recipe 6 serv (29.6 oz)	1377
apple crisp	1/2 cup (5 oz)	230
boston cream pie	1/8 cake (3.3 oz)	293
carrot w/ cream cheese icing	1/12 cake (3.9 oz)	484
carrot w/ cream cheese icing	1 cake 10 in diam	6175
cheesecake	1/12 cake (4.5 oz)	456
cheesecake w/ cherry topping	1/12 cake (5 oz)	359
chocolate cupcake creme filled w/ frosting	1 (1.8 oz)	188
chocolate w/o frosting	1/12 cake (3.3 oz)	340

FOOD	PORTION	CALS.
chocolate w/o frosting	2 layers (39.9 oz)	4067
coffeecake creme-filled chocolate frosting	1/6 cake (3.2 oz)	298
coffeecake crumb topped cinnamon	1/12 cake (2.1 oz)	240
cream puff w/ custard filling	1 (4.6 oz)	336
eclair	1 (3 oz)	262
fruitcake	1/36 cake (2.9 oz)	302
fruitcake dark	1 cake 7½ in x 2¼ in	5185
gingerbread	1/9 cake (2.6 oz)	264
pineapple upside down	1/9 cake (4 oz)	367
pound	1 loaf 8½ in x 3½ in	1935
pound cake	1 slice (1 oz)	120
sheet cake w/ white frosting	1 cake 9 in sq	4020
sheet cake w/ white frosting	1/9 cake	445
sheet cake w/o frosting	1 cake 9 in sq	2830
sheet cake w/o frosting	1/9 cake	315
shortcake	1 (2.3 oz)	225
sponge	1/12 cake (2.2 oz)	140
white w/ coconut frosting	1/12 cake (3.9 oz)	399
white w/o frosting	1/12 cake (2.6 oz)	264
yellow w/o frosting	2 layers (28.7 oz)	2947
yellow w/o frosting	1/12 cake (2.4 oz)	245
MIX		
angelfood	10 in cake (20.9 oz)	1535
angelfood	1/12 cake (1.8 oz)	129
carrot w/o frosting	2 layers (29.6 oz)	2886
carrot w/o frosting	1/12 cake (2.5 oz)	239
cheesecake no-bake	1/8 cake (3.5 oz)	271
chocolate pudding type w/o frosting	1/12 cake (2.7 oz)	270
chocolate pudding type w/o frosting	2 layers (32.4 oz)	3234
chocolate w/o frosting	1/12 cake (2.3 oz)	198
chocolate w/o frosting	2 layers (26.8 oz)	2393
chocolate w/o frosting low sodium	1/10 cake (1.3 oz)	116
coffeecake crumb topped cinnamon	1/8 cake (2 oz)	178
devil's food w/o frosting	1/12 cake (2.3 oz)	198
devil's food w/ chocolate frosting	1 cake 9 in diam	3755
devil's food w/ chocolate frosting	1/16 cake	235
fudge w/o frosting	1/12 cake (2.3 oz)	198
german chocolate pudding type w/ coconut nut frosting	1/12 cake (3.9 oz)	404
gingerbread	1 cake 8 in sq	1575
gingerbread	1/9 cake (2.4 oz)	207
lemon w/o frosting no sugar low sodium	1/10 cake (1.3 oz)	118
marble pudding type w/o frosting	2 layers (30.6 oz)	3021
marble pudding type w/o frosting	1/12 cake (2.6 oz)	253

FOOD	PORTION	CALS.
white pudding type w/o frosting	2 layers (29 oz)	2915
white pudding type w/o frosting	1/12 cake (2.4 oz)	244
white w/o frosting	1/12 cake (2.2 oz)	190
white w/o frosting	2 layer cake (26 oz)	2265
white w/o frosting no sugar low sodium	1/10 cake (1.3 oz)	118
yellow pudding-type w/o frosting	2 layers (31 oz)	3084
yellow pudding-type w/o frosting	1/12 cake (2.6 oz)	257
yellow w/ chocolate frosting	1/16 cake	235
yellow w/o frosting	2 layers (26.5 oz)	2415
yellow w/o frosting	1/12 cake (2.2 oz)	202
yellow w/ chocolate frosting	1 cake 9 in diam	3895
Aunt Jemima		
Coffee Cake Easy Mix	1/3 cup (1.4 oz)	170
Betty Crocker		
Angel Food Confetti	1/12 cake	150
Angel Food Traditional	1/12 cake	130
Angel Food White	1/12 cake	150
Apple Streusel MicroRave	1/6 cake	240
Apple Streusel MicroRave No Cholesterol Recipe	1/6 cake	210
Butter Chocolate	1/12 cake	280
Butter Pecan SuperMoist	1/12 cake	250
Butter Yellow	1/12 cake	260
Carrot	1/12 cake	250
Carrot No Cholesterol Recipe	1/12 cake	210
Cherry Chip	1/12 cake	190
Chocolate Chocolate Chip	1/12 cake	260
Chocolate Pudding Classic Dessert	1/6 cake	230
Chocolate Chip	1/12 cake	290
Chocolate Chip No Cholesterol Recipe	1/12 cake	220
Chocolate Fudge	1/12 cake	260
Cinnamon Pecan Streusel Microwave	1/6 cake	280
Cinnamon Pecan Streusel Microwave No Cholesterol	1/6 cake	230
Devil's Food	1/12 cake	260
Devil's Food Chocolate Frosting MicroRave	1/6 cake	310
Devil's Food No Cholesterol Recipe	1/12 cake	220
Devils Food SuperMoist Light	1/12 cake	200
Devils Food SuperMoist Light No Cholesterol Recipe	1/12 cake	180
Devils Food With Chocolate Frosting MicroRave Single	1	440
German Chocolate	1/12 cake	260

FOOD	PORTION	CALS.
Betty Crocker (CONT.)		
German Chocolate Chocolate Frosting MicroRave	1/6 cake	320
German Chocolate No Cholesterol Recipe	1/12 cake	220
Gingerbread Classic Dessert	1/9 cake	22
Gingerbread Classic Dessert No Cholesterol Recipe	1/9 cake	210
Golden Pound Classic Dessert	1/12 cake	200
Golden Vanilla	1/12 cake	280
Golden Vanilla No Cholesterol Recipe	1/12 cake	220
Golden Vanilla Rainbow Chip Frosting MicroRave	1/6 cake	320
Lemon	1/12 cake	260
Lemon Chiffon Classic Dessert	1/12 cake	200
Lemon No Cholesterol Recipe	1/12 cake	220
Lemon Pudding Classic Dessert	1/6 cake	230
Marble	1/12 cake	260
Marble No Cholesterol Recipe	1/12 cake	220
Milk Chocolate	1/12 cake	260
Milk Chocolate No Cholesterol Recipe	1/12 cake	210
Pineapple Upsidedown Classic Dessert	1/9 cake	250
Rainbow Chip	1/12 cake	250
Sour Cream Chocolate	1/12 cake	260
Sour Cream Chocolate No Cholesterol Recipe	1/12 cake	220
Sour Cream White	1/12 cake	180
Spice	1/12 cake	260
Spice No Cholesterol Recipe	1/12 cake	220
White	1/12 cake	240
White No Cholesterol Recipe	1/12 cake	220
White SuperMoist Light	1/12 cake	180
Yellow	1/12 cake	260
Yellow SuperMoist Light	1/12 cake	200
Yellow SuperMoist Light No Cholesterol Recipe	1/12 cake	190
Bisquick		
Mix	½ cup (2 oz)	240
Reduced Fat	½ cup (2 oz)	210
Dromedary		
Carrot	1/12 cake	232
Cobbler Apple Crumb	1/8 cake	237
Cobbler Cherry Crumb	1/8 cake	231
Date Nut	1/12 cake	183
Date Nut Roll	½ in slice	80

FOOD	PORTION	CALS.
Dromedary (CONT.)		
Gingerbread	1 piece (2 in x 2 in)	100
Pound	½ in slice	150
Duncan Hines		
Angel Food	1/12 pkg (1.3 oz)	140
Cupcake Yellow With Chocolate Frosting	1	180
Devil's Food Moist Deluxe	1/12 cake (1.5 oz)	290
French Vanilla Moist Deluxe	1/12 cake (1.5 oz)	250
Fudge Marble Moist Deluxe	1/12 cake (1.5 oz)	250
Lemon Supreme Moist Deluxe	1/12 cake (1.5 oz)	250
Yellow Moist Deluxe	1/12 cake (1.5 oz)	250
Estee		
Lite White as prep	1/5 cake (1.7 oz)	200
Lite Chocolate	1/5 cake (1.7 oz)	190
Lite Pound as prep	1/5 cake (1.7 oz)	200
Hain		
Whole Wheat Baking Mix	1½ oz	150
Jell-O		
Cheesecake	⅛ cake	277
Cheesecake New York Style	⅛ cake	283
Jiffy		
Devil's Food as prep	1/5 cake	220
Golden Yellow as prep	1/5 cake	220
White as prep	1/5 cake	210
Pillsbury		
Apple Cinnamon Coffee Cake	⅛ cake	240
Banana Quick Bread	1/12 loaf	170
Blueberry Nut Quick Bread	1/12 loaf	150
Butter Recipe	1/12 cake	260
Cherry Nut Quick Bread	1/12 loaf	180
Chocolate Microwave	⅛ cake	210
Chocolate With Chocolate Frosting	⅛ cake	300
Chocolate With Vanilla Frosting	⅛ cake	300
Cranberry Quick Bread	1/12 loaf	160
Date Quick Bread	1/12 loaf	160
Devil's Food	1/12 cake	270
Double Chocolate Supreme Microwave	⅛ cake	330
Double Lemon Supreme Microwave	⅛ cake	300
Fudge Marble	1/12 cake	270
German Chocolate	1/12 cake	250
Gingerbread	3 in sq	190
Lemon	1/12 cake	250
Lemon Microwave	⅛ cake	220
Lemon With Lemon Frosting	⅛ cake	300

FOOD	PORTION	CALS.
Pillsbury (CONT.)		
Nut Quick Bread	1/12 loaf	170
Strawberry	1/12 cake	260
Streusel Swirl Cinnamon	1/16 cake	260
Streusel Swirl Cinnamon Microwave	1/8 cake	240
Streusel Swirl Lemon	1/16 cake	270
Tunnel of Fudge Bundt	1/16 cake	270
Tunnel of Fudge Bundt Microwave	1/8 cake	290
White	1/12 cake	240
Yellow	1/12 cake	260
Yellow Microwave	1/8 cake	220
Yellow With Chocolate Frosting	1/8 cake	300
Royal		
Cheese Cake Lite No-Bake	1/8 pie	130
Cheese Cake Real No-Bake	1/8 pie	160
Wanda's		
Double Chocolate	1/4 cup mix per serv (1.4 oz)	170
READY-TO-EAT		
angelfood	1 cake (11.9 oz)	876
angelfood	1/12 cake (1 oz)	73
bakewell tart	1 slice (3 oz)	410
battenburg cake	1 slice (2 oz)	204
cheesecake	1/6 cake (2.8 oz)	256
cheesecake	1 cake 9 in diam	3350
cherry fudge w/ chocolate frosting	1/8 cake (2.5 oz)	187
chocolate w/ chocolate frosting	1/8 cake (2.2 oz)	235
coffeecake cheese	1/6 cake (2.7 oz)	258
coffeecake crumb topped cheese	1/6 cake (2.7 oz)	258
coffeecake crumb topped cinnamon	1/9 cake (2.2 oz)	263
coffeecake fruit	1/8 cake (1.8 oz)	156
crumpets toasted	2 (4 oz)	119
eccles cake	1 slice (2 oz)	285
eclair	1 (1.4 oz)	149
fruitcake	1 piece (1.5 oz)	139
madeira cake	1 slice (1 oz)	98
panettone dal forno	1/9 cake (1.9 oz)	212
pound	1/10 cake (1 oz)	117
pound fat free	1 oz	80
pound fat free	1 cake (12 oz)	961
pound cake	1 cake (8½ x 3½ x 3 in)	1935
pound cake	1 slice (1 oz)	110
sour cream pound	1/10 cake (1 oz)	117
sponge	1/12 cake (1.3 oz)	110

FOOD	PORTION	CALS.
strudel apple	1 piece (2½ oz)	195
tiramisu	1 piece (5.1 oz)	409
tiramisu	1 cake (4.4 lbs)	5732
treacle tart	1 slice (2.5 oz)	258
vanilla slice	1 slice (2½ oz)	248
white w/ white frosting	1 cake 9 in diam	4170
white w/ white frosting	1/16 cake	260
yellow w/ chocolate frosting	1 cake 9 diam	3895
yellow w/ chocolate frosting	1/8 cake (2.2 oz)	242
Baker Maid		
Creole Royal Pineapple Apricot	1 slice (1.7 oz)	90
Creole Royal Pineapple Apricot	3 slices (5 oz)	270
Dutch Mill		
Dessert Shells Chocolate Covered	1 (0.5 oz)	80
Entenmann's		
Apple Puffs	1 (3 oz)	280
Apple Strudel Old Fashioned	1 serving (1.5 oz)	120
Cheese Topped Buns	1 (2.3 oz)	240
Cinnamon Buns	1 (2.1 oz)	230
Cinnamon Filbert Ring	1 serving (1.5 oz)	190
Coffee Cake Cheese	1 serving (1.6 oz)	150
Coffee Cake Cheese Filled Crumb	1 serving (1.4 oz)	130
Coffee Cake Crumb	1 serving (1.3 oz)	160
Danish Ring	1 serving (1.5 oz)	180
Danish Ring Pecan	1 serving (1.5 oz)	190
Danish Ring Walnut	1 serving (1.5 oz)	190
Danish Twist Lemon	1 serving (1.2 oz)	140
Danish Twist Raspberry	1 serving (1.2 oz)	140
Devil's Food Cake Fudge Iced	1 serving (1.2 oz)	130
French Crumb Cake All Butter	1 serving (1.6 oz)	180
Louisiana Crunch Cake	1 serving (1.7 oz)	180
Pound Loaf All Butter	1 serving (1 oz)	110
Pound Loaf Sour Cream	1 serving (1 oz)	120
Thick Fudge Golden Cake	1 serving (1.2 oz)	130
Freihofer's		
Angel Food	1/5 cake (2 oz)	150
Cinnamon Swirl Buns	1 (2.8 oz)	290
Coffee Cake Cinnamon Pecan	1/8 cake (2 oz)	220
Crumb	1/8 cake (2 oz)	240
Homestyle Golden Loaf	1/8 cake (1.8 oz)	200
Pound	1/5 cake (2.8 oz)	330
Hostess		
Angel Food Ring	1/6 cake (1.6 oz)	150
Fruit Cake Holiday	1/6 cake (5.3 oz)	490

FOOD	PORTION	CALS.
Hostess (CONT.)		
Pound Cake	⅕ cake (3.2 oz)	350
Perugina		
Pannettone Au Beurre	⅙ cake (2.9 oz)	310
Sinbad		
Baklava	1 piece (2 oz)	337
Thomas'		
Date Nut Loaf	1 oz	90
REFRIGERATED		
Baby Watson		
Cheesecake	1 slice (3.8 oz)	390
Cheesecake Light	1/16 cake (3.9 oz)	280
Pillsbury		
Apple Turnovers	1	170
Cherry Turnovers	1	170
Coffee Cake Cinnamon Swirl	⅛ of cake	180
Coffee Cake Pecan Struesel	⅛ of cake	180
Pastry Pockets	1	240
SNACK		
devil's food cupcake w/ chocolate frosting	1	120
devil's food w/ creme filling	1 (1 oz)	105
sponge w/ creme filling	1 (1.5 oz)	155
toaster pastry apple	1 (1¾ oz)	204
toaster pastry blueberry	1 (1¾ oz)	204
toaster pastry brown sugar cinnamon	1 (1¾ oz)	206
toaster pastry cherry	1 (1¾ oz)	204
toaster pastry strawberry	1 (1¾ oz)	204
Drake's		
Coffee Cake	1 (1.1 oz)	140
Coffee Cake Chocolate Crumb	1 (2.5 oz)	245
Coffee Cake Cinnamon Crumb	1/12 cake (1.3 oz)	150
Coffee Cake Small	1 (2 oz)	220
Devil Dog	1 (1.5 oz)	160
Funny Bones	1 (1.25 oz)	150
Light & Fruity Apple	1 (1.2 oz)	90
Light & Fruity Blueberry	1 (1.2 oz)	90
Light & Fruity Cinnamon Raisin	1 (1.2 oz)	90
Pound Cake	1	110
Ring Ding	1 (1.5 oz)	180
Ring Ding Mint	1 (1.5 oz)	190
Sunny Doodle	1 (1 oz)	100
Yankee Doodle	1 (1 oz)	100
Yodel's	1 (1 oz)	150

FOOD	PORTION	CALS.
Greenfield		
Blondie Apple Spice	1 (1.4 oz)	120
Blondie Chocolate Chip	1 (1.4 oz)	120
Hostess		
Apple Twist	1 (2.5 oz)	220
Baseball Yellow Cakes	1 (1.6 oz)	160
Choco Licious	1 (1.5 oz)	170
Choco-Diles	1 (1.8 oz)	210
Cinnaminis Original	5 (2.4 oz)	300
Cinnamon Roll	1 (2.3 oz)	220
Crumb Cake	1 (1.9 oz)	210
Crumb Cake Light	1 (1.8 oz)	150
Cup Cakes Chocolate	1 (1.6 oz)	170
Cup Cakes Chocolate Light	1 (1.4 oz)	120
Cup Cakes Orange	1 (1.5 oz)	160
Dessert Cups	1 (1 oz)	90
Ding Dongs	1 (1.3 oz)	160
Fruit Loaf	1 (3.8 oz)	350
Ho Ho's	1 (1 oz)	130
Holiday Cakes	1 (1.6 oz)	160
Honey Bun Glazed	1 (2.7 oz)	320
Honey Bun Iced	1 (3.4 oz)	390
Hopper Cakes	1 (1.6 oz)	160
Lil Angels	1 (1 oz)	90
Pecan Spinners	1 (1 oz)	110
Sno Balls	1 (1.6 oz)	160
Suzy Q's	1 (2 oz)	220
Suzy Q's Banana	1 (2 oz)	220
Swirls Caramel Pecan	1 (2 oz)	140
Tiger Tails	1 (1.5 oz)	160
Twinkies	1 (1.4 oz)	140
Twinkies Banana	2 (2.7 oz)	300
Twinkies Devil Food	2 (2.7 oz)	300
Twinkies Lights	1 (1.4 oz)	120
Twinkies Strawberry Fruit 'n Creme	1 (1.6 oz)	150
Kellogg's		
Pop-Tarts Apple Cinnamon	1 (1.8 oz)	210
Pop-Tarts Blueberry	1 (1.8 oz)	210
Pop-Tarts Brown Sugar Cinnamon	1 (1.8 oz)	220
Pop-Tarts Cherry	1 (1.8 oz)	200
Pop-Tarts Chocolate Graham	1 (1.8 oz)	210
Pop-Tarts Frosted Blueberry	1 (1.8 oz)	200
Pop-Tarts Frosted Brown Sugar Cinnamon	1 (1.8 oz)	210
Pop-Tarts Frosted Cherry	1 (1.8 oz)	200

FOOD	PORTION	CALS.
Kellogg's (CONT.)		
Pop-Tarts Frosted Chocolate Vanilla Creme	1 (1.8 oz)	200
Pop-Tarts Frosted Chocolate Fudge	1 (1.8 oz)	200
Pop-Tarts Frosted Grape	1 (1.8 oz)	200
Pop-Tarts Frosted Raspberry	1 (1.8 oz)	210
Pop-Tarts Frosted S'mores	1 (1.8 oz)	200
Pop-Tarts Frosted Strawberry	1 (1.8 oz)	200
Pop-Tarts Strawberry	1 (1.8 oz)	200
Pop-Tarts Minis Frosted Chocolate	1 pkg (1.5 oz)	170
Pop-Tarts Minis Frosted Grape	1 pkg (1.5 oz)	170
Pop-Tarts Minis Frosted Strawberry	1 pkg (1.5 oz)	170
Rice Krispies Treats	1 (0.8 oz)	90
Lance		
Apple Oatmeal	1 pkg (51 g)	200
Dunking Sticks	1 (39 g)	190
Fig Cake	1 pkg (60 g)	210
Honey Buns	1 (85 g)	330
Oatmeal Cake	1 (57 g)	240
Pecan Twirls	1 pkg (57 g)	220
Raisin Cake	1 (57 g)	230
Little Debbie		
Apple Delights	1 pkg (1.2 oz)	140
Apple-Roos	1 pkg (1.5 oz)	150
Banana Nut Muffin Loaves	1 pkg (1.9 oz)	210
Banana Twins	1 pkg (2.2 oz)	250
Be My Valentine	1 pkg (2.2 oz)	280
Cherry Cordials	1 pkg (1.3 oz)	160
Choc-o-Jel	1 pkg (1.2 oz)	150
Choco-Cakes	1 pkg (2.2 oz)	240
Choco-Cakes	1 pkg (2.1 oz)	250
Chocolate	1 pkg (3 oz)	360
Chocolate Chip	1 pkg (2.4 oz)	290
Chocolate Twins	1 pkg (2.4 oz)	240
Christmas Tree Cakes	1 pkg (1.5 oz)	190
Coconut	1 pkg (2.1 oz)	270
Coconut	1 pkg (2.4 oz)	300
Coconut Rounds	1 pkg (1.2 oz)	140
Coffee Cake Apple	1 pkg (1.9 oz)	220
Coffee Cake Apple Streusel	1 pkg (2 oz)	220
Devil Cremes	1 pkg (1.6 oz)	190
Devil Cremes	1 pkg (3.2 oz)	380
Devil Squares	1 pkg (2.2 oz)	260
Easter Basket Cakes	1 pkg (2.5 oz)	310
Fancy Cakes	1 pkg (2.4 oz)	300

FOOD	PORTION	CALS.
Little Debbie (CONT.)		
Fudge Crispy	1 pkg (1.1 oz)	170
Fudge Round	1 pkg (2.5 oz)	290
Fudge Round	1 pkg (3 oz)	350
Fudge Rounds	1 pkg (1.2 oz)	140
Golden Cremes	1 pkg (1.5 oz)	170
Golden Cremes	1 pkg (3 oz)	330
Holiday Cake Chocolate	1 pkg (2.4 oz)	290
Holiday Cake Vanilla	1 pkg (2.5 oz)	310
Honey Bun	1 pkg (4 oz)	510
Honey Bun	1 pkg (3 oz)	380
Jelly Rolls	1 pkg (2.1 oz)	230
Lemon Stix	1 pkg (1.5 oz)	210
Marshmallow Supremes	1 pkg (1.1 oz)	130
Mint Sprints	1 pkg (1.5 oz)	230
Nutty Bar	1 pkg (2 oz)	290
Pecan Twins	1 pkg (2 oz)	220
Pumpkin Delights	1 pkg (1.1 oz)	130
Smiley Faces Cherry	1 pkg (1.2 oz)	140
Smiley Faces Pumpkin	1 pkg (1 oz)	130
Snack Cake Chocolate	1 pkg (2.5 oz)	300
Snack Cake Vanilla	1 pkg (2.6 oz)	320
Spice	1 pkg (2.5 oz)	300
Star Crunch	1 pkg (1.1 oz)	140
Star Crunch	1 pkg (2.6 oz)	330
Swiss Rolls	1 pkg (2.1 oz)	250
Swiss Rolls	1 pkg (3.2 oz)	380
Swiss Rolls	1 pkg (2.7 oz)	320
Teddy Berries	1 pkg (1.2 oz)	130
Vanilla	1 pkg (3 oz)	370
Vanilla Cremes	1 pkg (1.4 oz)	170
Zebra Cakes	1 pkg (2.6 oz)	150
Nabisco		
Frosted Strawberry	1 (1.7 oz)	190
Pepperidge Farm		
Toaster Tart Apple Cinnamon	1	170
Toaster Tart Cheese	1	190
Toaster Tart Strawberry	1	190
Rice Krisples		
Cereal Bar Chocolate Chip	1 (1 oz)	120
Sara Lee		
All Butter Pound	1	200
Chocolate Fudge Cake	1	190
Classic Cheesecake	1	200

FOOD	PORTION	CALS.
Sara Lee (CONT.)		
Coffee Cake Apple Cinnamon	1	290
Coffee Cake Butter Streusel	1	230
Coffee Cake Pecan	1	280
Deluxe Carrot Cake	1	180
Tastykake		
Butter Cream Cream Filled Cupcake	1 (32 g)	120
Chocolate Cream Filled Cupcake	1 (34 g)	130
Chocolate Cupcake	1 (30 g)	100
Creamies Banana Treat	1	138
Creamies Chocolate	1	174
Creamies Vanilla	1	182
Honeybun Glazed	1 pkg (92 g)	360
Honeybun Iced	1 pkg (92 g)	350
Junior Chocolate	1 pkg (94 g)	340
Junior Coconut	1 pkg (94 g)	300
Junior Lemon	1 pkg (94 g)	310
Junior Orange	1 pkg (94 g)	340
Kandy Kake Chocolate	1 (19 g)	80
Kandy Kake Coconut	1 (19 g)	80
Kandy Kake Peanut Butter	1 (19 g)	90
Koffee Kake Cream Filled	1 (29 g)	110
Koffee Kake Junior	1 pkg (71 g)	260
Kreme Kup	1 (25 g)	90
Krimpet Butterscotch	1 (28 g)	100
Krimpet Jelly	1 (28 g)	90
Krimpet Strawberry	1 (28 g)	100
Pastry Pocket Apple	1 (85 g)	320
Pastry Pocket Cheese	1 (85 g)	330
Pastry Pocket Cherry	1 (85 g)	330
Pecan Twirls	1 (28 g)	110
Royale Chocolate Cupcake	1 (46 g)	170
Tasty Too Chocolate Cream Filled Cupcake	1 (32 g)	100
Tasty Too Vanilla Cream Filled Cupcake	1 (32 g)	100
Tasty Twists	1 (4 g)	18
Toast-R-Cakes		
Blueberry	1	110
Bran	1	103
Corn	1	120
Toastettes		
Frosted Blueberry	1 (1.7 oz)	190
Frosted Brown Sugar Cinnamon	1 (1.7 oz)	190
Frosted Cherry	1 (1.7 oz)	190
Frosted Fudge	1 (1.7 oz)	190

FOOD	PORTION	CALS.
Toastettes (CONT.)		
Strawberry	1 (1.7 oz)	190
Well-Bred Loaf		
Banana Bread	1 slice (3.5 oz)	330
Banana Nut	1 slice (4.3 oz)	440
Blueberry	1 slice (4.3 oz)	440
Carrot	1 slice (4.3 oz)	480
Carrot Traditional	1 slice (4.3 oz)	440
Chocolate Chip	1 slice (4.3 oz)	490
Cinnamon Walnut	1 slice (4.3 oz)	480
Coconut Rum	1 slice (4.3 oz)	490
Cranberry	1 slice (4.3 oz)	460
Marble	1 slice (4.3 oz)	530
Pound All Butter	1 slice (4.3 oz)	470
Pound Mandarin Orange	1 slice (4 oz)	460
Raisin	1 slice (4.3 oz)	460
TAKE-OUT		
baklava	1 oz	126
strudel	1 piece (4.1 oz)	272
trifle w/ cream	6 oz	291

CALZONE

TAKE-OUT		
cheese	1 (12 oz)	1020

CANADIAN BACON

unheated	2 slices (1.9 oz)	89
Hormel		
Canadian Bacon	2 oz	70
Jones		
Slices	1	30
Oscar Mayer		
Canandian Bacon	2 slices (1.6 oz)	50

CANDY

(*see also* MARSHMALLOW)		
boiled sweets	¼ lb	327
butterscotch	1 piece (6 g)	24
butterscotch	1 oz	112
candied cherries	1 (4 g)	12
candied citron	1 oz	89
candied lemon peel	1 oz	90
candied orange peel	1 oz	90
candied pineapple slice	1 slice (2 oz)	179
candy corn	1 oz	105

FOOD	PORTION	CALS.
caramels	1 piece (8 g)	31
caramels	1 pkg (2.5 oz)	271
caramels chocolate	1 bar (2.3 oz)	231
caramels chocolate	1 piece (6 g)	22
carob bar	1 (3.1 oz)	453
crisped rice bar almond	1 bar (1 oz)	130
crisped rice bar chocolate chip	1 bar (1 oz)	115
dark chocolate	1 oz	150
fondant chocolate coated	1 sm (0.4 oz)	40
fondant chocolate coated	1 lg (1.2 oz)	128
fondant mint	1 oz	105
fruit pastilles	1 tube (1.4 oz)	101
gumdrops	10 sm (0.4 oz)	135
gumdrops	10 lg (3.8 oz)	420
hard candy	1 oz	106
jelly beans	10 sm (0.4 oz)	40
jelly beans	10 lg (1 oz)	104
lollipop	1 (6 g)	22
marzipan	3½ oz	497
milk chocolate	1 bar (1.55 oz)	226
milk chocolate crisp	1 bar (1.45 oz)	203
milk chocolate w/ almonds	1 bar (1.45 oz)	215
nougat nut cream	3½ oz	342
peanut bar	1 (1.4 oz)	209
peanuts chocolate covered	1 cup (5.2 oz)	773
peanuts chocolate covered	10 (1.4 oz)	208
pretzels chocolate covered	1 oz	130
pretzels chocolate covered	1 (0.4 oz)	50
sesame crunch	1 oz	146
sesame crunch	20 pieces (1.2 oz)	181
sweet chocolate	1 bar (1.45 oz)	201
sweet chocolate	1 oz	143
100 Grand		
Bar	1 bar (1.5 oz)	200
3 Musketeers		
Bar	2 fun size (1.2 oz)	140
Bar	1 (2.1 oz)	260
5th Avenue		
Bar	1 (2.1 oz)	290
After Eight		
Dark Chocolate Wafer Thin Mints	1	35
Almond Joy		
Bar	1 (1.76 oz)	250

FOOD	PORTION	CALS.
Baby Ruth		
Bar	1 (2.1 oz)	280
Fun Size	2 pieces	200
Bar None		
Candy	1 (1.5 oz)	240
Bit-O-Honey		
Candy	1.7 oz	200
Bits O Brickle		
Candy	1 tbsp (0.5 oz)	80
Bonus		
Bar	1 bar (2.1 oz)	290
Breath Savers		
Sugar Free Mint Cinnamon	1 piece (2 g)	10
Sugar Free Peppermint	1 piece (2 g)	10
Sugar Free Spearmint	1 piece (2 g)	10
Sugar Free Wintergreen	1 piece (2 g)	10
Brock		
Butterscotch Discs	3 pieces (0.6 oz)	70
Candy Corn	21 pieces (1.4 oz)	150
Candy Rolls	2 rolls (0.5 oz)	50
Caramel Dots	3 pieces (1.3 oz)	140
Cinnamon Discs	3 pieces (0.6 oz)	70
Circus Peanuts	11 pieces (2.5 oz)	260
Coconut Mountains	4 pieces (1.4 oz)	170
Fruit Basket	3 pieces (0.6 oz)	60
Fruit Kisses	3 pieces (0.6 oz)	70
Glitters	2 pieces (0.5 oz)	50
Gummy Bears	5 pieces (1.4 oz)	130
Gummy Squirms	5 pieces (1.3 oz)	120
Jelly Beans	12 pieces (1.4 oz)	140
Lemon Drops	3 pieces (0.6 oz)	60
Orange Slices	4 pieces (1.5 oz)	140
Party Mints	9 pieces (0.5 oz)	60
Peanut Butter Crunch	3 pieces (0.6 oz)	80
Pops Assorted	2 (0.5 oz)	60
Sour Balls	3 pieces (0.6 oz)	70
Sour Sharks	23 pieces (2.5 oz)	30
Spearmint Starlights	3 pieces (0.6 oz)	60
Spice Drops	12 pieces (1.4 oz)	130
Starlight Mints	3 pieces (0.6 oz)	60
Toffee	6 pieces (1.5 oz)	170
Butterfinger		
BB's	1 pkg (1.7 oz)	230
Bar	1 (2.1 oz)	280

FOOD	PORTION	CALS.
Butterfinger (CONT.)		
Fun Size	2 bars (1.6 oz)	200
Caramello		
Candy	1 (1.6 oz)	220
Cellas		
Chocolate Covered Cherries Dark Chocolate	2 pieces (1 oz)	100
Chocolate Covered Cherries Milk Chocolate	2 pieces (1 oz)	110
Certs		
Breath Mints	1 piece (1.67 g)	6
Mini Sugar Free	1 piece (0.365 g)	1
Sugar Free	1 piece (1.67 g)	7
Charleston Chew		
Candy	1 pkg (1.9 oz)	230
Chocolate	½ bar	120
Strawberry	½ bar	120
Vanilla	½ bar	120
Charms		
Blow Pop	1 (0.7 oz)	80
Pop	1 (0.6 oz)	70
Chuckles		
Candy	4 pieces (1.4 oz)	140
Chunky		
Bar	1 (1.4 oz)	200
Clorets		
Mints	1 piece (1.67 g)	6
Crunch		
Fun Size	4 bars (1.5 oz)	200
Dove		
Dark Chocolate	¼ bar (1.5 oz)	230
Dark Chocolate	1 bar (1.3 oz)	200
Dark Chocolate Minatures	7 (1.5 oz)	220
Milk Chocolate	¼ bar (1.5 oz)	230
Milk Chocolate	1 bar (1.3 oz)	200
Milk Chocolate Miniatures	7 (1.5 oz)	230
Truffles	3 (1.2 oz)	200
Dream		
Caramel & Nougat In Milk Chocolate	1 bar (1 oz)	90
Estee		
Caramels Chocolate & Vanilla No Sugar Added	5 (1.3 oz)	150
Dark Chocolate	½ bar (1.4 oz)	200
Gum Drops Assorted Fruit Sugar Free	23 (1.4 oz)	140

FOOD	PORTION	CALS.
Estee (CONT.)		
Gum Drops Licorice	23 (1.4 oz)	140
Gummy Bears Sugar Free	16 (1.4 oz)	140
Hard Candies Assorted Fruit Sugar Free	5 (0.5 oz)	60
Hard Candies Assorted Mint Sugar Free	5 (0.5 oz)	60
Hard Candies Butterscotch Sugar Free	2 (0.4 oz)	50
Hard Candies Peppermint Swirls Sugar Free	3 (0.5 oz)	60
Hard Candies Tropical Fruit Sugar Free	5 (0.5 oz)	60
Lollipops Assorted Fruit Sugar Free	2 (0.5 oz)	60
Milk Chocolate	½ bar (1.4 oz)	230
Milk Chocolate With Almonds	½ bar (1.4 oz)	230
Milk Chocolate With Crisp Rice	1 bar (2.3 oz)	370
Milk Chocolate With Fruit & Nuts	½ bar (1.4 oz)	220
Mint Chocolate	½ bar (1.4 oz)	200
Peanut Brittle No Sugar Added	⅓ box (1.5 oz)	210
Peanut Butter Cups	1 (0.3 oz)	40
Peanut Butter Cups	5 (1.3 oz)	200
Toffee Sugar Free	5 (0.5 oz)	60
Ferrero Rocher		
Candy	2 pieces (0.9 oz)	150
Franklin		
Crunch 'N Munch Candied	1.25 oz	170
Crunch 'N Munch Caramel	1.25 oz	160
Crunch 'N Munch Maple Walnut	1.25 oz	160
Crunch 'N Munch Toffee	1.25 oz	160
Glenny's		
Brown Rice Treats Carob & Mint With Oat Bran	1 bar (1.75 oz)	180
Brown Rice Treats Cinnamon & Raisin	1 bar (1.75 oz)	170
Brown Rice Treats Peanut & Raisin	1 bar (2 oz)	210
Brown Rice Treats Plain & Fancy	1 bar (1.25 oz)	120
Brown Rice Treats Toasted Almond With Oat Bran	1 bar (1.75 oz)	200
Fruit Drops Black Cherry	1	6
Fruit Drops Gentle Mint	1	6
Fruit Drops Mandarin Orange	1	6
Fruit Drops Mixed Fruit	1	6
Fruit Drops Twist Of Lemon	1	6
Hard Candies Fruit	1	19
Hard Candies Peppermint	1	19
Lollipops C Pops	1	35
Lollipops Fruit	1	21
Moist & Chewy Coconut Almondine Bar	1 bar (1.5 oz)	190

FOOD	PORTION	CALS.
Glenny's (CONT.)		
Moist & Chewy Oatmeal Raisin Bar	1 bar (1.5 oz)	160
Moist & Chewy Peanut Bar	1 bar (1.5 oz)	180
Moist & Chewy Sunflower Bar	1 bar (1.5 oz)	180
Snack Bar Fat-Free Apple-Cinnamon	1 (125 oz)	120
Snack Bar Fat-Free Caramel	1 (1.25 oz)	120
Snack Bar Fat-Free Chocolate	1 (1.25 oz)	120
Snack Bar Fat-Free Raspberry	1 (1.25 oz)	120
Godiva		
Almond Butter Dome	3 pieces (1.5 oz)	240
Bouchee Au Chocolat	1 piece (1.5 oz)	210
Bouchee Ivory Raspberry	1 pieces (1 oz)	160
Gold Ballotin	3 pieces (1.5 oz)	210
Truffle Amaretto Di Saronno	2 pieces (1.5 oz)	210
Truffle Deluxe Liqueur	2 pieces (1.5 oz)	210
Golden Almond		
Bar	½ bar	260
Golden III		
Bar	½ bar	250
Goldenberg's		
Peanut Chews	3 pieces (1.3 oz)	180
Goo Goo Supreme		
With Pecans	1 pkg (1.5 oz)	188
Goobers		
Peanuts	1 pkg (1.38 oz)	210
Good & Fruity		
Candy	1 box (1.8 oz)	140
Good & Plenty		
Snacksize	3 boxes (1.5 oz)	140
Heath		
Bar	1 (1.4 oz)	210
Hershey		
Amazin'Fruit Gummy Candy	2 snack pkg (1.4 oz)	130
Bar	1 (1.55 oz)	240
Bar With Almonds	1 (1.45 oz)	230
Kisses	9 pieces (1.46 oz)	220
Special Dark Sweet Chocolate Bar	1 (1.45)	220
Jolly Rancher		
Candies	3 pieces (0.6 oz)	60
Joyva		
Halvah	1.5 oz	240
Halvah Chocolate Covered	1 bar (2 oz)	380
Jells Raspberry	3 pieces (1.6 oz)	200
Joys Raspberry	1 (1.6 oz)	200

FOOD	PORTION	CALS.
Joyva (CONT.)		
Marshmallow Twists Chocolate Covered	2 (1.5 oz)	190
Rings Orange & Raspberry	3 pieces (1.5 oz)	190
Sesame Crunch	3 pieces (0.5)	80
Sticks Orange	3 pieces (1.6 oz)	200
Twists Vanilla & Cherry	2 pieces (1.5 oz)	190
Juicefuls		
Candy	3 pieces (0.5 oz)	60
Junior Mints		
Candies	1 pkg (1.6 oz)	190
Just Born		
Jelly Beans	1 oz	108
Sugar Coated	1½ oz	148
Toasted Coconut	1⅜ oz	140
Kit Kat		
Bar	1 (1.625 oz)	250
Krackel		
Bar	1 (1.55 oz)	230
Kraft		
Butter Mints	7 (0.5 oz)	60
Caramels	5 (1.4 oz)	170
Fudgies	5 (1.4 oz)	180
Party Mints	7 (0.5 oz)	60
Peanut Brittle	5 pieces (1.3 oz)	170
Laffy Taffy		
Apple Chews	1 oz	110
Banana Chews	1 oz	110
Grape Chews	1 oz	110
Passion Punch Chews	1 oz	110
Strawberry Chews	1 oz	110
Sweet & Sour Cherry Chews	1 oz	110
Watermelon Chews	1 oz	110
Lance		
Chocolaty Peanut Bar	1 (57 g)	320
Peanut Bar	1 pkg (50 g)	260
Popscotch	1 pkg (35 g)	160
Lifesavers		
Big Tablet Candy Cane	4 pieces (0.5 oz)	60
Cards 'N Candy	4 pieces (0.4 oz)	40
Christmas Tin	4 pieces (0.5 oz)	60
Egg-Sortment	1 roll (0.4 oz)	40
Fruit Juicers Lollipops	1	40
Gummi Bunnies	3 pkg (1.6 oz)	140
Gummi Savers Five Flavor	1 roll (1.5 oz)	130

FOOD	PORTION	CALS.
Lifesavers (CONT.)		
Gummi Savers Five Flavor	1 pkg (1.8 oz)	160
Gummi Savers Mixed Berry	1 roll (1.5 oz)	130
Gummi Savers Mixed Berry	1 pkg (1.8 oz)	160
Gummi Savers Tangy Fruits	1 roll (1.5 oz)	130
Gummi Savers Tangy Fruits	1 pkg (1.8 oz)	160
Gummi Savers Variety	2 pkg (1.3 oz)	120
Gummi Savers Wacky Frootz	1 roll (1.5 oz)	130
Gummi Savers Wacky Frootz	1 pkg (1.8 oz)	160
Holes Five Flavor	20 pieces (5 g)	20
Holes Island Fruit	20 pieces (5 g)	20
Holes Sour 'N Sweet	16 pieces (5 g)	20
Holes Sunshine Fruits	20 pieces (0.2 oz)	20
Holes Super Tart	20 pieces (5 g)	20
Holes Tangerine	1 candy	2
Holes Wild Fruits	20 pieces (5 g)	20
Lollipops Candy Cane	1 (0.4 oz)	40
Lollipops Christmas	1 (0.4 oz)	40
Lollipops Easter	1 (0.4 oz)	40
Lollipops Fruit Flavors	1 (0.4 oz)	45
Lollipops Swirled Flavors	1 (0.4 oz)	40
Lollipops Valentine	1 (0.4 oz)	40
Roll Butter Rum	2 pieces (5 g)	20
Roll Candy Cane	4 pieces (0.4 oz)	40
Roll Cryst-O-Mint	2 pieces (5 g)	20
Roll Five Flavor	2 pieces (5 g)	20
Roll Fruits On Fire	2 pieces (5 g)	20
Roll Pep-O-Mint	3 pieces (5 g)	20
Roll Spear-O-Mint	3 pieces (5 g)	20
Roll Sunshine Fruits	2 pieces (5 g)	20
Roll Tangy Fruit Swirl	2 pieces (5 g)	20
Roll Tangy Fruit Watermelon	1 pieces (5 g)	20
Roll Tangy Fruits	2 pieces (5 g)	20
Roll Tropical Fruits	2 pieces (5 g)	20
Roll Wild Cherry	1 pieces (5 g)	20
Roll Wild Flavors	2 pieces (5 g)	20
Roll Wild Sour Berries	2 pieces (5 g)	20
Roll Wint-O-Green	3 pieces (5 g)	20
Sack'it Butter Rum	4 pieces (0.5 oz)	60
Sack'it Five Flavor	4 pieces (0.5 oz)	60
Sack'it Holiday Tin	4 pieces (0.5 oz)	60
Sack'it Pep-O-Mint	4 pieces (0.5 oz)	60
Sack'it Tangy Fruits	4 pieces (0.5 oz)	60
Sack'it Wild Cherry	4 pieces (0.5 oz)	60

FOOD	PORTION	CALS.
Lifesavers (CONT.)		
Sack'it Wint-O-Green	4 pieces (0.5 oz)	60
Sugar Free Iced Mint	1 pieces (2 g)	10
Sugar Free Vanilla Mint	1 pieces (2 g)	10
Valentine Book	2 pieces (5 g)	20
M&M's		
Almond	1 pkg (1.3 oz)	200
Almond	1.5 oz	220
Mint	1.5 oz	200
Mint	1 pkg (1.7 oz)	230
Peanut	½ bag king size (1.6 oz)	240
Peanut	1 pkg (1.7 oz)	250
Peanut	1 fun size (0.7 oz)	110
Peanut	1.5 oz	220
Peanut Butter	1 pkg (1.6 oz)	240
Peanut Butter	1 fun size (0.7 oz)	110
Peanut Butter	1.5 oz	220
Plain	1 pkg fun size (0.7 oz)	100
Plain	1.5 oz	200
Plain	1 pkg (1.7 oz)	230
Plain	½ pkg king size (1.6 oz)	220
Mars		
Almond Bar	2 fun size (1.3 oz)	190
Almond Bar	1 bar (1.8 oz)	240
Mayfair		
Mints	5 pieces (1.3 oz)	180
Milk Duds		
Pieces	1 box (1.8 oz)	230
Snack Size	4 boxes (1.3 oz)	160
Milkshake		
Bar	1 bar (1.8 oz)	220
Milky Way		
Bar	2 fun size (1.4 oz)	180
Bar	⅓ king size (1.2 oz)	160
Bar	1 (2.1 oz)	280
Dark	1 bar (1.8 oz)	220
Dark	1 fun size (0.7 oz)	90
Miniature	5 (1.5 oz)	190
Mounds		
Bar	1 (1.9 oz)	260
Mr. Goodbar		
Candy	1 (1.75 oz)	290
NECCO		
Mint	1 piece	12

FOOD	PORTION	CALS.
Natural Touch		
Caroby Almond Bar	4 sections (28 g)	150
Caroby Milk Bar	4 sections (28 g)	150
Caroby Milk Free Bar	4 sections (28 g)	160
Caroby Mint Bar	4 sections (28 g)	150
Nestle		
Areo Bar	1 bar (1.45 oz)	210
Buncha Crunch	1 pkg (1.4 oz)	90
Crunch	1 bar (1.55 oz)	230
Milk Chocolate	1 bar (1.45 oz)	220
Turtles Pecan Caramel Candy	2 pieces (1.2 oz)	160
Nips		
Butter Rum	2 pieces (0.5 oz)	60
Caramel	2 pieces (0.5 oz)	60
Chocolate Mint	2 pieces (0.5 oz)	60
Chocolate Parfait	2 pieces (0.5 oz)	60
Peanut Butter Parfait	2 pieces (0.5 oz)	60
Ocean Spray		
Fruit Waves Assorted	3 pieces (0.3 oz)	35
Oh Henry!		
Bar	1 (1.8 oz)	230
PayDay		
Bar	1 (1.85 oz)	240
Pearson		
Licorice	2 pieces (0.5 oz)	60
Pez		
Candy	1 roll (0.3 oz)	30
Planters		
Original Peanut Bar	1 pkg (1.6 oz)	230
Pom Pom		
Candies	1 pkg (1.6 oz)	200
Raisinets		
Raisins	1 pkg (1.58 oz)	200
Reese's		
Peanut Butter Cups	1 (1.8 oz)	280
Pieces	1.85 oz	260
Riesen		
Candy	5 pieces (1.4 oz)	180
Rolo		
Carmels In Milk Chocolate	8 pieces (1.93 oz)	270
Russell Stover		
Assorted Creams	3 pieces (1.4 oz)	180
Skittles		
Original	2 pkg fun size (1.6 oz)	180

FOOD	PORTION	CALS.
Skittles (CONT.)		
Original	1.5 oz	170
Original	1 pkg (2.8 oz)	250
Original	½ king size (1.3 oz)	150
Tropical	1.5 oz	170
Tropical	2 bags fun size (1.4 oz)	160
Tropical	1 bag (2.2 oz)	250
Wild Berry	1 bag (2.2 oz)	250
Wild Berry	1.5 oz	170
Wild Berry	2 bags fun size (1.4 oz)	160
Skor		
Toffee Bar	1 (1.4 oz)	220
Snickers		
Bar	1 bar (2.1 oz)	280
Bar	2 bars fun size (1.4 oz)	190
Bar	½ king size (1.2 oz)	170
Miniatures	4 (1.3 oz)	170
Munch Bar	1 (1.4 oz)	230
Peanut Butter	1 bar (2 oz)	310
Sno Caps		
Candies	1 pkg (2.3 oz)	300
Solitaires		
Candies	½ bag	260
Sour Punch		
Candy Straws Sour Apple	6 pieces (1.4 oz)	130
Spice Stix		
And Drops	14 pieces (1.6 oz)	140
Starburst		
California Fruits	8 pieces (1.4 oz)	160
California Fruits	1 stick (2.1 oz)	240
Original Fruits	½ king size (1.2 oz)	140
Original Fruits	8 pieces (1.4 oz)	160
Orignal Fruits	1 stick (2.1 oz)	240
Strawberry Fruits	8 pieces (1.4 oz)	160
Strawberry Fruits	1 stick (2.1 oz)	240
Tropical Fruits	8 pieces (1.4 oz)	160
Tropical Fruits	1 stick (2.1 oz)	240
Sugar Babies		
Candies	1 pkg (1.7 oz)	190
Tidbits	1 pkg	180
Sugar Daddy		
Candies	1 pkg (1.7 oz)	200
Swedish Red Fish		
Candy	19 pieces (1.4 oz)	150

FOOD	PORTION	CALS.
Sweet Escapes		
Triple Chocolate Wafer Bars	1 (0.7 oz)	80
Switzer		
Cherry Bites	12 pieces (1.6 oz)	50
Licorice Bites	12 pieces (1.6 oz)	46
Symphony		
Almond/ Butterchips	1 (1.4 oz)	220
Milk Chocolate	1 (1.4 oz)	220
Terry's		
Orange Milk Chocolate	5 pieces (1.5 oz)	240
Tootsie Roll		
Candy	1 (1 oz)	110
Dots	12 (1.5 oz)	160
Midgees	6 (1.4 oz)	160
Pop	1 (0.6 oz)	60
Twix		
Caramel	1 fun size (0.5 oz)	80
Caramel	1 (1 oz)	140
Caramel	1 pkg (2 oz)	280
Caramel	1 king size (0.8 oz)	120
Peanut Butter	1 (0.9 oz)	130
Twizzlers		
Candy	4 pieces (1.4 oz)	130
Pull-N-Peel Cherry	1 piece (1.1 oz)	110
Velamints		
Cocoamint	1 piece (1.7 g)	5
Peppermint	1 piece (1.7 g)	5
Spearmint	1 piece (1.7 g)	5
Wintergreen	1 piece (1.7 g)	5
Very Special		
Chocolate Bottles Liquor Filled	3 pieces (1 oz)	150
Whatchamacallit		
Bar	1 (1.8 oz)	260
Whitman's		
Assorted	3 pieces (1.4 oz)	190
Dark Chocolate	3 pieces (1.4 oz)	200
Little Ambassadors	7 pieces (1.4 oz)	190
Pecan Delight	1 bar (2 oz)	310
Pecan Roll	1 bar (2 oz)	300
Sampler	3 pieces (1.4 oz)	200
Whoppers		
Candy	1 pkg (1.8 oz)	230
Y&S		
Bites Cherry	1 oz	100

FOOD	PORTION	CALS.
York		
Peppermint Patty	1 snack size (0.5 oz)	57
Peppermint Patty	1 (1.5 oz)	180
Zero		
Bar	2 pieces (1.4 oz)	170
HOME RECIPE		
divinity	1 (11 g)	38
divinity	1 recipe 48 pieces (19 oz)	1891
fondant	1 recipe 60 pieces (32.6 oz)	3327
fondant	1 piece (0.6 oz)	57
fudge brown sugar w/ nuts	1 piece (0.5 oz)	56
fudge brown sugar w/ nuts	1 recipe 60 pieces (30.7 oz)	3453
fudge chocolate	1 piece (0.6 oz)	65
fudge chocolate	1 recipe 48 pieces (29 oz)	3161
fudge chocolate marshmallow	1 piece (0.7 oz)	84
fudge chocolate marshmallow	1 recipe (43.1 oz)	5182
fudge chocolate marshmallow w/ nuts	1 piece (0.8 oz)	96
fudge chocolate marshmallow w/ nuts	1 recipe 60 pieces (43.1 oz)	5182
fudge chocolate marshmallow w/ nuts	1 recipe 60 pieces (46.1 oz)	5742
fudge chocolate w/ nuts	1 piece (0.7 oz)	81
fudge chocolate w/ nuts	1 recipe 48 pieces (32.7 oz)	3967
fudge peanut butter	1 recipe 36 pieces (20.4 oz)	2161
fudge peanut butter	1 piece (0.6 oz)	59
fudge vanilla	1 piece (0.6 oz)	59
fudge vanilla	1 recipe 48 pieces (27.5 oz)	2893
fudge vanilla w/ nuts	1 piece (0.5 oz)	62
fudge vanilla w/ nuts	1 recipe 60 pieces (31 oz)	3666
peanut brittle	1 recipe (17.6 oz)	2288
peanut brittle	1 oz	128
praline	1 recipe 23 pieces (31.8 oz)	4116
praline	1 piece (1.4 oz)	177
taffy	1 piece (0.5 oz)	56
taffy	1 recipe 48 pieces (25 oz)	2677

FOOD	PORTION	CALS.
toffee	1 piece (0.4 oz)	65
toffee	1 recipe 48 pieces (19.4 oz)	2997
truffles	1 recipe 49 pieces (21.5 oz)	2985
truffles	1 piece (0.4 oz)	59

CANTALOUPE
FRESH

cubed	1 cup	57
half	½	94

Chiquita

Fresh	1 cup	70

Dole

Cantaloup	¼	50

FROZEN

Big Valley

Balls	¾ cup (4.9 oz)	40

CAPERS
Progresso

Capers (drained)	1 tsp (5 g)	0

Reese

Capers	1 tsp (5 g)	0

CARAMBOLA

fresh	1	42

CARAWAY

seed	1 tsp	7

CARDAMOM

ground	1 tsp	6

CARDOON

fresh cooked	3½ oz	22
raw shredded	½ cup	36

CARIBOU

roasted	3 oz	142

CARISSA

fresh	1	12

CAROB

carob mix	3 tsp	45
carob mix as prep w/ whole milk	9 oz	195
flour	1 tbsp	14
flour	1 cup	185

FOOD	PORTION	CALS.
CARP		
fresh cooked	3 oz	138
fresh cooked	1 fillet (6 oz)	276
raw	3 oz	108
roe raw	3½ oz	130
CARROT JUICE		
canned	6 oz	73
Hain		
Juice	6 fl oz	80
Hollywood		
Juice	6 fl oz	80
Odwalla		
Juice	8 fl oz	70
CARROTS		
CANNED		
slices	½ cup	17
slices low sodium	½ cup	17
Allen		
Sliced	½ cup (4.5 oz)	35
Crest Top		
Sliced	½ cup (4.5 oz)	35
Del Monte		
Cut	½ cup (4.3 oz)	35
Sliced	½ cup (4.3 oz)	35
S&W		
Diced Fancy	½ cup	30
Julienne French Style Fancy	½ cup	30
Sliced Fancy	½ cup	30
Sliced Water Pack	½ cup	30
Whole Tiny Fancy	½ cup	30
Seneca		
Diced	½ cup	30
Sliced	½ cup	30
FRESH		
baby raw	1 (½ oz)	6
raw	1 (2.5 oz)	31
raw shredded	½ cup	24
slices cooked	½ cup	35
Dole		
Medium	1	40
FROZEN		
slices cooked	½ cup	26

FOOD	PORTION	CALS.
Big Valley		
Carrots	½ cup (3 oz)	35
Birds Eye		
Baby Whole Deluxe	½ cup	40
Polybag Sliced	¾ cup	35
Fresh Like		
Carrots	3.5 oz	42
Green Giant		
Harvest Fresh Baby	½ cup	18
Hanover		
Crinkle Sliced	½ cup	35
CASABA		
cubed	1 cup	45
fresh	1/10	43
CASHEWS		
cashew butter w/o salt	1 tbsp	94
dry roasted	1 oz	163
dry roasted salted	1 oz	163
oil roasted	1 oz	163
oil roasted salted	1 oz	163
Beer Nuts		
Cashews	1 pkg (1 oz)	170
Fisher		
Honey Roasted Halves	1 oz	150
Honey Roasted Whole	1 oz	150
Oil Roasted Halves	1 oz	170
Oil Roasted Whole	1 oz	170
Frito Lay		
Cashews	1 oz	170
Guy's		
Whole Salted	1 oz	170
Hain		
Cashew Butter Raw	2 tbsp	190
Cashew Butter Raw Unsalted	2 tbsp	210
Cashew Butter Toasted	2 tbsp	210
Lance		
Cashews	1 pkg (32 g)	190
Planters		
Fancy Oil Roasted	1 oz	170
Fancy Oil Roasted	1 pkg (2 oz)	340
Halves Lightly Salted Oil Roasted	1 oz	160
Halves Oil Roasted	1 oz	170
Honey Roasted	1 oz	150

FOOD	PORTION	CALS.
Planters (CONT.)		
Honey Roasted	1 pkg (2 oz)	310
Munch'N Go Honey Roasted	1 pkg (2 oz)	310
Munch'N Go Singles Oil Roasted	1 pkg (2 oz)	330
Oil Roasted	1 pkg (1 oz)	160
Oil Roasted	1 pkg (1.5 oz)	250

CASSAVA
raw	3½ oz	120

CATFISH
channel breaded & fried	3 oz	194
channel raw	3 oz	99

CATSUP
(*see* KETCHUP)

CAULIFLOWER
FRESH

broccoflower raw	½ cup (1.8 oz)	16
cooked	½ cup (2.2 oz)	14
flowerets cooked	3 (2 oz)	12
flowerets raw	3 (2 oz)	14
green cooked	½ cup (2.2 oz)	20
raw	½ cup (1.8 oz)	13
Dole		
Cauliflower	⅙ med head	18
Green	⅕ head	35
FROZEN		
cooked	½ cup	17
Big Valley		
Florets	¾ cup (3 oz)	25
Birds Eye		
Frzn	⅔ cup	25
Polybag	½ cup	20
With Cheese Sauce	½ pkg	90
Fresh Like		
Cauliflower	3.5 oz	26
Green Giant		
Cuts	½ cup	12
In Cheese Sauce	½ cup	60
One Serve In Cheese Sauce	1 pkg	80
Hanover		
Cauliflower	½ cup	20

FOOD	PORTION	CALS.
Hanover (CONT.)		
Florets	½ cup	20
JARRED		
Vlasic		
Hot & Spicy	1 oz	4
Sweet	1 oz	35
CAVIAR		
black granular	1 tbsp	40
black granular	1 oz	71
red granular	1 oz	71
red granular	1 tbsp	40
CELERIAC		
fresh cooked	3½ oz	25
raw	½ cup	31
CELERY		
DRIED		
seed	1 tsp	8
FRESH		
diced cooked	½ cup	13
raw	1 stalk (1.3 oz)	6
raw diced	½ cup	10
Dole		
Stalks	2 med	20
FROZEN		
Fresh Like		
Celery	3.5 oz	14
CELTUCE		
raw	3½ oz	22
CEREAL		
COOKED		
corn grits instant	1 pkg (0.8 oz)	82
corn grits quick	1 cup	146
corn grits quick not prep	1 cup	579
corn grits quick not prep	1 tbsp	36
corn grits regular	1 cup	146
corn grits regular not prep	1 cup	579
farina	¾ cup	87
farina not prep	1 tbsp	40
oatmeal	1 cup	145
oatmeal instant cooked w/o salt	1 cup	145
oatmeal not prep	1 cup	311

FOOD	PORTION	CALS.
oatmeal quick cooked w/o salt	1 cup	145
oatmeal regular cooked w/o salt	1 cup	145
Albers		
Hominy Quick Grits uncooked	¼ cup	140
Arrowhead		
4 Grain + Flax	¼ cup (1.6 oz)	150
7 Grain	⅓ cup (1.4 oz)	140
Bear Mush	¼ cup (1.6 oz)	160
Oat Flakes Rolled	⅓ cup (1.2 oz)	130
Oat Groats	¼ cup (1.5 oz)	160
Oatmeal Instant Original	1 oz	100
Rice & Shine	¼ cup (1.5 oz)	150
Wheat Flakes Rolled	⅓ cup (1.2 oz)	110
Aunt Jemima		
Enriched White Hominy Grits Regular	3 tbsp	101
Erewhon		
Barley Plus	1 oz	110
Brown Rice Cream	1 oz	110
Oat Bran With Toasted Wheat Germ	1 oz	115
Oatmeal Instant Apple Cinnamon	1.25 oz	145
Oatmeal Instant Apple Raisin	1.3 oz	150
Oatmeal Instant Dates & Walnuts	1.2 oz	130
Oatmeal Instant Maple Spice	1.2 oz	140
Oatmeal Instant With Added Oat Bran	1.25 oz	125
Good Shepherd		
Spelt	1 oz	90
H-O		
Farina Instant	1 pkg	110
Farina not prep	3 tbsp	120
Oatmeal Instant	1 pkg	110
Oatmeal Instant	½ cup	130
Oatmeal Instant Apple Cinnamon	1 pkg	130
Oatmeal Instant Maple Brown Sugar	1 pkg	160
Oatmeal Instant Raisin & Spice	1 pkg	150
Oatmeal Instant Sweet 'n Mellow	1 pkg	150
Oats 'n Fiber	1 pkg	110
Oats 'n Fiber	⅓ cup	100
Oats 'n Fiber Apple & Bran	1 pkg	130
Oats 'n Fiber Raisin & Bran	1 pkg	150
Oats Gourmet	⅓ cup	100
Oats Quick	½ cup	130
Health Valley		
Oat Bran Natural Apples & Cinnamon	¼ cup (1 oz)	100
Oat Bran Natural Raisins & Spice	¼ cup	100

FOOD	PORTION	CALS.
Kashi		
5-Bran	2½ oz	281
Cereal	2 oz	177
Little Crow		
Coco Wheat	3 tbsp (36 g)	130
Maltex		
Cereal	1 oz	105
Maypo		
30 Second	1 oz	100
Vermont Style	1 oz	105
With Oat Bran	1 oz	130
McCann's		
Irish Oatmeal	1 oz	110
Mother's		
Oatmeal Instant	½ cup (1.4 oz)	150
Whole Wheat Natural	½ cup (1.4 oz)	130
Nabisco		
Cream Of Rice	1 oz	100
Cream Of Wheat Quick as prep	1 cup	120
Cream Of Wheat Regular as prep	1 cup	120
Mix'n Eat Cream Of Wheat Apple & Cinnamon	1 pkg (1¼ oz)	130
Mix'n Eat Cream Of Wheat Maple Brown Sugar	1 pkg (1¼ oz)	130
Mix'n Eat Cream Of Wheat Our Original	1 pkg (1¼ oz)	100
Pillsbury		
Farina	⅔ cup	80
Pritikin		
Apple Raisin Spice	1 pkg (1.6 oz)	170
Multigrain	1 pkg	160
Quaker		
Enriched White Hominy Grits Quick	3 tbsp	101
Enriched Yellow Hominy Quick Grits	3 tbsp	101
Instant Grits White Hominy	1 pkg	79
Instant Grits With Imitation Bacon Bits	1 pkg	101
Instant Grits With Imitation Ham Bits	1 pkg	99
Instant Grits With Real Cheddar Cheese	1 pkg	104
Multigrain	½ cup	130
Oatmeal Instant	1 pkg (1.2 oz)	130
Oatmeal Instant Apples & Cinnamon	1 pkg (1.2 oz)	130
Oatmeal Instant Cinnamon Graham Cookie	1 pkg (1.4 oz)	150
Oatmeal Instant Cinnamon Spice	1 pkg (1.6 oz)	170
Oatmeal Instant Cinnamon Toast	1 pkg (1.2 oz)	130
Oatmeal Instant Fruit & Cream Blueberry	1 pkg (1.2 oz)	130

FOOD	PORTION	CALS.
Quaker (CONT.)		
Oatmeal Instant Honey Nut	1 pkg (1.2 oz)	130
Oatmeal Instant Kids Choice Radical Raspberry	1 pkg (1.4 oz)	150
Oatmeal Instant Maple Brown Sugar	1 pkg (1.5 oz)	160
Oatmeal Instant Peaches & Cream	1 pkg (1.2 oz)	130
Oatmeal Instant Raisin & Walnut	1 pkg (1.3 oz)	140
Oatmeal Instant Raisin Date Walnut	1 pkg (1.3 oz)	130
Oatmeal Instant Raisin Spice	1 pkg (1.5 oz)	160
Oatmeal Instant Strawberries & Cream	1 pkg (1.2 oz)	130
Oatmeal Instant Strawberries 'N Stuff	1 pkg (1.4 oz)	150
Oats Old Fashion	½ cup	150
Oats Quick	½ cup	150
Ralston		
Corn Flakes	1¼ cup (1.1 oz)	120
Roman Meal		
Apple Cinnamon	1.2 oz	105
Cream Of Rye	1.3 oz	111
Oats Wheat Dates Raisins Almonds	1.3 oz	129
Oats Wheat Honey Coconuts Almonds	1.3 oz	155
Original	1 oz	83
Original With Oats	1.2 oz	108
Stone-Buhr		
4 Grain	⅓ cup (1.6 oz)	140
Cracked Wheat	¼ cup (2.4 oz)	210
Manna Golden	6 tsp (1.6 oz)	160
Rolled Oats Old Fashion	6 tsp (1.6 oz)	150
Scotch Oats	¼ cup (1.6 oz)	150
Uncle Roy's		
Muesli Swiss Style	½ cup (1.6 oz)	170
Wheatena		
Cereal	⅓ cup (1.4 oz)	150
READY-TO-EAT		
all bran	½ cup (1 oz)	76
bran flakes	¾ cup (1 oz)	90
corn flakes	1¼ cup (1 oz)	110
corn flakes low sodium	1 cup	100
crispy rice	1 cup	111
fortified oat flakes	1 cup	177
puffed rice	1 cup	57
puffed wheat	1 cup	44
shredded wheat	1 biscuit	83
sugar-coated corn flakes	¾ cup (1 oz)	110

FOOD	PORTION	CALS.
Arrowhead		
Amaranth Flakes	1 cup (1.2 oz)	130
Apple Corns	1 cup (1.5 oz)	150
Bran Flakes	1 cup (1 oz)	100
Kamut Flakes	1 cup (1.1 oz)	120
Maple Corns	1 cup (1.9 oz)	190
Multi Grain Flakes	1 cup (1.2 oz)	140
Nature O's	1 cup (1.1 oz)	130
Oat Bran Flakes	1 cup (1.2 oz)	110
Puffed Corn	1 cup (0.8 oz)	80
Puffed Kamut	1 cup (0.6 oz)	50
Puffed Millet	1 cup (0.9 oz)	90
Puffed Rice	1 cup (0.8 oz)	90
Puffed Wheat	1 cup (0.9)	90
Spelt Flakes	1 cup (1.1 oz)	100
Cap'n Crunch		
Crunchberries	¾ cup	113
Original	¾ cup	113
Peanut Butter Crunch	¾ cup	119
Chex		
Corn	1¼ cup (1 oz)	110
Double	1¼ cup (1 oz)	120
Graham	1 cup (1.8 oz)	210
Rice	1 cup (1.1 oz)	120
Wheat	¾ cup (1.8 oz)	190
Erewhon		
Aztec	1 oz	100
Crispy Brown Rice	1 oz	110
Fruit 'n Wheat	1 oz	100
Raisin Bran	1 oz	100
Super-O's	1 oz	110
Wheat Flakes	1 oz	100
Estee		
Corn Flakes	1 pkg (1 oz)	90
Raisin Bran	1 pkg (1 oz)	90
General Mills		
Basic 4	¾ cup	130
Body Buddies Natural Fruit	1 cup (1 oz)	110
Booberry	1 cup (1 oz)	110
Cheerios	1¼ cup (1 oz)	110
Cheerios Apple Cinnamon	¾ cup (1 oz)	110
Cheerios Honey Nut	¾ cup (1 oz)	110
Cheerios-to-Go	1 pkg (0.75 oz)	80
Cheerios-to-Go Apple Cinnamon	1 pkg (1 oz)	110

FOOD	PORTION	CALS.
General Mills (CONT.)		
Cheerios-to-Go Honey Nut	1 pkg (1 oz)	110
Cinnamon Toast Crunch	¾ cup (1 oz)	120
Clusters	½ cup (1 oz)	110
Cocoa Puffs	1 cup (1 oz)	110
Count Chocula	1 cup (1 oz)	110
Country Corn Flakes	1 cup (1 oz)	110
Crispy Wheats 'N Raisins	¾ cup (1 oz)	100
Fiber One	½ cup (1 oz)	60
Frankenberry	1 cup (1 oz)	110
Fruity Yummy Mummy	1 cup (1 oz)	110
Golden Grahams	¾ cup (1 oz)	110
Kaboom	1 cup (1 oz)	110
Kix	1½ cup (1 oz)	110
Lucky Charms	1 cup (1 oz)	110
Oatmeal Crisp	½ cup (1 oz)	110
Oatmeal Raisin Crisp	½ cup (1.2 oz)	130
Raisin Nut Bran	½ cup (1 oz)	110
S'Mores Grahams	¾ cup (1 oz)	120
Sun Crunchers	1 cup (1.9 oz)	210
Total	1 cup (1 oz)	100
Total Corn Flakes	1 cup (1 oz)	110
Total Raisin Bran	1 cup (1.5 oz)	140
Triples	¾ cup (1 oz)	110
Trix	1 cup (1 oz)	110
Wheaties	1 cup (1 oz)	100
Glenny's		
Maple Frosted Corn	1 oz	109
Oat Mini Puffs	1 oz	108
Oat Mini Puffs No Salt No Sugar	1 oz	108
Rice Mini Puffs	1 oz	109
Good Shepherd		
Millet Rice Flakes Wheat Free	1 oz	95
Spelt Flakes	1 oz	100
Grist Mill		
Apple Cinnamon Natural	½ cup (1.9 oz)	260
Bran	½ cup (1.9 oz)	250
Oat & Honey Natural	½ cup (1.9 oz)	270
Oat Honey & Raisin Natural	½ cup (1.9 oz)	260
Health Valley		
100% Natural Bran With Apples & Cinnamon	¼ cup (1 oz)	100
Blue Corn Flakes 100% Organic	½ cup (1 oz)	90
Bran Cereal With Dates 100% Organic	¼ cup (1 oz)	100

FOOD	PORTION	CALS.
Health Valley (CONT.)		
Bran Cereal With Raisins 100% Organic	¼ cup (1 oz)	100
Fiber 7 Flakes 100% Organic	½ cup (1 oz)	90
Fiber 7 Flakes With Raisins 100% Organic	½ cup (1 oz)	90
Fruit & Fitness	1 cup (2 oz)	220
Fruit Lites Corn	½ cup (0.5 oz)	45
Fruit Lites Rice	½ cup (0.5 oz)	45
Fruit Lites Wheat	½ cup (0.5 oz)	45
Healthy Crunch Almond Date	¼ cup (1 oz)	110
Healthy Crunch Apple Cinnamon	¼ cup (1 oz)	110
Healthy O's 100% Organic	¾ cup (1 oz)	90
Lites Puffed Corn	½ cup (1 oz)	50
Lites Puffed Rice	½ cup (1 oz)	50
Lites Puffed Wheat	½ cup (1 oz)	50
Oat Bran Flakes 100% Organic	½ cup (1 oz)	100
Oat Bran Flakes Almonds/Dates 100% Organic	½ cup (1 oz)	100
Oat Bran Flakes With Raisins 100% Organic	½ cup (1 oz)	100
Oat Bran O'S 100% Organic	½ cup (1 oz)	110
Oat Bran O'S Fruit & Nuts	½ cup (1 oz)	110
Orangeola Almonds & Dates	¼ cup	110
Orangeola Bananas & Hawaiian Fruit	¼ cup (1 oz)	120
Raisin Bran Flakes 100% Organic	½ cup (1 oz)	100
Real Oat Bran Almond Crunch	¼ cup (1 oz)	110
Real Oat Bran Hawaiian Fruit	¼ cup (1 oz)	130
Real Oat Bran Raisin Nut	¼ cup (1 oz)	130
Rice Bran O's	½ cup	110
Rice Bran With Almonds & Dates	½ cup (1 oz)	110
Sprouts 7 Bananas & Hawaiian Fruit	¼ cup (1 oz)	90
Sprouts 7 Raisin	¼ cup	90
Swiss Breakfast Raisin Nut	¼ cup (1 oz)	100
Swiss Breakfast Tropical Fruit	¼ cup (1 oz)	100
Healthy Choice		
Multi-Grain Flakes	1 cup (1.1 oz)	100
Multi-Grain Squares	1¼ cup (2 oz)	190
Heartland		
Coconut	1 oz	130
Plain	1 oz	130
Raisin	1 oz	130
Kashi		
Brittles Sesame/Maple	3½ oz	473
Puffed	¾ oz	74

FOOD	PORTION	CALS.
Kellogg's		
All-Bran	½ cup (1 oz)	80
All-Bran With Extra Fiber	½ cup (1 oz)	50
Apple Cinnamon Rice Krispies	¾ cup (1 oz)	110
Apple Cinnamon Squares	¾ cup (1.9 oz)	180
Apple Jacks	1 cup (1 oz)	110
Apple Raisin Crisp	1 cup (1.9 oz)	180
Blueberry Squares	¾ cup (1.9 oz)	180
Bran Buds	⅓ cup (1 oz)	70
Cinnamon Mini Buns	¾ cup (1 oz)	120
Cocoa Krispies	¾ cup (1 oz)	120
Common Sense Oat Bran	¾ cup (1 oz)	110
Complete Bran Flakes	¾ cup (1 oz)	100
Corn Flakes	1 cup (1 oz)	110
Corn Pops	1 cup (1 oz)	110
Cracklin' Oat Bran	¾ cup (1.9 oz)	230
Crispix	1 cup (1 oz)	110
Double Dip Crunch	¾ cup (1 oz)	110
Froot Loops	1 cup (1 oz)	120
Frosted Mini-Wheats	1 cup (1.9 oz)	190
Frosted Mini-Wheats Bite Size	1 cup (1.9 oz)	190
Frosted Bran	¾ cup (1 oz)	100
Frosted Flakes	¾ cup (1 oz)	120
Frosted Krispies	¾ cup (1 oz)	110
Fruitful Bran	1¼ cup (1.9 oz)	170
Fruity Marshmallow Krispies	¾ cups (1 oz)	110
Just Right Crunchy Nuggets	1 cup (1.9 oz)	200
Just Right Fruit & Nut	1 cup (1.9 oz)	210
Mueslix Golden Crunch	¾ cup (1.9 oz)	210
Nut & Honey Crunch	1¼ cup (1.9 oz)	220
Oatbake Raisin Nut	⅓ cup (1 oz)	110
Pop-Tart Crunch Frosted Strawberry	¾ cup (1 oz)	120
Product 19	1 cup (1 oz)	110
Raisin Bran	1 cup (1.9 oz)	170
Raisin Squares	¾ cup (1.9 oz)	180
Rice Krispies	1¼ cup (1 oz)	110
Special K	1 cup (1 oz)	110
Strawberry Squares	¾ cup (1.9 oz)	180
Temptations French Vanilla Almond	¾ cup (1 oz)	120
Temptations Honey Roasted Pecan	1 cup (1 oz)	120
LaLoma		
Ruskets Biscuits	2 biscuits (30 g)	110
Life		
Cinnamon	⅔ cup	101

FOOD	PORTION	CALS.
Life (CONT.)		
Original	⅔ cup	101
Mueslix		
Crispy Blend	⅔ cup (1.9 oz)	200
Nabisco		
100% Bran	⅓ cup (1 oz)	70
Fruit Wheats Apple	1 oz	90
Shredded Wheat 'n Bran	⅔ cup (1 oz)	90
Shredded Wheat Spoon Size	⅔ cup (1 oz)	90
Shredded Wheat With Oat Bran	⅔ cup (1 oz)	100
Nut & Honey		
Crunch O's	¾ cup (1 oz)	120
Nutri-Grain		
Almond Raisin	1¼ cup (2 oz)	200
Golden Wheat	¾ cup (1.1 oz)	100
Golden Wheat & Raisin	1¼ cup (2 oz)	180
Post		
Alpha-Bits	1 cup (1 oz)	111
Alpha-Bits Marshmallow Sweetened Letter Shaped Oats	1 cup	110
Cocoa Pebbles	⅞ cup (1 oz)	113
Crispy Critters	1 cup (1 oz)	110
Fruit & Fibre Dates Raisins Walnuts With Oat Clusters	⅔ cup	120
Fruit & Fibre Tropical Fruit With Oat Clusters	⅔ cup	125
Fruity Pebbles	⅞ cup	113
Grape-Nuts	¼ cup (1 oz)	105
Grape-Nuts Raisin	¼ cup (1 oz)	102
Honey Bunches Of Oats Honey Roasted	⅔ cup (1 oz)	111
Honey Bunches Of Oats With Almonds	⅔ cup (1 oz)	115
Honeycomb	1 ⅓ cups (1 oz)	110
Natural Bran Flakes	⅔ cup (1 oz)	88
Oat Flakes	⅔ cup (1 oz)	107
Post Toasties Corn Flakes	1¼ cup (1 oz)	111
Raisin Bran	⅔ cup (40 g)	122
Super Golden Crisp	⅞ cup (1 oz)	104
Quaker		
100% Natural	¼ cup	127
100% Natural Apples & Cinnamon	¼ cup	126
100% Natural Raisin & Date	¼ cup	123
Crunchy Bran	⅔ cup	89
Crunchy Not Oh!s	1 cup	127
Honey Graham Oh!s	1 cup	122

FOOD	PORTION	CALS.
Quaker (CONT.)		
King Vitaman	1½ cup	110
Oat Squares	½ cup	105
Popeye Sweet Crunch	1 cup	113
Puffed Rice	1 cup	54
Puffed Wheat	1 cup	50
Shredded Wheat	2 biscuits	132
Ralston		
Almond Delight	1 cup (1.8 oz)	210
Bran Flakes	¾ cup (1.1 oz)	110
Chex Multi-Bran	1¼ cup (2 oz)	220
Cocoa Crispy Rice	1 cup (1.8 oz)	200
Cocoa Crunchies	¾ cup (1.1 oz)	120
Cookie Crisp	1 cup (1 oz)	120
Crisp Crunch	¾ cup (1.1 oz)	120
Crisp Rice	1¼ cup (1.2 oz)	130
Frosted Flakes	¾ cup (1.1 oz)	120
Fruit Rings	¾ cup (0.9 oz)	100
Magic Stair	¾ cup (1.1 oz)	120
Muesli Blueberry	1 cup (1.9 oz)	200
Muesli Cranberry	¾ cup (1.9 oz)	200
Muesli Peach	¾ cup (1.9 oz)	200
Muesli Raspberry	¾ cup (2 oz)	220
Muesli Strawberry	1 cup (1.9 oz)	210
Multi Vitamin Whole Grain Flakes	1 cup (1.1 oz)	120
Nutty Nuggets	½ cup (1.7 oz)	180
Raisin Bran	¾ cup (1.9 oz)	190
Tasteeos	1¼ cup (1.1 oz)	130
Tasteeos Apple Cinnamon	1 cup (1.2 oz)	130
Tasteeos Honey Nut	1 cup (1.2 oz)	130
Rice Krispies		
Treats	¾ cup (1 oz)	120
Smacks		
Cereal	¾ cup (1 oz)	110
Stone-Buhr		
7 Grain	⅓ cup (1.6 oz)	140
Bran Flakes	¼ cup (0.6 oz)	64
Sunbelt		
Muesli	1.9 oz	210
Team		
Cereal	1 cup	110
US Mills		
Poppets	1 oz	110
Uncle Sam	1 oz	110

FOOD	PORTION	CALS.
Weetabix		
Cereal	2 (1.3 oz)	142
CHAMPAGNE		
sekt german champagne	3.5 fl oz	84
Andre		
Blush	1 fl oz	22
Brut	1 fl oz	21
Cold Duck	1 fl oz	25
Extra Dry	1 fl oz	23
Ballatore		
Spumante	1 fl oz	23
Eden Roc		
Brut	1 fl oz	21
Brut Rose'	1 fl oz	22
Extra Dry	1 fl oz	21
Tott's		
Blanc de Noir	1 fl oz	22
Brut	1 fl oz	20
Extra Dry	1 fl oz	21
CHAYOTE		
fresh cooked	1 cup	38
raw	1 (7 oz)	49
raw cut up	1 cup	32
CHEESE		
(*see also* CHEESE DISHES, CHEESE SUBSTITUTES, COTTAGE CHEESE, CREAM CHEESE)		
NATURAL		
bel paese	3½ oz	391
blue	1 oz	100
blue crumbled	1 cup	477
brick	1 oz	105
brie	1 oz	95
cacio di roma sheep's milk cheese	1 oz	130
caerphilly	1.4 oz	150
camembert	1 oz	85
camembert	1 wedge (1⅓ oz)	114
caraway	1 oz	107
cheddar	1 oz	114
cheddar low fat	1 oz	49
cheddar low sodium	1 oz	113
cheddar reduced fat	1.4 oz	104
cheddar shredded	1 cup	455

FOOD	PORTION	CALS.
cheshire	1 oz	110
cheshire reduced fat	1.4 oz	108
colby	1 oz	112
colby low fat	1 oz	49
colby low sodium	1 oz	113
derby	1.4 oz	161
edam	1 oz	101
edam reduced fat	1.4 oz	92
emmentaler	3½ oz	403
feta	1 oz	75
fontina	1 oz	110
fromage frais	1.6 oz	51
gjetost	1 oz	132
gloucester double	1.4 oz	162
goat hard	1 oz	128
goat semi-soft	1 oz	103
goat soft	1 oz	76
gorgonzola	3½ oz	376
gouda	1 oz	101
gruyere	1 oz	117
lancashire	1.4 oz	149
leicester	1.4 oz	160
limburger	1 oz	93
lymeswold	1.4 oz	170
monterey	1 oz	106
mozzarella	1 lb	1276
mozzarella	1 oz	80
mozzarella low moisture	1 oz	90
mozzarella low moisture part skim	1 oz	79
mozzarella part skim	1 oz	72
muenster	1 oz	104
parmesan grated	1 oz	129
parmesan grated	1 tbsp	23
parmesan hard	1 oz	111
port du salut	1 oz	100
provolone	1 oz	100
quark 20% fat	3½ oz	116
quark 40% fat	3½ oz	167
quark made w/ skim milk	3½ oz	78
queso anego	1 oz	106
queso asadero	1 oz	101
queso chichuahua	1 oz	106
ricotta	1 cup	428
ricotta	½ cup	216

FOOD	PORTION	CALS.
ricotta part skim	1 cup	340
ricotta part skim	½ cup	171
romadur 40% fat	3½ oz	289
romano	1 oz	110
roquefort	I oz	105
stilton blue	1.4 oz	164
stilton white	1.4 oz	145
swiss	1 oz	107
tilsit	1 oz	96
wensleydale	1.4 oz	151
whey cheese	3.5 oz	440
yogurt cheese	1 oz	20
Alouette		
Brie Baby	1 oz	110
Brie Baby With Herbs	1 oz	110
Alpine Lace		
Cheddar Reduced Fat	1 piece (1 oz)	80
Colby Reduced Fat	1 piece (1 oz)	80
Feta Reduced Fat	1 piece (1 oz)	60
Mozzarella Reduced Sodium Part Skim	1 piece (1 oz)	70
Muenster Reduced Sodium	1 piece (1 oz)	100
Provolone Smoked Reduced Fat	1 piece (1 oz)	70
Swiss Reduced Fat	1 piece (1 oz)	90
Armour		
Cheddar	1 oz	110
Cheddar Lower Salt	1 oz	110
Colby Lower Salt	1 oz	110
Monterey Jack	1 oz	110
Monterey Jack Lower Salt	1 oz	110
BabyBel		
Mini Light	1 (0.7 oz)	45
Bongrain		
Chavrie	2 tbsp (0.8 oz)	40
Montrachet	1 oz	70
Montrachet Chive	1 oz	70
Montrachet Classic	1 oz	70
Montrachet Classic Herb	1 oz	70
Montrachet Herbs & Garlic	1 oz	70
Montrachet In Oil drained	1 oz	70
Montrachet With Ash	1 oz	70
Breakstone		
Ricotta	¼ cup (2.2 oz)	110
Bresse		
Brie	1 oz	110

FOOD	PORTION	CALS.
Bresse (CONT.)		
Brie Light	1 oz	70
Brie With Herbs	1 oz	110
Creme De Brie	2 tbsp (1 oz)	90
Creme De Brie Herb	2 tbsp (1 oz)	90
Brier Run		
Cherve	1 oz	61
Quark	1 oz	34
Bristol Gold		
Cheddar Light	1 oz	70
French Onion Light	1 oz	70
Garlic & Herb Light	1 oz	70
Horseradish Light	1 oz	70
Smoke Light	1 oz	70
Wine Light	1 oz	70
Cabot		
Cheddar	1 oz	110
Monterey Jack	1 oz	80
Vitalait	1 oz	70
Vitalait Jalapeno	1 oz	70
Churney		
Feta	1 oz	80
Cracker Barrel		
Cheddar Sharp Reduced Fat	1 oz	80
Cheddar Sharp Reduced Fat Shredded	¼ cup (0.9 oz)	80
Delice De France		
Cheese	1 oz	110
With Herbs	1 oz	110
Di Giorno		
Parmesan	2 tsp (5 g)	20
Parmesan Grated	2 tsp (5 g)	20
Parmesan Shredded	2 tsp (5 g)	20
Romano	2 tsp (5 g)	20
Romano Grated	2 tsp (5 g)	25
Romano Shredded	2 tsp (5 g)	20
Dorman		
Cheda-Jack Reduced Fat Low Sodium	1 oz	80
Cheddar	1 oz	110
Cheddar Reduced Fat Low Sodium	1 oz	80
Colby	1 oz	110
Edam	1 oz	100
Gouda	1 oz	100
Monterey Reduced Fat Low Sodium	1 oz	80
Monterey Jack	1 oz	100

FOOD	PORTION	CALS.
Dorman (CONT.)		
Mozzarella Park Skim	1 oz	90
Mozzarella Reduced Fat Low Sodium	1 oz	80
Muenster	1 oz	110
Muenster Low Sodium	1 oz	110
Muenster Reduced Fat Low Sodium	1 oz	80
Parmesan	1 oz	110
Provolone	1 oz	90
Provolone Reduced Fat Low Sodium	1 oz	80
Romano	1 oz	100
Swiss	1 oz	100
Swiss No Salt Added	1 oz	100
Swiss Reduced Fat Low Sodium	1 oz	90
Father Time		
Cheddar Extra-Sharp Premium	1 oz	110
Friendship		
Farmer	2 tbsp (1 oz)	50
Farmer No Salt Added	2 tbsp (1 oz)	50
Hoop	2 tbsp (1 oz)	20
Frigo		
Asiago	1 oz	110
Blue	1 oz	100
Cheddar	1 oz	110
Cheddar Lite	1 oz	80
Feta	1 oz	100
Impastata	1 oz	60
Mozzarella Part Skim Low Moisture	1 oz	80
Mozzarella Whole Milk Low Moisture	1 oz	90
Mozzarella Lite Whole Milk Low Moisture	1 oz	60
Parmazest	1 oz	120
Parmesan Dry Grated	1 oz	130
Parmesan Grated	1 oz	110
Parmesan Whole	1 oz	110
Pizza Shredded	1 oz	65
Provolone	1 oz	100
Provolone Lite	1 oz	70
Ricotta Low Fat Low Salt	1 oz	30
Ricotta Part Skim	1 oz	40
Ricotta Whole Milk	1 oz	60
Romano Dry Grated	1 oz	130
Romano Grated	1 oz	110
Romano Whole	1 oz	110
String	1 oz	80
String Lite	1 oz	60

FOOD	PORTION	CALS.
Frigo (CONT.)		
Swiss	1 oz	110
Taco Shredded	1 oz	110
Gerard		
Brie	1 oz	90
Healthy Choice		
Cheddar Fancy Shreds	¼ cup (1 oz)	45
Cheddar Shreds	¼ cup (1 oz)	45
Mexican Shreds	¼ cup (1 oz)	45
Mozzarella	1 oz	45
Mozzarella Shreds	¼ cup (1 oz)	45
Mozzarella String Cheese	1 stick (1 oz)	45
Pizza Fancy Shreds	¼ cup (1 oz)	45
Pizza String	1 stick (1 oz)	45
Heluva Good Cheese		
Cheddar Curds Snack	1 oz	113
Cheddar Extra-Sharp	1 oz	110
Cheddar Mild	1 oz	110
Cheddar Mild Reduced Fat	1 oz	80
Cheddar Mild White	1 oz	110
Cheddar Sharp	1 oz	110
Cheddar Sharp White	1 oz	110
Cheddar Shredded	¼ cup (1 oz)	110
Cheddar Very Low Sodium	1 oz	110
Cheddar White Extra-Sharp	1 oz	110
Cheddar White Very Low Sodium	1 oz	110
Cheddar White Shredded	¼ cup (1 oz)	110
Colby	1 oz	117
Colby-Jack	1 oz	110
Monterey Jack	1 oz	100
Monterey Jack Shredded	¼ cup (1 oz)	100
Monterey Jack With Jalapenos	1 oz	100
Mozzarella Part Skim Low Moisture Shredded	¼ cup (1 oz)	80
Mozzarella Whole Milk	1 oz	80
Muenster	1 oz	100
Swiss	1 oz	112
Washed Curd Cheese	1 oz	110
Holland Farm		
Edam	1 oz	97
Farmer	1 oz	102
Gouda	1 oz	103
Monterey Jack	1 oz	102
Muenster	1 oz	102

FOOD	PORTION	CALS.
Hollow Road Farms		
Sheep's Milk	1 oz	45
Keller's		
Chub	2 tbsp (1 oz)	100
Kraft		
Baby Swiss	1 oz	110
Blue	1 oz	100
Blue Crumbles	1 oz	100
Brick	1 oz	110
Cheddar	1 oz	110
Cheddar Fat Free Shredded	¼ cup (1 oz)	45
Cheddar Mild Reduced Fat	1 oz	80
Cheddar Mild Reduced Fat Shredded	¼ cup (1.1 oz)	90
Cheddar Nacho Blend With Peppers	1 oz	110
Cheddar Sharp Reduced Fat	1 oz	80
Cheddar Shredded Finely	¼ cup (0.8 oz)	90
Colby	1 oz	110
Colby Reduced Fat	1 oz	80
Colby And Monterey Jack	1 oz	110
Colby And Monterey Jack Shredded	¼ cup (1 oz)	120
Colby And Monterey Jack Shredded Reduced Fat Light	1 oz	80
Farmers	1 oz	100
Gouda	1 oz	110
Havarti	1 oz	120
House Italian ⅓ Less Fat Grated	2 tsp (0.2 oz)	25
Italian Blend Grated	2 tsp (0.2 oz)	25
Limburger	1 oz	90
Monterey Jack	1 oz	110
Monterey Jack Reduced Fat	1 oz	80
Monterey Jack Shredded	¼ cup (1 oz)	110
Monterey Jack With Jalapeno Peppers	1 oz	110
Monterey Jack With Peppers Reduced Fat	1 oz	80
Mozzarella Fat Free Shredded	¼ cup (1 oz)	50
Mozzarella Low Moisture Part Skim Reduced Fat Shredded	¼ cup (1.1 oz)	80
Mozzarella Low Moisture Part Skim Shredded	¼ cup (1 oz)	90
Mozzarella Low Moisture Part Skim Shredded Finely	¼ cup (0.8 oz)	70
Mozzarella Low Moisture Whole Milk Shredded	¼ cup (1 oz)	90
Mozzarella Part Skim Low Moisture	1 oz	80
Mozzarella String Cheese Low Moisture Part Skim	1 stick (1 oz)	80

FOOD	PORTION	CALS.
Kraft (CONT.)		
Muenster	1 oz	110
Parmesan Grated	2 tsp (0.2 oz)	20
Parmesan Shredded	2 tsp (0.2 oz)	20
Pizza Four Cheeses Shredded	¼ cup (0.9 oz)	90
Pizza Mild Cheddar & Mozzarella Shredded	¼ cup (0.9 oz)	90
Pizza Mozzarella & Cheddar	¼ cup (0.9 oz)	100
Pizza Mozzarella & Provolone	¼ cup (0.9 oz)	90
Provolone Smoke Flavor	1 oz	100
Romano Grated	2 tsp (0.2 oz)	25
Shredded	¼ cup (1 oz)	120
String With Jalapeno Peppers	1 oz	80
Swiss	1 oz	110
Swiss Shredded	¼ cup (1 oz)	80
Taco Cheddar & Monterey Jack Shredded	¼ cup (0.9 oz)	100
Land O'Lakes		
Baby Swiss	1 oz	110
Brick	1 oz	100
Chedarella	1 oz	100
Cheddar Light	1 oz	70
Gouda	1 oz	110
Monterey Jack	1 oz	110
Mozzarella	1 oz	80
Muenster	1 oz	100
Provolone	1 oz	100
Swiss	1 oz	110
Swiss Light	1 oz	80
Laughing Cow		
Babybel	1 oz	90
Babybel Mini	1 (0.7 oz)	70
Bonbel	1 oz	100
Bonbel Mini	1 (0.7 oz)	70
Gouda Mini	1 (0.7 oz)	80
Marin French Cheese		
Breakfast	1 oz	86
Brie	1 oz	86
Camembert	1 oz	86
Schloss	1 oz	86
MayBud		
Edam	1 oz	100
Gouda	1 oz	100
Gouda Round	1 oz	100

FOOD	PORTION	CALS.
New Holland		
Cheese	1 oz	90
Garlic	1 oz	90
Havarti Lower Fat Garden Vegetable	1 oz	80
Jalapeno	1 oz	80
Natural Vegetable	1 oz	80
Northfield		
Naturally Slender	1 oz	90
Polly-O		
Mozzarella Free	1 oz	35
Mozzarella Lite	1 oz	60
Mozzarella Part Skim	1 oz	70
Mozzarella Part Skim Shredded	¼ cup	80
Mozzarella Shredded Free	¼ cup	45
Mozzarella Shredded Lite	¼ cup	60
Mozzarella Whole Milk	1 oz	80
Mozzarella Whole Milk Shredded	¼ cup	90
Ricotta Free	¼ cup	50
Ricotta Lite	¼ cup	70
Ricotta Part Skim	¼ cup	90
Ricotta Whole Milk	¼ cup	110
String	1 oz	80
Quaker		
Chub	2 tbsp (1 oz)	100
Sargento		
4 Cheese Mexican Recipe Blend Shredded	¼ cup (1 oz)	110
6 Cheese Italian Recipe Blend Shredded	¼ cup (1 oz)	90
Blue Crumbled	¼ cup (1 oz)	100
Cheddar	1 slice (1 oz)	110
Cheddar Mild Shredded Classic Supreme	¼ cup (1 oz)	110
Cheddar Mild Shredded Fancy Supreme	¼ cup (1 oz)	110
Cheddar Mild Shredded Preferred Light	¼ cup (1 oz)	70
Cheddar Mild White Shredded Classic Supreme	¼ cup (1 oz)	110
Cheddar New York Sharp Shredded Classic Supreme	¼ cup (1 oz)	110
Cheddar Sharp Shredded Classic Supreme	¼ cup (1 oz)	110
Cheddar Sharp Shredded Fancy Supreme	¼ cup (1 oz)	110
Cheese For Nachos & Tacos Shredded	¼ cup (1 oz)	110
Cheese For Pizza Shredded	¼ cup (1 oz)	90
Cheese For Tacos Shredded	¼ cup (1 oz)	110
Cheese For Tacos Shredded Preferred Light	¼ cup (1 oz)	70
Colby	1 slice (1 oz)	110

FOOD	PORTION	CALS.
Sargento (CONT.)		
Colby-Jack Shredded Fancy Supreme	¼ cup (1 oz)	110
Gourmet Parm	1 tbsp	20
Jarlsberg	1 slice (1.2 oz)	120
Monterey Jack	1 slice (1 oz)	100
MooTown Snackers Cheddar	1 piece (0.8 oz)	100
MooTown Snackers Cheddar Mild Light	1 piece (0.8 oz)	60
MooTown Snackers Cheese & Pretzels	1 pkg (1 oz)	90
MooTown Snackers Colby-Jack	1 piece (0.8 oz)	90
MooTown Snackers Pizza Cheese & Sticks	1 pkg (1 oz)	100
MooTown Snackers String Light	1 piece (0.8 oz)	60
Mozzarella	1 slice (1.5 oz)	130
Mozzarella Preferred Light	1 slice (1.5 oz)	100
Mozzarella Shredded Classic Supreme	¼ cup (1 oz)	80
Mozzarella Shredded Fancy Supreme	¼ cup (1 oz)	80
Mozzarella Shredded Preferred Light	¼ cup (1 oz)	70
Muenster	1 slice (1 oz)	100
Parmesan Fresh	1 oz	111
Parmesan Shredded	¼ cup (1 oz)	110
Parmesan & Romano Shredded	¼ cup (1 oz)	110
Pizza Double Cheese Shredded	¼ cup (1 oz)	90
Provolone	1 slice (1 oz)	100
Ricotta Light	¼ cup (2.2 oz)	60
Ricotta Old Fashioned	¼ cup (2.2 oz)	90
Ricotta Part Skim	¼ cup (2.2 oz)	80
Swiss	1 slice (0.7 oz)	80
Swiss Preferred Light	1 slice (1 oz)	80
Swiss Shredded Fancy Supreme	¼ cup (1 oz)	110
Swiss Wafer Thin	2 slices (1 oz)	110
Treasure Cave		
Blue Crumbled	1 oz	110
Feta Crumbled	1 oz	80
Tree Of Life		
Cheddar 33% Reduced Fat Organic Milk	1 oz	90
Cheddar Low Sodium Raw Milk	1 oz	110
Cheddar Mild Organic Milk	1 oz	110
Cheddar Mild Raw Milk	1 oz	110
Cheddar Razor Sharp Raw Milk	1 oz	110
Cheddar Sharp Organic Milk	1 oz	110
Cheddar Sharp Raw Milk	1 oz	110
Colby Organic Milk	1 oz	120
Colby Raw Milk	1 oz	110
Farmer Part-Skim Organic Milk	1 oz	90
Jalapeno Jack Organic Milk	1 oz	110

FOOD	PORTION	CALS.

Tree Of Life (CONT.)

Jalapeno Jack Semi-Soft Organic Milk	1 oz	110
Monterey Jack 35% Reduced Fat Organic Milk	1 oz	80
Monterey Jack Organic Milk	1 oz	100
Monterey Jack Semi-Soft Raw Milk	1 oz	110
Mozzarella Low Moisture Part Skim	1 oz	80
Mozzarella Low Moisture Part Skim Organic Milk	1 oz	80
Muenster Organic Milk	1 oz	100
Muenster Semi-Soft Raw Milk	1 oz	100
Provolone	1 oz	100
Swiss Raw Milk	1 oz	110

Weight Watchers

Cheddar Mild Yellow	1 oz	80
Cheddar Sharp Yellow	1 oz	80
Fat Free Grated Parmesan	1 tbsp	15
Low Sodium Cheddar Mild	1 oz	80
Monterey Jack	1 oz	80

White Clover

Cheddar Light With Simplesse	1 oz	80
Colby Light With Simplesse	1 oz	80
Monterey Jack Light With Simplesse	1 oz	70
Muenster Light With Simplesse	1 oz	70

PROCESSED

american	1 oz	93
american cheese food	1 pkg (8 oz)	745
american cheese spread	1 oz	82
american cheese spread	1 jar (5 oz)	412
american cold pack	1 pkg (8 oz)	752
pimento	1 oz	106
swiss	1 oz	95
swiss cheese food	1 pkg (8 oz)	734

Alouette

French Onion	2 tbsp (0.8 oz)	70
Garlic	2 tbsp (0.8 oz)	70
Light Dill	2 tbsp (0.8 oz)	50
Light Garlic	2 tbsp (0.8 oz)	50
Light Herb	2 tbsp (0.8 oz)	50
Light Herbs & Garlic	2 tbsp (0.8 oz)	50
Light Spring Vegetable	2 tbsp (0.8 oz)	50
Salmon	2 tbsp (0.8 oz)	60
Scallions	2 tbsp (0.8 oz)	70
Spinach	2 tbsp (0.8 oz)	60

FOOD	PORTION	CALS.
Alpine Lace		
American	1 slice (0.66 oz)	50
American Fat Free	1 piece (1 oz)	45
American Hot Pepper Less Fat Less Sodium	1 piece (1 oz)	80
American Less Fat Less Sodium	1 piece (1 oz)	80
Cheddar Fat Free	1 piece (1 oz)	45
Fat Free For Parmesan Lovers	2 tsp (5 g)	10
Fat Free Mexican Macho	2 tbsp (1 oz)	30
Fat Free Singles	1 slice (0.66 oz)	25
Mozzarella Fat Free	1 piece (1 oz)	45
Borden		
American Slices	1 oz	110
American Very Sharp	1 oz	110
Lite Line Mozzarella	1 oz	50
Lite Line Sharp Cheddar	1 oz	50
Lite Line Swiss	1 oz	50
Swiss Slices	1 oz	100
Cheez Whiz		
Light	2 tbsp (1.2 oz)	80
Spread	2 tbsp (1.2 oz)	90
Spread Hot Salsa	2 tbsp (1.2 oz)	90
Spread Jalapeno Peppers	2 tbsp (1.2 oz)	90
Spread Mild Salsa	2 tbsp (1.2 oz)	90
Squeezable	2 tbsp (1.2 oz)	100
Zap-A-Pack Cheese Sauce	2 tbsp (1.2 oz)	90
Zap-A-Pack Cheese Sauce With Mild Salsa	2 tbsp (1.2 oz)	90
Churney		
Diet Snack Cheddar Flavored	1 oz	70
Diet Snack Port Wine Flavored	1 oz	70
Cracker Barrel		
Cheddar Extra Sharp	2 tbsp (1.1 oz)	100
Cheddar Sharp	2 tbsp (1.1 oz)	100
Delico		
Alouette Cajun	2 tbsp (0.8 oz)	70
Alouette French Onion	2 tbsp (0.8 oz)	70
Alouette Garden Vegetable	2 tbsp (0.8 oz)	60
Alouette Garlic	2 tbsp (0.8 oz)	70
Alouette Horseradish & Chive	2 tbsp (0.8 oz)	60
Alouette Spinach	2 tbsp (0.8 oz)	60
Dorman's		
Lo-Chol Cheddar	1 oz	100
Lo-Chol Colby	1 oz	100
Lo-Chol Mozzarella	1 oz	90

FOOD	PORTION	CALS.
Dorman's (CONT.)		
Lo-Chol Muenster	1 oz	100
Lo-Chol Swiss	1 oz	100
Easy Cheese		
Spread American	2 tbsp (1.2 oz)	100
Spread Cheddar	2 tbsp (1.2 oz)	100
Spread Cheddar'n Bacon	2 tbsp (1.2 oz)	100
Spread Nacho	2 tbsp (1.2 oz)	100
Spread Sharp Cheddar	2 tbsp (1.2 oz)	100
Formagg		
Formaggio D'Oro	1 oz	70
Handi-Snacks		
Cheez'n Breadsticks	1 pkg (1.1 oz)	130
Cheez'n Pretzels	1 pkg (1 oz)	110
Mozzarella String Cheese	1 stick (1 oz)	80
Harvest Moon		
American	1 slice (0.7 oz)	70
American	0.7 oz	50
Spread American	0.7 oz	60
Healthy Choice		
American Singles White	1 slice (0.7 oz)	30
American Singles Yellow	1 slice (0.7 oz)	30
Loaf	1 in cube (1 oz)	35
Heluva Good Cheese		
American	1 slice (0.7)	45
Cold Pack Cheddar Sharp	2 tbsp (1 oz)	90
Cold Pack Cheddar Sharp With Bacon	2 tbsp (1 oz)	90
Cold Pack Cheddar Sharp With Horseradish	2 tbsp (1 oz)	90
Cold Pack Cheddar Sharp With Jalapenos	2 tbsp (1 oz)	90
Cold Pack Cheddar Sharp With Port Wine	2 tbsp (1 oz)	90
Hoffman		
American Yellow	1 oz	110
Hot Pepper	1 oz	90
Super Sharp	1 oz	110
Kraft		
American Grated	1 tbsp (0.2 oz)	25
American Shredded	¼ cup (0.9 oz)	110
Cheese With Garlic	1 oz	90
Cheese With Jalapeno Peppers	1 oz	60
Deluxe 25% Less Fat American	0.7 oz	70
Deluxe American	1 oz	100
Deluxe American	1 slice (0.7 oz)	70
Deluxe American	1 slice (1 oz)	110

FOOD	PORTION	CALS.
Kraft (CONT.)		
Deluxe American White	1 oz	100
Deluxe American White	1 slice (0.7 oz)	70
Deluxe American White	1 slice (1 oz)	110
Deluxe Pimento	1 slice (1 oz)	100
Deluxe Swiss	1 slice (1 oz)	90
Deluxe Swiss	1 slice (0.7 oz)	70
Free Singles	1 slice (0.7 oz)	30
Free Singles Sharp Cheddar	1 slice (0.7 oz)	30
Free Singles Swiss	1 slice (0.7 oz)	30
Free Singles White	1 slice (0.7 oz)	30
Singles ⅓ Less Fat American	0.7 oz	40
Singles ⅓ Less Fat American White	0.7 oz	50
Singles ⅓ Less Fat Sharp Cheddar	0.7 oz	50
Singles ⅓ Less Fat Swiss	0.7 oz	50
Singles American	1 slice (0.7 oz)	70
Singles American	1 slice (1.2 oz)	110
Singles American White	1 slice (0.7 oz)	70
Singles Mild Mexican Jalapeno Peppers	1 slice (0.7 oz)	70
Singles Monterey	1 slice (0.7 oz)	70
Singles Pimento	1 slice (0.7 oz)	60
Singles Sharp	1 slice (0.7 oz)	70
Singles Swiss	1 slice (0.7 oz)	70
Spread Jalapeno Pepper	1 oz	80
Spread Olive & Pimento	2 tbsp (1.1 oz)	70
Spread Pimento	2 tbsp (1.1 oz)	80
Spread Pineapple	2 tbsp (1.1 oz)	70
Lactaid		
American	3.5 oz	328
Land O'Lakes		
American	1 oz	110
American	2 slices (1 oz)	100
American	1 slice (0.75 oz)	80
American Less Salt	1 oz	110
American Light	1 oz	70
American Sharp	1 oz	110
American & Swiss	1 oz	100
Jalapeno Light	1 oz	70
Laughing Cow		
Assorted Wedge	1 (1 oz)	70
Cheesebits	6 pieces (1 oz)	70
Original Wedge	1 (1 oz)	70
Wedge Light	1 (1 oz)	50

FOOD	PORTION	CALS.
Light N'Lively		
Singles 50% Less Fat American	0.7 oz	50
Singles 50% Less Fat American White	0.7 oz	50
Mohawk Valley		
Spread Limburger	2 tbsp (1.1 oz)	80
Old English		
American Sharp	1 oz	100
Spread Sharp	2 tbsp (1.1 oz)	70
Price's		
Cheese & Bacon Spread	2 tbsp (1.1 oz)	90
Jalapeno Nacho Dip Hot	2 tbsp (1.1 oz)	80
Jalapeno Nacho Dip Mild	2 tbsp (1.1 oz)	80
Pimento Cheese Spread	2 tbsp (1.1 oz)	80
Pimento Cheese Spread Light	2 tbsp (1.1 oz)	60
Vegetable Garden	2 tbsp (1.1 oz)	70
Roka		
Spread Blue	2 tbsp (1.1 oz)	80
Rondele		
Light Soft Spreadable Garlic & Herb	2 tbsp (0.9 oz)	60
Soft Spreadable Garlic & Herbs	2 tbsp (1 oz)	100
Smart Beat		
American	1 slice (0.6 oz)	35
Low Sodium	1 slice (0.6 oz)	35
Sharp	1 slice (0.6 oz)	35
Spreadery		
Medium Cheddar	2 tbsp (1.1 oz)	80
Pimento Spread	2 tbsp (1.1 oz)	100
Sharp Cheddar	2 tbsp (1.1 oz)	80
Vermont Sharp White Cheddar	2 tbsp (1.1 oz)	80
Squeez-A-Snak		
Spread Sharp	2 tbsp (1.1 oz)	90
Velveeta		
Cheese	1 slice (0.7 oz)	60
Cheese	1 slice (1.2 oz)	100
Cheese	1 slice (0.8 oz)	70
Hot Mexican With Jalapeno Peppers Shredded	¼ cup (1.3 oz)	130
Light	1 oz	60
Mild Mexican With Jalapeno Peppers Shredded	¼ cup (1.3 oz)	130
Shredded	¼ cup (1.3 oz)	130
Spread	1 oz	80
Spread Hot Mexican Jalapeno Pepper	1 oz	80
Spread Italiana	1 oz	60

FOOD	PORTION	CALS.
Velveeta (CONT.)		
Spread Mild Mexican With Jalapeno Pepper	1 oz	80
Weight Watchers		
Fat Free Sharp Cheddar	2 slices (0.75 oz)	30
Fat Free Swiss	2 slices (0.75 oz)	30
Fat Free White	2 slices (0.75 oz)	30
Fat Free Yellow	2 slices (0.75 oz)	30
Reduced Sodium American White	2 slices (0.75 oz)	30
Reduced Sodium American Yellow	2 slices (0.75 oz)	30
WisPride		
Chunk	1 oz	110
Garlic & Herb Cup	2 tbsp (1.1 oz)	100
Hickory Smoked Cup	2 tbsp (1.1 oz)	100
Port Wine Ball	2 tbsp (1.1 oz)	100
Port Wine Cup	2 tbsp (1.1 oz)	100
Port Wine Light Cup	2 tbsp (1.1 oz)	80
Sharp Ball	2 tbsp (1.1 oz)	100
Sharp Cheddar Ball	2 tbsp (1.1 oz)	100
Sharp Cup	2 tbsp (1.1 oz)	100
Sharp Light Cup	2 tbsp (1.1 oz)	80
Swiss Ball	2 tbsp (1.1 oz)	110

CHEESE DISHES

FROZEN
Stouffer's

Welsh Rarebit	¼ cup (1.1 oz)	120
HOME RECIPE		
welsh rarebit as prep w/ 1 white toast	1 slice	228
TAKE-OUT		
cheese omelette as prep w/ 2 eggs	1 (6.8 oz)	519
fondue	1 cup (7.5 oz)	492
fondue	½ cup (3.8 oz)	247
macaroni & cheese	6.3 oz	320

CHEESE SUBSTITUTES

mozzarella	1 oz	70
Borden		
Taco-Mate	1 oz	100
Formagg		
American White	1 slice (0.66 oz)	60
American Yellow	1 slice (0.66 oz)	60
Caesar's Italian Garden American	1 oz	60
Cheddar	1 slice (0.66 oz)	60
Cheddar Shredded	1 oz	60

FOOD	PORTION	CALS.
Formagg (CONT.)		
Classic American	1 oz	60
Macaroni And Cheese Sauce	⅔ cup (5 oz)	190
Mozzarella Shredded	1 oz	60
Old World Mozzarella	1 oz	60
Parmesan Grated	2 tsp (5 g)	15
Swiss	1 oz	60
Swiss White	1 slice (0.66 oz)	60
Vintage Provolone	1 oz	60
Zesty Jalapeno American	1 oz	60
Frigo		
Imitation Cheddar	1 oz	90
Imitation Mozzaralla	1 oz	90
Georgio's		
Imitation Cheddar Shredded	¼ cup (1 oz)	90
Imitation Mozzarella Shredded	¼ cup (1 oz)	90
Golden Image		
American	0.7 oz	70
Harvest Moon		
American Shredded	¼ cup (1.3 oz)	120
Cheddar Shredded	¼ cup (1.3 oz)	120
Mozzarella Shredded	¼ cup (1.3 oz)	110
Lunchwagon		
American	1 slice (0.7 oz)	70
Sargento		
Classic Supreme Cheddar Shredded	¼ cup (1 oz)	90
Classic Supreme Mozzarella Shredded	¼ cup (1 oz)	80
Fancy Supreme Cheddar Shredded	¼ cup (1 oz)	90
White Wave		
Soy A Melt Cheddar	1 oz	80
Soy A Melt Fat Free Cheddar	1 oz	40
Soy A Melt Fat Free Mozzarella	1 oz	40
Soy A Melt Garlic Herb	1 oz	80
Soy A Melt Jalapeno Jack	1 oz	80
Soy A Melt Monterey Jack	1 oz	80
Soy A Melt Mozzarella	1 oz	80
Soy A Melt Singles American	1 slice (¾ oz)	60
Soy A Melt Singles Mozzarella	1 slice (¾ oz)	60

CHERIMOYA

fresh	1	515

CHERRIES
CANNED

sour in heavy syrup	½ cup	232

FOOD	PORTION	CALS.
sour in light syrup	½ cup	189
sour water packed	1 cup	87
sweet in heavy sirup	½ cup	107
sweet in light syrup	½ cup	85
sweet juice pack	½ cup	68
sweet water pack	½ cup	57
Del Monte		
Dark Pitted In Heavy Syrup	½ cup (4.2 oz)	120
Sweet Dark Whole Unpitted In Heavy Syrup	½ cup (4.2 oz)	120
DRIED		
Chukar		
Bing	2 oz	160
Rainer	2 oz	160
Tart	2 oz	170
Tart 'n Sweet	2 oz	180
Sonoma		
Pitted	¼ cup (1.4 oz)	140
FRESH		
sour	1 cup	51
sweet	10	49
Dole		
Cherries	1 cup	90
FROZEN		
sour unsweetened	1 cup	72
sweet sweetened	1 cup	232
Big Valley		
Dark Sweet	¾ cup (4.9 oz)	90

CHERRY JUICE

FOOD	PORTION	CALS.
After The Fall		
Black Cherry	1 can (12 oz)	170
Hi-C		
Box	8.45 fl oz	140
Drink	8 fl oz	130
Juice Works		
Drink	6 oz	100
Juicy Juice		
Drink	1 box (8.45 fl oz)	130
Drink	1 bottle (6 fl oz)	90
Kool-Aid		
Black Cherry	8 oz	98
Drink	8 oz	98
Koolers	1 (8.45 oz)	142

FOOD	PORTION	CALS.
Kool-Aid (CONT.)		
Sugar Free	8 oz	3
Sipps		
Wild Cherry	8.45 oz	130
Smucker's		
Black Cherry	8 oz	130
Black Cherry Sparkler	10 oz	120
Tang		
Fruit Box	8.45 oz	121
Tree Of Life		
Concentrate	8 tsp (1.4 oz)	110

CHERVIL

seed	1 tsp	1

CHESTNUTS

chinese cooked	1 oz	44
chinese dried	1 oz	103
chinese raw	1 oz	64
chinese roasted	1 oz	68
cooked	1 oz	37
dried peeled	1 oz	105
japanese cooked	1 oz	16
japanese dried	1 oz	102
japanese raw	1 oz	44
japanese roasted	1 oz	57
raw peeled	1 oz	56
roasted	1 cup	350
roasted	1 oz	70

CHEWING GUM

bubble gum	1 block (8 g)	27
stick	1 (3 g)	10
Bazooka		
Fruit Chunk	1 piece (6 g)	25
Fruit Soft	1 piece (6 g)	25
Gum	1 piece (4 g)	15
Gum	1 piece (6 g)	25
Beech-Nut		
Peppermint	1 stick (3 g)	10
Spearmint	1 stick (3 g)	10
Big Red		
Stick	1	10
Brock		
Bubble Gum	1 piece (0.2 oz)	20

FOOD	PORTION	CALS.
Bubble Yum		
Bananaberry Split	1 piece (0.3 oz)	25
Cotton Candy	1 piece (0.3 oz)	25
Grape	1 piece (0.3 oz)	25
Luscious Lime	1 piece (0.3 oz)	25
Regular	1 piece (0.3 oz)	25
Sour Apple	1 piece (0.3 oz)	25
Sour Cherry	1 piece (0.3 oz)	25
Sugarless	1 piece (0.2 oz)	15
Sugarless Grape	1 piece (0.2 oz)	15
Sugarless Strawberry	1 piece (0.2 oz)	15
Sugarless Variety	1 piece (0.2 oz)	15
Variety Pack	1 piece (0.3 oz)	25
Watermelon	1 piece (0.3 oz)	25
Wild Strawberry	1 piece (0.3 oz)	25
Bubblicious		
Gum	1 piece (7.9 g)	25
*Care*Free*		
Bubble Gum Sugarless	1 stick (3 g)	10
Sugarless Cinnamon	1 piece (3 g)	5
Sugarless Peppermint	1 piece (3 g)	5
Sugarless Spearmint	1 piece (3 g)	5
Wild Cherry Sugarless	1 stick (3 g)	10
Chiclets		
Original	1 piece (1.59 g)	6
Tiny Size	8 pieces (0.13 g)	tr
Clorets	1 piece (1.59 g)	6
Dentyne		
Cinn-A-Burst	1 piece (3.2 g)	9
Gum	1 piece (1.88 g)	6
Sugar Free	1 piece (1.88 g)	5
Doublemint		
Chewing Gum	1 piece	10
Extra Sugar Free		
Cinnamon	1 piece	8
Spearmint & Peppermint	1 stick	8
Winter Fresh	1 piece	8
Freedent		
Spearmint Peppermint & Cinnamon	1 stick	10
Freshen-Up		
Gum	1 piece (4.2 g)	13
Fruit Stripe		
Variety Pack Chewing & Bubble Gum	1 stick (3 g)	10

FOOD	PORTION	CALS.
Hubba Bubba		
Bubble Gum Cola	1 piece	23
Bubble Gum Sugarfree Grape	1 piece	13
Bubble Gum Sugarfree Original	1 piece	14
Original	1 piece	23
Strawberry Grape Raspberry	1 piece	23
Juicy Fruit		
Stick	1	10
Rain-Blo		
Bubble Gum Balls	1 piece (2 g)	5
Stick*Free		
Sugarless Peppermint	1 stick (3 g)	10
Sugarless Spearmint	1 stick (3 g)	10
Swell		
Bubble Gum	1 piece (3 g)	10
Trident		
Gum	1 piece (1.88 g)	5
Soft Bubble Gum	1 piece (3.3 g)	9
Wrigley's		
Spearmint	1 stick	10

CHIA SEEDS

dried	1 oz	134

CHICKEN

(see also CHICKEN DISHES, CHICKEN SUBSTITUTES, DINNER, HOT DOGS)

CANNED		
chicken spread	1 oz	55
chicken spread	1 tbsp	25
chicken spread barbeque flavored	1 oz	55
w/ broth	1 can (5 oz)	234
w/ broth	½ can (2.5 oz)	117
Hormel		
Chunk	2 oz	70
Chunk Breast	2 oz	60
No Salt Chunk Breast	2 oz	60
Swanson		
Chunk Style Mixin' Chicken	2½ oz	130
White	2½ oz	100
White & Dark	2½ oz	100
Underwood		
Chunky	2.08 oz	150
Chunky Light	2.08 oz	80
Smoky	2.08 oz	150

FOOD	PORTION	CALS.
FRESH		
broiler/fryer back w/ skin batter dipped & fried	½ back (2.5 oz)	238
broiler/fryer back w/ skin floured & fried	1.5 oz	146
broiler/fryer back w/ skin roasted	1 oz	96
broiler/fryer back w/ skin stewed	½ back (2.1 oz)	158
broiler/fryer back w/o skin fried	½ back (2 oz)	167
broiler/fryer breast w/ skin batter dipped & fried	2.9 oz	218
broiler/fryer breast w/ skin batter dipped & fried	½ breast (4.9 oz)	364
broiler/fryer breast w/ skin roasted	2 oz	115
broiler/fryer breast w/ skin roasted	½ breast (3.4 oz)	193
broiler/fryer breast w/ skin stewed	½ breast (3.9 oz)	202
broiler/fryer breast w/o skin fried	½ breast (3 oz)	161
broiler/fryer breast w/o skin roasted	½ breast (3 oz)	142
broiler/fryer breast w/o skin stewed	2 oz	86
broiler/fryer dark meat w/ skin batter dipped & fried	5.9 oz	497
broiler/fryer dark meat w/ skin floured & fried	3.9 oz	313
broiler/fryer dark meat w/ skin roasted	3.5 oz	256
broiler/fryer dark meat w/ skin stewed	3.9 oz	256
broiler/fryer dark meat w/o skin fried	1 cup (5 oz)	334
broiler/fryer dark meat w/o skin roasted	1 cup (5 oz)	286
broiler/fryer dark meat w/o skin stewed	3 oz	165
broiler/fryer dark meat w/o skin stewed	1 cup (5 oz)	269
broiler/fryer drumstick w/ skin batter dipped & fried	1 (2.6 oz)	193
broiler/fryer drumstick w/ skin floured & fried	1 (1.7 oz)	120
broiler/fryer drumstick w/ skin roasted	1 (1.8 oz)	112
broiler/fryer drumstick w/ skin stewed	1 (2 oz)	116
broiler/fryer drumstick w/o skin fried	1 (1.5 oz)	82
broiler/fryer drumstick w/o skin roasted	1 (1.5 oz)	76
broiler/fryer drumstick w/o skin stewed	1 (1.6 oz)	78
broiler/fryer leg w/ skin batter dipped & fried	1 (5.5 oz)	431
broiler/fryer leg w/ skin floured & fried	1 (3.9 oz)	285
broiler/fryer leg w/ skin roasted	1 (4 oz)	265
broiler/fryer leg w/ skin stewed	1 (4.4 oz)	275
broiler/fryer leg w/o skin fried	1 (3.3 oz)	195
broiler/fryer leg w/o skin roasted	1 (3.3 oz)	182
broiler/fryer leg w/o skin stewed	1 (3.5 oz)	187
broiler/fryer light meat w/ skin batter dipped & fried	4 oz	312

FOOD	PORTION	CALS.
broiler/fryer light meat w/ skin floured & fried	2.7 oz	192
broiler/fryer light meat w/ skin roasted	2.8 oz	175
broiler/fryer light meat w/ skin stewed	3.2 oz	181
broiler/fryer light meat w/o skin fried	1 cup (5 oz)	268
broiler/fryer light meat w/o skin roasted	1 cup (5 oz)	242
broiler/fryer light meat w/o skin stewed	1 cup (5 oz)	223
broiler/fryer neck w/ skin stewed	1 (1.3 oz)	94
broiler/fryer neck w/o skin stewed	1 (.6 oz)	32
broiler/fryer skin batter dipped & fried	from ½ chicken (6.7 oz)	748
broiler/fryer skin batter dipped & fried	4 oz	449
broiler/fryer skin floured & fried	1 oz	166
broiler/fryer skin floured & fried	from ½ chicken (2 oz)	281
broiler/fryer skin roasted	from ½ chicken (2 oz)	254
broiler/fryer skin stewed	from ½ chicken (2.5 oz)	261
broiler/fryer thigh w/ skin batter dipped & fried	1 (3 oz)	238
broiler/fryer thigh w/ skin floured & fried	1 (2.2 oz)	162
broiler/fryer thigh w/ skin roasted	1 (2.2 oz)	153
broiler/fryer thigh w/ skin stewed	1 (2.4 oz)	158
broiler/fryer thigh w/o skin fried	1 (1.8 oz)	113
broiler/fryer thigh w/o skin roasted	1 (1.8 oz)	109
broiler/fryer thigh w/o skin stewed	1 (1.9 oz)	107
broiler/fryer w/ skin floured & fried	½ chicken (11 oz)	844
broiler/fryer w/ skin floured & fried	½ breast (3.4 oz)	218
broiler/fryer w/ skin fried	½ chicken (16.4 oz)	1347
broiler/fryer w/ skin roasted	½ chicken (10.5 oz)	715
broiler/fryer w/ skin stewed	½ chicken (11.7 oz)	730
broiler/fryer w/ skin neck & giblets batter dipped & fried	1 chicken (2.3 lbs)	2987
broiler/fryer w/ skin neck & giblets roasted	1 chicken (1.5 lbs)	1598
broiler/fryer w/ skin neck & giblets stewed	1 chicken (1.6 lbs)	1625
broiler/fryer w/o skin fried	1 cup	307
broiler/fryer w/o skin roasted	1 cup (5 oz)	266
broiler/fryer w/o skin stewed	1 cup (5 oz)	248
broiler/fryer w/o skin fried	1 oz	54
broiler/fryer wing w/ skin batter dipped & fried	1 (1.7 oz)	159
broiler/fryer wing w/ skin floured & fried	1 (1.1 oz)	103
broiler/fryer wing w/ skin roasted	1 (1.2 oz)	99
broiler/fryer wing w/ skin stewed	1 (1.4 oz)	100
capon w/ skin neck & giblets roasted	1 chicken (3.1 lbs)	3211
cornish hen w/o skin & bone roasted	½ hen (2 oz)	72
cornish hen w/o skin & bone roasted	1 hen (3.8 oz)	144
cornish hen w/skin roasted	1 hen (8 oz)	595

FOOD	PORTION	CALS.
cornish hen w/skin roasted	½ hen (4 oz)	296
roaster dark meat w/o skin roasted	1 cup (5 oz)	250
roaster light meat w/o skin roasted	1 cup (5 oz)	214
roaster w/ skin neck & giblets roasted	1 chicken (2.4 lbs)	2363
roaster w/ skin roasted	½ chicken (1.1 lbs)	1071
roaster w/o skin roasted	1 cup (5 oz)	469
stewing dark meat w/o skin stewed	1 cup (5 oz)	361
stewing w/ skin neck & giblets stewed	1 chicken (1.3 lbs)	1636
stewing w/ skin stewed	6.2 oz	507
stewing w/ skin stewed	½ chicken (9.2 oz)	744
Perdue		
Boneless Breasts Cooked	3 oz	120
Boneless Breast Tenderloins Cooked	3 oz	100
Boneless Thighs Roasted	2 (3.5 oz)	200
Breast Quarters Cooked	3 oz	180
Burger Cooked	1 (3 oz)	170
Chicken Breast Seasoned Barbecue Cooked	3 oz	110
Chicken Breast Seasoned Italian Cooked	3 oz	100
Chicken Breast Seasoned Lemon Pepper Cooked	3 oz	90
Chicken Breast Seasoned Oriental Cooked	3 oz	100
Cornish Hen Split Dark Meat Roasted	1 half (6.5 oz)	210
Cornish Hen White Meat Cooked	3 oz	170
Drumsticks Roasted	1 (2 oz)	110
Drumsticks Skinless Roasted	2 (3.5 oz)	150
Ground Cooked	3 oz	180
Jumbo Drumsticks Roasted	1 (2 oz)	110
Jumbo Split Breast Roasted	1 (7 oz)	370
Jumbo Thighs Roasted	1 (3 oz)	240
Jumbo Whole Leg Roasted	2 (5.5 oz)	360
Jumbo Wings Roasted	2 (3 oz)	210
Leg Quarters Cooked	3 oz	210
Oven Stuffer Boneless Breast Cooked	3 oz	120
Oven Stuffer Boneless Breast Thin Sliced Cooked	1 slice (2 oz)	80
Oven Stuffer Boneless Thighs Roasted	1 (3.5 oz)	170
Oven Stuffer Dark Meat Roasted	3 oz	200
Oven Stuffer Drumstick Roasted	1 (3.5 oz)	190
Oven Stuffer White Meat Roasted	3 oz	160
Oven Stuffer Whole Breast Cooked	3 oz	150
Oven Stuffer Wing Drummettes Roasted	2 (2.5 oz)	170
Split Breast Skinless Roasted	1 (6 oz)	250
Split Breasts Roasted	1 (7 oz)	370

FOOD	PORTION	CALS.
Perdue (CONT.)		
Thighs Roasted	1 (3 oz)	240
Thighs Skinless Roasted	1 (2.5 oz)	160
Whole White Meat Cooked	3 oz	160
Whole Leg Roasted	1 (5.5 oz)	360
Wingettes Roasted	3 (3 oz)	200
Wings Roasted	2 (3 oz)	210
Tyson		
Breast	3 oz	116
Cornish Hen	3.5 oz	250
Drumstick	3 oz	131
Thigh	3 oz	152
Whole	3 oz	134
Wing	3 oz	147
Wampler Longacre		
Ground raw	1 oz	50
FROZEN		
Tyson		
Boneless Breasts	3.5 oz	210
Boneless Skinless Breast	3.5 oz	130
Boneless Skinless Thighs	3.5 oz	200
Drums & Thighs	3.5 oz	270
Skinless Breast Tenders	3.5 oz	120
FROZEN PREPARED		
Banquet		
Country Fried	1 serv (3 oz)	270
Drum Snackers	2.25 oz	190
Fried Breast	1 piece (4.45 oz)	240
Fried Chicken Thigh & Drumsticks	1 serv (3 oz)	260
Hot & Spicy Nuggets	2.5 oz	230
Hot Popcorn Chicken	1 pkg (3 oz)	290
Nuggets	3 oz	240
Nuggets Chicken & Cheddar	2.7 oz	280
Nuggets Chicken & Mozzarella	6 (2.8 oz)	210
Nuggets Southern Fried	6 (4.5 oz)	340
Nuggets Sweet & Sour	6 (4.5 oz)	320
Patties	1 (2.5 oz)	180
Patties Southern Fried	1 (2.5 oz)	190
Skinless Fried	1 serv (3 oz)	210
Skinless Fried Honey BBQ	1 serv (3 oz)	210
Southern Fried	1 serv (3 oz)	270
Tenders	3 pieces (3 oz)	260
Tenders Southern Fried	3 pieces (3 oz)	260
Wings Hot & Spicy	4 pieces (5 oz)	230

FOOD	PORTION	CALS.
Country Skillet		
Chicken Chunks	5 (3.1 oz)	270
Chicken Nuggets	10 (3.3 oz)	280
Chicken Patties	2.5 oz	190
Southern Fried Chicken Chunks	5 (3.1 oz)	250
Southern Fried Chicken Patties	1 (2.5 oz)	190
Empire		
Nuggets	5 (3 oz)	180
Stix	4 (3.1 oz)	180
Ozark Valley		
Nuggets	4 (2.9 oz)	210
Patties	1 (3 oz)	210
Sensible Chef		
Fried Breast	1 (3 oz)	200
Swanson		
Chicken Nibbles	3¼ oz	300
Chicken Nuggets	3 oz	230
Fried Chicken Breast Portion	4½ oz	360
Pre-Fried Chicken Parts	3¼ oz	270
Thighs & Drumsticks	3¼ oz	290
Tyson		
BBQ Breast Fillets	3 oz	110
Breaded Patties	3 oz	300
Breast Chunks	3 oz	240
Breast Fillets	3 oz	190
Breast Patties	2.6 oz	220
Breast Tenders	3 oz	220
Chick'n Cheddar	2.6 oz	220
Chick'n Chunks	2.6 oz	220
Cordon Blue Mini	1	90
Diced	3 oz	130
Grilled Sandwich	3.5 oz	200
Hors D'Oeuvres Mesquite Chunks	3.5 oz	100
Hot BBQ Breast Tenders	2.75 oz	110
Mesquite Breast Fillets	2.75 oz	100
Mesquite Breast Strips	2.75 oz	100
Mesquite Breast Tenders	2.75 oz	110
Microwave Chunks	3.5 oz	220
Microwave Tenders	3.5 oz	230
Roasted Breast Fillets	1 oz	50
Roasted Breasts	1 oz	50
Roasted Drumsticks	1 oz	50
Roasted Half Chicken	1 oz	60
Roasted Thighs	1 oz	70

FOOD	PORTION	CALS.
Tyson (CONT.)		
Roasted Whole Chicken	1 oz	60
Southern Fried Breast Fillets	3 oz	220
Southern Fried Breast Patties	2.6 oz	220
Southern Fried Chick'n Chunks	2.6 oz	220
Thick & Crispy Patties	2.6 oz	220
Weaver		
Batter Dipped Breast	4.4 oz	310
Batter Dipped Drums & Thighs	3 oz	210
Batter Dipped Wings	4 oz	400
Breast Fillets	4.5 oz	270
Breast Fillets Strips	3.3 oz	200
Breast Patties	3 oz	205
Chicken Nuggets	2.6 oz	190
Crispy Dutch Frye Assorted	3.6 oz	290
Crispy Dutch Frye Breasts	4.5 oz	350
Crispy Dutch Frye Drums & Thighs	3.5 oz	290
Crispy Dutch Frye Wings	4 oz	400
Crispy Light Skinless	2.9 oz	170
Croquettes	2 pieces	280
Croquettes With Gravy	2 pieces + ½ cup gravy	282
Honey Batter Tenders	3 oz	220
Hot Wings	2.7 oz	170
Mini Drums Crispy	3 oz	210
Mini Drums Herbs & Spice	3 oz	200
Premium Tenders	3 oz	170
Rondelets Cheese	1 (2.6 oz)	190
Rondelets Italian	1 (2.6 oz)	190
Rondelets Original	1 (3 oz)	190
READY-TO-USE		
chicken roll light meat	2 oz	90
chicken roll light meat	1 pkg (6 oz)	271
poultry salad sandwich spread	1 tbsp (13 g)	109
poultry salad sandwich spread	1 oz	238
Carl Buddig		
Chicken	1 oz	50
Chicken By George		
Cajun	1 breast (4 oz)	120
Caribbean Grill	1 breast (4 oz)	150
Garlic & Herb	1 breast (4 oz)	120
Italian Bleu Cheese	1 breast (4 oz)	130
Lemon Herb	1 breast (4 oz)	120
Lemon Oregano	1 breast (4 oz)	130
Mesquite Barbecue	1 breast (4 oz)	120

FOOD	PORTION	CALS.
Chicken By George (CONT.)		
Mustard Dill	1 breast (4 oz)	140
Roasted	1 breast (4 oz)	110
Teriyaki	1 breast (4 oz)	130
Tomato Herb With Basil	1 breast (4 oz)	140
Empire		
Barbarcue Whole	5 oz	280
Battered & Breaded Cutlets	1 (3.3 oz)	200
Battered & Breaded Nuggets	5 (3 oz)	200
Bologna	3 slices (1.8 oz)	200
Fried Drum & Thigh	3 oz	240
Falls		
BBQ	3 oz	150
Healthy Choice		
Deli-Thin Oven Roasted Breast	6 slices (2 oz)	45
Deli-Thin Smoked Breast	6 slices (2 oz)	60
Fresh-Trak Oven Roasted Breast	1 slice (1 oz)	30
Oven Roasted Breast	1 slice (1 oz)	25
Smoked Breast	1 slice (1 oz)	35
Hebrew National		
Deli Thin Oven Roasted	1.8 oz	45
Hillshire		
Deli Select Oven Roasted Breast	1 slice	10
Deli Select Smoked Breast	1 slice	10
Flavor Pack 90-99% Fat Free Smoked Breast	1 slice (0.75 oz)	20
Lunch 'N Munch Smoked Chicken/ Monterey Jack	1 pkg (4.5 oz)	350
Lunch 'N Munch Smoked Chicken/ Monterey/ Snickers	1 pkg (4.25 oz)	400
Louis Rich		
Deli-Thin Oven Roasted Breast	4 slices (1.8 oz)	60
Deluxe Oven Roasted Breast	1 slice (1 oz)	40
Hickory Smoked Breast	1 slice (1 oz)	30
Oven Roasted Breast	1 slice (1 oz)	40
Mr. Turkey		
Deli Cuts Hardwood Smoked	3 slices	30
Deli Cuts Oven Roasted	3 slices	25
Oscar Mayer		
Deli-Thin Honey Glazed Breast	4 slices (1.8 oz)	60
Free Oven Roasted Breast	4 slices (1.8 oz)	45
Healthy Favorites Oven Roasted Breast	4 slices (1.8 oz)	40
Lunchables Chicken/Monterey Jack	1 pkg (4.5 oz)	350
Lunchables Deluxe Chicken/Turkey	1 pkg (5.1 oz)	380

FOOD	PORTION	CALS.
Oscar Mayer (CONT.)		
Lunchables Dessert Chocolate Pudding/ Chicken/ Jack	1 pkg (6.2 oz)	370
Smoked Breast	1 slice (1 oz)	25
Perdue		
Cornish Hen Dark Meat Cooked	3 oz	200
Cornish Hen Split White Meat Roasted	½ hen (6.5 oz)	200
Nuggets Chicken & Cheese	5 (3 oz)	220
Nuggets Chik-Tac-Toe Cooked	5 (3 oz)	200
Nuggets Football Basketball Baseball	4 (3 oz)	230
Nuggets Original	5 (3 oz)	200
Nuggets Star & Drumstick	4 (3 oz)	200
Original Tenderloins Cooked	3 oz	160
Original Cutlets Cooked	1 (3.5 oz)	230
Oven Roasted Breast	1 (5 oz)	190
Oven Roasted Drumsticks	2 (2.5 oz)	100
Oven Roasted Half Dark Meat	3 oz	170
Oven Roasted Half White Meat	3 oz	140
Oven Roasted Thighs	1 (3 oz)	170
Oven Roasted Whole Chicken Dark Meat	3 oz	170
Oven Roasted Whole Chicken White Meat	3 oz	140
Perdue Done It! Nuggets Original	1 (.67 oz)	48
Short Cuts Italian	3 oz	110
Short Cuts Lemon Pepper	3 oz	110
Short Cuts Mesquite	3 oz	110
Short Cuts Oven Roasted	3 oz	110
Wings Barbecued	3 oz	200
Wings Hot & Spicy	3 oz	190
Tyson		
Bologna	1 slice	44
Hickory Smoked Breast	1 slice	25
Honey Flavored Breast	1 slice	25
Oven Roasted Breast	1 slice	25
Oven Roasted Mesquite Breast	1 slice	25
Roll	1 slice	26
Wings Barbecue	6-7 (3.5 oz)	218
Wings Hot & Spicy	6-7 (3.5 oz)	218
Wings Roasted	6-7 (3.5 oz)	218
Wings Teriyaki	6-7 (3.5 oz)	218
Wampler Longacre		
Breast	1 oz	35
Chef's Select Breast	1 oz	35
Premium Oven Roasted Breast	1 oz	50
Roll	1 oz	65

FOOD	PORTION	CALS.
Wampler Longacre (CONT.)		
Roll Sliced	1 slice (0.8 oz)	50
Weaver		
Roasted Wings	1 oz	70
Weight Watchers		
Roasted & Smoked Breast	2 slices (¾ oz)	25
TAKE-OUT		
boneless breaded & fried w/ barbecue sauce	6 pieces (4.6 oz)	330
boneless breaded & fried w/ honey	6 pieces (4 oz)	339
boneless breaded & fried w/ mustard sauce	6 pieces (4.6 oz)	323
boneless breaded & fried w/ sweet & sour sauce	6 pieces (4.6 oz)	346
breast & wing breaded & fried	2 pieces (5.7 oz)	494
drumstick breaded & fried	2 pieces (5.2 oz)	430
oven roasted breast of chicken	2 oz	60
thigh breaded & fried	2 pieces (5.2 oz)	430

CHICKEN DISHES

(*see also* CHICKEN SUBSTITUTES, DINNER)

FOOD	PORTION	CALS.
CANNED		
Dinty Moore		
Chicken Stew	1 cup (7.5 oz)	180
Microwave Cup Chicken & Dumpling	1 cup (7.5 oz)	190
Stew	1 cup (8.5 oz)	220
Swanson		
Chicken & Dumplings	7½ oz	220
Chicken Ala King	5¼ oz	190
Chicken Stew	7⅝ oz	160
FROZEN		
Croissant Pocket		
Stuffed Sandwich Chicken Broccoli & Cheddar	1 piece (4.5 oz)	300
Hot Pocket		
Stuffed Sandwich Chicken & Cheddar With Broccoli	1 (4.5 oz)	300
Jimmy Dean		
Grilled Breast Sandwich	1 (5.5 oz)	330
Lean Pockets		
Stuffed Sandwich Chicken Fijita	1 (4.5 oz)	260
Stuffed Sandwich Chicken Parmesan	1 (4.5 oz)	260
Stuffed Sandwich Glazed Chicken Supreme	1 (4.5 oz)	240
Luigino's		
Chicken A La King With Noodles	1 pkg (8 oz)	240

FOOD	PORTION	CALS.
Luigino's (CONT.)		
Noodles With Chicken Peas & Carrots	1 cup (6.3 oz)	260
Noodles With Chicken Peas & Carrots	1 pkg (8 oz)	300
Sweet & Sour Chicken With Rice	1 pkg (8 oz)	300
MicroMagic		
Chicken Sandwich	1 pkg (4.5 oz)	390
Ovenstuffs		
Chicken Turnover	1 (4.75 oz)	350
Tyson		
Microwave Breast Sandwich	4.25 oz	328
Weight Watchers		
Chicken, Broccoli & Cheese Pocket Sandwich	1 (5 oz)	250
Grilled Chicken Sandwich	1 (4 oz)	210
White Castle		
Grilled Chicken Sandwich	2 (4 oz)	250
Grilled Chicken Sandwich w/ Sauce	2 (4.8 oz)	290
MIX		
Skillet Chicken Helper		
Cheesy Broccoli as prep	⅕ pkg (7.5 oz)	270
Creamy Chicken as prep	⅕ pkg (8.25 oz)	290
Creamy Mushroom as prep	⅕ pkg (8 oz)	280
Fettucine Alfredo as prep	⅕ pkg (7.5 oz)	270
Stir-Fried Chicken as prep	⅕ pkg (7 oz)	330
READY-TO-USE		
Spreadables		
Chicken Salad	¼ can	100
Wampler Longacre		
Cacciatore	1 serv (4 oz)	118
Salad	1 oz	70
Salad Lite	1 oz	45
Smokey Barbecue	1 serv (4 oz)	175
Sweet N Sour	1 serv (4 oz)	106
Szechwan With Peanuts	1 serv (4 oz)	112
SHELF-STABLE		
Dinty Moore		
American Classics Chicken & Noodles	1 bowl (10 oz)	260
American Classics Chicken With Mashed Potatoes	1 bowl (10 oz)	220
Lunch Bucket		
Dumplings'n Chicken	1 pkg (7.5 oz)	140
Light'n Healthy Chicken Fiesta	1 pkg (7.5 oz)	170
Top Shelf		
Chicken Cacciatore	1 bowl (10 oz)	210

FOOD	PORTION	CALS.
Top Shelf (CONT.)		
Chicken Acapulco Fiesta Chicken	1 bowl (10 oz)	420
Chicken Ala King	1 bowl (10 oz)	380
Glazed Breast Of Chicken	1 bowl (10 oz)	200
TAKE-OUT		
chicken & dumplings	¾ cup	256
chicken & noodles	1 cup	365
chicken a la king	1 cup	470
chicken pie w/ top crust	1 slice (5.6 oz)	472
fillet sandwich plain	1	515
fillet sandwich w/ cheese lettuce mayonnaise & tomato	1	632

CHICKEN SUBSTITUTES

FOOD	PORTION	CALS.
Harvest Direct		
TVP Poultry Chunks	3.5 oz	280
TVP Poultry Ground	3.5 oz	280
Jaclyn's		
Salsa Chicken Style Dinner	11.5 oz	325
Sesame Chicken Style Dinner	11.5 oz	345
Knox Mountain Farm		
Chick'N Wheat Mix	1 serv (1/9 pkg)	110
LaLoma		
Chicken Supreme not prep	¼ cup (16 g)	50
Chik Nuggets	5 nuggets (85 g)	270
Fried Chicken	1 piece (57 g)	180
Fried Chicken w/ Gravy	2 piece (85 g)	140
White Wave		
Meatless Sandwich Slices	2 slices (1.6 oz)	80
Worthington		
Chick-ketts	½ cup (84 g)	160
ChickStiks	1 (47 g)	110
Chicken Sliced	2 slices (57 g)	130
CrispyChik	6 nuggets (85 g)	280
CrispyChik	1 patty (71 g)	220
Cutlets	1.5 slices (92 g)	100
Diced Chik	¼ cup (60 g)	90
FriChik	2 pieces (90 g)	180
Golden Croquettes	5 pieces (106 g)	280
Savory Slices	2 slices (60 g)	90
Vegetarian Chicken Pie	1 (227 g)	380

CHICKPEAS

FOOD	PORTION	CALS.
CANNED		
chickpeas	1 cup	285

FOOD	PORTION	CALS.
Allen		
Garbanzo	½ cup (4.4 oz)	120
East Texas Fair		
Garbanzo	½ cup (4.4 oz)	120
Eden		
Organic	½ cup (4.1 oz)	110
Goya		
Spanish Style	7.5 oz	150
Green Giant		
Garbanzo	½ cup	90
Hanover		
Chickpeas	½ cup	100
Old El Paso		
Garbanzo	½ cup (4.6 oz)	120
Progresso		
Chick Peas	½ cup (4.6 oz)	120
S&W		
Garbanzo Lite 50% Less Salt	½ cup	110
Garbanzo Premium Large	½ cup	110
Garbanzo Water Pack	½ cup	105
DRIED		
cooked	1 cup	269
Bean Cuisine		
Garbanzo	½ cup	115

CHICORY

greens raw chopped	½ cup	21
root raw	1 (2.1 oz)	44
roots raw cut up	½ cup (1.6 oz)	33
witloof head raw	1 (1.9 oz)	9
witloof raw	½ cup (1.6 oz)	8

CHILI

CANNED		
chili w/ beans	1 cup	286
Allen		
Mexican Chili Beans	½ cup (4.5 oz)	120
Armour		
Chili No Beans	1 cup (8.7 oz)	470
Chili With Beans	1 cup (8.9 oz)	440
Chili With Beans Hot	1 cup (8.9 oz)	440
Chili With Beans Western Style	1 cup (8.8 oz)	460
Brown Beauty		
Mexican Chili Beans	½ cup (4.5 oz)	120

FOOD	PORTION	CALS.
Chi-Chi's		
San Antonio	1 cup (8.5 oz)	240
Del Monte		
Sauce	1 tbsp (0.6 oz)	20
Dennison's		
Chili Beans In Chili Gravy	7.5 oz	180
Chili Con Carne w/ Beans	7.5 oz	310
Chili Con Carne w/ Beans	7.5 oz	300
Chunky Chili w/ Beans	7.5 oz	310
Cook-off Chili w/ Beans	7.5 oz	340
Hot Chili Con Carne w/ Beans	7.5 oz	310
Gebhardt		
Hot With Beans	1 cup	470
Plain	1 cup	530
With Beans	1 cup	495
Hain		
Spicy Tempeh	7½ oz	160
Spicy Vegetarian	7½ oz	160
Spicy Vegetarian Reduced Sodium	7½ oz	170
Spicy With Chicken	7½ oz	130
Health Valley		
Mild Vegetarian With Beans	5 oz	160
Mild Vegetarian With Beans No Salt Added	5 oz	160
Mild Vegetarian With Lentils	5 oz	140
Mild Vegetarian With Lentils No Salt Added	5 oz	140
Spicy Vegetarian With Beans	5 oz	160
Hormel		
Chili Mac	1 can (7.5 oz)	200
Chili No Beans	1 cup (8.3 oz)	410
Chili With Beans	1 cup (8.7 oz)	340
Chunky Chili With Beans	1 cup (8.7 oz)	330
Hot Chili No Beans	1 cup (8.3 oz)	410
Hot Chili With Beans	1 cup (8.7 oz)	340
Hot With Beans	1 can (7.5 oz)	250
No Beans	1 can (7.5 oz)	390
Turkey Chili With Beans	1 cup (8.7 oz)	220
Turkey Chili No Beans	1 cup (8.3 oz)	190
With Beans	1 can (7.5 oz)	250
Hunt's		
Chili Beans	4 oz	100
Just Rite		
Hot With Beans	4 oz	195
With Beans	4 oz	200

FOOD	PORTION	CALS.
Just Rite (CONT.)		
Without Beans	4 oz	180
Luck's		
Hot Chili Beans	7.5 oz	200
Natural Touch		
Vegetarian	⅔ cup (190 g)	230
Old El Paso		
Chili With Beans	1 cup (8 oz)	200
S&W		
Chili Beans	½ cup	130
Chili Makin's Original	½ cup	100
Van Camp's		
Chilee Beanee Weenee	1 can (8 oz)	240
Chili With Beans	1 cup (8.9 oz)	350
Wolf Brand		
Chili-Mac	7.5 oz	317
Extra Spicy With Beans	7.5 oz	324
Extra Spicy Without Beans	7.5 oz	363
Plain	7.5 oz	330
With Beans	7.5 oz	345
Without Beans	1 cup	387
Worthington		
Chili	⅔ cup (141 g)	190
DRIED		
powder	1 tsp	8
Gebhardt		
Chili Powder	1 tsp	15
Chili Quik Seasoning	1 tsp	10
Hain		
Hot Chili	¼ pkg	30
Medium Chili	¼ pkg	30
Mild Chili	¼ pkg	30
Nile Spice		
Chili'n Beans Original	1 pkg	150
Chili'n Beans Spicy	1 pkg	150
Old El Paso		
Chili Seasoning Mix	1 tbsp (0.3 oz)	25
Watkins		
Chili Seasoning	1¼ tsp (4 g)	15
Powder	¼ tsp (0.5 g)	0
FROZEN		
Lean Cuisine		
Three Bean	1 pkg (9 oz)	210

FOOD	PORTION	CALS.
Lightlife		
Chili	4.3 oz	110
Luigino's		
Chili-Mac	1 pkg (8 oz)	230
Stouffer's		
With Beans	1 pkg (8.75 oz)	270
Swanson		
Homestyle Chili Con Carne	8¼ oz	270
Tabatchnick		
Vegetarian	7.5 oz	210
Tyson		
Chicken Chili	3.5 oz	105
SHELF-STABLE		
Lunch Bucket		
Chili With Beans	1 pkg (7.5 oz)	300
Micro Cup Meals		
Chili Mac	1 cup (7.5 oz)	200
Chili No Beans	1 cup (7.5 oz)	290
Chili With Beans	1 cup (7.5 oz)	250
Chili With Beans	1 cup (10.4 oz)	410
Hot Chili With Beans	1 cup (7.5 oz)	250
Wampler Longacre		
Turkey	1 serv (4 oz)	118
TAKE-OUT		
con carne w/ beans	8.9 oz	254

CHINESE CABBAGE
(*see* CABBAGE)

CHINESE FOOD
(*see* ORIENTAL FOOD)

CHINESE PRESERVING MELON
cooked	½ cup	11

CHIPS
(*see also* POPCORN, PRETZELS, SNACKS)
CORN

barbecue	1 oz	148
barbecue	1 bag (7 oz)	1036
cones nacho	1 oz	152
cones plain	1 oz	145
onion	1 oz	142
plain	1 oz	153
plain	1 bag (7 oz)	1067
puffs cheese	1 oz	157

FOOD	PORTION	CALS.
puffs cheese	1 bag (8 oz)	1256
twists cheese	1 oz	157
twists cheese	1 bag (8 oz)	1256
Energy Food Factory		
Corn Pops Fat Free	½ oz	50
Corn Pops Nacho	½ oz	50
Corn Pops Original	½ oz	50
Fritos		
Chili Cheese	34 pieces (1 oz)	160
Chips	34 pieces (1 oz)	150
Crisp 'N Thin	18 pieces (1 oz)	160
Dip Size	13 pieces (1 oz)	150
Non-Stop Nacho Cheese	34 pieces (1 oz)	150
Rowdy Rustlers Bar-B-Q	34 pieces (1 oz)	150
Wild 'N Mild	32 pieces (1 oz)	160
Health Valley		
Chips	1 oz	160
No Salt Added	1 oz	160
With Cheddar Cheese	1 oz	160
Lance		
BBQ	1 pkg (50 g)	260
Chips	1 pkg (50 g)	270
Planters		
Corn Chips	34 chips (1 oz)	170
King Size	17 chips (1 oz)	160
Snacks To Go	1 pkg (1.5 oz)	240
Snyder's		
BBQ	1 oz	160
Chips	1 oz	160
Wise		
Corn	1 oz	160
Corn Crunchies	1 oz	160
Crispy Corn	1 oz	160
Crispy Corn Nacho Cheese	1 oz	160
MULTIGRAIN		
Sunchips		
Chips	12 pieces (1 oz)	150
French Onion	12 pieces (1 oz)	140
POTATO		
barbecue	1 bag (7 oz)	971
barbecue	1 oz	139
cheese	1 bag (6 oz)	842
cheese	1 oz	140
light	1 bag (6 oz)	801

FOOD	PORTION	CALS.
light	1 oz	134
potato	1 oz	152
potato	1 pkg (8 oz)	1217
potato	1 oz	152
potato	1 bag (8 oz)	1217
sour cream & onion	1 bag (7 oz)	1051
sour cream & onion	1 oz	150
sticks	½ cup (0.6 oz)	94
sticks	1 oz	148
sticks	1 pkg (1 oz)	148
sticks	½ cup	94
Barrel O' Fun		
Barbeque	1 oz	145
Chips	1 oz	150
Sour Cream & Onion	1 oz	150
Butterfield		
Sticks	⅔ cup (1 oz)	150
Sticks	1 pkg (1.7 oz)	250
Cape Cod		
Chips	19 chips (1 oz)	150
Cottage Fries		
No Salt Added	1 oz	160
Energy Food Factory		
Potato Pops Au Gratin	½ oz	60
Potato Pops Fat Free	½ oz	50
Potato Pops Herb & Garlic	½ oz	50
Potato Pops Mesquite	½ oz	50
Potato Pops Original	½ oz	50
Potato Pops Salt N' Vinegar	½ oz	50
Health Valley		
Country Ripple	1 oz	160
Country Ripple No Salt Added	1 oz	160
Dip Chips	1 oz	160
Dip Chips No Salt Added	1 oz	160
Natural	1 oz	160
Natural No Salt Added	1 oz	160
Kelly's		
Bar-B-Q	1 oz	150
Chips	1 oz	150
Crunchy	1 oz	150
Rippled	1 oz	150
Sour Cream n' Onion	1 oz	150
Unsalted	1 oz	150

FOOD	PORTION	CALS.
Lance		
BBQ	1 pkg (32 g)	190
Cajun Style	1 pkg (32 g)	160
Chips	1 pkg (32 g)	190
Hot Fries	1 pkg (28 g)	160
Ripple	1 pkg (32 g)	190
Sour Cream & Onion	1 pkg (32 g)	190
Lay's		
Bar-B-Q	17 pieces (1 oz)	150
Cheddar Cheese	17 pieces (1 oz)	150
Chips	17 pieces (1 oz)	150
Crunch Tators	16 pieces (1 oz)	150
Crunch Tators Amazin' Cajun	16 pieces (1 oz)	150
Crunch Tators Hoppin' Jalapeno	16 pieces (1 oz)	140
Crunch Tators Mighty Mesquite	16 pieces (1 oz)	150
Crunch Tators Supreme Sour Cream	16 pieces (1 oz)	150
Flamin' Hot	17 pieces (1 oz)	150
Kansas City Style Bar-B-Q	17 pieces (1 oz)	150
Salt & Vinegar	17 pieces (1 oz)	150
Sour Cream & Onion	17 pieces (1 oz)	160
Tangy Ranch	17 pieces (1 oz)	160
Unsalted	17 pieces (1 oz)	150
Louise's		
"1g" Mesquite BBQ	1 oz	110
"1g" Original	1 oz	110
70% Less Fat Mesquite BBQ	1 oz	110
70% Less Fat Original	1 oz	110
Fat-Free Maui Onion	1 oz	110
Fat-Free Mesquite BBQ	1 oz	110
Fat-Free No Salt	1 oz	110
Fat-Free Original	1 oz	110
Fat-Free Vinegar & Salt	1 oz	110
Mr. Phipps		
Tater Crisps Bar-B-Que	21 (1 oz)	130
Tater Crisps Original	23 (1 oz)	120
Tater Crisps Sour Cream 'n Onion	22 (1 oz)	130
New York Deli		
Chips	1 oz	160
Old Dutch Foods		
Augratin	1 oz	150
BBQ	1 oz	140
Chips	1 oz	150
Dill Flavored	1 oz	150
Onion & Garlic	1 oz	150

FOOD	PORTION	CALS.
Old Dutch Foods (CONT.)		
Ripple	1 oz	150
Sour Cream & Onion	1 oz	150
Pringles		
BBQ	14 chips (1 oz)	150
Cheez-ums	14 chips (1 oz)	150
Original	14 chips (1 oz)	160
Ranch	14 chips (1 oz)	150
Ridges Cheddar & Sour Cream	12 chips (1 oz)	150
Ridges Mesquite BBQ	12 chips (1 oz)	150
Ridges Original	12 chips (1 oz)	150
Right BBQ	16 chips (1 oz)	140
Right Original	16 chips (1 oz)	140
Right Ranch	16 chips (1 oz)	140
Right Sour Cream 'N Onion	16 chips (1 oz)	140
Rippled Original	10 chips (1 oz)	160
Sour Cream N'Onion	14 chips (1 oz)	160
Ruffles		
Cheddar Cheese & Sour Cream	18 chips (1 oz)	160
Chips	18 chips (1 oz)	150
Light	18 chips (1 oz)	130
Light Sour Cream & Onion	18 chips (1 oz)	130
Mesquite Grille B-B-Q	18 chips (1 oz)	160
Monterey Jack Cheese Attack	18 chips (1 oz)	160
Ranch	18 chips (1 oz)	160
Sour Cream & Onion	18 chips (1 oz)	160
Snyder's		
BBQ	1 oz	150
Cheddar Bacon	1 oz	150
Chips	1 oz	150
Coney Island	1 oz	150
Grilled Steak & Onion	1 oz	150
Hot Buffalo Wings	1 oz	150
Kosher Dill	1 oz	150
No Salt	1 oz	150
Salt & Vinegar	1 oz	150
Sausage Pizza	1 oz	150
Sour Cream & Onion	1 oz	150
Sour Cream & Onion Unsalted	1 oz	150
State Line		
Chips	1 pkg (0.5 oz)	80
Suprimos		
Cheddar & Jack	1 oz	140
Cool Onion	1 oz	140

FOOD	PORTION	CALS.
Weight Watchers		
Barbecue Curls	1 pkg (0.5 oz)	60
Wise		
Natural	1 oz	160
Ridgies Barbecue	1 oz	150
TORTILLA		
nacho	1 oz	141
nacho	1 bag (8 oz)	1131
nacho light	1 bag (6 oz)	757
nacho light	1 oz	126
plain	1 bag (7.5 oz)	1067
plain	1 oz	142
ranch	1 oz	139
ranch	1 bag (7 oz)	969
taco	1 bag (8 oz)	1089
taco	1 oz	136
Barrel O' Fun		
Nacho	1 oz	140
Tostada Yellow	1 oz	140
White	1 oz	140
Doritos		
Lightly Salted	16 chips (1 oz)	150
Frito Lay		
Salsa 'N Cheese	16 (1 oz)	150
Guiltless Gourmet		
Baked	22-26 chips (1 oz)	110
Hain		
Sesame	1 oz	140
Sesame Cheese	1 oz	160
Sesame No Salt Added	1 oz	140
Taco Style	1 oz	160
La FAMOUS		
No Salt Added	1 oz	140
Tortilla	1 oz	140
Lance		
Jalapeno Cheese	1 pkg (1⅛ oz)	160
Nacho	1 pkg (32 g)	160
Louise's		
95% Fat-Free	1 oz	120
Mr. Phipps		
Nacho	28 (1 oz)	130
Original	28 (1 oz)	130
Old El Paso		
NACHIPS	9 chips (1 oz)	150

FOOD	PORTION	CALS.
Old El Paso (CONT.)		
White Corn	11 chips (1 oz)	140
Santitas		
Cantina Style	1 oz	140
Cantina Style Fajita	1 oz	140
Chips	1 oz	140
Strips	1 oz	140
Snyder's		
Chips	1 oz	140
Enchilada	1 oz	140
Nacho Cheese	1 oz	140
No Salt	1 oz	140
Ranch	1 oz	140
Tostitos		
Baked	1 oz	110
Baked Cool Ranch	1 oz	130
Baked Unsalted	1 oz	110
Bite Size	16 pieces (1 oz)	150
Chips	11 pieces (1 oz)	140
Restaurant Style Lime 'N Chili	7 pieces (1 oz)	150
Restaurant Style White Corn	7 pieces (1 oz)	150
Tyson		
Nacho Cheese	1 oz	140
Ranch Flavor	1 oz	140
Traditional	1 oz	140
Unsalted	1 oz	140
Wise		
Bravos	1 oz	150
VEGETABLE		
taro	10 (0.8 oz)	115
taro	1 oz	141
Eden		
Vegetable Chips	50 (1 oz)	130
Wasabi Chip Hot & Spicy	50 (1 oz)	130
Hain		
Carrot Chips	1 oz	150
Carrot Chips Barbecue	1 oz	140
Carrot Chips No Salt Added	1 oz	150
Health Valley		
Carrot Lites	0.5 oz	75
Terra Chips		
Sweet Potato	1 oz	140
Sweet Potato Spiced	1 oz	140
Taro Spiced	1 oz	130

FOOD	PORTION	CALS.
Terra Chips (CONT.)		
Vegetable	1 oz	140
Top Banana		
Plantain Chips	1 oz	150

CHITTERLINGS

pork, simmered	3 oz	258

CHIVES

freeze-dried	1 tbsp	1
fresh chopped	1 tbsp	1
fresh chopped	1 tsp	0

CHOCOLATE

(*see also* CANDY, CAROB, COCOA, ICE CREAM TOPPINGS, MILK DRINKS)

FOOD	PORTION	CALS.
BAKING		
baking	1 oz	145
grated unsweetened	1 cup (4.6 oz)	690
liquid unsweetened	1 oz	134
squares unsweetened	1 square (1 oz)	148
Baker's		
German Sweet	¼ cup	200
German Sweet	1 oz	143
Semi-Sweet	1 oz	135
Unsweetened	1 oz	141
Hershey		
Premium Semi-Sweet	1 oz	140
Premium Unsweetened	1 oz	190
Nestle		
Choco Bake	½ oz	80
Premier White	½ oz	80
Semi-Sweet	½ oz	70
Unsweetened	½ oz	80
CHIPS		
milk chocolate	1 cup (6 oz)	862
semisweet	1 cup (6 oz)	804
semisweet	60 pieces (1 oz)	136
Baker's		
Big Milk Chocolate	¼ cup	239
Big Semi-Sweet	¼ cup	220
Chips	1 oz	143
Real Semi-Sweet	¼ cup	198
Semi-Sweet	¼ cup	197
Hershey		
Chunks Milk Chocolate	1 oz	160

FOOD	PORTION	CALS.
Hershey (CONT.)		
Chunks Semi-Sweet	1 oz	140
Milk Chocolate	1 oz	150
Mint Chocolate	¼ cup	230
Semi-Sweet	¼ cup (1.5 oz)	220
Semi-Sweet Miniature	¼ cup (1.5 oz)	220
M&M's		
Baking Bits Milk Chocolate	0.5 oz	70
Baking Bits Semi-Sweet	0.5 oz	70
Nestle		
Morsels Milk Chocolate	1 tbsp	70
Morsels Mint Chocolate	1 tbsp	70
Morsels Rainbow	1 tbsp	70
Morsels Mini Semi-Sweet	1 tbsp	70
Semi-Sweet Morsels	1 tbsp	40
MIX		
powder	2-3 heaping tsp	75
powder as prep w/ whole milk	9 oz	226
Crumpy		
Chocolate Hazelnut Spread	1 tbsp (0.5 oz)	80
Hershey		
Chocolate Milk Mix	3 tbsp	90

CHOCOLATE MILK
(*see* CHOCOLATE, COCOA, MILK DRINKS)

CHOCOLATE SYRUP

chocolate fudge	1 tbsp (0.7 oz)	73
chocolate fudge	1 cup (11.9 oz)	1176
syrup	1 cup	653
syrup	2 tbsp	82
syrup as prep w/ whole milk	9 oz	232
Estee		
Choco-Syp	2 tbsp (1.2 oz)	50
Hershey		
Syrup	2 tbsp	80
Marzetti		
Syrup	2 tbsp	40
Quik		
Chocolate	1 ⅔ tbsp	100
Red Wing		
Syrup	2 tbsp (1.4 oz)	110

CHUTNEY

apple	1.2 oz	68

FOOD	PORTION	CALS.
apple cranberry	1 tbsp	16
tomato	1.2 oz	54
Sonoma		
Dried Tomato	1 tbsp (0.7 g)	35
CILANTRO		
fresh	¼ cup	1
Watkins		
Dried	¼ tsp (0.5 oz)	0
CINNAMON		
ground	1 tsp	6
sticks	0.5 oz	39
Watkins		
Ground	¼ tsp (0.5 g)	0
CISCO		
raw	3 oz	84
smoked	3 oz	151
smoked	1 oz	50
CLAM JUICE		
Doxsee		
Canned	3 fl oz	4
CLAMS		
CANNED		
liquid only	1 cup	6
liquid only	3 oz	2
meat only	1 cup	236
meat only	3 oz	126
American Original		
Quahogs	4 oz	66
Doxsee		
Chopped	6.5 oz	90
Empress		
Whole Baby	4 oz	60
Gorton's		
Minced & Chopped	½ can	70
Progresso		
Minced	¼ cup (2 oz)	25
White Clam Sauce	½ cup (4.4 oz)	120
S&W		
Fancy Chopped	2 oz	28
Fancy Minced	2 oz	28
Whole Baby Chowder Clams	2 oz	33

FOOD	PORTION	CALS.
Snow's		
Minced	6.5 oz	90
FRESH		
cooked	3 oz	126
cooked	20 sm	133
raw	20 sm (180 g)	133
raw	9 lg (180 g)	133
raw	3 oz	63
FROZEN		
Gorton's		
Microwave Chrunchy Clam Strips	3.5 oz	330
Mrs. Paul's		
Fried	2½ oz	200
Microwave Fried Clams	2.5 oz	260
HOME RECIPE		
breaded & fried	3 oz	171
breaded & fried	20 sm	379
JARRED		
Progresso		
Creamy Clam	½ cup (4.2 oz)	100
Red Clam	½ cup (4.4 oz)	80
TAKE-OUT		
breaded & fried	¾ cup	451

CLOVES

ground	1 tsp	7

COCOA
(*see also* CHOCOLATE)

hot cocoa	1 cup	218
mix as prep w/ water	7 oz	103
mix w/ equal as prep w/ water	7 oz	48
powder unsweetened	1 tbsp (5 g)	11
powder unsweetened	1 cup (3 oz)	197
Carnation		
Hot Cocoa 70 Calorie	3 tsp (21 g)	70
Hot Cocoa Milk Chocolate	1 pkg or 4 heaping tsp (1 oz)	110
Hot Cocoa Natural Mint	1 pkg or 4 heaping tsp (1 oz)	110
Hot Cocoa Rich Chocolate	1 pkg or 4 heaping tsp (1 oz)	110
Hot Cocoa Rich Chocolate w/ Marshmallows	1 pkg or 4 heaping tsp (1 oz)	110
Hot Cocoa Sugar Free Mint	1 pkg or 4 heaping tsp (15 g)	50

FOOD	PORTION	CALS.
Carnation (CONT.)		
Hot Cocoa Sugar Free Rich Chocolate	1 pkg or 4 heaping tsp (15 g)	50
Hershey		
Cocoa	⅓ cup (1 oz)	120
European Cocoa	1 oz	90
Hills Bros.		
Hot Cocoa	6 oz	110
Hot Cocoa Sugar Free	6 oz	60
Nestle		
Cocoa	1 tbsp	15
Hot Cocoa Mix	1 oz	110
Hot Cocoa Mix With Marshmallows	1 oz	120
Hot Cocoa Mix With Marshmallows as prep w/ 2% milk	6 oz	220
Hot Cocoa Mix With Marshmallows as prep w/ skim milk	6 oz	190
Hot Cocoa Mix With Marshmallows as prep w/ whole milk	6 oz	240
Hot Cocoa Mix as prep w/ 2% milk	6 oz	210
Hot Cocoa Mix as prep w/ skim milk	6 oz	180
Hot Cocoa Mix as prep w/ whole milk	6 oz	230
Swiss Miss		
Cocoa Diet	6 oz	20
Hot Cocoa Bavarian Chocolate	6 oz	110
Hot Cocoa Double Rich	6 oz	110
Hot Cocoa Milk Chocolate	6 oz	110
Hot Cocoa With Mini Marshmallows	6 oz	110
Lite as prep	6 oz	70
Sugar Free With Sugar Free Marshmallows as prep	6 oz	50
Sugar Free as prep	6 oz	60
Ultra Slim-Fast		
Hot Cocoa as prep w/ water	8 oz	190
Weight Watchers		
Cocoa	1 pkg	60

COCONUT

FOOD	PORTION	CALS.
coconut water	1 cup	46
coconut water	1 tbsp	3
cream canned	1 tbsp	36
cream canned	1 cup	568
dried sweetened flaked	1 cup	351
dried sweetened flaked	7 oz pkg	944

FOOD	PORTION	CALS.
dried sweetened flaked canned	1 cup	341
dried sweetened shredded	7 oz pkg	997
dried sweetened shredded	1 cup	466
dried toasted	1 oz	168
dried unsweetened	1 oz	187
fresh	1 piece (1½ oz)	159
fresh shredded	1 cup	283
milk canned	1 cup	445
milk canned	1 tbsp	30
milk frozen	1 tbsp	30
milk frozen	1 cup	486
Baker's		
Angel Flake Toasted	⅓ cup	212
Premium Shred	⅓ cup	135
Coco Lopez		
Cream Of Coconut	2 tbsp	120

COD
CANNED
atlantic	3 oz	89
atlantic	1 can (11 oz)	327
roe	3.5 oz	118
DRIED
| atlantic | 3 oz | 246 |
FRESH
atlantic cooked	1 fillet (6.3 oz)	189
atlantic cooked	3 oz	89
pacific baked	3 oz	95
roe baked w/ butter & lemon juice	3.5 oz	126
roe raw	3½ oz	130
FROZEN
Gorton's		
Fishmarket Fresh	5 oz	110
Mrs. Paul's		
Light Fillets	1 fillet	240
Van De Kamp's		
Lightly Breaded Fillets	1 (4 oz)	220

COFFEE
(*see also* COFFEE BEVERAGES, COFFEE SUBSTITUTES)
INSTANT
cappuccino mix as prep	7 oz	62
decaffeinated	1 rounded tsp (1.8 g)	4
decaffeinated as prep	6 oz	4
french mix as prep	7 oz	57

FOOD	PORTION	CALS.
mocha mix as prep	7 oz	51
regular	1 rounded tsp	4
regular as prep	6 oz	4
regular w/ chicory	1 rounded tsp	6
regular w/ chicory as prep	6 oz	6
Kava		
Instant	1 tsp	2
REGULAR		
brewed	6 oz	4
Folgers		
Colombian Supreme	1 tbsp	16
Custom Roast	1 tbsp	16
Decaffeinated	1 tbsp	17
French Roast	1 tbsp	16
Gourmet Supreme	1 tbsp	16
Instant	1 tsp	8
Instant Decaffeinated	1 tsp	8
Singles	1 bag	21
Singles Decaffeinated	1 bag	21
Special Roast	1 tbsp	16
Vacuum Pack	1 tbsp	16
Maryland Club		
Ground	1 tbsp	16
TAKE-OUT		
cafe au lait	1 cup (8 fl oz)	77
cafe brulot	1 cup (4.8 fl oz)	48
cappuccino	1 cup (8 fl oz)	77
coffee con leche	1 cup (8 fl oz)	77
espresso	1 cup (3 fl oz)	2
irish coffee	1 serv (9 fl oz)	107
mocha	1 mug (9.6 fl oz)	202

COFFEE BEVERAGES
(*see also* COFFEE SUBSTITUTES)

Chock o'ccino		
Cinnamon	8 oz	120
Coffee	8 oz	120
Mocha	8 oz	120
General Foods		
International Coffee Cafe Amaretto	6 oz	51
International Coffee Cafe Francais	6 oz	55
International Coffee Cafe Irish Creme	6 oz	55
International Coffee Cafe Vienna	6 oz	59
International Coffee Irish Mocha Mint	6 oz	51

FOOD	PORTION	CALS.
General Foods (CONT.)		
International Coffee Orange Cappuccino	6 oz	59
International Coffee Sugar Free Cafe Francais	6 oz	35
International Coffee Sugar Free Cafe Irish Creme	6 oz	31
International Coffee Sugar Free Cafe Vienna	6 oz	29
International Coffee Sugar Free Irish Mocha Mint	6 oz	28
International Coffee Sugar Free Orange Cappuccino	6 oz	29
International Coffee Sugar Free Suisse Mocha	6 oz	29
International Coffee Suisse Mocha	6 oz	53

COFFEE SUBSTITUTES

powder	1 tsp	9
powder as prep	6 oz	9
powder as prep w/ milk	6 oz	121
Natural Touch		
Kaffree Roma	1 tsp	6
Postum		
Instant	6 oz	11
Instant Coffee Flavored	6 oz	11

COFFEE WHITENERS

(*see also* MILK SUBSTITUTES)

LIQUID		
nondairy frzn	1 tbsp	20
Coffee-Mate		
Liquid	1 tbsp (0.5 fl oz)	16
Hood		
Non Dairy	1 tbsp (0.5 oz)	20
International Delight		
Amaretto	1 tbsp (0.6 fl oz)	45
Cinnamon Hazelnut	1 tbsp (0.6 fl oz)	45
Irish Creme	1 tbsp (0.6 fl oz)	45
No Fat Amaretto	1 tbsp (0.5 fl oz)	30
No Fat French Vanilla Royale	1 tbsp (0.5 fl oz)	30
No Fat Hawaiian Macadamia	1 tbsp (0.5 fl oz)	30
No Fat Irish Creme	1 tbsp (0.5 fl oz)	30
Suisse Chocolate Mocha	1 tbsp (0.6 fl oz)	45
Mocha Mix		
Fat-Free	1 tbsp (0.5 fl oz)	10

FOOD	PORTION	CALS.
Mocha Mix (CONT.)		
Lite	1 tbsp (0.5 fl oz)	10
Lite	4 fl oz	80
Original	1 tbsp (0.5 fl oz)	20
Signature Flavors French Vanilla	1 tbsp (0.5 fl oz)	35
Signature Flavors Irish Creme	1 tbsp (0.5 fl oz)	35
Signature Flavors Kahlua	1 tbsp (0.5 fl oz)	35
Signature Flavors Mauna Loa Macadamia Nut	1 tbsp (0.5 fl oz)	35
POWDER		
nondairy	1 tsp	11
Coffee-Mate		
Powder	1 tsp (2 g)	10
Cremora		
Whitener	1 tsp	12
N-Rich Creamer		
Whitener	1 tsp	10

COLESLAW
(*see* CABBAGE)

COLLARDS
CANNED
Allen

Collards	½ cup (4.1 oz)	30
Sunshine		
Collards	½ cup (4.1 oz)	30
FRESH		
cooked	½ cup	17
raw chopped	½ cup	6
FROZEN		
chopped cooked	½ cup	31

COOKIES
(*see also* BROWNIE, CAKE, DOUGHNUT, PIE)
HOME RECIPE

chocolate chip as prep w/ butter	1 (0.42 oz)	78
chocolate chip as prep w/ margarine	1 (0.56 oz)	78
macaroons	1 (0.8 oz)	97
oatmeal	1 (0.5 oz)	67
oatmeal w/ raisins	1 (0.52 oz)	65
peanut butter	1 (0.7 oz)	95
shortbread as prep w/ butter	1 (0.38 oz)	60
shortbread as prep w/ margarine	1 (0.38 oz)	60
sugar as prep w/ butter	1 (0.49 oz)	66
sugar as prep w/ margarine	1 (0.49 oz)	66

FOOD	PORTION	CALS.
MIX		
chocolate chip	1 (0.56 oz)	79
oatmeal	1 (0.6 oz)	74
oatmeal raisin	1 (0.6 oz)	74
Betty Crocker		
Chocolate Chip Big Batch	2	120
Date Bar Classic Dessert	1	60
Estee		
Chocolate Chip	3	130
READY-TO-EAT		
animal	11 crackers (1 oz)	126
animal crackers	1 box (2.4 oz)	299
animal crackers	1 (2.5 g)	11
butter	1 (5 g)	23
chocolate chip	1 (0.4 oz)	48
chocolate chip	1 box (1.9 oz)	233
chocolate chip low fat	1 (0.25 oz)	45
chocolate chip low sugar low sodium	1 (0.24 oz)	31
chocolate chip soft-type	1 (0.5 oz)	69
chocolate w/ creme filling	1 (0.35 oz)	47
chocolate w/ creme filling chocolate coated	1 (0.60 oz)	82
chocolate w/ creme filling sugar free low sodium	1 (0.35 oz)	46
chocolate w/ extra creme filling	1 (0.46 oz)	65
chocolate wafer	1 (0.2 oz)	26
chocolate wafer cookie crumbs	½ cup (5.9 oz)	728
digestive biscuits plain	2	141
fig bars	1 (0.56 oz)	56
fortune	1 (0.28 oz)	30
fudge	1 (0.73 oz)	73
gingersnaps	1 (0.24 oz)	29
graham	1 squares (0.24 oz)	30
graham chocolate covered	1 (0.49 oz)	68
graham cracker crumbs	½ cup (4.4 oz)	540
graham honey	1 (0.24 oz)	30
ladyfingers	1 (0.38 oz)	40
marshmallow chocolate coated	1 (0.46 oz)	55
marshmallow pie chocolate coated	1 (1.4 oz)	165
molasses	1 (0.5 oz)	65
oatmeal	1 (0.52 oz)	71
oatmeal	1 (0.6 oz)	81
oatmeal soft-type	1 (0.5 oz)	61
oatmeal raisin	1 (0.6 oz)	81
oatmeal raisin low sugar no sodium	1 (0.24 oz)	31

FOOD	PORTION	CALS.
oatmeal raisin soft-type	1 (0.5 oz)	61
peanut butter sandwich	1 (0.5 oz)	67
peanut butter sandwich sugar free low sodium	1 (0.35 oz)	54
peanut butter soft-type	1 (0.5 oz)	69
raisin soft-type	1 (0.5 oz)	60
shortbread	1 (0.28 oz)	40
shortbread pecan	1 (0.49 oz)	79
sugar	1 (0.52 oz)	72
sugar low sugar sodium free	1 (0.24 oz)	30
sugar wafers w/ creme filling	1 (0.12 oz)	18
sugar wafers w/ creme filling sugar free sodium free	1 (0.14 oz)	20
vanilla sandwich	1 (0.35 oz)	48
vanilla wafers	1 (0.21 oz)	28
Archway		
Almond Crescents	2 (0.8 oz)	100
Apple N'Raisin	1 (1.1 oz)	130
Apricot Filled	1 (1 oz)	110
Bells And Stars	3 (1 oz)	150
Blueberry Filled	1 (1 oz)	110
Carrot Cake	1 (1 oz)	120
Cherry Filled	1 (1 oz)	110
Cherry Nougat	3 (1 oz)	150
Chocolate Chip	1 (1 oz)	130
Chocolate Chip Bag	3 (0.9 oz)	130
Chocolate Chip Drop	1 (1 oz)	140
Chocolate Chip Ice Box	1 (1 oz)	140
Chocolate Chip Mini	12 (1.1 oz)	150
Cinnamon Snaps	12 (1.1 oz)	150
Coconut Macaroon	1 (0.8 oz)	90
Cookie Jar Hermits	1 (1 oz)	110
Dark Chocolate	1 (1 oz)	110
Dutch Chocolate	1 (1 oz)	120
Fig Bars Low Fat	2 (1.1 oz)	100
Frosty Lemon	1 (1 oz)	120
Frosty Orange	1 (1 oz)	120
Fruit And Honey Bar	1 (1 oz)	110
Fruit Bar No Fat	1 (1 oz)	90
Fruit Cake	1 (1.1 oz)	140
Fudge Nut Bar	1 (1 oz)	110
Fun Chip Mini	12 (1.1 oz)	140
Gingersnaps	5 (1.1 oz)	130
Granola No Fat	1 (0.5 oz)	50

FOOD	PORTION	CALS.
Archway (CONT.)		
Holiday Pak	3 (1.1 oz)	150
Iced Gingerbread	3 (1.1 oz)	140
Iced Molasses	1 (1 oz)	110
Iced Oatmeal	1 (1 oz)	120
Lemon Snaps	12 (1.1 oz)	150
New Orleans Cake	1 (1 oz)	110
Nutty Nougat	3 (1.1 oz)	160
Oatmeal	1 (0.9 oz)	110
Oatmeal Apple Filled	1 (1 oz)	110
Oatmeal Date Filled	1 (1 oz)	110
Oatmeal Mini	12 (1.1 oz)	150
Oatmeal Pecan	1 (1 oz)	120
Oatmeal Raisin	1 (1 oz)	110
Oatmeal Raisin Bran	1 (1 oz)	110
Old Fashioned Molasses	1 (1 oz)	120
Old Fashioned Windmill	1 (0.7 oz)	100
Party Treats	3 (1.1 oz)	140
Peanut Butter	1 (1 oz)	140
Peanut Butter Nougat	3 (1.1 oz)	160
Pecan Crunch	6 (1.1 oz)	150
Pecan Ice Box	1 (1 oz)	140
Pecan Malted Nougat	3 (1.1 oz)	160
Pfeffernusse	2 (1.3 oz)	140
Pineapple Filled	1 (0.9 oz)	100
Raisin Oatmeal	1 (1 oz)	130
Raisin Oatmeal Bag	3 (1 oz)	130
Raspberry Filled	1 (1 oz)	110
Rocky Road	1 (1 oz)	130
Ruth's Golden Oatmeal	1 (1 oz)	120
Select Assortment	3 (0.9 oz)	130
Soft Molasses Drop	1 (1 oz)	110
Soft Sugar	1 (1 oz)	110
Strawberry Filled	1 (1 oz)	110
Sugar	1 (1 oz)	120
Vanilla Wafer	5 (1.1 oz)	130
Wedding Cakes	3 (1.1 oz)	160
Bakery Wagon		
Apple Walnut Raisin	1	100
Cobbler Apple Cranberry Fat Free	1	70
Cobbler Apple Fat Free	1	70
Cobbler Mixed Fruit Fat Free	1	70
Cobbler Raspberry Fat Free	1	70
Ginger Snaps	5	160

FOOD	PORTION	CALS.
Bakery Wagon (CONT.)		
Honey Fruit Bars	1	100
Iced Molasses	1	100
Iced Molasses Mini	3	130
Oatmeal Apple Filled	1	90
Oatmeal Chocolate Chunk	1	100
Oatmeal Date Filled	1	90
Oatmeal Raspberry Filled	1	100
Oatmeal Soft	1	100
Oatmeal Walnut Raisin	1	100
Vanilla Wafers Cholesterol Free	6	130
Baking On The Lite Side		
Oatmeal Crunchy	2 (0.6 oz)	60
Raspberry Linzer	1 (0.6 oz)	55
Barnum's		
Animal Crackers	12 (1.1 oz)	140
Biscos		
Sugar Wafers	8 (1 oz)	140
Waffle Cremes	4 (1.2 oz)	180
Chip-A-Roos		
Cookies	3 (1.3 oz)	190
Chips Ahoy!		
Bit Size Chocolate Chip	14 (1.1 oz)	170
Chewy Chocolate Chip	3 (1.3 oz)	170
Chunky Chocolate Chip	1 (0.5 oz)	80
Real Chocolate Chip	3 (1.1 oz)	160
Reduced Fat	3 (1.1 oz)	150
Sprinkled Real Chocolate Chip	3 (1.3 oz)	170
Striped Chocolate Chip	1 (0.5 oz)	80
Cookie Lover's		
Blue Ribbon Brownies	1 (0.8 oz)	90
Classic Shortbread	1 (0.8 oz)	110
Dutch Chocolate Chip	1 (0.8 oz)	90
Fancy Peanut Butter	1 (0.8 oz)	100
Grahams Cinnamon Honey	2 (1 oz)	110
Grahams Honey	2 (1 oz)	100
Old-Time Raisin	1 (0.8 oz)	90
Delacre		
Cookie Assortment	4 (1.1 oz)	130
Drake's		
Chocolate Chip	2 (1 oz)	140
Chocolate- Chocolate Chip	2 (1 oz)	130
Coconut	2 (1 oz)	130
Coconut Macaroon	1 (1 oz)	135

FOOD	PORTION	CALS.
Drake's (CONT.)		
Hermit	1 (2 oz)	230
Oatmeal	2 (1 oz)	120
Oatmeal Creme	1 (2 oz)	240
Peanut Butter Wafers	1 (2.25 oz)	324
Dutch Mill		
Chocolate Chip	3 (1.1 oz)	160
Coconut Macaroons	3 (1 oz)	120
Oatmeal Raisin	3 (1 oz)	130
Entenmann's		
Chocolate Chip	3 (0.9 oz)	140
Estee		
Chocolate Chip	4 (1.1 oz)	150
Coconut	4 (1 oz)	140
Creme Wafers Chocolate	7 (1.1 oz)	160
Creme Wafers Lemon	5 (1.2 oz)	170
Creme Wafers Peanut Butter	5 (1.2 oz)	170
Creme Wafers Triple Decker Banana Split	3 (0.9 oz)	140
Creme Wafers Triple Decker Chocolate Caramel & Peanut Butter	3 (0.9 oz)	140
Creme Wafers Vanilla	7 (1.1 oz)	160
Creme Wafers Vanilla & Strawberry	5 (1.2 oz)	170
Fig Bars Apple Low Fat	2 (1 oz)	100
Fig Bars Cranberry Low Fat	2 (1 oz)	100
Fig Bars Low Fat	2 (1 oz)	100
Fudge	4 (1 oz)	150
Lemon	4 (1 oz)	140
Oatmeal Raisin	4 (1 oz)	130
Sandwich Chocolate	3 (1.2 oz)	160
Sandwich Original	3 (1.2 oz)	160
Sandwich Peanut Butter	3 (1.2 oz)	160
Sandwich Vanilla	3 (1.2 oz)	160
Shortbread Reduced Fat	4 (1 oz)	130
Vanilla	4 (1 oz)	140
FFV		
Animal Crackers	9	110
Caramel Patties	2	150
Fig Bars Vanilla	1	60
Fig Bars Whole Wheat	1	60
Ginger Boys Calcium Enriched	6	120
Jelly Tarts	2	110
Mint Sandwich	2	160
Oatmeal Calcium Enriched	5	130
Peanut Butter Sandwich	2	170

FOOD	PORTION	CALS.
FFV (CONT.)		
Regal Grahams	2	140
Royal Dainty	2	120
T.C. Rounds	2	160
Tango	2	160
Trolley Cakes Devilsfood	2	120
Vanilla Wafers	8	120
Famous Amos		
Chocolate Chip	3 (1 oz)	140
Chocolate Chip Pecan	3 (1 oz)	150
Oatmeal Raisin	3 (1 oz)	134
Freihofer's		
Chocolate Chip	2 (0.9 oz)	120
Frito Lay		
Peanut Butter Bar	1.75 oz	270
Frookie		
7-Grain Oatmeal	1	45
Animal Frackers	6	60
Apple Cinnamon Oat Bran	1	45
Apple Cinnamon Oat Bran	1 lg	120
Apple Fruitins	1	60
Chocolate Chip	1 lg	120
Chocolate Chip	1	45
Chocolate Chip Mint	1	45
Fig Fruitins	1	60
Ginger Spice	1	45
Mandarin Chocolate Chip	1	45
Oat Bran Muffin	1	45
Oat Bran Muffin	1 lg	120
Oatmeal Raisin	1	45
Oatmeal Raisin	1 lg	120
General Mills		
Dunkaroos	1 pkg (1 oz)	130
FundaMiddles Vanilla Creme In Chocolate Graham Shells	1 pkg (0.8 oz)	110
Glenny's		
Noah'N Friends Animal Peanut Butter	0.5 oz	65
Noah'N Friends Animal Vanilla	0.5 oz	65
Noah'N Friends Animal Wheat-Free Oatmeal	0.5 oz	65
Nookie Bar	1 (1.15 oz)	138
Sesame Nookie	1 (0.5 oz)	60
Sesame Nookie	1 pkg (1.5 oz)	180

FOOD	PORTION	CALS.
Golden Fruit		
Apple	1 (0.7 oz)	80
Cranberry	1 (0.7 oz)	70
Cranberry Low Fat	1 (0.7 oz)	70
Raisin	1 (0.7 oz)	80
Grandma's		
Animal Cookies Candied	5 (1 oz)	140
Chocolate Chip	2 (2.75 oz)	370
Chocolate Chip Rich'N Chewy	3 (1 oz)	140
Fudge Chocolate Chip	2 (2.75 oz)	350
Grab Cookie Bits Chocolate	8 (1 oz)	140
Grab Cookie Bits Peanut Butter	8 (1 oz)	140
Grab Cookie Bits Vanilla	8 (1 oz)	140
Oatmeal Apple Spice	2 (2.75 oz)	330
Old Time Molasses	2 (2.75 oz)	320
Peanut Butter	2 (2.75 oz)	410
Raisin Soft	2 (2.75 oz)	320
Health Valley		
Amaranth Cookies	1	70
Fancy Fruit Chunks Apricot Almond	2	90
Fancy Fruit Chunks Date Pecan	2	90
Fancy Fruit Chunks Raisin Oat Bran	2	70
Fancy Fruit Chunks Tropical Fruit	2	90
Fancy Peanut Chunks	2	90
Fat Free Apple Spice	3	75
Fat Free Apricot Delight	3	75
Fat Free Date Delight	3	75
Fat Free Jumbos Apple Raisin	1	70
Fat Free Jumbos Raisin	1	70
Fat Free Jumbos Raspberry	1	70
Fat Free Raisin Oatmeal	3	75
Fiber Jumbos Blueberry Nut	1	100
Fiber Jumbos Chunky Pecan	1	100
Fiber Jumbos Raisin Nut	1	100
Fruit & Fitness	5	200
Fruit Jumbos Almond Date	1	70
Fruit Jumbos Oat Bran	1	70
Fruit Jumbos Raisin Nut	1	70
Fruit Jumbos Tropical Fruit	1	70
Graham Amaranth	7	110
Graham Honey	7	100
Graham Oat Bran	7	120
Honey Jumbos Crisp Cinnamon	1	70
Honey Jumbos Crisp Peanut Butter	1	70

FOOD	PORTION	CALS.
Health Valley (CONT.)		
Honey Jumbos Fancy Oat Bran	2	130
Oat Bran Animal Cookies	7	110
Oat Bran Fruit & Nut	2	110
The Great Tofu	2	90
The Great Wheat Free	2	80
Heyday		
Caramel & Peanut	1 (0.8 oz)	110
Fudge	1 (0.8 oz)	110
Honey Maid		
Cinnamon Grahams	10 (1.1 oz)	140
Honey Grahams	8 (1 oz)	120
Hydrox		
Original	3	150
Reduced Fat	3 (1.1 oz)	130
Keebler		
Buttercup	3	70
Chocolate Fudge Sandwich	1	80
Commodore	1	60
Cookies Mates	2	50
French Vanilla Creme	1	80
Graham Honey Fiber Enriched	2	90
Graham Kitchen Rich	2	60
Homeplate	1	60
Keebies	1	80
Krisp Kreem Wafers	2	50
Old Fashion Chocolate Chip	1	80
Old Fashion Double Fudge	1	80
Old Fashion Oatmeal	1	80
Old Fashion Peanut Butter	1	80
Old Fashion Sugar	1	80
Pitter Patter	1	90
Vanilla Wafers	4	80
LU		
Chocolatiers	4 (1.1 oz)	170
Chocolatiers Dipped	3 (1 oz)	170
Little Schoolboy Dark Chocolate	2 (0.9 oz)	130
Little Schoolboy Milk Chocolate	2 (0.9 oz)	130
Marie Lu	3 (1.2 oz)	170
Truffle Lu	4 (1.2 oz)	180
La Choy		
Fortune	1	15
Lance		
Choc-O-Lunch	1 pkg (37 g)	180

FOOD	PORTION	CALS.
Lance (CONT.)		
Choc-O-Mint	1 pkg (35 g)	180
Chocolate Chip Fudge	1 (28 g)	130
Chocolate Chip Soft	1 (28 g)	130
Coated Graham	1 pkg (50 g)	200
Fig Bar	1 pkg (42 g)	150
Lem-O-Lunch	1 pkg (48 g)	240
Lemon Nekot	1 pkg (42 g)	220
Malt	1 pkg (35 g)	190
Nut-O-Lunch	1 oz	140
Oatmeal	1 (57 G)	130
Peanut Butter Creme Filled Wafer	1 pkg (50 g)	240
Van-O-Lunch	1 pkg (37 g)	180
Little Debbie		
Animal	1 pkg (1.5 oz)	190
Caramel Cookie Bars	1 pkg (1.2 oz)	160
Chocolate Chip Chewy	1 pkg (2 oz)	370
Chocolate Chip Crisp	1 pkg (1.5 oz)	210
Cookie Wreaths	1 pkg (0.6 oz)	90
Creme Filled Chocolate	1 pkg (1.8 oz)	260
Creme Filled Chocolate	1 pkg (1.2 oz)	180
Easter Puffs	1 pkg (1.2 oz)	140
Figaroos	1 pkg (1.5 oz)	160
Figaroos	1 pkg (2 oz)	200
Fudge Macaroons	1 pkg (1 oz)	140
Ginger	1 pkg (0.7 oz)	90
Oatmeal Crisp	1 pkg (1.5 oz)	210
Oatmeal Lights	1 pkg (1.3 oz)	140
Oatmeal Raisin	1 pkg (2.7 oz)	320
Peanut Butter	1 pkg (1.5 oz)	210
Peanut Butter Bars	1 pkg (1.9 oz)	270
Peanut Clusters	1 pkg (1.4 oz)	190
Pecan Spinwheels	1 pkg (1 oz)	110
Pecan Shortbread	1 pkg (1.5 oz)	220
Lorna Doone		
Cookies	4 (1 oz)	140
Mallomars		
Cookies	2 (0.9 oz)	120
Mallopuffs		
Cookies	1 (0.6 oz)	70
Manischewitz		
Macaroons Chocolate	2 (0.9 oz)	90
Mother's		
Almond Shortbread	3	180

FOOD	PORTION	CALS.
Mother's (CONT.)		
Butter	5	140
Checkerboard Wafers	8	150
Chocolate Chip	2	160
Chocolate Chip Angel	3	180
Chocolate Chip Bag	4	140
Chocolate Chip Parade	4	130
Circus Animals	6	140
Cocadas	5	150
Cookie Parade	4	140
Dinosaur Grrrahams	2	130
Double Fudge	3	170
Duplex Creme	3	170
English Tea	2	180
Fig Bar	2	130
Fig Bar Fat Free	1	70
Fig Bar Whole Wheat	2	130
Fig Bar Whole Wheat Fat Free	1	70
Flaky Flix Fudge	2	140
Flaky Flix Vanilla	2	140
Frosted Holiday	4	130
Fudge Bowl Crowns	2	140
Fudge Bowl Nuggets	2	140
Gaucho Peanut Butter	2	190
Gingerbread Man	6	140
Iced Oatmeal	2	120
Iced Oatmeal Bag	4	120
Iced Raisin	2	180
MLB Double Header Duplex	3	170
Macaroon	2	150
Marias	3	170
North Poles	2	140
Oatmeal	2	110
Oatmeal Chocolate Chip	2	120
Oatmeal Raisin	5	150
Oatmeal Walnut Chocolate Chip	2	130
Pecan Goldens	2	170
Rainbow Wafers	8	150
Striped Shortbread	3	170
Sugar	2	140
Taffy	2	180
Triplet Assortment	2	140
Vanilla Wafers	6	150
Walnut Fudge	2	130

FOOD	PORTION	CALS.
Mother's (CONT.)		
Zoo Pals	14	140
Mystic Mint		
Cookies	1 (0.5 oz)	90
Nabisco		
Brown Edge Wafers	5 (1 oz)	140
Bugs Bunny Chocolate Graham	13 (1.1 oz)	140
Bugs Bunny Cinnamon Graham	13 (1.1 oz)	140
Bugs Bunny Graham	13 (1.1 oz)	140
Cameo	2 (1 oz)	130
Chocolate Grahams	3 (1.1 oz)	160
Chocolate Chip Snaps	7 (1.1 oz)	150
Chocolate Snaps	7 (1.1 oz)	140
Cookie Break	3 (1.1 oz)	160
Danish Imported	5 (1.1 oz)	170
Family Favorites Fudge Covered Grahams	3 (1 oz)	140
Family Favorites Fudge Striped Shortbread	3 (1.1 oz)	160
Family Favorites Oatmeal	1 (0.5 oz)	80
Family Favorites Vanilla Sandwich	3 (1.2 oz)	170
Famous Chocolate Wafers	5 (1.1 oz)	140
Ginger Snaps Old Fashioned	4 (1 oz)	120
Grahams	8 (1 oz)	120
Marshmallow Puffs	1 (0.75 oz)	90
Marshmallow Twirls	1 (1 oz)	130
Nilla Wafers	8 (1.1 oz)	140
Pecan Passion	1 (0.5 oz)	90
Pinwheels	1 (1 oz)	130
National		
Arrowroot	1 (5 g)	20
Newtons		
Apple Fat Free	2 (1 oz)	100
Cranberry Fat Free	2 (1 oz)	100
Fig	2 (1.1 oz)	110
Fig Fat Free	1 (1 oz)	100
Raspberry Fat Free	2 (1 oz)	100
Strawberry Fat Free	2 (1 oz)	100
Nutra/Balance		
Chocolate Chip	1 (2 oz)	260
Oatmeal Raisin	1 (2 oz)	240
Nutter Butter		
Bites Peanut Butter Sandwich	10 (1.1 oz)	150
Peanut Butter Sandwich	2 (1 oz)	130
Peanut Creme Patties	5 (1.1 oz)	160

FOOD	PORTION	CALS.
Oreo		
Cookies	3 (1.2 oz)	160
Double Stuf	2 (1 oz)	140
Fudge Covered	1 (0.75 oz)	110
Halloween Treats	2 (1 oz)	140
Reduced Fat	3 (1.2 oz)	140
White Fudge Covered	1 (0.75 oz)	110
Pally		
Butter	4 (0.88 oz)	100
Pepperidge Farm		
Beacon Hill Chocolate Chocolate Walnut	1	120
Blondie Chocolate Chip Fat Free	1 (1.4 oz)	120
Bordeaux	2	70
Brownie Chocolate Nut	2	110
Brownie Nut Large	1	140
Brussels	2	110
Brussels Mint	2	130
Butter Chessman	2	90
Cappucino	1	50
Capri	1	80
Champagne	2	110
Chantilly	1	80
Cheasapeake Chocolate Chunk Pecan	1	120
Cheyenne Peanut Butter Milk Chocolate Chunk	1	110
Chocolate Chip	2	100
Chocolate Chip Large	1	130
Chocolate Chunk Pecan	1	70
Dakota Milk Chocolate Oatmeal	1	110
Date Pecan	2	110
Fruit Filled Apricot- Raspberry	2	100
Fruit Filled Strawberry	2	100
Geneva	2	130
Gingerman	2	70
Hazelnut	2	110
Irish Oatmeal	2	90
Lemon Nut Crunch	2	110
Lido	1	90
Linzer	1	120
Milano	2	120
Milk Chocolate Macadamia	2	140
Mint Milano	2	150
Molasses Crisps	2	70
Nantucket Chocolate Chunk	1	120

FOOD	PORTION	CALS.
Pepperidge Farm (CONT.)		
Nassau	1	80
Oatmeal Large	1	120
Oatmeal Raisin	2	110
Old Fashioned Chocolate Chip	2	100
Orange Milano	2	150
Orleans	3	90
Orleans Sandwich	2	120
Paris	2	100
Pecan Shortbread	1	70
Pirouettes Chocolate Laced	2	70
Pirouettes Original	2	70
Raisin Bran	2	110
Ripple Milk Chocolate Fat Free	1 (0.6 oz)	60
Sante Fe Oatmeal Raisin	1	100
Sausalito Milk Chocolate Macadamia	1	120
Seville	2	100
Shortbread	2	150
Southport	2	170
Sugar	2	100
Tahiti	1	90
Zurich	1	60
Ritz		
Chocolate Covered	3 (1 oz)	150
Salerno		
Dinosaur Grrrahams Chocolate	1 pkg (1.25 oz)	167
Dinosaur Grrrahams Cinnamon	1 pkg (1.25 oz)	165
Dinosaur Grrrahams Original	1 pkg (1.25 oz)	156
Sargento		
MooTown Snackers Cookies & Creme Honey Graham Sticks & Vanilla Creme With Sprinkles	1 pkg (1.1 oz)	140
MooTown Snackers Cookies & Creme Vanilla Sticks & Chocolate Fudge Creme	1 pkg (1.1 oz)	140
SnackWell's		
Fat Free Cinnamon Grahams	20 (1 oz)	110
Fat Free Devil's Food	1 (0.5 oz)	50
Fat Free Double Fudge	1 (0.5 oz)	50
Reduced Fat Chocolate Sandwich With Chocolate Creme	2 (0.9 oz)	100
Reduced Fat Oatmeal Raisin	2 (1 oz)	110
Reduced Fat Vanilla Sandwich	2 (0.9 oz)	110
Social Tea		
Cookies	6 (1 oz)	120

FOOD	PORTION	CALS.
Stella D'Oro		
Almond Toast Mandel	1	60
Angel Bars	1	80
Angel Wings	1	70
Angelica Goodies	1	110
Anginetti	1	30
Anisette Sponge	1	50
Anisette Toast	1	50
Anisette Toast Jumbo	1	110
Apple Pastry Low Sodium	1	80
Biscottini Cashews	1	110
Breakfast Treats	1	100
Castelets Chocolate	1	60
Chinese Dessert Cookies	1	170
Como Delight	1	150
Deep Night Fudge	1	65
Dutch Apple Bars	1	110
Egg Biscuits Low Sodium	3	120
Egg Biscuits Sugared	1	80
Egg Jumbo	1	50
Fruit Delight Apple Cinnamon Fat Free	1	70
Fruit Delight Peach Apricot Fat Free	1	70
Fruit Delight Raspberry Fat Free	1	70
Fruit Slices	1	60
Fruit Slices Fat Free	1	50
Golden Bars	1	110
Holiday Rings & Stars	1	47
Holiday Trinkets	1	40
Hostess Assortment	1	40
Indulgent Cashew Biscottini	1 (1.1 oz)	150
Kichel Low Sodium	21	150
Lady Stella Assortment	1	40
Margherite Chocolate	1	70
Margherite Vanilla	1	70
Peach Apricot Pastry Sodium Free	1	80
Pfeffernusse Spice Drops	1	40
Prune Pastry Dietetic	1	90
Roman Egg Biscuits	1	140
Royal Nuggets	1	2
Sesame Regina	1	50
Swiss Fudge	1	70
Sunshine		
Almond Crescents	4 (1.1 oz)	150
Animal Crackers	1 box (2 oz)	260

FOOD	PORTION	CALS.
Sunshine (CONT.)		
Animal Crackers	14 (1.1 oz)	140
Classics Chocolate Chip With Pecans	1 (0.7 oz)	110
Classics Chocolate Chip With Walnuts	1 (0.7 oz)	100
Classics Premier Chocolate Chip	1 (0.7 oz)	100
Dixie Vanilla	2 (0.9 oz)	120
Fig Bars	2 (1 oz)	110
Fudge Family Bears Vanilla	2 (1 oz)	140
Fudge Mint Patties	2 (0.8 oz)	130
Fudge Striped Shortbread	3 (1.1 oz)	160
Ginger Snaps	7 (1 oz)	130
Grahams Cinnamon	2 (1.1 oz)	140
Grahams Fudge Dipped	4 (1.2 oz)	170
Grahams Honey	2 (1 oz)	120
Grahamy Bears	1 pkg (2 oz)	260
Grahamy Bears	10 (1.1 oz)	140
Iced Gingerbread	5 (1 oz)	130
Iced Oatmeal	2 (0.9 oz)	120
Jingles	6 (1.1 oz)	150
Lemon Coolers	5 (1 oz)	140
Mini Chocolate Chip Cookies	5 (1.1 oz)	160
Mini Fudge Royals	15 (1.1 oz)	160
Oatmeal Chocolate Chip	3 (1.3 oz)	170
Oatmeal Country Style	3 (1.2 oz)	170
School House Cookies	20 (1.1 oz)	140
Sugar Wafers Chocolate	3 (0.9 oz)	130
Sugar Wafers Peanut Butter	4 (1.1 oz)	170
Sugar Wafers Vanilla	3 (0.9 oz)	130
Tru Blu Chocolate	1 (0.6 oz)	80
Tru Blu Lemon	1 (0.6 oz)	80
Tru Blu Vanilla	1 (0.5 oz)	80
Vanilla Wafers	7 (1.1 oz)	150
Vienna Fingers	2 (1 oz)	140
Tastykake		
Chocolate Chip Bar	1 (43 g)	190
Chocolate Chunk Macadamia Nut	1 pkg (56 g)	310
Fudge Bar	1 (50 g)	200
Oatmeal Raisin Bar	1 (50 g)	210
Soft'n Chewy Chocolate Chip	1 (39 g)	170
Soft'n Chewy Oatmeal Raisin	1 (39 g)	160
Vanilla Sugar Wafer	1 (6 g)	36
Teddy Grahams		
Chocolate	24 (1 oz)	140
Cinnamon	24 (1 oz)	140

FOOD	PORTION	CALS.
Teddy Grahams (CONT.)		
Honey	24 (1 oz)	140
Tree Of Life		
Creme Supremes	2 (0.9 oz)	120
Creme Supremes Mint	2 (0.9 oz)	120
Fat Free Classic Carrot Cake	1 (0.8 oz)	60
Fat Free Devil's Food Chocolate	1 (0.8 oz)	70
Fat Free Golden Oatmeal Raisin	1 (0.8 oz)	70
Fat Free Harvest Fruit & Nut	1 (0.8 oz)	70
Fat Free Toasted Almond Butter	1 (0.8 oz)	70
Fruit Bars Apple Spice	2 (1.3 oz)	120
Fruit Bars Fat Free Fig	1 (0.8 oz)	70
Fruit Bars Fat Free Peach Apricot	1 (0.8 oz)	70
Fruit Bars Fat Free Wildberry	1 (0.8 oz)	70
Fruit Bars Fig	2 (1.3 oz)	120
Fruit Bars Peach Apricot	2 (1.3 oz)	120
Honey-Sweet Colossal Carrot Cake	1 (0.8 oz)	110
Honey-Sweet Lemon Burst	1 (0.8 oz)	110
Honey-Sweet Oh-So-Oatmeal	1 (0.8 oz)	110
Honey-Sweet Pecans-A-Plenty	1 (0.8 oz)	125
Monster Fat Free Carrot Cake	¼ cookie (0.9 oz)	60
Monster Fat Free Devil's Food Chocolate	¼ cookie (0.9 oz)	80
Monster Fat Free Gingerbread	¼ cookie (0.9 oz)	80
Monster Fat Free Maple Pecan	¼ cookie (0.9 oz)	90
Royal Vanilla	2 (0.9 oz)	120
Small World Animal Grahams	7 (1 oz)	120
Small World Chocolate Chip	7 (1 oz)	120
Soft-Bake Chocolate Chip	1 (0.8 oz)	125
Soft-Bake Double Fudge	1 (0.8 oz)	110
Soft-Bake Maui Macaroon	1 (0.8 oz)	135
Soft-Bake Oatmeal	1 (0.8 oz)	115
Soft-Bake Peanut Butter	1 (0.8 oz)	125
Wheat-Free American Oatmeal	1 (0.8 oz)	90
Wheat-Free California Carob	1 (0.8 oz)	105
Wheat-Free Georgia Peanut Butter	1 (0.8 oz)	95
Wheat-Free Mountain Maple Walnut	1 (0.8 oz)	100
Vienna Fingers		
Low Fat	2 (1 oz)	130
Weight Watchers		
Apple Raisin Bar	1 (0.75 oz)	70
Chocolate Sandwich	2 (1.06)	140
Fruit Filled Fig	1 (0.7 oz)	70
Fruit Filled Raspberry	1 (0.7 oz)	70
Oatmeal Raisin	2 (1.06 oz)	120

FOOD	PORTION	CALS.
Weight Watchers (CONT.)		
Vanilla Sandwich	2 (1.06 oz)	140
REFRIGERATED		
chocolate chip	1 (0.42 oz)	59
chocolate chip unbaked	1 oz	126
oatmeal	1 (0.4 oz)	56
oatmeal raisin	1 (0.4 oz)	56
peanut butter	1 (0.4 oz)	60
peanut butter dough	1 oz	130
sugar	1 (0.42 oz)	58
sugar dough	1 oz	124
Pillsbury		
Chocolate Chip	1	70
Oatmeal Raisin	1	60
Peanut Butter	1	70
Sugar	1	70
TAKE-OUT		
biscotti with nuts chocolate dipped	1 (1.3 oz)	117

CORIANDER

FOOD	PORTION	CALS.
leaf dried	1 tsp	2
leaf fresh	¼ cup	1
seed	1 tsp	5

CORN

(*see also* BRAN, CEREAL, CORNMEAL, FLOUR)

FOOD	PORTION	CALS.
CANNED		
cream style	½ cup	93
w/ red & green peppers	½ cup	86
white	½ cup	66
yellow	½ cup	66
Del Monte		
Cream Style Golden	½ cup (4.4 oz)	90
Cream Style Golden 50% Less Salt	½ cup (4.4 oz)	90
Cream Style Golden No Salt Added	½ cup (4.4 oz)	90
Cream Style Supersweet Golden	½ cup (4.4 oz)	60
Cream Style White	½ cup (4.4 oz)	100
Whole Kernel Golden	½ cup (4.4 oz)	90
Whole Kernel Golden Supersweet 50% Less Salt	½ cup (4.4 oz)	60
Whole Kernel Golden Supersweet No Salt Added	½ cup (4.4 oz)	60
Whole Kernel Golden Supersweet No Sugar	½ cup (4.4 oz)	60
Whole Kernel Golden Supersweet Vacuum Packed	½ cup (3.7 oz)	70

FOOD	PORTION	CALS.
Del Monte (CONT.)		
Whole Kernel Golden Supersweet Vacuum Packed No Salt Added	½ cup (3.7 oz)	70
Whole Kernel White Sweet	½ cup (4.4 oz)	80
Green Giant		
50% Less Salt No Sugar Added	½ cup	50
Corn	½ cup	70
Cream Style	½ cup	100
Deli Corn	½ cup	80
Golden Kernel 50% Less Salt	½ cup	70
Golden Vacuum Packed	½ cup	80
Mexi Corn	½ cup	80
No Salt No Sugar	½ cup	80
Sweet Select	½ cup	60
White Vacuum Packed	½ cup	80
Ka-Me		
Baby	½ cup (4.5 oz)	20
Stir Fry	½ cup (4.5 oz)	20
Owatonna		
Cream Style	½ cup	100
Whole Kernel In Brine	½ cup	90
Whole Kernel Vacuum Pack	½ cup	100
S&W		
Cream Style Premium Homestyle	½ cup	105
Sweet 'N Natural	½ cup	90
Whole Kernel Tender Young	½ cup	90
Whole Kernel Water Pack	½ cup	80
Seneca		
Cream Style	½ cup	80
Whole Kernel	½ cup	90
Whole Kernel Natural Pack	½ cup	80
FRESH		
on-the-cob w/ butter cooked	1 ear	155
white cooked	½ cup	89
white raw	½ cup	66
yellow cooked	1 ear (2.7 oz)	83
yellow cooked	½ cup	89
yellow raw	½ cup	66
yellow raw	1 ear (3 oz)	77
FROZEN		
cooked	½ cup	67
on-the-cob cooked	1 ear (2.2 oz)	59
Birds Eye		
Big Ears	1 ear	160

FOOD	PORTION	CALS.
Birds Eye (CONT.)		
In Butter Sauce	½ cup	90
Little Ears	2 ears	130
On The Cob	1 ear	120
Polybag Cut	½ cup	80
Polybag Deluxe Tender Sweet	½ cup	80
Sweet	½ cup	80
Fresh Like		
Cob Corn	1 ear (5 in)	96
Cob Corn	1 ear (3 in)	96
Cut	3.5 oz	85
Green Giant		
Cream Style	½ cup	110
Harvest Fresh Niblets	½ cup	80
Harvest Fresh White Shoepeg	½ cup	90
In Butter Sauce	½ cup	100
Nibblers Corn On The Cob	2 ears	120
Niblet Ears	1 ear	120
Niblets	½ cup	90
One Serve Niblets In Butter Sauce	1 pkg	120
One Serve On The Cob	1 pkg	120
Super Sweet Nibblers Corn On The Cob	2 ears	90
Super Sweet Niblet Ears	1 ear	90
Super Sweet Niblet Select	½ cup	60
White In Butter Sauce	½ cup	100
White Select	½ cup	90
Hanover		
White Shoepeg	½ cup	80
White Sweet	½ cup	80
Yellow Sweet	½ cup	80
Mrs. Paul's		
Fritters	2	240
Ore Ida		
Cob Corn	1 ear (6.1 oz)	180
Cob Corn Mini-Gold	1 ear (3.1 oz)	90
Stouffer's		
Souffle	½ cup (2.4 oz)	170
Tree Of Life		
Corn	⅔ cup (3.2 oz)	80
SHELF-STABLE		
Pantry Express		
Golden Whole Kernel	½ cup	60
TAKE-OUT		
fritters	1 (1 oz)	62
scalloped	½ cup	258

FOOD	PORTION	CALS.
CORN CHIPS		
(see CHIPS)		
CORNISH HENS		
(see CHICKEN)		
CORNMEAL		
(see also POLENTA)		
corn grits cooked	1 cup	146
corn grits uncooked	1 cup	579
degermed	1 cup	506
self-rising degermed	1 cup	489
whole grain	1 cup	442
Albers		
White	3 tbsp	110
Yellow	3 tbsp	110
Arrowhead		
Yellow	¼ cup (1.2 oz)	120
Aunt Jemima		
White	3 tbsp	102
Yellow	3 tbsp	102
Quaker		
White	3 tbsp	102
Yellow	3 tbsp	102
HOME RECIPE		
hush puppies	5 (2.7 oz)	256
hush puppies	1 (¾ oz)	74
MIX		
Arrowhead		
Corn Bread	¼ cup (1.2 oz)	120
Aunt Jemima		
Bolded White Mix	3 tbsp	99
Buttermilk Self Rising White Mix	3 tbsp	101
Self Rising White Mix	3 tbsp	98
Self Rising Yellow Mix	3 tbsp	100
Golden Dipt		
Corny Dog Batter Mix	1 oz	100
Hush Puppy Deluxe Mix	1¼ oz	120
Hush Puppy Jalapeno Mix	1¼ oz	120
Hush Puppy With Onion	1¼ oz	120
Hodgson Mill		
Yellow Self Rising	¼ cup (1 oz)	90
Yellow	¼ cup (1 oz)	100
Kentucky Kernal		
White Corn Meal Mix	¼ cup (1 oz)	100

FOOD	PORTION	CALS.
Miracle Maize		
Complete as prep	1 piece (1.5 oz)	193
Country Style as prep	1 piece 2 in x 2 in (1.8 oz)	230
Sweet as prep	1 piece 2 in x 2 in (1.8 oz)	236
Stone-Buhr		
Yellow Corn Meal	¼ cup (1 oz)	100
READY-TO-USE		
Aurora		
Polenta	½ cup (5 oz)	110
CORNSALAD		
raw	1 cup	12
CORNSTARCH		
cornstarch	⅓ cup	164
Argo		
Cornstarch	1 tbsp (8 g)	30
Cornstarch	1 cup (128 g)	460
Hodgson Mill		
Cornstarch	2 tsp (0.4 oz)	35
Kingsford's		
Cornstarch	1 tbsp (8 g)	30
Cornstarch	1 cup (128 g)	460
COTTAGE CHEESE		
creamed	1 cup	217
creamed	4 oz	117
creamed w/ fruit	4 oz	140
dry curd	1 cup	123
dry curd	4 oz	96
lowfat 1%	1 cup	164
lowfat 1%	4 oz	82
lowfat 2%	4 oz	101
lowfat 2%	1 cup	203
Axelrod		
Nonfat	½ cup (4.4 oz)	90
Borden		
4%	½ cup	120
Dry Curd 0.5%	½ cup	80
Unsalted 4%	½ cup	120
Breakstone		
2% Fat Large Curd	½ cup (4.2 oz)	90
2% Fat Small Curd	½ cup (4.2 oz)	90

FOOD	PORTION	CALS.
Breakstone (CONT.)		
4% Fat Large Curd	½ cup (4.2 oz)	120
4% Fat Small Curd	½ cup (4.2 oz)	120
Dry Curd ½% Fat	¼ cup (1.9 oz)	45
Cabot		
Cottage Cheese	4 oz	120
Light	4 oz	90
Friendship		
California Style	½ cup (4 oz)	115
Lowfat No Salt Added	½ cup (4 oz)	90
Lowfat Pineapple	½ cup (4 oz)	120
Lowfat 1%	½ cup (4 oz)	90
Nonfat	½ cup (4 oz)	80
Nonfat Plus Peach	½ cup (4 oz)	110
Pot Style	½ cup (4 oz)	90
With Pineapple	½ cup (4 oz)	140
Hood		
1% Fat	½ cup (4 oz)	90
1% Fat Chive & Onion	½ cup (4 oz)	90
1% Fat No Salt Added	½ cup (4 oz)	90
1% Fat Pepper & Herb	½ cup (4 oz)	90
1% Fat Pineapple Cherry	½ cup (4 oz)	110
4% Fat	½ cup (4 oz)	120
4% Fat Chive	½ cup (4 oz)	130
4% Fat Pineapple	½ cup (4 oz)	130
Nonfat	½ cup (4 oz)	80
Nonfat Pineapple	½ cup (4 oz)	110
Knudsen		
1.5% Fat Peach	4 oz	110
1.5% Fat Pineapple	4 oz	110
1.5% Fat Strawberry	4 oz	110
1.5% Fat Tropical Fruit	4 oz	120
2% Fat Small Curd	½ cup (4.2 oz)	100
4% Fat Large Curd	½ cup (4.5 oz)	130
4% Fat Small Curd	½ cup (4.3 oz)	120
Free	½ cup (4.3 oz)	80
Lactaid		
1%	4 oz	72
Light N'Lively		
1% Fat	½ cup (4 oz)	80
1% Fat Garden Salad	½ cup (4.2 oz)	90
1% Fat Peach & Pineapple	½ cup (4.3 oz)	120
Free	½ cup (4.4 oz)	80

FOOD	PORTION	CALS.
Lite Line		
Lowfat 1 ½%	½ cup	90
Sealtest		
2% Fat Small Curd	½ cup (4.2 oz)	90
4% Fat Large Curd	½ cup (4.2 oz)	120
4% Fat Small Curd	½ cup (4.2 oz)	120
Viva		
Nonfat	½ cup	70
Weight Watchers		
1%	½ cup	90
2%	½ cup	90

COTTONSEED

kernels roasted	1 tbsp	51

COUGH DROPS

Halls		
Cough Drops	1 (3.8 g)	15
Plus	1 (4.7 g)	18
With Vitamin C	1 (3.8 g)	14
Lifesavers		
Menthol	2 (0.5 oz)	60

COUSCOUS

cooked	½ cup	101
dry	½ cup	346
Casbah		
Almond Chicken Vegetarian	1 pkg (1.5 oz)	160
Asparagus Au Gratin Organic	1 pkg (1.5 oz)	150
Cheddar Broccoli	1 pkg (1.3 oz)	130
Hearty Harvest Zestful Organic as prep	1 pkg (10 fl oz)	180
Moroccan Stew	1 pkg (2 oz)	180
Pilaf as prep	1 cup	200
Tomato Parmesan	1 pkg (1.8 oz)	170
Kitchen Del Sol		
Aegean Citrus as prep	½ cup (1.1 oz)	110
Moroccan Ginger as prep	½ cup (1.1 oz)	120
Spicy Vegetable as prep	½ cup (1.1 oz)	120
Tomato & Olive	½ cup (1 oz)	120
Near East		
As Prep	1¼ cup	260

COWPEAS

catjang dried cooked	1 cup	200
common canned	1 cup	184
frozen cooked	½ cup	112

FOOD	PORTION	CALS.
leafy tips chopped cooked	1 cup	12
leafy tips raw chopped	1 cup	10
CRAB		
CANNED		
blue	3 oz	84
blue	1 cup	133
S&W		
Dungeness Crab	3.25 oz	81
FRESH		
alaska king cooked	1 leg (4.7 oz)	129
alaska king cooked	3 oz	82
alaska king raw	1 leg (6 oz)	144
alaska king raw	3 oz	71
blue cooked	3 oz	87
blue cooked	1 cup	138
blue raw	3 oz	74
blue raw	1 crab (.7 oz)	18
dungeness raw	3 oz	73
dungeness raw	1 crab (5.7 oz)	140
queen steamed	3 oz	98
FROZEN		
Mrs. Paul's		
Deviled Crab	1 cake	180
Deviled Crab Miniatures	3½ oz	240
READY-TO-USE		
crab cakes	1 cake (2.1 oz)	93
TAKE-OUT		
baked	1 (3.8 oz)	160
cake	1 (2 oz)	160
soft-shell fried	1 (4.4 oz)	334
CRACKER CRUMBS		
cracker meal	1 cup (4 oz)	440
Golden Dipt		
Cracker Meal	1 oz	100
Honey Maid		
Graham Cracker	0.5 oz	70
Keebler		
Cracker Meal	1 cup	100
Graham Crumbs	1 cup	520
Zesty Meal	1 cup	85
Kellogg's		
Corn Flake Crumbs	2 tbsp (0.4 oz)	40

FOOD	PORTION	CALS.
Lance		
Cracker Meal	1 oz	100
Nabisco		
Nilla Cookie Crumbs	2 tbsp (0.5 oz)	70
Oreo		
Cookie Crumbs	2 tbsp (0.5 oz)	80
Premium		
Fat Free Cracker Crumbs	¼ cup (1 oz)	100
Ritz		
Cracker Crumbs	⅓ cup (1 oz)	140
Sunshine		
Graham	3 tbsp (0.6 oz)	80

CRACKERS

(*see also* CRACKER CRUMBS)

FOOD	PORTION	CALS.
cheese	1 (1 in sq) (1 g)	5
cheese	14 (½ oz)	71
cheese low sodium	1 (1 in sq) (1 g)	5
cheese low sodium	14 (½ oz)	71
cheese w/ peanut butter filling	1 (0.24 oz)	34
crispbread	3	61
crispbread rye	1 (0.35 oz)	37
crispbread rye	3	77
melba toast plain	1 (5 g)	19
melba toast pumpernickel	1 (5 g)	19
melba toast rye	1 (5 g)	19
melba toast wheat	1 (5 g)	19
milk	1 (0.42 oz)	55
oyster cracker	1 (1 g)	4
peanut butter sandwich	1 (7 g)	34
rusk toast	1 (0.35 oz)	41
rye w/ cheese filling	1 (0.24 oz)	34
rye wafers plain	1 (0.9 oz)	84
rye wafers seasoned	1 (0.8 oz)	84
saltines	1 (3 g)	13
saltines fat free low sodium	3 (0.5 oz)	59
saltines fat free low sodium	6 (1 oz)	118
saltines low salt	1 (3 g)	13
snack cracker	1 (3 g)	15
snack cracker low salt	1 (3 g)	15
snack cracker w/ cheese filling	1 (7 g)	33
soup cracker	1 (1 g)	4
water biscuits	3	92
wheat w/ cheese filling	1 (0.24 oz)	35

FOOD	PORTION	CALS.
wheat w/ peanut butter filling	1 (0.24 oz)	35
wheat thins	1 (2 g)	9
wheat thins	7 (0.5 oz)	67
wheat thins low salt	7 (0.5 oz)	67
whole wheat	1 (4 g)	18
whole wheat low salt	1 (4 g)	18
zwieback	3½ oz	374
Adrienne's		
Gourmet Flatbread Caraway & Rye	2	20
Gourmet Flatbread Classic Island	2	20
Gourmet Flatbread Slightly Onion	2	20
Gourmet Flatbread Ten Grain	2	20
American Heritage		
Sesame	9 (1.1 oz)	160
Wheat & Bran	9 (1 oz)	140
Better Cheddars		
Crackers	22 (1 oz)	70
Low Sodium	22 (1 oz)	150
Reduced Fat	24 (1 oz)	140
Burns & Ricker		
Bagel Crisps Garlic	5 (1 oz)	100
Cheez-It		
Crackers	27 (1 oz)	160
Crackers	1 pkg (2 oz)	290
Crackers	1 pkg (1.5 oz)	220
Hot & Spicy	26 (1 oz)	160
Hot & Spicy	1 pkg (1.5 oz)	220
Low Sodium	27 (1 oz)	160
Party Mix	½ cup (1 oz)	140
Reduced Fat	30 (1 oz)	130
White Cheddar	26 (1 oz)	160
White Cheddar	1 pkg (1.5 oz)	220
Crown Pilot		
Crackers	1 (0.5 oz)	70
Devonsheer		
Melba Rounds Garlic	½ oz	56
Melba Rounds Honey Bran	½ oz	52
Melba Rounds Onion	½ oz	51
Melba Rounds Plain	½ oz	53
Melba Rounds Plain Unsalted	½ oz	52
Melba Rounds Rye	½ oz	53
Melba Rounds Sesame	½ oz	57
Eden		
Brown Rice	5 (1 oz)	120

FOOD	PORTION	CALS.
Escort		
Crackers	3 (0.5 oz)	70
Estee		
Unsalted	1 (0.5 oz)	70
FFV		
Cheddar Thins	7	70
Double Cheddar	7	70
Ham & Cheese Crispy Wafers	7	70
Ocean Crisp	1	60
Sesame Crisp	2	120
Stoned Wheat	4	60
Wheat Crispy Wafers	6	70
Frito Lay		
Cheese Filled	6 (1.5 oz)	210
Cracker Snacks Cheddar	13-16 (1 oz)	70
Cracker Snacks Zesty Italian	13-16 (1 oz)	70
Peanut Butter Filled	6 (1.5 oz)	210
Goya		
Butter Crackers	1	40
Crackers	1	30
Hain		
Cheese	1 oz	130
Onion	1 oz	130
Onion No Salt Added	1 oz	130
Rich	1 oz	130
Rich No Salt Added	1 oz	130
Rye	1 oz	120
Rye No Salt Added	1 oz	120
Sesame	1 oz	140
Sesame No Salt Added	1 oz	140
Sour Cream & Chive	1 oz	130
Sour Cream & Chive No Salt Added	1 oz	130
Sourdough	½ oz	65
Sourdough Low Salt	1 oz	130
Vegetable	1 oz	130
Vegetable No Salt Added	1 oz	130
Harvest Crisps		
5 Grain	13 (1.1 oz)	130
Oat	13 (1.1 oz)	140
Health Valley		
Herb Stoned Wheat	13	55
Herb Stoned Wheat No Salt	13	55
Rice Bran	7	130
Sesame Stoned Wheat	13	55

FOOD	PORTION	CALS.
Health Valley (CONT.)		
Sesame Stoned Wheat No Salt Added	13	55
Seven Grain Vegetable Stoned Wheat	13	55
Seven Grain Vegetable Stoned Wheat No Salt Added	13	55
Stoned Wheat	13	55
Stoned Wheat No Salt Added	13	55
Healthy Choice		
Bread Crisps Garlic Herb	11 (1 oz)	110
Hi Ho		
Butter Flavored	9 (1.1 oz)	160
Cracked Pepper	9 (1.1 oz)	160
Crackers	9	160
Low Salt	9 (1.1 oz)	160
Multi Grain	9 (1.1 oz)	160
Reduced Fat	10 (1.1 oz)	140
Whole Wheat	9 (1.1 oz)	150
Ideal Crispbread		
Extra Thin	3	48
Fiber Thins	2	41
Oatbran Thins	2	50
J.J. Flats		
Breadflats Caraway	1	52
Breadflats Caraway And Salt	1	51
Breadflats Cinnamon	1	53
Breadflats Flavorall	1	52
Breadflats Garlic	1	52
Breadflats Oat Bran	1	49
Breadflats Onion	1	53
Breadflats Plain	1	53
Breadflats Poppy	1	53
Breadflats Sesame	1	55
Kavli		
Crackers	1 piece	40
Keebler		
Club	2	30
Melba Toast Garlic	2	25
Melba Toast Long	2	30
Melba Toast Onion	2	25
Melba Toast Plain	2	25
Melba Toast Sesame	2	25
Oyster Crackers Large	26	80
Oyster Crackers Small	50	80
Snack Crackers Toasted Rye	2	30

FOOD	PORTION	CALS.
Keebler (CONT.)		
Snack Crackers Toasted Sesame	2	30
Snack Crackers Toasted Wheat	2	30
Toasted Snack Bacon	2	30
Toasted Snack Onion	2	30
Toasted Snack Pumpernickel	2	30
Wholegrain Wheat	2	30
Krispy		
Cracked Pepper	5 (0.5 oz)	60
Fat Free	5 (0.5 oz)	60
Mild Cheddar	5 (0.5 oz)	60
Original	5 (0.5 oz)	60
Soup & Oyster Crackers	17 (0.5 oz)	60
Unsalted Tops	5 (0.5 oz)	60
Whole Wheat	5 (0.5 oz)	60
Lance		
Bonnie	1 pkg (34 g)	160
Captain Wafers	2	30
Captain Wafers Very Low Sodium	2	30
Captain Wafers w/ Cream Cheese & Chives	1 pkg (37 g)	170
Cheese-On-Wheat	1 pkg (37 g)	180
Lanchee	1 pkg (35 g)	180
Melba Toast Oblong	2	30
Melba Toast Plain	2	20
Melba Toast Round Garlic	2	20
Melba Toast Round Onion	2	20
Melba Toast Sesame	2	25
Nekot	1 pkg (42 g)	210
Nip-Chee	1 pkg (37 g)	180
Oyster Crackers	1 pkg (14 g)	70
Peanut Butter Wheat	1 pkg (37 g)	190
Rye Twins	2	30
Rye-Chee	1 pkg (41 g)	190
Saltines	2	25
Saltines Slug Pack	4 crackers	50
Sesame Twins	2	40
Toastchee	1 pkg (39 g)	190
Toasty	1 pkg (35 g)	180
Wheat Twins	2	30
Wheatswafer	2	30
Lavash		
Bread Crisp Original	2 (0.5 oz)	60
Bread Crisp Sesame	2 (0.5 oz)	60

FOOD	PORTION	CALS.
Little Debbie		
Cheese Crackers With Peanut Butter	1 pkg (1.4 oz)	210
Cheese Crackers With Peanut Butter	1 pkg (0.9 oz)	140
Toasty Crackers With Peanut Butter	1 pkg (0.9 oz)	140
Toasty Crackers With Peanut Butter	1 pkg (1.4 oz)	200
Wheat Crackers With Cheddar Cheese	1 pkg (0.9 oz)	140
Manischewitz		
Tam Tams	10	147
Tam Tams No Salt	10	138
Tams Garlic	10	153
Tams Onion	10	150
Tams Wheat	10	150
McCrackens		
Cracker Crisp Country Butter	1 oz	140
Cracker Crisp Sour Cream & Chives	1 oz	140
Cracker Crisp Tangy Cheddar	1 oz	140
Cracker Crisp Toasted Wheat	1 oz	140
NABS		
Cheese Peanut Butter Sandwich	6 (1.4 oz)	190
Peanut Butter Toast Sandwich	6 (1.4 oz)	190
Nabisco		
Bacon Flavored	15 (1.1 oz)	160
Chicken In A Biskit	14 (1 oz)	160
Garden Crisps	15 (1 oz)	130
Oat Thins	18 (1 oz)	140
Royal Lunch	1 (0.4 oz)	50
Swiss	15 (1 oz)	140
Tid-Bit Cheese	32 (1 oz)	150
Vegetable Thins	14 (1.1 oz)	160
Wheat Thins Original	16 (1 oz)	140
Wheat Thins Reduced Fat	18 (1 oz)	120
Zings!	1 pkg (1.8 oz)	240
Nips		
Cheese	29 (1 oz)	150
Old London		
Melba Toast Pumpernickel	½ oz	54
Melba Toast Rye	½ oz	52
Melba Toast Sesame	½ oz	55
Melba Toast Sesame Unsalted	½ oz	55
Melba Toast Wheat	½ oz	51
Melba Toast White	½ oz	51
Melba Toast White Unsalted	½ oz	51
Melba Toast Whole Grain	½ oz	52
Melba Toast Whole Grain Unsalted	½ oz	53

FOOD	PORTION	CALS.
Old London (CONT.)		
Rounds Bacon	½ oz	53
Rounds Garlic	½ oz	56
Rounds Onion	½ oz	52
Rounds Rye	½ oz	52
Rounds Sesame	½ oz	56
Rounds White	½ oz	48
Rounds Whole Grain	½ oz	54
Oysterettes		
Crackers	19 (0.5 oz)	60
Pepperidge Farm		
Butter Thins	4	70
Cracked Wheat	3	100
Crispy Graham	4	70
English Water Biscuits	4	70
Flutters Garden Herb	¾ oz	100
Flutters Golden Sesame	¾ oz	110
Flutters Original Butter	¾ oz	100
Flutters Toasted Wheat	¾ oz	110
Garden Vegetable	5	60
Goldfish Cheddar Cheese	1 pkg (1½ oz)	190
Goldfish Cheddar Cheese	1 oz	120
Goldfish Cheese Thins	4	50
Goldfish Original	1 oz	130
Goldfish Parmesan Cheese	1 oz	120
Goldfish Pizza Flavored	1 oz	130
Goldfish Pretzel	1 oz	110
Hearty Wheat	4	100
Multi Grain	4	70
Sesame	4	80
Snack Mix Classic	1 oz	140
Snack Mix Lightly Smoked	1 oz	150
Snack Sticks Cheese	8	130
Snack Sticks Pretzel	8	120
Snack Sticks Pumpernickel	8	140
Snack Sticks Sesame	8	140
Spicy Lightly Smoked	1 oz	140
Toasted Rice	4	60
Toasted Wheat With Onion	4	80
Planters		
Cheese Peanut Butter Sandwiches	1 pkg (1.4 oz)	190
Toast Peanut Butter Sandwiches	1 pkg (1.4 oz)	190
Premium		
Saltine Fat Free	5 (0.5 oz)	50

FOOD	PORTION	CALS.
Premium (CONT.)		
Saltine Low Sodium	5 (0.5 oz)	60
Saltine Original	5 (0.5 oz)	60
Saltine Unsalted Tops	5 (0.5 oz)	60
Soup & Oyster	23 (0.5 oz)	60
Ralston		
Oat Bran Krisp	2	60
Ritz		
Bits	48 (1 oz)	160
Bits Sandwiches With Peanut Butter	13 (1 oz)	150
Bits Sanwiches With Real Cheese	14 (1.1 oz)	160
Crackers	5 (0.5 oz)	80
Low Sodium	5 (0.5 oz)	80
Sandwiches With Real Cheese	1 pkg (1.4 oz)	210
Rykrisp		
Natural	2	40
Seasoned	2	45
Seasoned Twindividuals	2	45
Sesame	2	50
Ryvita		
Crisp Bread Dark Finn Crisp	2	38
Crisp Bread Dark Rye	1	26
Crisp Bread Dark w/ Caraway Seeds Finn Crisp	2	38
Crisp Bread High Fiber	1	23
Crisp Bread Light Rye	1	26
Crisp Bread Toasted Sesame Rye	1	31
Snackbread High Fiber	1	14
Snackbread Original Wheat	1	20
Sesmark		
Brown Rice	15 (1 oz)	120
Cheese Thins	15 (1 oz)	130
Rice Thins Original	15 (1 oz)	130
Rice Thins Teriyaki Flavored	13 (1 oz)	130
Savory Thins Original	15 (1 oz)	125
Sesame Thins Cheddar	9 (1 oz)	150
Sesame Thins Garlic	9 (1 oz)	150
Sesame Thins Original	9 (1 oz)	150
Sesame Thins Unsalted	11 (1 oz)	150
SnackWell's		
Cracked Pepper	7 (0.5 oz)	60
Fat Free Wheat	5 (0.5 oz)	60
Reduced Fat Cheese	38 (1 oz)	130
Reduced Fat Classic Golden	6 (0.5 oz)	60

FOOD	PORTION	CALS.
Snorkles		
Cheddar	56 (1 oz)	140
Sociables		
Crackers	7 (0.5 oz)	80
Sunshine		
Saltines Cracked Pepper	5 (0.5 oz)	60
Town House		
Crackers	2	35
Tree Of Life		
Bite Size Fat Free Corn & Salsa	12	60
Bite Size Fat Free Cracked Pepper	12	55
Bite Size Fat Free Garden Vegetable	12	55
Bite Size Fat Free Garlic & Herb	12	55
Bite Size Fat Free Soya Nut	12	60
Bite Size Fat Free Toasted Onion	12	60
Bite Size Fat Free Whole Wheat	12	60
Fat Free Oyster	40 (0.5 oz)	60
Saltine Cracked Pepper Fat Free	4 (0.5 oz)	60
Saltine Fat Free	4 (0.5 oz)	50
Triscuit		
Crackers	7 (1.1 oz)	140
Deli-Style Rye	7 (1.1 oz)	140
Garden Herb	6 (1 oz)	130
Low Sodium	7 (1.1 oz)	150
Reduced Fat	8 (1.1 oz)	130
Wheat 'n Bran	7 (1.1 oz)	140
Tuscany		
Pita Crisps	1 oz	90
Pita Crisps Sesame	1 oz	96
Toast	1 oz	95
Toast Pepato	1 oz	93
Toast Pesto	1 oz	96
Toast Tomato	1 oz	95
Twigs		
Sesame & Cheese Sticks	15 (1 oz)	150
Uneeda Biscuit		
Unsalted Tops	2 (0.5 oz)	60
Venus		
Armenian Thin Bread	2 (0.9 oz)	100
Bran Wafers Salt Free	5 (0.5 oz)	60
Corn Crackers Salt Free	5 (0.5 oz)	60
Cracked Wheat Wafers Salt Free	5 (0.5 oz)	60
Cracker Bread	5 (0.5 oz)	60
Hors D'oeuvre	3 (0.5 oz)	60

FOOD	PORTION	CALS.
Venus (CONT.)		
Oat Bran Wafers	5 (0.5 oz)	60
Oat Bran Wafers Salt Free	5 (0.5 oz)	60
Old Brussels Cheddar Waferettes	5 (0.5 oz)	80
Old Brussels Jalapeno Waferettes	5 (0.5 oz)	80
Rye Wafers Low Salt	5 (0.5 oz)	60
Stoned Wheat Wafers Bite Size	7 (0.5 oz)	60
Water Crackers Fat Free	5 (0.5 oz)	55
Wheat Wafers Low Salt	5 (0.5 oz)	60
Waldorf		
Sodium Free	2	30
Wasa Crispbread		
Breakfast	1	50
Extra Crisp	1	25
Falu Rye	1	30
Fiber Plus	1	35
Golden Rye	1	30
Hearty Rye	1	50
Light Rye	1	25
Royal	½	26
Savory Sesame	1	30
Sesame Rye	1	30
Sesame Wheat	1	60
Toasted Wheat	1	50
Waverly		
Crackers	5 (0.5 oz)	70
Wheat Thins		
Low Salt	16 (1 oz)	140
Multi-Grain	17 (1 oz)	130
Wheatworth		
Stone Ground	5 (0.5 oz)	80
Zesta		
Saltine	2	25
Saltine Unsalted Top	2	25
Zwieback		
Crackers	1 (8 g)	35

CRANBERRIES
CANNED

cranberry sauce sweetened	½ cup	209
Ocean Spray		
CranFruit Cranberry Raspberry Sauce	2 oz	100
CranFruit Cranberry Strawberry Sauce	2 oz	100
Cranberry Sauce Jellied	2 oz	90

FOOD	PORTION	CALS.
Ocean Spray (CONT.)		
Whole Berry Sauce	2 oz	90
S&W		
Cranberry Sauce Jellied Old Fashioned	½ cup	90
Cranberry Sauce Whole Berry Old Fashioned	½ cup	90
DRIED		
Ocean Spray		
Craisins	⅓ cup (1.4 oz)	130
FRESH		
chopped	1 cup	54
Ocean Spray		
Fresh	½ cup	25

CRANBERRY BEANS

FOOD	PORTION	CALS.
CANNED		
cranberry beans	1 cup	216
DRIED		
cooked	1 cup	240
Bean Cuisine		
Dried	½ cup	115

CRANBERRY JUICE

FOOD	PORTION	CALS.
cocktail	1 cup	147
cranberry juice cocktail	6 oz	108
cranberry juice cocktail low calorie	6 oz	33
cranberry juice cocktail frzn	12 oz can	821
cranberry juice cocktail frzn as prep	6 oz	102
After The Fall		
Cape Cod Cranberry	1 bottle (10 oz)	130
Cranberry Ginger Ale	1 can (12 oz)	140
Apple & Eve		
Juice	6 fl oz	100
Ocean Spray		
Cocktail	8 fl oz	140
Cocktail Reduced Calorie	8 fl oz	50
Lightstyle Low Calorie Cranberry Juice Cocktail	8 fl oz	40
Seneca		
Cocktail frzn as prep	8 fl oz	140
Smucker's		
Juice Sparkler	10 oz	140
Snapple		
Cranberry Royal	10 fl oz	150
Tree Of Life		
Concentrate	8 tsp (1.4 oz)	110

FOOD	PORTION	CALS.
Tropicana		
Twister Ruby Red	1 bottle (10 fl oz)	150
Twister Ruby Red	8 fl oz	120
Veryfine		
Drink	8 oz	160

CRAYFISH
(*see also* LOBSTER)

cooked	3 oz	97
raw	3 oz	76
raw	8	24

CREAM
(*see also* SOUR CREAM, SOUR CREAM SUBSTITUTES, WHIPPED TOPPINGS)

LIQUID

half & half	1 tbsp	20
half & half	1 cup	315
heavy whipping	1 tbsp	52
light coffee	1 cup	496
light coffee	1 tbsp	29
light whipping	1 tbsp	44
Farmland		
Half & Half	2 tbsp	40
Light Cream	2 tbsp	30
Hood		
Half & Half	2 tbsp (1 oz)	40
Heavy	1 tbsp (0.5 oz)	50
Light	1 tbsp (0.5 oz)	30
Whipping Cream	1 tbsp (0.5 oz)	45
Parmalat		
Half & Half	2 tbsp (1 oz)	40

WHIPPED

heavy whipping	1 cup	411
light whipping	1 cup	345

CREAM CHEESE

cream cheese	1 oz	99
cream cheese	1 pkg (3 oz)	297
Alpine Lace		
Fat Free Garden Vegetable	2 tbsp (1 oz)	30
Fat Free Garlic & Herbs	2 tbsp (1 oz)	30
Breakstone		
Temp-Tee Whipped	3 tbsp (1.2 oz)	110
Fleur De Lait		
Bermuda Onion & Chives	2 tbsp (0.9 oz)	90

FOOD	PORTION	CALS.
Fleur De Lait (CONT.)		
Cinnamon Raisin	2 tbsp (0.9 oz)	90
Date Nut Rum	2 tbsp (0.9 oz)	90
Fresh Cut Garden Vegetable	2 tbsp (0.9 oz)	80
Garden Vegetable	2 tbsp (0.9 oz)	80
Garlic & Spice	2 tbsp (0.9 oz)	90
Herb & Spice	2 tbsp (0.9 oz)	90
Irish Creme	2 tbsp (0.9 oz)	100
Lemon	2 tbsp (0.9 oz)	90
Lox	2 tbsp (0.9 oz)	90
Mandarin Orange	2 tbsp (0.9 oz)	90
Peach	2 tbsp (0.9 oz)	90
Pineapple	2 tbsp (0.9 oz)	90
Plain	2 tbsp (1 oz)	100
Strawberry	2 tbsp (0.9 oz)	90
Toasted Onion	2 tbsp (0.9 oz)	90
Wildberry	2 tbsp (0.9 oz)	90
Fresh Cut		
Bac'n & Horseradish	2 tbsp (0.9 oz)	90
Bermuda Onion & Chives	2 tbsp (0.9 oz)	90
Date Nut & Rum	2 tbsp (0.9 oz)	90
Garlic & Spice	2 tbsp (0.9 oz)	90
Herb & Spice	2 tbsp (0.9 oz)	90
Lox	2 tbsp (0.9 oz)	90
Peaches & Cream	2 tbsp (0.9 oz)	90
Strawberry	2 tbsp (0.9 oz)	90
Friendship		
NY Style Reduced Fat	2 tbsp (1 oz)	50
Healthy Choice		
Herbs & Garlic	2 tbsp (1 oz)	25
Plain	2 tbsp (1 oz)	25
Strawberry	2 tbsp (1 oz)	30
Heluva Good Cheese		
Cream Cheese	1 tbsp (1 oz)	100
Philadelphia		
Free	1 oz	25
Free Soft	2 tbsp (1.2 oz)	30
Light Soft	2 tbsp (1.1 oz)	70
Philadelphia		
	1 oz	100
Soft	2 tbsp (1 oz)	100
Soft Herb & Garlic	2 tbsp (1.1 oz)	110
Soft Olive & Pimento	2 tbsp (1.1 oz)	100
Soft Pineapple	2 tbsp (1.1 oz)	100
Soft Smoked Salmon	2 tbsp (1.1 oz)	100

FOOD	PORTION	CALS.
Philadelphia (CONT.)		
Soft Strawberries	2 tbsp (1.1 oz)	100
Soft With Chives & Onions	2 tbsp (1.1 oz)	110
Whipped	3 tbsp (1.1 oz)	110
Whipped Smoked Salmon	3 tbsp (1.1 oz)	100
With Chives	1 oz	90
With Pimentos	1 oz	90
Ultra Delight		
Cheddar Cream Cheese	2 tbsp (0.9 oz)	60
Chive	2 tbsp (0.9 oz)	60
Garlic	2 tbsp (0.9 oz)	60
Mixed Berry	2 tbsp (0.9 oz)	70
Nacho	2 tbsp (0.9 oz)	60
Salsa	2 tbsp (0.9 oz)	60
Shrimp	2 tbsp (0.9 oz)	60
Strawberry	2 tbsp (0.9 oz)	60
Vegetable	2 tbsp (0.9 oz)	50
Weight Watchers		
Light	2 tbsp	40

CREAM CHEESE SUBSTITUTES

Tofutti

Better Than Cream Cheese French Onion	1 oz	80
Better Than Cream Cheese Herb & Chive	1 oz	80
Better Than Cream Cheese Plain	1 oz	80

CREAM OF TARTAR

cream of tartar	1 tsp	8

CREPES

basic crepe unfilled	1	75

CRESS

(*see also* WATERCRESS)

garden cooked	½ cup	16
garden raw	½ cup	8

CROAKER

atlantic breaded & fried	3 oz	188
atlantic raw	3 oz	89

CROISSANT

apple	1 (2 oz)	145
cheese	1 (2 oz)	236
plain	1 (2 oz)	232
plain	1 mini (1 oz)	115

FOOD	PORTION	CALS.
Pepperidge Farm		
Croissant Sandwich Quartet	1	170
Petite All Butter	1	120
Rudy's Farm		
Ham & Swiss Sandwich	1 (3.4 oz)	310
Sara Lee		
All Butter	1	170
All Butter Petite Size	1	120
TAKE-OUT		
w/ egg & cheese	1	369
w/ egg cheese & bacon	1	413
w/ egg cheese & ham	1	475
w/ egg cheese & sausage	1	524

CROUTONS

FOOD	PORTION	CALS.
plain	1 cup (1 oz)	122
seasoned	1 cup (1.4 oz)	186
Arnold		
Crispy Cheddar Romano	½ oz	64
Crispy Cheese Garlic	½ oz	60
Crispy Fine Herbs	½ oz	50
Crispy Italian	½ oz	60
Crispy Onion & Garlic	½ oz	60
Crispy Seasoned	½ oz	60
Brownberry		
Ceasar Salad	½ oz	62
Cheddar Cheese	½ oz	63
Onion & Garlic	½ oz	60
Seasoned	½ oz	59
Toasted	½ oz	56
Pepperidge Farm		
Cheddar & Romano Cheese	½ oz	60
Cheese & Garlic	½ oz	70
Onion & Garlic	½ oz	70
Seasoned	½ oz	70
Sour Cream & Chive	½ oz	70

CUCUMBER

FOOD	PORTION	CALS.
FRESH		
raw	1 (11 oz)	38
raw sliced	½ cup (1.8 oz)	7
JARRED		
Rosoff's		
Salad	3 slices (1 oz)	12

FOOD	PORTION	CALS.
Schorr's		
Cucumber Garden Salad	3 slices (1 oz)	12
TAKE-OUT		
cucumber salad	3.5 oz	50
CUMIN		
seed	1 tsp	8
CURRANT JUICE		
black currant nectar	3½ oz	55
red currant nectar	3½ oz	54
CURRANTS		
black fresh	½ cup	36
zante dried	½ cup	204
CUSK		
fillet baked	3 oz	106
CUSTARD		
HOME RECIPE		
baked	½ cup (5 oz)	148
baked	1 recipe 4 serv (19.8 oz)	549
flan	½ cup (5.4 oz)	220
flan	1 recipe 10 serv (53.7 oz)	2206
MIX		
as prep w/ 2% milk	½ cup (4.7 oz)	148
as prep w/ 2% milk	1 recipe 4 serv (18.7 oz)	595
as prep w/ whole milk	1 recipe 4 serv (18.7 oz)	652
as prep w/ whole milk	½ cup (4.7 oz)	163
flan as prep w/ 2% milk	1 recipe 4 serv (18.7 oz)	542
flan as prep w/ 2% milk	½ cup (4.7 oz)	135
flan as prep w/ whole milk	1 recipe 4 serv (18.7 oz)	600
flan as prep w/ whole milk	½ cup (4.7 oz)	150
Jell-O		
Flan	½ cup	151
Golden Egg Americana as prep	½ cup	160
Royal		
Custard	mix for 1 serving	60
Flan Caramel Custard	mix for 1 serving	60
TAKE-OUT		
baked	½ cup (5 oz)	148
zabaione	½ cup (57.2 g)	135
CUTTLEFISH		
steamed	3 oz	134

FOOD	PORTION	CALS.

DANDELION GREENS

FOOD	PORTION	CALS.
fresh cooked	½ cup	17
raw chopped	½ cup	13

DANISH PASTRY

FROZEN

Morton

FOOD	PORTION	CALS.
Honey Buns	1 (2.28 oz)	250
Honey Buns Mini	1 (1.23 oz)	160

Pepperidge Farm

FOOD	PORTION	CALS.
Apple	1	220
Cheese	1	240
Cinnamon Raisin	1	250
Raspberry	1	220

Sara Lee

FOOD	PORTION	CALS.
Apple	1	120
Apple Free & Light	1 slice (2 oz)	130
Cheese	1	130
Cheese Danish Twist	1 slice (1.9 oz)	200
Cinnamon Raisin	1	150
Raspberry Danish Twist	1 slice (1.9 oz)	200

READY-TO-EAT

FOOD	PORTION	CALS.
plain ring	1 (12 oz)	1305

Hostess

FOOD	PORTION	CALS.
Apple	1 (3.8 oz)	400
Apple Fruit Roll	1 (2 oz)	180
Coffee Cake Raspberry	1 (1.2 oz)	110

REFRIGERATED

Pillsbury

FOOD	PORTION	CALS.
Caramel Danish w/ Nuts	1	160
Cinnamon Raisin Danish w/ Icing	1	150
Orange Danish w/ Icing	1	150

TAKE-OUT

FOOD	PORTION	CALS.
almond	1 (4¼ in) (2.3 oz)	280
apple	1 (4¼ in) (2.5 oz)	264
cheese	1 (3 oz)	353
cheese	1 (4¼ in) (2.5 oz)	266
cinnamon	1 (3 oz)	349
cinnamon	1 (4¼ in) (2.3 oz)	262
cinnimon nut	1 (4¼ in) (2.3 oz)	280
fruit	1 (3.3 oz)	335
lemon	1 (4¼ in) (2.5 oz)	264
raisin	1 (4¼ in) (2.5 oz)	264
raisin nut	1 (4¼ in) (2.3 oz)	280

FOOD	PORTION	CALS.
raspberry	1 (4¼ in) (2.5 oz)	264
strawberry	1 (4¼ in) (2.5 oz)	264

DATES
DRIED
California Deglet Noor	10	240
chopped	1 cup	489
whole	10	228
Bordo		
Diced	2 oz	203
Dole		
Chopped	½ cup	230
Pitted	½ cup	280
Dromedary		
Chopped	¼ cup	130
Pitted	5	100
Sonoma		
Dried	5-6 (1.4 oz)	110

DEER
(*see* VENISON)

DELI MEATS/COLD CUTS
(*see also* CHICKEN, HAM, MEAT SUBSTITUTES, TURKEY)

barbecue loaf pork & beef	1 oz	49
beerwurst beef	1 slice (2¾ in x ¹⁄₁₆ in)	20
beerwurst beef	1 slice (4 in x ⅛ in)	75
beerwurst pork	1 slice (2¾ in x ¹⁄₁₆ in)	14
beerwurst pork	1 slice (4 in x ⅛ in)	55
berliner pork & beef	1 oz	65
blood sausage	1 oz	95
bologna beef	1 oz	88
bologna beef & pork	1 oz	89
bologna pork	1 oz	70
braunschweiger pork	1 oz	102
braunschweiger pork	1 slice (2½ in x ¼ in)	65
corned beef loaf	1 oz	43
dried beef	1 oz	47
dried beef	5 slices (21 g)	35
dutch brand loaf pork & beef	1 oz	68
headcheese pork	1 oz	60
honey loaf pork & beef	1 oz	36
honey roll sausage beef	1 oz	42
lebanon bologna beef	1 oz	60
liver cheese pork	1 oz	86

FOOD	PORTION	CALS.
liverwurst pork	1 oz	92
luncheon meat beef	1 oz	87
luncheon meat pork & beef	1 oz	100
luncheon meat pork canned	1 oz	95
luncheon sausage pork & beef	1 oz	74
luxury loaf pork	1 oz	40
mortadella beef & pork	1 oz	88
mother's loaf pork	1 oz	80
new england sausage pork & beef	1 oz	46
olive loaf pork	1 oz	67
peppered loaf pork & beef	1 oz	42
pepperoni pork & beef	1 slice (0.2 oz)	27
pepperoni pork & beef	1 (9 oz)	1248
pickle & pimiento loaf pork	1 oz	74
picnic loaf pork & beef	1 oz	66
salami cooked beef & pork	1 oz	71
salami hard pork	1 pkg (4 oz)	460
salami hard pork	1 slice (⅓ oz)	41
salami hard pork & beef	1 slice (⅓ oz)	42
salami hard pork & beef	1 pkg (4 oz)	472
sandwich spread pork & beef	1 tbsp	35
sandwich spread pork & beef	1 oz	67
summer sausage thuringer cervelat	1 oz	98
Armour		
Beef Bologna Lower Salt	1 oz	90
Bologna Lower Salt	1 oz	90
Salami Lower Salt	1 oz	80
Carl Buddig		
Beef	1 oz	40
Corned Beef	1 oz	40
Pastrami	1 oz	40
DiLusso		
Genoa	1 oz	100
Hansel n'Gretel		
Healthy Deli Bologna Beef & Pork	1 oz	41
Healthy Deli Cooked Corn Beef	1 oz	35
Healthy Deli Italian Roast Beef	1 oz	31
Healthy Deli Pastrami Round	1 oz	34
Healthy Deli Regular Roast Beef	1 oz	30
Healthy Deli St Paddy's Corned Beef	1 oz	24
Healthy Choice		
Bologna	1 slice (1 oz)	30
Bologna Beef	1 slice (1 oz)	35
Deli-Thin Bologna	4 slices (1.8 oz)	60

FOOD	PORTION	CALS.
Healthy Choice (CONT.)		
Well-Pack Bologna	1 slice (1 oz)	30
Hebrew National		
Bologna Beef	2 oz	180
Bologna Beef Reduced Fat	2 oz	130
Bologna Lean Chub	2 oz	90
Bologna Midget	2 oz	180
Deli Pastrami	2 oz	80
Deli Express Corned Beef	2 oz	80
Deli Express Tongue Sliced	2 oz	120
Salami Beef	2 oz	170
Salami Beef Reduced Fat	2 oz	110
Salami Sean Chub	2 oz	90
Salami Midget	2 oz	170
Hillshire		
Bologna Large	1 oz	90
Bologna Ring	1 oz	90
Brunschweiger	1 oz	95
Deli Select Corned Beef	1 slice	10
Deli Select Light Bologna	1 slice	12
Deli Select Oven Roasted Cured Beef	1 slice	10
Deli Select Pastrami	1 slice	10
Deli Select Roast Beef	1 slice	10
Deli Select Smoked Beef	1 slice	10
Flavor Pack 90-99% Fat Free Light Bologna	1 slice (0.73 oz)	30
Flavor Pack 90-99% Fat Free Pastrami	1 slice (0.6 oz)	18
Lunch 'N Munch Bologna/ American/ Snickers	1 pkg (4.25 oz)	490
Lunch 'N Munch Bologna/ American/ Snickers/Hi-C	1 pkg (4.25 oz + 6 fl oz)	590
Lunch 'N Munch Bologna/American	1 pkg (4.5 oz)	480
Lunch 'N Munch Cotto Salami/ Monterey Jack	1 pkg (4.5 oz)	440
Lunch 'N Munch Pepperoni/ American	1 pkg (4.5 oz)	570
Pepperoni	1 oz	110
Salami Hard	1 oz	100
Salami Hard	1 oz	90
Summer Sausage	2 oz	180
Summer Sausage Beef	2 oz	190
Summer Sausage Light	2 oz	150
Summer Sausage w/Cheddar Cheese	2 oz	200
Homeland		
Hard Salami	1 oz	110

FOOD	PORTION	CALS.
Hormel		
Liverwurst Spread	4 tbsp (2 oz)	130
Pepperoni Chunk	1 oz	140
Pepperoni Sliced	15 slices (1 oz)	140
Pepperoni Twin	1 oz	140
Pillow Pack Genoa Salami	4 slices (1.1 oz)	120
Pillow Pack Pepperoni	16 slices (1 oz)	140
Pillow Pack Pepperoni	1 oz	140
Jones		
Liver Sausage	1 slice	80
Liver Sausage Chub	1 slice	80
Oscar Mayer		
Bologna Beef	1 slice (1 oz)	90
Bologna Garlic	1 slice (1.4 oz)	110
Bologna Light	1 slice (1 oz)	60
Bologna Light Beef	1 slice (1 oz)	60
Bologna Pork & Chicken & Beef	1 slice (1 oz)	90
Bologna Wisconsin Made Ring	2 oz	140
Braunschweiger	1 slice (1 oz)	100
Brunschweiger	2 oz	190
Brunschweiger German Brand	2 oz	200
Cotto Salami	2 slices (1.6 oz)	100
Cotto Salami Beef	2 slices (1.6 oz)	90
Free Bologna	2 slices (1.6 oz)	35
Genoa Salami	3 slices (1 oz)	100
Hard Salami	3 slices (1 oz)	100
Head Cheese	1 slice (1 oz)	50
Healthy Favorites Bologna	2 slices (1.6 oz)	45
Honey Loaf	1 slice (1 oz)	35
Liver Cheese	1 slice (1.3 oz)	120
Lunchables Bologna/American	1 pkg (4.5 oz)	450
Lunchables Deluxe Turkey/Ham	1 pkg (5.1 oz)	360
Lunchables Dessert Jello/Honey Turkey/ Cheddar	1 pkg (5.7 oz)	320
Lunchables Fun Pack Bologna/Wild Cherry	1 pkg (11.2 oz)	530
Lunchables Fun Pack Ham/Fruit Punch	1 pkg (11.2 oz)	450
Lunchables Ham/Swiss	1 pkg (4.5 oz)	320
Lunchables Pepperoni/ American	1 pkg (4.5 oz)	480
Lunchables Salami/American	1 pkg (4.5 oz)	430
Luncheon Loaf Spiced	1 slice (1 oz)	70
New England Brand Sausage	2 slices (1.6 oz)	60
Old Fashioned Loaf	1 slice (1 oz)	60
Olive Loaf	1 slice (1 oz)	70
Peppered Loaf	1 slice (1 oz)	39

FOOD	PORTION	CALS.
Oscar Mayer (CONT.)		
Pickle And Pimiento Loaf	1 slice (1 oz)	70
Salami For Beer	1 slices (1.6 oz)	110
Salami Machaich Brand Beef	2 slices (1.6 oz)	120
Sandwich Spread	2 oz	140
Summer Sausage	2 slices (1.6 oz)	140
Summer Sausage Beef	2 slices (1.6 oz)	140
Russer		
Bologna	2 oz	180
Bologna Jalapeno Pepper	2 oz	170
Bologna Wunderbar German Brand	2 oz	190
Bologna Beef	2 oz	180
Bologna Garlic	2 oz	180
Bologna Italian Brand Sweet Red Pepper	2 oz	180
Braunschweiger	2 oz	170
Cooked Salami	2 oz	120
Dutch Brand	2 oz	130
Hot Cooked Salami	2 oz	110
Italian Brand Loaf	2 oz	130
Jalapeno Loaf With Monterey Jack Cheese	2 oz	160
Kielbasa Loaf	2 oz	120
Light Bologna	2 oz	120
Light Bologna Beef	2 oz	120
Light Braunschweiger	2 oz	120
Light Old Fashioned Loaf	2 oz	90
Light P&P Loaf	2 oz	100
Light Salami Cooked	2 oz	90
Olive Loaf	2 oz	160
P&P Loaf	2 oz	160
Pepper Loaf	2 oz	90
Polish Loaf	2 oz	140
Sara Lee		
Pastrami Beef	2 oz	100
Peppered Beef	2 oz	70
Shofar		
Salami Beef	2 oz	160
Spam		
Less Salt	2 oz	170
Lite	2 oz	110
Original	2 oz	170
Underwood		
Liverwurst	2.08 oz	180
Weight Watchers		
Bologna	2 slices (¾ oz)	35

FOOD	PORTION	CALS.
TAKE-OUT		
corned beef	2 oz	70
corned beef brisket	2 oz	90
submarine w/ salami ham, cheese lettuce tomato onion & oil	1	456

DIETING AIDS

(*see* NUTRITIONAL SUPPLEMENTS)

DILL

seed	1 tsp	6
sprigs fresh	5	0
sprigs fresh	1 cup	4
weed dry	1 tsp	3
Watkins		
Liquid Spice	1 tbsp (0.5 oz)	120

DINNER

(*see also* PASTA DISHES, POT PIES, ORIENTAL FOOD, SPANISH FOODS)

FROZEN

Armour		
Classics Chicken Parmigiana	1 meal (10.75 oz)	360
Classics Chicken & Noodles	1 meal (11 oz)	280
Classics Chicken Mesquite	1 meal (9.5 oz)	280
Classics Chicken w/ Wine & Mushroom	1 meal (10 oz)	260
Classics Glazed Chicken	1 meal (10.75 oz)	280
Classics Meatloaf	1 meal (11.25 oz)	300
Classics Salisbury Steak	1 meal (11.25 oz)	330
Classics Swedish Meatballs	1 meal (10 oz)	300
Classics Turkey and Dressing	1 meal (11.25 oz)	270
Classics Veal Parmigiana	1 meal (11.25 oz)	400
Classics Lite Beef Pepper	1 meal (11 oz)	210
Classics Lite Chicken Burgundy	1 meal (10 oz)	210
Classics Lite Salisbury Steak	1 meal (11.5 oz)	260
Classics Lite Shrimp Creole	1 meal (10 oz)	220
Classics Lite Sweet & Sour Chicken	1 meal (11 oz)	220
Banquet		
BBQ Style Chicken	1 meal (9 oz)	320
Beef	1 meal (9 oz)	240
Chicken Parmigiana	1 pkg (9.5 oz)	290
Chicken & Dumplings	1 meal (10 oz)	260
Chicken Fried Steak	1 pkg (10 oz)	400
Chicken Nuggets	1 pkg (6.75 oz)	410
Extra Helping All White Chicken	1 meal (18 oz)	820
Extra Helping Chicken Parmigiana	1 meal (19 oz)	650

FOOD	PORTION	CALS.
Banquet (CONT.)		
Extra Helping Chicken Fried Steak	1 meal (18.5 oz)	800
Extra Helping Fried Chicken	1 meal (18 oz)	790
Extra Helping Meatloaf	1 meal (19 oz)	650
Extra Helping Mexican Style	1 meal (22 oz)	820
Extra Helping Salisbury Steak	1 meal (19 oz)	740
Extra Helping Southern Fried Chicken	1 meal (17.5 oz)	750
Extra Helping Turkey Dinner	1 meal (18.8 oz)	560
Family Entree Beef Stew	1 serv (8.13 oz)	160
Family Entree Chicken Parmigiana	1 serv (4.67 oz)	240
Family Entree Chicken & Dumplings	1 serv (7.47 oz)	290
Family Entree Gravy & Sliced Turkey	1 serv (4.8 oz)	100
Family Entree Gravy w/ Charbroiled Beef	1 serv (4.67 oz)	180
Family Entree Onion Gravy w/ Beef	1 serv (4.67 oz)	180
Family Entree Salisbury Steak	1 serv (4.67 oz)	200
Family Entree Veal Parmigiana	1 serv (4.67 oz)	230
Family Entrees Dumplings & Chicken	7 oz	280
Family Entrees Gravy & Sliced Beef	1 serv (5.6 oz)	100
Family Entrees Gravy & Sliced Turkey	6 oz	120
Fried Chicken	1 meal (9 oz)	470
Gravy w/ Beef Patty	1 pkg (9.5 oz)	300
Hot Sandwich Toppers Chicken Ala King	1 pkg (4.5 oz)	100
Hot Sandwich Toppers Creamed Chipped Beef	1 pkg (4 oz)	100
Hot Sandwich Toppers Gravy & Sliced Beef	1 pkg (4 oz)	70
Hot Sandwich Toppers Gravy & Sliced Turkey	1 pkg (5 oz)	90
Hot Sandwich Toppers Salisbury Steak	1 pkg (5 oz)	220
Hot Sandwich Toppers Sloppy Joe	1 meal (4 oz)	140
Meatloaf	1 meal (9.5 oz)	280
Mexican Style Combo Meal	1 pkg (11 oz)	380
Mexican Style Meal	1 pkg (11 oz)	340
Oriental Style Chicken	1 pkg (9 oz)	260
Salisbury Steak	1 meal (9.5 oz)	310
Southern Fried Chicken Meal	1 pkg (8.75 oz)	260
Turkey	1 meal (9.25 oz)	270
Veal Parmagiana	1 pkg (9 oz)	530
Western Style Meal	1 meal (9.5 oz)	210
White Meat Chicken Meal	1 pkg (8.75 oz)	470
Birds Eye		
Easy Recipe Beef Burgundy not prep	½ pkg	120
Easy Recipe Beef Fajitas not prep	½ pkg	80

FOOD	PORTION	CALS.
Budget Gourmet		
Beef Cantonese	1 meal (9.1 oz)	270
Beef Stroganoff	1 meal (8.75 oz)	260
Chicken And Egg Noodles	1 meal (10 oz)	440
Chicken Au Gratin	1 meal (9.1 oz)	230
Chicken Breast Parmigiana	1 pkg (11 oz)	270
Chicken Marsala	1 meal (9 oz)	260
Chicken With Fettucini	1 meal (10 oz)	400
Chinese Style Vegetables & Chicken	1 meal (10 oz)	280
French Recipe Chicken	1 meal (10 oz)	220
Glazed Turkey	1 meal (9 oz)	260
Ham & Asparagus Au Gratin	1 meal (8.7 oz)	300
Herbed Chicken Breast With Fettucini	1 pkg (11 oz)	240
Italian Style Vegetables & Chicken	1 meal (10.25 oz)	310
Mandarin Chicken	1 meal (10 oz)	240
Mesquite Chicken Breast	1 pkg (11 oz)	250
Orange Glazed Chicken	1 meal (9 oz)	270
Oriental Beef	1 meal (10 oz)	290
Oriental Chicken With Vegetables	1 meal (9 oz)	280
Pepper Steak With Rice	1 meal (10 oz)	300
Pot Roast Beef	1 meal (10.5 oz)	230
Roast Chicken With Homestyle Gravy	1 meal (11 oz)	280
Roast Sirloin Supreme	1 meal (9 oz)	320
Sirloin Salisbury Steak	1 meal (9 oz)	220
Sirloin Salisbury Steak	1 meal (11 oz)	280
Sirloin Cheddar Melt	1 meal (9.4 oz)	380
Sirloin Of Beef In Herb Sauce	1 meal (9.5 oz)	250
Sirloin Of Beef In Wine Sauce	1 pkg (11 oz)	280
Sirloin Tips And Country Vegetables	1 meal (10 oz)	290
Special Recipe Sirloin Of Beef	1 meal (11 oz)	250
Stuffed Turkey Breast	1 pkg (11 oz)	250
Swedish Meatballs With Noodles	1 meal (10 oz)	590
Sweet And Sour Chicken	1 meal (10 oz)	340
Teriyaki Beef	1 pkg (10.75 oz)	260
Teriyaki Chicken Breast	1 meal (11 oz)	300
Healthy Choice		
Beef & Peppers Cantonese	1 meal (11.5 oz)	270
Beef Pepper Steak Oriental	1 meal (9.5 oz)	250
Beef Tips Francais	1 meal (9.5 oz)	280
Beef Tips With Sauce	1 meal (11 oz)	290
Chicken Cantonese	1 meal (11.25)	210
Chicken Parmigiana	1 meal (11.5 oz)	300
Chicken & Vegetables Marsala	1 meal (11.5 oz)	220
Chicken Bangkok	1 meal (9.5 oz)	270

FOOD	PORTION	CALS.
Healthy Choice (CONT.)		
Chicken Dijon	1 meal (11 oz)	280
Chicken Imperial	1 meal (9 oz)	230
Chicken Picante	1 meal (11.25 oz)	220
Chicken Teriyaki	1 meal (12.25 oz)	270
Classics Beef Broccoli Beijing	1 meal (12 oz)	330
Classics Cacciatore Chicken	1 meal (12.5 oz)	260
Classics Chicken Fransesca	1 meal (12.5 oz)	360
Classics Country Inn Roast Turkey	1 meal (10 oz)	250
Classics Ginger Chicken Hunan	1 meal (12.6 oz)	350
Classics Mesquite Beef Barbecue	1 meal (11 oz)	310
Classics Salisbury Steak	1 meal (11 oz)	260
Classics Sesame Chicken Shanghai	1 meal (12 oz)	310
Classics Shrimp & Vegetables Maria	1 meal (12.5 oz)	260
Country Glazed Chicken	1 meal (8.5 oz)	200
Country Herb Chicken	1 meal (11.5 oz)	270
Country Roast Turkey With Mushroom	1 meal (8.5 oz)	220
Country Turkey & Pasta	1 meal (12.6 oz)	300
Homestyle Turkey With Vegetables	1 meal (9.5 oz)	260
Honey Mustard Chicken	1 meal (9.5 oz)	260
Lemon Pepper Fish	1 meal (10.7 oz)	290
Mandarin Chicken	1 meal (10 oz)	280
Mesquite Chicken Barbecue	1 meal (10.5 oz)	320
Shrimp Marinara	1 meal (10.5 oz)	220
Smoky Chicken Barbecue	1 meal (12.75 oz)	380
Southwestern Glazed Chicken	1 meal (12.5 oz)	300
Sweet & Sour Chicken	1 meal (11.5 oz)	310
Traditional Breast Of Turkey	1 meal (10.5 oz)	280
Traditional Meat Loaf	1 meal (12 oz)	320
Traditional Beef Tips	1 meal (11.25 oz)	260
Tradtional Salisbury Steak	1 meal (11.5 oz)	320
Yankee Pot Roast	1 meal (11 oz)	280
Kid Cuisine		
Chicken Sandwiche	1 pkg (9.43 oz)	480
Chicken Nuggets	1 pkg (9.1 oz)	440
Fish Sticks	1 pkg (8.25 oz)	370
Fried Chicken	1 pkg (10.1 oz)	440
Hot Dogs w/ Buns	6.7 oz	450
Macaroni & Beef	1 pkg (9.6 oz)	370
Le Menu		
Beef Sirlion Tips	11½ oz	400
Beef Stroganoff	10 oz	430
Chicken Parmigiana	11¾ oz	410
Chicken A La King	10¼ oz	330

FOOD	PORTION	CALS.
Le Menu (CONT.)		
Chicken Cordon Bleu	11 oz	460
Chicken In Wine Sauce	10 oz	280
Chopped Sirloin Beef	12¼ oz	430
Entree LightStyle Chicken A La King	8¼ oz	240
Entree LightStyle Chicken Dijon	8 oz	240
Entree LightStyle Empress Chicken	8¼ oz	210
Entree LightStyle Glazed Turkey	8¼ oz	260
Entree LightStyle Herb Roast Chicken	7¾ oz	260
Entree LightStyle Swedish Meatballs	8 oz	260
Entree LightStyle Traditional Turkey	8 oz	200
Ham Steak	10 oz	300
LightStyle Glazed Chicken Breast	10 oz	230
LightStyle Herb Roasted Chicken	10 oz	240
LightStyle Salisbury Steak	10 oz	280
LightStyle Sliced Turkey	10 oz	210
LightStyle Sweet & Sour Chicken	10 oz	250
LightStyle Turkey Divan	10 oz	260
LightStyle Veal Marsala	10 oz	230
Pepper Steak	11½ oz	370
Salisbury Steak	10½ oz	370
Sliced Breast Of Turkey w/ Mushroom Gravy	10½ oz	300
Sweet & Sour Chicken	11¼ oz	400
Veal Parmigiana	11½ oz	390
Yankee Pot Roast	10 oz	330
Lean Cuisine		
Baked Chicken	1 meal (8 oz)	240
Beef Pot Roast	1 meal (9 oz)	210
Chicken Italiano	1 pkg (9 oz)	270
Chicken & Vegetables	1 meal (10.5 oz)	240
Chicken A L'Orange	1 meal (8 oz)	260
Chicken In Peanut Sauce	1 pkg (9 oz)	280
Chicken In Honey Barbecue Sauce	1 pkg (8.75 oz)	250
Chicken Marsala	1 meal (8.1 oz)	180
Chicken Oriental	1 pkg (9 oz)	260
Chicken Parmesan	1 meal (10.9 oz)	220
Chicken Pie	1 meal (9.5 oz)	320
Fiesta Chicken	1 pkg (8.5 oz)	240
Fish Divan	1 pkg (10.4 oz)	210
Glazed Chicken	1 meal (8.5 oz)	240
Homestyle Turkey	1 pkg (9.4 oz)	230
Honey Mustard Chicken	1 pkg (7.5 oz)	250
Meatloaf	1 pkg (9.4 oz)	270

FOOD	PORTION	CALS.
Lean Cuisine (CONT.)		
Oriental Beef	1 meal (9 oz)	250
Roasted Turkey Breast	1 pkg (9.75 oz)	290
Salisbury Steak With Macaroni & Cheese	1 meal (9.5 oz)	200
Stuffed Cabbage	1 meal (9.5 oz)	220
Swedish Meatballs	1 pkg (9.1 oz)	290
Sweet & Sour Chicken	1 pkg (10.4 oz)	260
Turkey Pie	1 pkg (9.5 oz)	300
Life Choice		
Garden Potato Casserole	1 meal (13.4 oz)	160
Morton		
Breaded Chicken Pattie	1 meal (6.75 oz)	280
Chicken Nugget	1 meal (7 oz)	320
Fried Chicken	1 meal (9 oz)	420
Meatloaf	1 meal (9 oz)	250
Mexican	1 meal (10 oz)	260
Salisbury Steak	1 meal (9 oz)	210
Turkey	1 meal (9 oz)	230
Veal Parmagiana	1 meal (8.75 oz)	280
Western	1 meal (9 oz)	290
Patio		
Chili	1 cup (8 oz)	260
Ranchera	1 pkg (13 oz)	410
Stouffer's		
Chicken A La King	1 pkg (9.5 oz)	320
Chicken Divan	1 pkg (8 oz)	210
Creamed Chicken	1 pkg (6.5 oz)	280
Creamed Chipped Beef	½ cup (4.5 oz)	150
Creamed Chipped Beef Over Country Biscuit	1 pkg (9 oz)	460
Escalloped Chicken & Noodles	1 pkg (10 oz)	440
Green Pepper Steak	1 pkg (10.5 oz)	330
Ham & Asparagus Bake	1 pkg (9.5 oz)	520
Homestyle Beef Pot Raost	1 pkg (8.9 oz)	270
Homestyle Breaded Chicken Tenders	1 pkg (6.6 oz)	380
Homestyle Chicken Parmigiana	1 pkg (10.9 oz)	320
Homestyle Chicken & Noodles	1 pkg (10 oz)	310
Homestyle Chicken Monterey	1 pkg (9.4 oz)	410
Homestyle Fish Filet With Macaroni & Cheese	1 pkg (9 oz)	430
Homestyle Fried Chicken	1 pkg (7.1 oz)	330
Homestyle Meatloaf	1 pkg (9.9 oz)	380
Homestyle Roast Turkey	1 pkg (7.9 oz)	280
Homestyle Salisbury Steak	1 pkg (9.6 oz)	370

FOOD	PORTION	CALS.
Stouffer's (CONT.)		
Homestyle Sliced Beef & Potatoes	1 pkg (8.1 oz)	270
Homestyle Veal Parmigiana	1 pkg (11.9 oz)	420
Honestyle Baked Chicken	1 pkg (8.9 oz)	270
Lunch Express Chicken With Garden Vegetables	1 pkg (9.9 oz)	340
Lunch Express Mandarin Chicken	1 pkg (9.75 oz)	270
Lunch Express Mexican Style Rice With Chicken	1 pkg (9 oz)	270
Lunch Express Oriental Beef	1 pkg (6.2 oz)	260
Lunch Express Stir-Fry Rice & Chicken	1 pkg (9 oz)	280
Stuffed Pepper	1 pkg (10 oz)	200
Swedish Meatballs	1 pkg (9.25 oz)	440
Swanson		
Beans & Franks	10½ oz	440
Beef	11¼ oz	310
Beef In Barbecue Sauce	11 oz	460
Chicken Duet Gourmet Nuggets Pizza Style	3 oz	210
Chopped Sirloin Beef	10¾ oz	340
Fish 'n' Chips	10 oz	500
Fried Chicken Dark Meat	9¾ oz	560
Fried Chicken White Meat	10¼ oz	550
Homestyle Chicken Cacciatore	10.95 oz	260
Homestyle Chicken Nibbles	4¼ oz	340
Homestyle Fish & Fries	6½ oz	340
Homestyle Fried Chicken	7 oz	390
Homestyle Salisbury Steak	10 oz	320
Homestyle Scalloped Potatoes & Ham	9 oz	300
Homestyle Seafood Creole With Rice	9 oz	240
Homestyle Sirloin Tips In Burgundy Sauce	7 oz	160
Homestyle Turkey With Dressing & Potatoes	9 oz	290
Homestyle Veal Parmigiana	10 oz	330
Hungry-Man Boneless Chicken	17¾ oz	700
Hungry-Man Chopped Beef Steak	16¾ oz	640
Hungry-Man Fried Chicken Dark Meat	14¼ oz	860
Hungry-Man Fried Chicken White Meat	14¼ oz	870
Hungry-Man Salisbury Steak	16½ oz	680
Hungry-Man Sliced Beef	15¼ oz	450
Hungry-Man Veal Parmigiana	18¼ oz	590
Loin Of Pork	10¾ oz	280
Macaroni & Beef	12 oz	370
Meatloaf	10¾ oz	360

FOOD	PORTION	CALS.
Swanson (CONT.)		
Noodles & Chicken	10½ oz	280
Salisbury Steak	10¾ oz	400
Swiss Steak	10 oz	350
Swedish Meatballs	8½ oz	360
Turkey	11½ oz	350
Turkey	8¾ oz	270
Veal Parmigiana	12¼ oz	430
Western Style	11½ oz	430
Tyson		
Beef Champignon	1 pkg (10.5 oz)	370
Chicken Picante	1 pkg (9 oz)	250
Chicken Supreme	1 pkg (9 oz)	230
Francais	1 pkg (9.5 oz)	280
Glazed Chicken With Sauce	1 pkg (9.25 oz)	240
Grilled Chicken	1 pkg (7.75 oz)	220
Grilled Italian Chicken	1 pkg (9 oz)	210
Healthy Portions BBQ Chicken	1 pkg (12.5 oz)	400
Healthy Portions Chicken Marinara	1 pkg (13.75 oz)	340
Healthy Portions Herb Chicken	1 pkg (13.75 oz)	340
Healthy Portions Honey Mustard Chicken	1 pkg (13.75 oz)	390
Healthy Portions Italian Style Chicken	1 pkg (13.75 oz)	310
Healthy Portions Mesquite Chicken	1 pkg (13.25 oz)	330
Healthy Portions Salsa Chicken	1 pkg (13.75 oz)	370
Healthy Portions Sesame Chicken	1 pkg (13.5 oz)	400
Honey Roasted Chicken	1 pkg (9 oz)	220
Kiev	1 pkg (9.25 oz)	450
Marsala	1 pkg (9 oz)	200
Mexquite	1 pkg (9 oz)	320
Picatta	1 pkg (9 oz)	200
Roasted Chicken	1 pkg (9 oz)	200
Sweet & Sour	1 pkg (11 oz)	420
Turkey With Gravy	1 pkg (9.5 oz)	320
Ultra Slim-Fast		
Beef Pepper Steak	12 oz	270
Chicken Fettucini	12 oz	380
Chicken & Vegetable	12 oz	290
Country Style Vegetable & Beef Tips	12 oz	230
Mesquite Chicken	12 oz	360
Roasted Chicken In Mushroom Sauce	12 oz	280
Shrimp Creole	12 oz	240
Shrimp Marinara	12 oz	290
Sweet & Sour Chicken	12 oz	330
Turkey Medallions In Herb Sauce	12 oz	280

FOOD	PORTION	CALS.
Weight Watchers		
Barbecue Glazed Chicken	1 pkg (7.4 oz)	190
Chicken Mirabella	1 pkg (9.2 oz)	170
Chicken Parmigiana	1 pkg (9.1 oz)	230
Chicken Cordon Bleu	1 pkg (9 oz)	220
Chicken Marsala	1 pkg (9 oz)	150
Fiesta Chicken	1 pkg (8.5 oz)	220
Fried Filet Of Fish	1 pkg (7.7 oz)	230
Grilled Salisbury Steak	1 pkg (8.5 oz)	250
Honey Mustard Chicken	1 pkg (8.5 oz)	200
Lemon Herb Chicken Picante	1 pkg (8.5 oz)	190
Roast Glazed Chicken	1 pkg (8.9 oz)	200
Roast Turkey Madallions	1 pkg (8.5 oz)	190
Shrimp Marinara	1 pkg (9 oz)	190
Southern Fried Chicken	1 pkg (8 oz)	280
Stuffed Turkey Breast	1 pkg (8.75 oz)	240
Swedish Meatballs	1 pkg (9 oz)	280
Tex-Mex Chicken	1 pkg (8.3 oz)	260
SHELF-STABLE		
My Own Meal		
Beef Stew	1 pkg (10 oz)	260
Chicken Mediterranean	1 pkg (10 oz)	270
Chicken Noodles	1 pkg (10 oz)	270
Chicken & Black Beans	1 pkg (10 oz)	240
Old World Stew	1 pkg (10 oz)	310
DIP		
Breakstone		
Sour Cream Bacon & Onion	2 tbsp (1.1 oz)	60
Sour Cream Chesapeake Clam	2 tbsp (1.1 oz)	50
Sour Cream French Onion	2 tbsp (1.1 oz)	50
Sour Cream Jalapeno Cheddar	2 tbsp (1.1 oz)	60
Sour Cream Toasted Onion	2 tbsp (1.1 oz)	50
Chi-Chi's		
Fiesta Bean	2 tbsp (0.9 oz)	35
Fiesta Cheese	2 tbsp (0.9 oz)	40
Durkee		
Sour Cream as prep	2 tbsp	25
Frito Lay		
Cheddar Cheese	1 oz	45
French Onion	1 oz	50
Jalapeno Bean	1 oz	30
Picante Sauce	1 oz	10
Guiltless Gourmet		
Black Bean Mild	1 oz	25

FOOD	PORTION	CALS.
Guiltless Gourmet (CONT.)		
Black Bean Spicy	1 oz	25
Pinto Bean	1 oz	25
Hain		
Hot Bean	4 tbsp	70
Mexican Bean	4 tbsp	60
Onion Bean	4 tbsp	70
Taco Dip & Sauce	4 tbsp	25
Heluva Good Cheese		
Bacon Horseradish	2 tbsp (1.1 oz)	60
Clam	2 tbsp (1.1 oz)	50
French Onion	2 tbsp (1.1 oz)	50
Homestyle Onion	2 tbsp (1.1 oz)	60
Light French Onion	2 tbsp (1.1 oz)	35
Light Jalapeno Cheddar	2 tbsp (1.1 oz)	40
Ranch	2 tbsp (1.1 oz)	60
Knudsen		
Nacho Cheese	2 tbsp (1.1 oz)	60
Sour Cream Bacon & Onion	2 tbsp (1.1 oz)	60
Sour Cream French Onion	2 tbsp (1.1 oz)	50
Kraft		
Avocado	2 tbsp (1.1 oz)	60
Bacon & Horseradish	2 tbsp (1.1 oz)	60
Clam	2 tbsp (1.1 oz)	60
French Onion	2 tbsp (1.1 oz)	60
Green Onion	2 tbsp (1.1 oz)	60
Jalapeno	2 tbsp (1.1 oz)	60
Jalapeno Cheese	2 tbsp (1.1 oz)	60
Premium Bacon & Horseradish	2 tbsp (1.1 oz)	50
Premium Bacon & Onion	2 tbsp (1.1 oz)	60
Premium Blue Cheese	2 tbsp (1.1 oz)	45
Premium Clam	2 tbsp (1.1 oz)	45
Premium Creamy Cucumber	2 tbsp (1.1 oz)	50
Premium Creamy Onion	2 tbsp (1.1 oz)	45
Premium French Onion	2 tbsp (1.1 oz)	50
Premium Nacho Cheese	2 tbsp (1.1 oz)	60
Ranch	2 tbsp (1.1 oz)	60
Louise's		
Fat Free Honey Mustard	1 oz	40
Fat Free Sour Cream & Onion	1 oz	25
Fat Free White Cheese Peppercorn	1 oz	25
Marzetti		
Blue Cheese Veggie	2 tbsp	200
Lemon Dill Veggie	2 tbsp	140

FOOD	PORTION	CALS.
Marzetti (CONT.)		
Light Ranch Veggie	2 tbsp	60
Ranch Veggie	2 tbsp	140
Sour Cream & Onion	2 tbsp	130
Southwestern Veggie	2 tbsp	130
Spinach Veggie	2 tbsp	130
Old El Paso		
Black Bean	2 tbsp (1 oz)	20
Cheese 'n Salsa Medium	2 tbsp (1 oz)	40
Cheese 'n Salsa Mild	2 tbsp (1 oz)	40
Chunky Salsa Medium	2 tbsp (1 oz)	15
Chunky Salsa Mild	2 tbsp (1 oz)	15
Jalapeno	2 tbsp (1 oz)	30
Sealtest		
French Onion	2 tbsp (1.1 oz)	50
Snyder's		
Mustard Pretzel	2 tbsp (1.2 oz)	90
Wise		
Jalapeno Bean	2 tbsp	25
Taco	2 tbsp	12
DOCK		
fresh cooked	3½ oz	20
raw chopped	½ cup	15
DOGFISH		
raw	3½ oz	193
DOLPHINFISH		
fresh baked	3 oz	93
fresh fillet baked	5.6 oz	174
DOUGHNUTS		
(see also DUNKIN' DONUTS, WINCHELL'S)		
cake type unsugared	1 (1.6 oz)	198
chocolate glazed	1 (1.5 oz)	175
chocolate sugared	1 (1.5 oz)	175
chocolate coated	1 (1.5 oz)	204
creme filled	1 (3 oz)	307
french cruller glazed	1 (1.4 oz)	169
frosted	1 (1.5 oz)	204
honey bun	1 (2.1 oz)	242
jelly	1 (3 oz)	289
old fashioned	1 (1.6 oz)	198
sugared	1 (1.6 oz)	192
wheat glazed	1 (1.6 oz)	162

FOOD	PORTION	CALS.
wheat sugared	1 (1.6 oz)	162
yeast glazed	1 (2.1 oz)	242
Drake's		
Old Fashion Donuts	1 (1.7 oz)	182
Powdered Sugar Donut Delites	7 (2.5 oz)	300
Dutch Mill		
Cider	1 (2.1 oz)	240
Cinnamon	1 (1.8 oz)	210
Donut Holes Double-Dipped Chocolate	3 (1.4 oz)	220
Donut Holes Shootin' Stars	3 (1.4 oz)	190
Double-Dipped Chocolate	1 (2.1 oz)	280
Glazed	1 (2.1 oz)	250
Glazed Chocolate	1 (2.4 oz)	270
Plain	1 (1.8 oz)	210
Sugared	1 (1.8 oz)	220
Earth Grains		
Cinnamon Apple	1	310
Devil's Food	1	330
Glazed Old Fashioned	1	310
Powdered Old Fashioned	1	290
Entenmann's		
Crumb Topped	1 (2.1 oz)	260
Devil's Food Crumb	1 (2.1 oz)	250
Rich Frosted	1 (2 oz)	280
Freihofer's		
Assorted	1 (2 oz)	270
Hostess		
Assorted Regular	1 (1.6 oz)	200
Cinnamon Family Pack	1 (1 oz)	110
Cinnamon Swirl	1 (1.6 oz)	180
Crumb Regular	1 (1 oz)	130
Frosted Regular	1 (1.4 oz)	180
Gem Donettes Cinnamon	6 (3 oz)	320
Gem Donettes Frosted	6 (3 oz)	390
Gem Donettes Frosted Strawberry Filled	3 (3 oz)	240
Gem Donettes Powdered	6 (3 oz)	350
Gem Donettes Powdered Strawberry Filled	3 (3 oz)	210
Glazed Party	1 (2.3 oz)	260
Jumbo Frosted	1 (2 oz)	260
Jumbo Plain	1 (1.1 oz)	140
Jumbo Powdered	1 (1.3 oz)	160
Mini Chocolate	5 (2 oz)	220
O's Raspberry Filled Powdered	1 (2.2 oz)	230
Old Fashioned Glazed	1 (2.1 oz)	250

FOOD	PORTION	CALS.
Hostess (CONT.)		
Old Fashioned Glazed Honey Wheat	1 (2.1 oz)	250
Old Fashioned Plain	1 (1.5 oz)	170
Plain Regular	1 (1 oz)	120
Powdered Family Pack	1 (1 oz)	110
Little Debbie		
Donut Sticks	1 pkg (1.6 oz)	210
Donut Sticks	1 pkg (3 oz)	390
Donut Sticks	1 pkg (2.5 oz)	320
Donut Sticks	1 pkg (2 oz)	250
Tastykake		
Cinnamon	1 (47 g)	180
Frosted Rich	1 (57 g)	260
Frosted Rich Mini	1 (14 g)	44
Honey Wheat	1 (57 g)	210
Honey Wheat Mini	1 (12 g)	40
Orange Glazed	1 (57 g)	210
Plain	1 (47 g)	190
Powdered Sugar	1 (46 g)	180
Powdered Sugar Mini	1 (12 g)	40

DRESSING
(*see* STUFFING/DRESSING)

DRINK MIXERS
(*see also* SODA, MINERAL/BOTTLED WATER)

FOOD	PORTION	CALS.
whiskey sour mix	2 oz	55
whiskey sour mix as prep	3.6 oz	169
Bacardi		
Margarita Mix w/ rum	8 fl oz	160
Margarita Mix w/o liquor	8 fl oz	100
Pina Colada	8 fl oz	140
Rum Runner	8 fl oz	140
Strawberry Daiquiri w/o liquor	8 fl oz	140
Canada Dry		
Collins Mixer	8 fl oz	120
Sour Mixer	8 fl oz	90
Libby		
Bloody Mary Mix	6 oz	40
McIlhenny		
Tabasco Bloody Mary Mix	8 fl oz	56
Schweppes		
Collins Mixer	8 fl oz	100
Tabasco		
Bloody Mary Mix Extra Spicy	8 fl oz	58

FOOD	PORTION	CALS.
DRUM		
freshwater fillet baked	5.4 oz	236
freshwater baked	3 oz	130
DUCK		
FRESH		
w/ skin roasted	½ duck (13.4 oz)	1287
w/ skin roasted	6 oz	583
w/o skin roasted	3.5 oz	201
w/o skin roasted	½ duck (7.8 oz)	445
wild breast w/o skin raw	½ breast (2.9 oz)	102
wild w/ skin raw	½ duck (9.5 oz)	571
DUMPLING		
FROZEN		
Pepperidge Farm		
Apple Dumpling	1 (3 oz)	260
DURIAN		
fresh	3½ oz	141
EEL		
fresh cooked	1 fillet (5.6 oz)	375
fresh cooked	3 oz	200
raw	3 oz	156
smoked	3.5 oz	330
EGG		
(*see also* EGG DISHES, EGG SUBSTITUTES)		
CHICKEN		
fried w/ margarine	1	91
frozen	1 cup	363
frozen	1	75
hard cooked	1	77
hard cooked chopped	1 cup	210
poached	1	74
raw	1	75
scrambled plain	2	200
scrambled w/ whole milk & margarine	1 cup	365
scrambled w/ whole milk & margarine	1	101
white only	1	17
white only	1 cup	121
OTHER POULTRY		
duck raw	1	130
goose raw	1	267
quail raw	1	14
turkey raw	1	135

FOOD	PORTION	CALS.

EGG DISHES

FROZEN

Chefwich

Cheese Omelet	5 oz	380
Ham & Cheese Omelet	5 oz	340
Sausage & Cheese Omelet	5 oz	400
Western Style Omelet	5 oz	350

Downyflake

Scrambled Eggs With Ham & Hash Browns	1 pkg (6.25 oz)	360
Scrambled Eggs With Ham & Pecan Twirl	1 pkg (6.25 oz)	470
Scrambled Eggs With Hash Browns & Sausage	1 pkg (6.25 oz)	420
Scrambled Eggs With Sausage & Pecan Twirl	1 pkg (6.25 oz)	510

Great Starts

Egg Sausage & Cheese	5½ oz	460
Omelets With Cheese & Ham	7 oz	390
Reduced Cholesterol Eggs With Mini Oatbran Muffins	4¾ oz	250
Scrambled Eggs & Bacon With Home Fries	5.6 oz	340
Scrambled Eggs & Home Fries	4.6 oz	260
Scrambled Eggs & Sausage With Hash Browns	6½ oz	430

Quaker

Scrambled Eggs & Sausage With Hash Browns	1 pkg (5.7 oz)	290
Scrambled Eggs & Sausage With Pancakes	1 pkg (5.2 oz)	270

Weight Watchers

Classic Omelet Sandwich	1 (3.8 oz)	220
Garden Omelet Sandwich	1 (3.6 oz)	220
Handy Ham & Cheese Omelet	1 (4 oz)	230

TAKE-OUT

deviled	2 halves	145
salad	½ cup	307
sandwich w/ cheese	1	340
sandwich w/ cheese & ham	1	348
scotch egg	1 (4.2 oz)	301

EGG ROLLS

(*see also* ORIENTAL FOODS)

egg roll wrapper fresh	1	83

Chun King

Chicken	8 (4.4 oz)	270

FOOD	PORTION	CALS.
Chun King (CONT.)		
Pork & Shrimp	8 (4.4 oz)	290
Shrimp	8 (4.4 oz)	260
Empire		
Large	1 (3 oz)	190
Miniature	6 (4.8 oz)	280
La Choy		
Almond Chicken Restaurant Style	1 (3 oz)	170
Chicken Mini	14 (7.25 oz)	430
Chicken Restaurant Style	1 (3 oz)	170
Lobster Mini	14 (7.25 oz)	410
Meat & Shrimp Mini	15 (3.75 oz) .	240
Mu Sho Pork Restaurant Style	1 (3 oz)	190
Pork Restaurant Style	1 (3 oz)	150
Pork & Shrimp Mini	14 (7.25 oz)	430
Shrimp Mini	14 (7.25 oz)	410
Shrimp Restaurant Style	1 (3 oz)	150
Sweet & Sour Restaurant Style	1 (3 oz)	180
Lo-An		
White Meat Chicken	1 (2.7 oz)	140
Luigino's		
Chicken	1 pkg (6 oz)	360
Pork & Shrimp	1 pkg (6 oz)	340
Shrimp	1 pkg (6 oz)	350
Sweet & Sour Chicken	1 pkg (6 oz)	400
Sweet & Sour Pork	1 pkg (6 oz)	360
Szechwan Vegetable	1 pkg (6 oz)	350
TAKE-OUT		
lobster	1 (4.8 oz)	270
meat & shrimp	1 (4.8 oz)	320
pork & shrimp	1 (5 oz)	300
shrimp	1 (3 oz)	170
spicy pork	1 (3 oz)	200
vegetable	1 (3 oz)	170

EGG SUBSTITUTES

frozen	¼ cup	96
frozen	1 cup	384
liquid	1 cup	211
liquid	1½ oz	40
powder	0.7 oz	88
powder	0.35 oz	44
Egg Beaters		
Eggs Substitute	¼ cup	25

FOOD	PORTION	CALS.
Egg Beaters (CONT.)		
Omelette Cheese	½ cup	110
Omelette Vegetable	½ cup	50
Egg Watchers		
Egg Substitute	2 oz	50
Healthy Choice		
Cholesterol Free	¼ cup (2 oz)	25
LaLoma		
Scramblers Links Muffins	1 pkg (4 oz)	220
Morningstar Farms		
Better'n Eggs	¼ cup (57 g)	30
Scramblers	¼ cup (57 g)	60
Scramblers Links Hash Browns	1 pkg (5 oz)	240
Scramblers Sandwich w/ Cheese	1 (3.5 oz)	220
Scramblers Sandwich w/ Pattie	1 (4.5 oz)	300
Scramblers Sandwich w/ Pattie Cheese	1 (5 oz)	350
Second Nature		
No Cholesterol	2 fl oz	60
No Fat	2 fl oz	40
No Fat With Garden Vegetables	2.5 fl oz	40
Simply Eggs		
Egg Substitue	1.75 fl oz	35
EGGNOG		
eggnog	1 cup	342
eggnog	1 qt	1368
eggnog flavor mix as prep w/ milk	9 oz	260
Borden		
Eggnog	4 fl oz	160
Light	½ cup	130
Hood		
Fat Free	4 fl oz	100
Golden	4 fl oz	180
Light	4 fl oz	120
Select	4 fl oz	210
EGGPLANT		
CANNED		
Progresso		
Appetizer	2 tbsp (1 oz)	30
FRESH		
cubed cooked	½ cup	13
raw cut up	½ cup (1.4 oz)	11
slices cooked	4 (7 oz)	38
whole peeled raw	1 (1 lb)	117

FOOD	PORTION	CALS.
FROZEN		
Mrs. Paul's		
Parmigiana	5 oz	240
TAKE-OUT		
baba ghannouj	¼ cup	55
ELDERBERRIES		
fresh	1 cup	105
ELDERBERRY JUICE		
elderberry	3½ oz	38
ELK		
roasted	3 oz	124
ENDIVE		
fresh	3½ oz	9
raw chopped	½ cup	4
ENGLISH MUFFIN		
FROZEN		
Great Starts		
Egg Beefsteak & Cheese	5.9 oz	360
Egg Canadian Bacon & Cheese	4.1 oz	290
Weight Watchers		
Sandwich	1 (4 oz)	230
HOME RECIPE		
cinnamon raisin	1	186
english muffin	1	158
honey bran	1	153
whole wheat	1	167
READY-TO-EAT		
apple cinnamon	1	138
granola	1	155
mixed grain	1	155
plain	1	134
plain toasted	1	133
raisin cinnamon	1	138
sourdough	1	134
wheat	1	127
whole wheat	1	134
Arnold		
Extra Crisp	1	130
Sourdough	1	130
Matthew's		
9 Grain & Nut	1	140

FOOD	PORTION	CALS.
Matthew's (cont.)		
Cinnamon Raisin	1	160
Golden White	1	140
Whole Wheat	1	150
Pepperidge Farm		
Cinnamon Apple	1	140
Cinnamon Chip	1	160
Cinnamon Raisin	1	150
Plain	1	140
Sourdough	1	135
Roman Meal		
English Muffin	1 (2.2 oz)	135
Tastykake		
Cinnamon Raisin	1 (64 g)	150
English Muffin	1 (57 g)	130
Sourdough	1 (57 g)	130
Thomas'		
Honey Wheat	1	128
Oat Bran	1	116
Raisin Cinnamon	1	151
Regular	1	130
Sandwich Size	1 (92 g)	210
Sour Dough	1	131
Wonder		
English Muffin	1 (2 oz)	120
Raisin Rounds	1 (2.1 oz)	150
Sourdough	1 (2 oz)	120
REFRIGERATED		
Roman Meal		
English Muffin	½ muffin (1.1 oz)	66
Honey Nut Oat Bran	½ muffin (1.1 oz)	81
TAKE-OUT		
w/ butter	1	189
w/ cheese & sausage	1	394
w/ egg cheese & bacon	1	487
w/ egg cheese & canadian bacon	1	383

EPPAW

raw	½ cup	75

FALAFEL

MIX		
Casbah		
as prep	5	130

FOOD	PORTION	CALS.
Near East		
As Prep	2½ patties	230
TAKE-OUT		
falafel	3 (1.8 oz)	170
falafel	1 (1.2 oz)	57

FAST FOODS
(*see individual names in Part II*)

FAT
(*see also* BUTTER, BUTTER BLENDS, BUTTER SUBSTITUTES, MARGARINE, OIL)

FOOD	PORTION	CALS.
beef cooked	1 oz	193
beef suet	1 oz	242
beef tallow	1 tbsp (13 g)	115
chicken	1 cup	1846
chicken	1 tbsp	115
cocoa butter	1 tbsp	120
duck	1 tbsp	115
goose	1 tbsp	115
goose	3.5 oz	900
lamb new zealand raw	1 oz	182
lard	1 tbsp (13 g)	115
lard	1 cup (205 g)	1849
nutmeg butter	1 tbsp	120
pork backfat	1 oz	230
pork cured	1 oz	164
pork cured roasted	1 oz	167
salt pork	1 oz	212
shortening	1 tbsp	113
shortening	1 cup	1812
turkey	1 tbsp	115
ucuhuba butter	1 tbsp	120
Crisco		
Butter Flavor	1 tbsp	110
Shortening	1 tbsp	110
Shortening	1 tbsp (0.4 oz)	110
Sticks	1 tbsp (0.4 oz)	110
Sticks Butter Flavor	1 tbsp (0.4 oz)	110
Empire		
Chicken Fat Rendered	1 tbsp (0.5 oz)	120
Wesson		
Shortening	1 tbsp	100

FAVA BEANS
CANNED
Progresso

FOOD	PORTION	CALS.
Fava Beans	½ cup (4.6 oz)	110

FOOD	PORTION	CALS.
FEIJOA		
fresh	1 (1.75 oz)	25
puree	1 cup	119
FENNEL		
fresh bulb	1 (8.2 oz)	72
fresh sliced	1 cup	27
leaves	3.5 oz	24
seed	1 tsp	7
FENUGREEK		
seed	1 tsp	12
FIBER		
Delta		
Natural Fiber	½ cup (1 oz)	20
FIGS		
CANNED		
in heavy syrup	3	75
in light syrup	3	58
water pack	3	42
S&W		
Kadota Figs Whole Fancy	½ cup	100
DRIED		
California	½ cup (3.5 oz)	200
cooked	½ cup	140
whole	10	477
Sonoma		
White Misson	3-4 (1.4 oz)	110
FRESH		
fig	1 med	50
FISH		
(*see also individual names,* FISH SUBSTITUTES, SUSHI)		
CANNED		
Holmes		
Finest Kippered Snacks drained	1 can (3.2 oz)	135
Port Clyde		
Fish Steaks In Louisiana Hot Sauce	1 can (3.75 oz)	150
Fish Steaks In Mustard Sauce	1 can (3.75 oz)	140
Fish Steaks In Soybean Oil With Hot Chilies drained	1 can (3.3 oz)	155
Fish Steaks In Soybean Oil drained	1 can (3.3 oz)	220
FROZEN		
breaded fillet	1 (2 oz)	155
sticks	1 stick (1 oz)	76

FOOD	PORTION	CALS.
Cajun Cookin'		
Seafood Gumbo	17 oz	330
Gorton's		
Crispy Batter Dipped Fillets	2	290
Crispy Batter Sticks	4	260
Crunch Fillets	2	230
Crunchy Sticks	4	210
Light Recipe Lightly Breaded Fish Fillets	1 fillet	180
Light Recipe Tempura Fillets	1 fillet	200
Microwave Crispy Batter Large Cut Fillets	1	320
Microwave Entree Fillets In Herb Butter	1 pkg	190
Microwave Larger Cut Fillets	1	320
Microwave Larger Cut Ranch Fillet	1	330
Microwave Sticks	6	340
Potato Crisp Fillets	2	300
Potato Crisp Sticks	4	260
Value Pack Portions	1 portion	180
Value Pack Sticks	4	190
Kineret		
Fish Sticks	5 pieces (4 oz)	280
Mrs. Paul's		
Buttered Fillet Microwave	1 fillet	80
Entree Light Seafood Dijon	8¾ oz	200
Entree Light Seafood Florentine	8 oz	220
Entree Light Seafood Mornay	9 oz	230
Fillet Sandwich Microwave	1	280
Fillets Microwave	1 fillet	280
Fish Cakes	2	190
Fish Fillets Batter Dipped	2 fillets	330
Fish Fillets Crispy Crunchy	2 fillets	220
Fish Fillets Crunchy Batter	2 fillets	280
Fish Sticks 40 Crunchy	4 (2.75 oz)	200
Fish Sticks Crispy Crunchy	4 sticks	190
Fish Sticks Microwave	5	290
In Butter Sauce Light Fillets	1 fillet	140
Portions Battered Fish	2 portions	300
Portions Crispy Crunchy Breaded Fish	2 portions	230
Seafood Platter Combination	9 oz	600
Sticks Battered Fish	4 sticks	210
Sticks Crispy Crunchy Breaded Fish	4 sticks	140
Van De Kamp's		
Battered Fish Fillets	1 (2.6 oz)	180
Battered Fish Nuggets	8 (4 oz)	280
Battered Fish Portions	2 pieces (5 oz)	350

FOOD	PORTION	CALS.
Van De Kamp's (CONT.)		
Battered Fish Sticks	6 (4 oz)	260
Breaded Fillets	2 (3.5 oz)	280
Breaded Fish Portions	3 pieces (4.5 oz)	330
Breaded Fish Sticks	6 (4 oz)	290
Breaded Mini Fish Sticks	13 (3.3 oz)	250
Crisp & Healthy Breaded Fillets	2 (3.5 oz)	150
Crisp & Healthy Fish Sticks	6 (4 oz)	180
Fish 'n Fries	1 pkg (6.6 oz)	380
MIX		
Golden Dipt		
Beer Batter Fry	1 oz	100
Cajun Style Fish Fry	⅔ oz	60
Fish & Chips Batter Mix	1¼ oz	120
Fish Fry	⅔ oz	60
Seafood Frying Mix	⅔ oz	60
Tempura Batter Mix	1 oz	100
TAKE-OUT		
fish cake	1 (4.7 oz)	166
kedgeree	5.6 oz	242
sandwich w/ tartar sauce	1	431
sandwich w/ tartar sauce & cheese	1	524
stew	1 cup (7.9 oz)	157
taramasalata	3.5 oz	446

FISH PASTE

fish paste	2 tsp	15

FISH SUBSTITUTES

FOOD	PORTION	CALS.
LaLoma		
Ocean Platter mix not prep	¼ cup (16 g)	50
Worthington		
Fillets	2 (85 g)	180
Tuno	2 oz (57 g)	100

FLAXSEED

FOOD	PORTION	CALS.
Arrowhead		
Flaxseed	3 tbsp (1 oz)	140
Stone-Buhr		
Flaxseed	1 tsp (1 oz)	150

FLOUNDER

FOOD	PORTION	CALS.
FRESH		
cooked	1 fillet (4.5 oz)	148
cooked	3 oz	99

FOOD	PORTION	CALS.
FROZEN		
Gorton's		
Fishmarket Fresh	5 oz	110
Microwave Entree Stuffed	1 pkg	350
Mrs. Paul's		
Crunchy Batter Fillets	2 fillets	220
Light Fillets	1 fillet	240
Van De Kamp's		
Lightly Breaded Fillets	1 (4 oz)	230
Natural Fillets	1 (4 oz)	110
TAKE-OUT		
battered & fried	3.2 oz	211
breaded & fried	3.2 oz	211
FLOUR		
corn masa	1 cup	416
corn whole grain	1 cup	422
cottonseed lowfat	1 oz	94
peanut defatted	1 cup	196
peanut defatted	1 oz	92
peanut lowfat	1 cup	257
potato	1 cup (6.3 oz)	628
rice brown	1 cup	574
rice white	1 cup	578
rye dark	1 cup	415
rye light	1 cup	374
rye medium	1 cup	361
sesame lowfat	1 oz	95
triticale whole grain	1 cup	440
white all-purpose	1 cup	455
white bread	1 cup	495
white cake	1 cup	395
white self-rising	1 cup	442
whole wheat	1 cup	407
Arrowhead		
Kamut	¼ cup (1.2 oz)	110
Pastry	⅓ cup (1.1 oz)	100
Rye Whole Grain	¼ cup (1.6 oz)	160
Spelt	¼ cup (1.2 oz)	100
Teff	¼ cup (1.4 oz)	140
Unbleached White	⅓ cup (1.6 oz)	160
Whole Grain Wheat	¼ cup (1.6 oz)	160
Whole Wheat	¼ cup (1.2 oz)	130
Aunt Jemima		
Self-Rising	3 tbsp	90

FOOD	PORTION	CALS.
Ballard		
All Purpose	1 cup	400
Self-Rising	1 cup	380
Ceresota		
All Purpose	1 cup	390
Whole Wheat	1 cup	400
General Mills		
Drifted Snow	1 cup	400
Softasilk	¼ cup	100
Gold Medal		
All Purpose	1 cup	400
La Pina	1 cup	390
Oat Blend	1 cup	390
Self-Rising	1 cup	380
Unbleached	1 cup	400
Whole Wheat	1 cup	350
Whole Wheat Blend	1 cup	380
Heckers		
All Purpose	1 cup	390
Whole Wheat	1 cup	400
Hodgson Mill		
50/50 Flour	¼ cup (1 oz)	100
Best For Bread	¼ cup (1 oz)	100
Buckwheat	⅓ cup (1.6 oz)	160
Oat Bran Blend	¼ cup (1 oz)	110
Oat Bran Flour	¼ cup (1 oz)	110
Rye	¼ cup (1 oz)	90
Seasoned Flour	¼ cup (1 oz)	90
White	¼ cup (1 oz)	100
Whole Wheat	¼ cup (1 oz)	100
King Arthur		
All Purpose Unbleached	¼ cup (1 oz)	100
Pillsbury		
All Purpose Best	1 cup	400
Bohemian Style Rye and Wheat Best	1 cup	400
Bread Best	1 cup	400
Rye Medium Best	1 cup	400
Self-Rising Best	1 cup	380
Shake & Blend Best	2 tbsp	50
Unbleached Best	1 cup	400
Whole Wheat Best	1 cup	400
Red Band		
All-Purpose	1 cup	390
Self-Rising	1 cup	380

FOOD	PORTION	CALS.
Robin Hood		
All Purpose	1 cup	400
Rye Stone Ground	1 cup	360
Self-Rising	1 cup	380
Unbleached	1 cup	400
Stone Ground Mills		
White Unbleached Organic	¼ cup (1.4 oz)	130
Whole Wheat 100% Stone Ground	3 tbsp (1 oz)	90
White Deer		
All-Purpose	1 cup	400
Wondra		
Flour	1 cup	400

FRANKFURTER
(*see* HOT DOG)

FRENCH BEANS
dried cooked	1 cup	228

FRENCH FRIES
(*see* POTATOES)

FRENCH TOAST

FROZEN		
french toast	1 slice (2 oz)	126
Aunt Jemima		
Cinnamon Swirl	2 pieces (4.1 oz)	240
Slices	2 pieces (4.1 oz)	240
Downyflake		
Extra Thick	1	150
French Toast	2 slices	270
Texas Style & Sausage	1 pkg (4.25 oz)	400
Great Starts		
Cinnamon Swirl With Sausage	5½ oz	390
French Toast With Sausage	5½ oz	380
Mini French Toast With Sausage	2½ oz	190
Oatmeal French Toast With Lite Links	4.65 oz	310
Healthy Starts		
French Toast With LeanLinks	6.5 oz	400
Quaker		
French Toast Sticks & Syrup	1 pkg (5.2 oz)	400
French Toast Wedges & Sausage	1 pkg (5.3 oz)	360
HOME RECIPE		
as prep w/ 2% milk	1 slice	149
as prep w/ whole milk	1 slice	151

FOOD	PORTION	CALS.
TAKE-OUT		
w/ butter	2 slices	356
FROG'S LEGS		
frog leg as prep w/ seasoned flour & fried	1 (0.8)	70
FROSTING		
(see CAKE)		
FRUCTOSE		
Estee		
Fructose	1 tsp (4 g)	15
Packet	1 pkg (3 g)	10
FRUIT DRINKS		
(see also LEMONADE)		
FROZEN		
citrus juice drink as prep	1 cup	114
citrus juice drink not prep	1 can (12 fl oz)	684
fruit punch as prep w/water	1 cup	113
fruit punch not prep	1 can (12 fl oz)	678
limeade	1 can (6 oz)	408
limeade as prep w/ water	1 cup	102
Bright & Early		
Fruit Punch	8 fl oz	130
Dole		
100% Juice Blend Country Raspberry as prep	8 fl oz	140
100% Juice Blend Orchard Peach as prep	8 fl oz	140
Mountain Cherry 100% Juice Blend as prep	8 fl oz	120
Pineapple Orange as prep	8 fl oz	120
Pineapple Orange Banana as prep	8 fl oz	130
Pineapple Orange Guava as prep	8 fl oz	120
Pineapple Passion Banana as prep	8 fl oz	120
Tropical Fruit as prep	8 fl oz	140
Five Alive		
Berry Citrus	8 fl oz	120
Citrus	8 fl oz	120
Tropical Citrus	8 fl oz	120
Minute Maid		
Berry Punch	8 fl oz	130
Citrus Punch	8 fl oz	120
Fruit Punch	8 fl oz	120
Limeade	8 fl oz	100
Pineapple Orange	8 fl oz	120

FOOD	PORTION	CALS.
Minute Maid (CONT.)		
Tropical Punch	8 fl oz	120
Seneca		
Cranberry-Apple Juice Cocktail frzn as prep	8 fl oz	140
Raspberry- Cranberry Juice Cocktail frzn as prep	8 fl oz	140
Tree Top		
Apple Citrus as prep	6 oz	90
Apple Cranberry as prep	6 oz	100
Apple Grape as prep	6 oz	100
Apple Pear as prep	6 oz	90
Apple Raspberry as prep	6 oz	80
MIX		
fruit punch as prep w/water	9 oz	97
Crystal Light		
Berry Blend Sugar Free	8 oz	3
Fruit Punch Sugar Free	8 oz	3
Lemon-Lime	8 oz	4
Tropic Quencher	8 oz	5
Kool-Aid		
Lemon-Lime	8 oz	98
Purplesaurus Rex	8 oz	98
Rainbow Punch	8 oz	98
Sharkleberry Fin	8 oz	98
Sugar Free Berry Blue	8 oz	3
Sugar Free Berry Punch	8 oz	3
Sugar Free Purplesaurus Rex	8 oz	3
Sugar Free Rainbow Punch	8 oz	4
Sugar Free Sharkleberry Fin	8 oz	3
Sugar Free Tropical Punch	8 oz	3
Sugar Sweetened Mountain Berry Punch	8 oz	98
Sugar Sweetened Purplesaurus Rex	8 oz	84
Sugar Sweetened Rainbow Punch	8 oz	84
Sugar Sweetened Sharkleberry Fin	8 oz	84
Sugar Sweetened Sunshine Punch	8 oz	83
Sugar Sweetened Surfin' Berry Punch	8 oz	79
Sugar Sweetened Tropical Punch	8 oz	84
Tropical Punch	8 oz	98
Unsweetened Berry Blue	8 oz	98
READY-TO-DRINK		
cranberry apple drink	6 fl oz	123
cranberry apricot drink	6 fl oz	118
fruit punch	6 fl oz	87

FOOD	PORTION	CALS.
orange grapefruit juice	8 fl oz	107
orange & apricot	8 fl oz	128
pineapple & grapefruit	8 fl oz	117
pineapple & orange drink	8 fl oz	125
After The Fall		
Amaretto Almond	1 can (12 oz)	170
American Pie Cherry	1 can (12 oz)	190
Apple Apricot	1 cup (8 oz)	100
Apple Raspberry	1 bottle (10 oz)	110
Apple Strawberry	1 bottle (10 oz)	120
Banana Casablanca	1 bottle (10 oz)	120
Berrymeister	1 can (12 oz)	160
Cranberry Meets Raspberry	1 bottle (10 oz)	120
Georgia Peach Blend	1 bottle (10 oz)	130
Mango Montage	1 bottle (10 oz)	140
Maui Grove	1 bottle (10 oz)	120
Nantucket Ginger Ale	1 can (12 oz)	140
Orange Icicle Cream	1 can (12 oz)	170
Oregon Berry	1 bottle (10 oz)	130
Passion Of The Islands	1 bottle (10 oz)	125
Peach Vanilla	1 can (12 oz)	170
Strawberry Vanilla	1 can (12 oz)	160
Twist O' Strawberry	1 can (12 oz)	190
Vanilla Bean Cream	1 can (12 oz)	170
Apple & Eve		
Apple Cranberry	6 fl oz	80
Apple Grape	6 fl oz	120
Cranberry Grape	6 fl oz	100
Fruit Punch	6 fl oz	78
Raspberry Cranberry	6 fl oz	90
BAMA		
Fruit Punch	8.45 fl oz	130
Boku		
White Grape Raspberry	16 fl oz	120
Chiquita		
Orange Banana	6 fl oz	90
Crystal Geyser		
Juice Squeeze Citrus Grape	1 bottle (12 fl oz)	145
Juice Squeeze Orange & Passion Fruit	1 bottle (12 fl oz)	130
Juice Squeeze Passion Fruit & Mango	1 bottle (12 fl oz)	125
Juice Squeeze Wild Berry	1 bottle (12 fl oz)	130
Dole		
Pineapple Orange	6 fl oz	90
Pineapple Orange Banana	6 fl oz	100

FOOD	PORTION	CALS.
Dole (CONT.)		
Pineapple Orange Guava	6 fl oz	100
Five Alive		
Citrus	1 bottle (16 fl oz)	120
Citrus	6 fl oz	90
Citrus	1 can (11.5 fl oz)	170
Citrus Chilled	8 fl oz	120
Hawaiian Punch		
Fruit Juicy Red	6 fl oz	90
Island Fruit Cocktail	6 fl oz	90
Lite Fruit Juicy Red	6 fl oz	60
Tropical Fruits	6 fl oz	90
Very Berry	6 fl oz	90
Wild Fruit	6 fl oz	90
Hi-C		
Boppin Berry Box	8.45 fl oz	140
Boppin' Berry	8 fl oz	130
Double Fruit Box	8.45 fl oz	130
Double Fruit Cooler	8 fl oz	130
Ecto Cooler	8 fl oz	130
Ecto Cooler	1 can (11.5 fl oz)	180
Ecto Cooler Box	8.45 fl oz	130
Fruit Punch	8 fl oz	130
Fruit Punch	1 can (11.5 fl oz)	190
Fruit Punch Box	8.45 fl oz	140
Fruity Bubble Gum	8 fl oz	120
Fruity Bubble Gum Box	8.45 fl oz	130
Hula Punch	8 fl oz	120
Hula Punch	1 can (11.5 fl oz)	170
Hula Punch Box	8.45 fl oz	120
Jammin' Apple Box	8.45 fl oz	130
Stompin' Banana Berry	8 fl oz	130
Stompin' Banana Berry Box	8.45 fl oz	130
Wild Berry	8 fl oz	120
Wild Berry Box	8.45 fl oz	130
Hood		
Natural Blenders Apple Cranberry Raspberry	1 cup (8 oz)	130
Natural Blenders Apple Grape Cherry	1 cup (8 oz)	130
Natural Blenders Apple Peach Pear	1 cup (8 oz)	120
Natural Blenders Pineapple Orange Kiwi	1 cup (8 oz)	120
Juice Works		
Appleberry	6 fl oz	100

FOOD	PORTION	CALS.
Juicy Juice		
Apple Grape	1 box (8.45 fl oz)	120
Berry	1 box (8.45 fl oz)	130
Berry	1 bottle (6 fl oz)	90
Punch	1 box (8.45 fl oz)	140
Punch	1 bottle (6 fl oz)	100
Tropical	1 bottle (6 fl oz)	110
Tropical	1 box (8.45 fl oz)	150
Kern's		
Apple Strawberry Nectar	6 fl oz	110
Apricot Pineapple Nectar	6 fl oz	110
Banana Pineapple Nectar	6 fl oz	110
Coconut Pineapple Nectar	6 fl oz	140
Orange Banana Nectar	6 fl oz	110
Strawberry Banana Nectar	6 fl oz	110
Tropical Nectar	6 fl oz	110
Kool-Aid		
Koolers Mountainberry Punch	1 pkg (8.45 fl oz)	142
Koolers Rainbow Punch	1 pkg (8.45 fl oz)	135
Koolers Sharkleberry Fin	1 pkg (8.45 fl oz)	140
Koolers Tropical Punch	1 pkg (8.45 fl oz)	132
Libby		
Strawberry Banana Nectar	1 can (11.5 fl oz)	220
Lifesavers		
Fruit Punch	8 fl oz	140
Lime Punch	8 fl oz	140
Mauna La'i		
Island Guava Hawaiian Guava Fruit Juice Drink	8 fl oz	130
Mango & Hawaiian Guava Fruit Juice Drink	8 fl oz	130
Paradise Guava Hawaiian Guava & Passion Fruit Juice Drink	8 fl oz	130
Minute Maid		
Berry Punch Box	8.45 fl oz	130
Berry Punch Chilled	8 fl oz	130
Citrus Punch Chilled	8 fl oz	130
Fruit Punch Box	8.45 fl oz	120
Fruit Punch Chilled	8 fl oz	120
Juices To Go Citrus Punch	1 can (11.5 fl oz)	180
Juices To Go Citrus Punch	1 bottle (10 fl oz)	160
Juices To Go Concord Punch	1 can (11.5 fl oz)	180
Juices To Go Concord Punch	1 bottle (10 fl oz)	160
Juices To Go Concord Punch	1 bottle (16 fl oz)	130
Juices To Go Fruit Punch	1 bottle (10 fl oz)	160

FOOD	PORTION	CALS.
Minute Maid (CONT.)		
Juices To Go Fruit Punch	1 can (11.5 fl oz)	180
Juices To Go Fruit Punch	1 bottle (16 fl oz)	120
Juices To Go Orange Blend	1 can (11.5 fl oz)	170
Juices To Go Orange Blend	1 bottle (10 fl oz)	150
Naturals Apple Cranberry	8 fl oz	170
Naturals Concord Medley	8 fl oz	130
Naturals Fruit Medley	8 fl oz	120
Naturals Orange Grape Medley	8 fl oz	120
Naturals Tropical Medley	8 fl oz	120
Tropical Punch Box	8.45 fl oz	130
Tropical Punch Chilled	8 fl oz	120
Mott's		
Apple Cranberry Blend	10 fl oz	180
Apple Cranberry From Concentrate as prep	8 fl oz	120
Apple Grape From Concentrate as prep	8 fl oz	120
Apple Raspberry Blend	10 fl oz	140
Apple Raspberry From Concentrate	8.45 fl oz	120
Fruit Basket Apple Raspberry Juice Cocktail as prep	8 fl oz	130
Fruit Basket Tropical Blend Juice Cocktail as prep	8 fl oz	120
Fruit Punch From Concentrate	8.45 fl oz	120
Fruit Punch From Concentrate	10 fl oz	170
Grape Apple	10 fl oz	170
Pineapple Orange	10 fl oz	170
Ocean Spray		
Cran.Blueberry	8 fl oz	160
Cran.Cherry	6 fl oz	160
Cran.Grape	8 fl oz	170
Cran.Raspberry	8 fl oz	140
Cran.Raspberry Reduced Calorie	8 fl oz	50
Cran.Strawberry	8 fl oz	140
Cranapple	8 fl oz	160
Cranapple Reduced Calorie	8 fl oz	50
Cranicot	8 fl oz	160
Crantastic	8 fl oz	150
Fruit Punch	8 fl oz	130
Lightstyle Low Calorie Cran.Grape	8 fl oz	40
Lightstyle Low Calorie Cran.Raspberry	8 fl oz	40
Refreshers Juice Drink Citrus Cranberry	8 fl oz	140
Refreshers Juice Drink Citrus Peach	8 fl oz	120
Refreshers Juice Drink Orange Cranberry	8 fl oz	130
Ruby Red & Tangerine Grapefruit Juice Cocktail	8 fl oz	130

FOOD	PORTION	CALS.
Odwalla		
Boyzenberry Mango	8 fl oz	140
C Monster	16 fl oz	300
Fruitshake Blackberry	8 fl oz	160
Guanaba Dabba Doo!	8 fl oz	130
Lotta Colada	8 fl oz	160
Mango Tango	8 fl oz	150
Mo Beta	16 fl oz	280
Raspberry Smoothie	8 fl oz	140
Strawberry Banana Smoothie	8 fl oz	100
Strawberry Go Man Go	8 fl oz	100
Super Protein	16 fl oz	400
Pek		
Mango Guava Ecstasy	1 bottle (20 fl oz)	110
Passionate Peach Grapefruit	8 fl oz	110
S&W		
Apricot Pineapple Nectar	6 fl oz	120
Apricot Pineapple Nectar Diet	6 fl oz	80
Sipps		
Fruit Punch	8.45 oz	130
Lemon Lime Cooler	8.45 oz	130
Mixed Berry	8.45 oz	130
Sunshine Punch	8.45 oz	130
Smucker's		
Apple Cranberry	8 oz	120
Orange Banana	8 oz	120
Snapple		
Diet Kiwi Strawberry	8 fl oz	13
Fruit Punch	8 fl oz	120
Kiwi Strawberry Cocktail	8 fl oz	130
Melonberry Cocktail	8 fl oz	120
Vitamin Supreme	10 fl oz	150
Squeezit		
Berry B. Wild	1 (6.75 fl oz)	90
Chucklin' Cherry	1 (6.75 fl oz)	90
Grumpy Grape	1 (6.75 fl oz)	90
Mean Green Puncher	1 (6.75 fl oz)	90
Silly Billy Strawberry	1 (6.75 fl oz)	90
Smarty Arty Orange	1 (6.75 fl oz)	90
Sunny Delight		
Drink	6 fl oz	90
Tang		
Mixed Fruit	8.45 fl oz	137

FOOD	PORTION	CALS.
Tree Top		
Apple Citrus	6 fl oz	90
Apple Cranberry	6 fl oz	100
Apple Grape	6 fl oz	100
Apple Pear	6 fl oz	90
Apple Raspberry	6 fl oz	80
Tropicana		
Berry Punch	8 fl oz	120
Citrus Punch	1 bottle (10 fl oz)	180
Citrus Punch	8 fl oz	140
Cranberry Punch	1 can (11.5 fl oz)	200
Cranberry Punch	1 bottle (10 fl oz)	170
Cranberry Punch	8 fl oz	140
Fruit Punch	1 bottle (10 fl oz)	150
Fruit Punch	1 can (11.5 fl oz)	170
Fruit Punch	8 fl oz	130
Fruit Punch	1 container (10 fl oz)	160
Orange Pineapple	8 fl oz	110
Orange Pineapple	1 bottle (10 fl oz)	130
Pineapple Punch	8 fl oz	120
Pineapple Punch	1 bottle (10 fl oz)	160
Season's Best Cranberry Medley	8 fl oz	120
Tropics Apple Cranberry Kiwi	8 fl oz	120
Tropics Orange Strawberry Banana	8 fl oz	110
Tropics Orange Kiwi Passion	8 fl oz	100
Tropics Orange Peach Mango	8 fl oz	110
Tropics Orange Pineapple	8 fl oz	110
Tropics Pineapple Passion	8 fl oz	120
Twister Apple Raspberry Blackberry	8 fl oz	120
Twister Apple Raspberry Blackberry	1 bottle (10 fl oz)	150
Twister Apple Raspberry Blackberry	1 can (11.5 fl oz)	180
Twister Cranberry Raspberry Strawberry	8 fl oz	120
Twister Cranberry Raspberry Strawberry	1 bottle (10 fl oz)	160
Twister Light Cranberry Raspberry Strawberry	8 fl oz	45
Twister Light Cranberry Raspberry Strawberry	1 container (10 fl oz)	50
Twister Light Orange Strawberry Banana	8 fl oz	35
Twister Light Orange Strawberry Banana	1 container (10 fl oz)	45
Twister Orange Strawberry Banana	1 container (10 fl oz)	140
Twister Strawberry Banana	1 bottle (10 fl oz)	140
Twister Strawberry Banana	8 fl oz	120

FOOD	PORTION	CALS.
Tropicana (CONT.)		
Twister Strawberry Banana	1 can (11.5 fl oz)	160
Twister Strawberry Guava	1 bottle (10 fl oz)	140
Twister Strawberry Guava	8 fl oz	110
Veryfine		
Apple Cherryberry	8 fl oz	130
Apple Cranberry	8 fl oz	130
Apple Raspberry	8 fl oz	110
Fruit Punch	8 fl oz	130
Guava Strawberry	8 fl oz	120
Lemon & Lime	8 fl oz	120
Papaya Punch	8 fl oz	120
Passionfruit Orange	8 fl oz	110
Pineapple Orange	8 fl oz	130
White House		
Apple Cherry	6 fl oz	90

FRUIT MIXED

(*see also individual names*)

CANNED

fruit cocktail in heavy syrup	½ cup	93
fruit cocktail juice pack	½ cup	56
fruit cocktail water pack	½ cup	40
fruit salad in heavy sirup	½ cup	94
fruit salad in light syrup	½ cup	73
fruit salad juice pack	½ cup	62
fruit salad water pack	½ cup	37
mixed fruit in heavy syrup	½ cup	92
tropical fruit salad in heavy sirup	½ cup	110
Del Monte		
Fruit Cocktail Fruit Naturals	½ cup (4.4 oz)	60
Fruit Cocktail In Heavy Syrup	½ cup (4.5 oz)	100
Fruit Cocktail Lite	½ cup (4.4 oz)	60
Lite Mixed Fruits Chunky	½ cup (4.4 oz)	60
Mixed Fruits Chunky Fruit Naturals	½ cup (4.4 oz)	60
Mixed Fruits Chunky In Heavy Syrup	½ cup (4.5 oz)	100
Snack Cups Mixed Fruit Fruit Naturals	1 serv (4.5 oz)	60
Snack Cups Mixed Fruit Fruit Naturals EZ-Open Lid	1 serv (4.5 oz)	60
Snack Cups Mixed Fruit In Heavy Syrup	1 serv (4.5 oz)	100
Snack Cups Mixed Fruit In Heavy Syrup EZ-Open Lid	1 serv (4.2 oz)	90
Snack Cups Mixed Fruit Lite	1 serv (4.5 oz)	60
Snack Cups Mixed Fruit Lite EZ-Open Lid	1 serv (4.5 oz)	60

FOOD	PORTION	CALS.
Dole		
Tropical Fruit Salad	½ cup	70
Hunt's		
Fruit Cocktail	4 oz	90
Libby		
Chunky Mixed Lite	½ cup (4.3 oz)	60
Fruit Cocktail Lite	½ cup (4.3 oz)	60
S&W		
Chunky Mixed Diet	½ cup	40
Chunky Mixed Natural Style	½ cup	90
Chunky Mixed Unsweetened	½ cup	40
Fruit Cocktail Diet	½ cup	40
Fruit Cocktail Heavy Syrup	½ cup	90
Fruit Cocktail Natural Lite	½ cup	60
Fruit Cocktail Natural Style	½ cup	90
Fruit Cocktail Unsweetened	½ cup	40
DRIED		
mixed	11 oz pkg	712
Del Monte		
Mixed	⅓ cup (1.4 oz)	110
Planters		
Fruit'n Nut Mix	1 oz	140
Sonoma		
Diced	⅓ cup (1.4 oz)	120
Mixed Fruit	5-8 pieces (1.4 oz)	120
FROZEN		
mixed fruit sweetened	1 cup	245
Big Valley		
Burst O' Berries	⅔ cup (4.9 oz)	70
California Tropics	⅔ cup (4.9 oz)	60
Cup A Fruit	1 pkg (4 oz)	50
Mixed	4.9 oz	60
Birds Eye		
Mixed Fruit	½ cup	120
Dole		
Applesauce Strawberry	1 pkg (4 oz)	60

FRUIT SNACKS

fruit leather	1 bar (0.8 oz)	81
fruit leather pieces	1 pkg (0.9 oz)	92
fruit leather pieces	1 oz	97
fruit leather rolls	1 lg (0.7 oz)	73
fruit leather rolls	1 sm (0.5 oz)	49
Crocker		
Berry 'N Blue	1 pkg (0.7 oz)	80

FOOD	PORTION	CALS.
Betty Crocker (CONT.)		
String Thing Cherry	1 pkg (0.7 oz)	80
String Thing Strawberry	1 pkg (0.7 oz)	80
Brock		
Beauty & The Beast	1 pkg (0.9 oz)	90
Cinderella	1 pkg (0.9 oz)	90
Dinosaurs	1 pkg (0.9 oz)	90
Ninja Trolls	1 pkg (0.9 oz)	90
Sharks	1 pkg (0.9 oz)	90
Del Monte		
Sierra Trail Mix	¼ cup (1.2 oz)	150
Sierra Trail Mix	1 pkg (1 oz)	120
Sierra Trail Mix	1 pkg (0.9 oz)	110
Fruit By The Foot		
Cherry	1	80
Grape	1	80
Strawberry	1	80
Fruit Roll-Ups		
Cherry	1 (½ oz)	50
Crazy Colors	1 (½ oz)	50
Fruit Punch	1 (½ oz)	50
Grape	1 (½ oz)	50
Raspberry	1 (½ oz)	50
Strawberry	1 (½ oz)	50
General Mills		
Garfield And Friends 1-2 Punch	1 pkg	100
Garfield And Friends Cat Cooler	1 pkg	100
Garfield And Friends Fat Cat Funnies	1 (½ oz)	50
Garfield And Friends Fruit Party	1 (½ oz)	50
Garfield And Friends Very Strawberry	1 pkg	100
Shark Bites & Berry Bears Assorted Fruit	1 pkg	100
Shark Bites & Berry Bears Fruit Punch	1 pkg	100
Surf's Up! Sun Splash	1 pkg	100
Surf's Up! Tutti Frutti	1 pkg	100
Thunder Jets Assorted Fruit Squadron	1 pkg	100
Thunder Jets Mach 1 Fruit Mix	1 pkg	100
Health Valley		
Bakes Apple	1 bar	100
Bakes Date	1 bar	100
Bakes Raisin	1 bar	100
Fat Free Fruit Bars 100% Organic Apple	1 bar	140
Fat Free Fruit Bars 100% Organic Date	1 bar	140
Fat Free Fruit Bars 100% Organic Raisin	1 bar	
Fruit & Fitness Bars	2 bars	

FOOD	PORTION	CALS.
Health Valley (CONT.)		
Oat Bran Bakes Apricot	1 bar	100
Oat Bran Bakes Fig & Nut	1 bar	110
Oat Bran Jumbo Fruit Bar Almond & Date	1 bar	170
Oat Bran Jumbo Fruit Bars Raisin & Cinnamon	1 bar	160
Rice Bran Jumbo Fruit Bars Almond & Date	1 bar	160
Sovex		
Fruit Bites Jungle Pals	1 pkg (0.9 oz)	90
Stretch Island		
Fruit Leather Berry Blackberry	2 pieces (1 oz)	90
Fruit Leather Chunky Cherry	2 pieces (1 oz)	90
Fruit Leather Great Grape	2 pieces (1 oz)	90
Fruit Leather Organic Apple	2 pieces (1 oz)	90
Fruit Leather Organic Grape	2 pieces (1 oz)	90
Fruit Leather Organic Raspberry	2 pieces (1 oz)	90
Fruit Leather Rare Raspberry	2 pieces (1 oz)	90
Fruit Leather Snappy Apple	2 pieces (1 oz)	90
Fruit Leather Tangy Apricot	2 pieces (1 oz)	90
Fruit Leather Truly Tropical	2 pieces (1 oz)	90
Sunbelt		
Fruit Boosters Apple	1 (1.3 oz)	130
Fruit Boosters Blueberry	1 (1.3 oz)	130
Fruit Jammers	1 (1 oz)	100
Sunkist		
Fruit Roll Apple	1 (0.7 oz)	70
Fruit Roll Apricot	1	76
Fruit Roll Apricot	1 (0.5 oz)	70
Fruit Roll Cherry	1 (0.7 oz)	70
Fruit Roll Cherry	1 (0.5 oz)	50
Fruit Roll Fruit Punch	1 (0.7 oz)	70
Fruit Roll Grape	1 (0.5 oz)	50
Fruit Roll Grape	1	76
Fruit Roll Grape	1 (0.7 oz)	80
Fruit Roll Raspberry	1 (0.7 oz)	70
Fruit Roll Raspberry	1 (0.5 oz)	45
Fruit Roll Strawberry	1 (0.5 oz)	45
Fruit Roll Strawberry	1	74
Fruit Roll Strawberry	1 (0.7 oz)	70
Weight Watchers		
Apple	1 pkg (0.5 oz)	50
Apple Chips	1 pkg (0.75 oz)	70
Cinnamon	1 pkg (0.5 oz)	50

FOOD	PORTION	CALS.
Weight Watchers (CONT.)		
Peach	1 pkg (0.5 oz)	50
Strawberry	1 pkg (0.5 oz)	50

GARBANZO
(*see* CHICKPEAS)

GARLIC

clove	1	4
powder	1 tsp	9
Watkins		
Garlic & Chive Seasoning	1 tbsp (7 g)	25
Garlic Lover's Herb Blend	¼ tsp (0.5 oz)	0
Liquid Spice	1 tbsp (0.5 oz)	120

GEFILTE FISH
READY-TO-USE

sweet	1 piece (1.5 oz)	35
Manischewitz		
Gefilte Fish	1 piece	107
Gefiltefish & Pike	1 piece	99
Gefiltefish & Pike Sweet	1 piece	129
Homestyle	1 piece	111
Sweet	1 piece	132

GELATIN
MIX

low calorie	½ cup	8
mix artificially sweetened as prep	½ cup (4.1 oz)	8
mix artificially sweetened as prep	1 pkg 4 serv (16.5 oz)	33
mix as prep	1 pkg 4 serv (19 oz)	319
mix as prep	½ cup (4.7 oz)	80
mix not prep	1 pkg (3 oz)	324
mix ▮▮fruit as prep	½ cup (3.7 oz)	73
mix ▮▮fruit as prep	1 pkg 8 serv (19 oz)	588
powder unsweetened	1 oz	94
powder unsweetened	1 pkg (7 g)	23
D-Zerta		
Cherry	½ cup	8
Lemon	½ cup	8
Lime	½ cup	9
Orange	½ cup	8
Raspberry	½ cup	8
Strawberry	½ cup	8
Emes		
Kosher-Jel	½ cup (4 fl oz)	60

FOOD	PORTION	CALS.
Emes (CONT.)		
Kosher-Jel Plain	1 tbsp (7 g)	21
Jell-O		
Apricot	½ cup	82
Black Cherry	½ cup	82
Black Raspberry	½ cup	82
Blackberry	½ cup	82
Cherry Sugar Free	½ cup	9
Concord Grape	½ cup	82
Hawaiian Pineapple Sugar Free	½ cup	8
Lemon	½ cup	82
Lemon Sugar Free	½ cup	8
Lime	½ cup	82
Lime Sugar Free	½ cup	9
Mixed Fruit	½ cup	82
Mixed Fruit Sugar Free	½ cup	8
Orange	½ cup	82
Orange Sugar Free	½ cup	8
Peach Sugar Free	½ cup	8
Raspberry Sugar Free	½ cup	8
Strawberry Banana Sugar Free	½ cup	9
Strawberry Sugar Free	½ cup	9
Triple Berry Sugar Free	½ cup	8
Wild Strawberry	½ cup	81
Kojel		
Diet	1 serv	10
Royal		
Apple	½ cup	80
Blackberry	½ cup	80
Cherry	½ cup	80
Cherry Sugar Free	½ cup	8
Concord Grape	½ cup	80
Fruit Punch	½ cup	80
Lemon	½ cup	80
Lemon-Lime	½ cup	80
Lime	½ cup	80
Lime Sugar Free	½ cup	8
Mixed Berry	½ cup	80
Orange	½ cup	80
Orange Sugar Free	½ cup	10
Peach	½ cup	80
Pineapple	½ cup	80
Raspberry	½ cup	80
Raspberry Sugar Free	½ cup	8

FOOD	PORTION	CALS.
Royal (cont.)		
Strawberry	½ cup	80
Strawberry Banana Sugar Free	½ cup	8
Strawberry Orange	½ cup	80
Strawberry Sugar Free	½ cup	8
Tropical Fruit	½ cup	80
READY-TO-USE		
Del Monte		
Gel Snack Cups Blue Berry	1 serv (3.5 oz)	70
Gel Snack Cups Cherry	1 serv (3.5 oz)	70
Gel Snack Cups Orange	1 serv (3.5 oz)	70
Gel Snack Cups Strawberry	1 serv (3.5 oz)	70

GIBLETS

capon simmered	1 cup (5 oz)	238
chicken floured & fried	1 cup (5 oz)	402
chicken simmered	1 cup (5 oz)	228
turkey simmered	1 cup (5 oz)	243

GINGER

ground	1 tsp (1.8 g)	6
root fresh	¼ cup	17
root fresh	5 slices	8
root fresh sliced	¼ cup	17
Ka-Me		
Crystallized Slices	5 pieces (1 oz)	100
Sliced	20 pieces (0.5 oz)	0

GINKGO NUTS

canned	1 oz	32
dried	1 oz	99
raw	1 oz	52

GIZZARDS

chicken simmered	1 cup (5 oz)	222
turkey simmered	1 cup (5 oz)	236

GOAT

roasted	3 oz	122

GOOSE

w/ skin roasted	6.6 oz	574
w/ skin roasted	½ goose (1.7 lbs)	2362
w/o skin roasted	5 oz	340
w/o skin roasted	½ goose (1.3 lbs)	1406

GOOSEBERRIES

fresh	1 cup	67

FOOD	PORTION	CALS.
CANNED		
in light sirup	½ cup	93

GRANOLA
BARS

almond	1 (0.8 oz)	117
almond	1 (1 oz)	140
chewy chocolate coated chocoate chip	1 (1 oz)	132
chewy chocolate coated chocolate chip	1 (1.25 oz)	165
chewy chocolate coated peanut butter	1 (1 oz)	144
chewy chocolate coated peanut butter	1 (1.3 oz)	187
chewy raisin	1 (1 oz)	127
chewy raisin	1 (1.5 oz)	191
chocolate chip	1 (1 oz)	124
chocolate chip	1 (0.8 oz)	103
chocolate chip chewy	1 (1.5 oz)	178
chocolate chip chewy	1 (1 oz)	119
chocolate chip, graham & marshmallow chewy	1 (1 oz)	121
nut & raisin chewy	1 (1 oz)	129
peanut	1 (1 oz)	136
peanut	1 (0.8 oz)	113
peanut butter	1 (0.8 oz)	114
peanut butter	1 (1 oz)	137
peanut butter chewy	1 (1 oz)	121
peanut butter & chocolate chip chewy	1 (1 oz)	122
plain	1 (1 oz)	134
plain	1 (0.9 oz)	115
plain chewy	1 (1 oz)	126
Carnation		
Chocolate Chunk	1 (1.26 oz)	140
Honey & Oats	1 (1.26 oz)	130
Fi-Bar		
Coconut	1	120
Peanut Butter	1	130
General Mills		
Nature Valley Cinnamon	1	120
Nature Valley Oat Bran Honey Graham	1	110
Nature Valley Oats N'Honey	1	120
Nature Valley Peanut Butter	1	120
Nature Valley Rice Bran Cinnamon Graham	1	90
Grist Mill		
Chewy Apple Cinnamon	1 (1 oz)	120
Chewy Chunky Nut & Raisin	1 (1 oz)	130

FOOD	PORTION	CALS.
Grist Mill (CONT.)		
Chewy Peanut Butter	1 (1 oz)	130
Chewy Peanut Butter Chocolate	1 (1 oz)	130
Chocolate Snack Chocolate Chip	1 (1.2 oz)	180
Chocolate Snack Nutty Fudge	1 (1.3 oz)	190
Crunchy Cinnamon	1 (0.8 oz)	110
Crunchy Oasts 'N Honey	1 (0.8 oz)	110
Hershey		
Chocolate Covered Chocolate Chip	1 (1.2 oz)	170
Chocolate Covered Cookies & Creme	1 (1.2 oz)	170
Kellogg's		
Low Fat Crunchy Almond & Brown Sugar	1 (0.7 oz)	80
Low Fat Crunchy Apple Spice	1 (0.7 oz)	80
Low Fat Crunchy Cinnamon Raisin	1 (0.7 oz)	80
Kudos		
Chocolate Chunk	1 (0.7 oz)	90
Chocolate Coated Chocolate Chip	1 (1 oz)	120
Chocolate Coated Milk & Cookies	1 (1 oz)	130
Chocolate Coated Nutty Fudge	1 (1 oz)	130
Chocolate Coated Peanut Butter	1 (1 oz)	130
Low Fat Blueberry	1 (0.7 oz)	90
Low Fat Strawberry	1 (0.7 oz)	80
New Country		
Chocolate Covered Cookies & Creme	1	200
Quaker		
Chewy Chocolate Chip	1	128
Chewy Chunky Nut & Raisin	1	131
Chewy Cinnamon Raisin	1	128
Chewy Honey & Oats	1	125
Chewy Peanut Butter	1	128
Chewy Peanut Butter Chocolate Chip	1	131
Dipps Caramel Nut	1	148
Dipps Chocolate Chip	1	139
Dipps Chocolate Fudge	1	160
Dipps Peanut Butter	1	170
Dipps Peanut Butter Chocolate Chip	1	174
Dipps Rocky Road	1	140
Sunbelt		
Chewy Chocolate Chip	1 (1.8 oz)	220
Chewy Oats & Honey	1 (1.7 oz)	210
Chewy With Almonds	1 (1.5 oz)	190
Chewy With Raisins	1 (1.2 oz)	150
Fudge Dipped Chewy Chocolate Chip	1 (1.5 oz)	190
Fudge Dipped Chewy Macaroo	1 bar (2 oz)	280

FOOD	PORTION	CALS.
Sunbelt (CONT.)		
Fudge Dipped Chewy Macaroo	1 (1.4 oz)	200
Fudge Dipped Chewy With Peanuts	1 bar (1.5 oz)	210
CEREAL		
granola	¼ cup	138
Erewhon		
Date Nut	1 oz	130
Honey Almond	1 oz	130
Maple	1 oz	130
Spiced Apple	1 oz	130
Sunflower Crunch	1 oz	130
With Bran	1 oz	130
General Mills		
Nature Valley Cinnamon & Raisin	⅓ cup (1 oz)	120
Nature Valley Fruit & Nut	⅓ cup (1 oz)	130
Nature Valley Toasted Oat	⅓ cup (1 oz)	130
Good Shepherd		
Crunchy	1 oz	130
Honey Almond	1 oz	120
Organic 5 Grain Muesli	1 oz	160
Organic Brown Rice	1 oz	130
Organic Wheat Free	1 oz	90
Organic Wheat Free Apple Cinnamon	1 oz	125
Organic Wheat Free Blueberry Amaranth	1 oz	110
Organic Wheat Free Strawberry Amaranth	1 oz	110
Grist Mill		
Low-Fat With Raisins	⅔ cup (1.9 oz)	220
Kellogg's		
Low Fat	½ cup (1.9 oz)	210
Low Fat With Raisins	⅔ cup (1.9 oz)	210
Post		
Post Hearty	¼ cup (1 oz)	128
Stone-Buhr		
Hot Apple	⅓ cup (1.6 oz)	153
Sun Country		
100% Natural With Almonds	¼ cup	130
100% Natural With Raisins & Dates	¼ cup	123
With Raisins	¼ cup	125
Sunbelt		
Banana Nut	1.9 oz	250
Fruit & Nut	1.9 oz	230
Low Fat	1.9 oz	200
Uncle Roy's		
Cashew Raisin	½ cup (1.6 oz)	180

FOOD	PORTION	CALS.
Uncle Roy's (CONT.)		
Fat Free Apple Cinnamon	½ cup (1.6 oz)	175
Fat Free Wild Cherry	½ cup (1.6 oz)	175
Fruit & Nut	½ cup (1.6 oz)	175
Low Fat Berries Jubilee	½ cup (1.6 oz)	175
Low Fat Crispy	½ cup (1.4 oz)	160
Low Fat Luscious Raspberry	½ cup (1.6 oz)	175
Low Fat True Blueberry	½ cup (1.6 oz)	175
Maple Date Nut	½ cup (1.6 oz)	180
Nut Butter & Almonds	½ cup (1.6 oz)	195
Organic Golden Honey	½ cup (1.6 oz)	190
Organic Maple Nut'N Rice	½ cup (1.4 oz)	170
Organic Maple Raisin	½ cup (1.6 oz)	190
GRAPE JUICE		
bottled	1 cup	155
frzn sweetened as prep	1 cup	128
frzn sweetened not prep	6 oz	386
grape drink	6 oz	84
BAMA		
Juice	8.45 fl oz	120
Bright & Early		
Frozen	8 fl oz	140
Hawaiian Punch		
Drink	6 oz	90
Hi-C		
Box	8.45 fl oz	130
Drink	1 can (11.5 fl oz)	180
Drink	8 fl oz	130
Juice Works		
Drink	6 oz	100
Juicy Juice		
Drink	1 bottle (6 fl oz)	90
Drink	1 box	130
Kool-Aid		
Drink	8 oz	98
Sugar Free	8 oz	3
Sugar Sweetened	8 oz	80
Lifesavers		
Grape Punch	8 fl oz	150
Minute Maid		
Chilled	8 fl oz	130
Grape Punch frzn	8 fl oz	130
Punch Chilled	8 fl oz	130

FOOD	PORTION	CALS.
Mott's		
Drink	10 fl oz	170
Fruit Basket Cocktail as prep	8 fl oz	130
S&W		
Concord Unsweetened	6 oz	100
Seneca		
Blush Grape Juice frzn as prep	8 fl oz	170
Fortified With Vitamin C frzn as prep	8 fl oz	170
Sweetened frzn as prep	8 fl oz	140
White Grape Juice frzn as prep	8 fl oz	140
Sippin' Pak		
100% Pure	8.45 fl	130
Sipps		
Juice	8.45 oz	130
Snapple		
Grapeade	8 fl oz	120
Tang		
Fruit Box	8.45 oz	131
Tree Top		
Juice	6 oz	120
Sparkling Juice	6 oz	120
Tropicana		
Season's Best	8 fl oz	160
Veryfine		
100%	8 oz	153
Grape Drink	8 oz	130

GRAPE LEAVES
Cedar's		
Grape Leaves Stuffed With Rice	6 pieces (4.9 oz)	180

GRAPEFRUIT
CANNED		
juice pack	½ cup	46
unsweetened	1 cup	93
water pack	½ cup	44
S&W		
Sections In Light Syrup	½ cup	80
Sections Natural Style	½ cup	40
FRESH		
pink	½	37
pink sections	1 cup	69
red	½	37
red sections	1 cup	69
white	½	39
white sections	1 cup	76

FOOD	PORTION	CALS.
Chiquita		
Ruby Red	½ fruit	40
Dole		
Grapefruit	½	50
Ocean Spray		
Pink	½ med	50
White	½ med	45
GRAPEFRUIT JUICE		
fresh	1 cup	96
frzn as prep	1 cup	102
frzn not prep	6 oz	302
sweetened	1 cup	116
After The Fall		
Pink	1 bottle (10 oz)	100
Crystal Geyser		
Juice Squeeze	1 bottle (12 fl oz)	150
Del Monte		
Juice	8 fl oz	100
Hood		
Select	1 cup (8 oz)	100
Minute Maid		
Frozen	8 fl oz	100
Juices To Go	1 can (11.5 fl oz)	140
Juices To Go	1 bottle (16 fl oz)	100
Juices To Go	1 bottle (10 fl oz)	120
Juices To Go Pink Cocktail	1 bottle (16 fl oz)	110
Juices To Go Pink Cocktail	1 bottle (10 fl oz)	140
Juices to Go Pink Cocktail	8 fl oz	160
Mott's		
From Concentrate as prep	8 fl oz	120
Ocean Spray		
100% Juice	8 oz	100
Lightstyle Low Calorie Pink Cocktail	8 fl oz	40
Pink Juice Cocktail	8 oz	110
Ruby Red Drink	8 oz	130
Odwalla		
Juice	8 fl oz	90
S&W		
Unsweetened	6 oz	80
Snapple		
Juice	10 fl oz	110
Pink Grapefruit Cocktail	8 fl oz	120
Tree Of Life		
Juice	8 fl oz	100

FOOD	PORTION	CALS.
Tree Top		
Juice	6 oz	80
Tropicana		
Juice	1 container (6 fl oz)	80
Juice	8 fl oz	90
Ruby Red	8 fl oz	100
Ruby Red	1 container (10 fl oz)	120
Season's Best	1 bottle (7 fl oz)	80
Season's Best	1 bottle (10 fl oz)	110
Season's Best	1 can (11.5 fl oz)	120
Season's Best	8 fl oz	90
Twister Light Pink	8 fl oz	40
Twister Light Pink	1 container (10 fl oz)	50
Twister Pink	1 can (11.5 fl oz)	160
Twister Pink	8 fl oz	110
Twister Pink	1 container (10 fl oz)	140
Veryfine		
100%	8 oz	101
Pink	8 oz	120

GRAPES

CANNED
thompson seedless in heavy sirup	½ cup	94
thompson seedless water pack	½ cup	48
S&W		
Thompson Seedless Premium	½ cup	100
FRESH		
grapes	10	36
Dole		
Grapes	1½ cup	85

GRAVY

(*see also* SAUCE)

CANNED
au jus	1 cup	38
beef	1 cup	124
beef	1 can (10 oz)	155
chicken	1 cup	189
mushroom	1 cup	120
turkey	1 cup	122
Franco-American		
Au Jus	2 oz	10
Beef	2 oz	25
Chicken	2 oz	45
Chicken Giblet	2 oz	30

FOOD	PORTION	CALS.
Franco-American (CONT.)		
Cream	2 oz	35
Mushroom	2 oz	25
Pork	2 oz	40
Turkey	2 oz	30
Gravymaster		
Seasoning	¼ tsp	3
Rudy's Farm		
Sausage Gravy	¼ cup (2 oz)	50
MIX		
au jus as prep w/ water	1 cup	32
brown as prep w/ water	1 cup	75
chicken as prep	1 cup	83
mushroom as prep	1 cup	70
onion as prep w/ water	1 cup	77
pork as prep	1 cup	76
turkey as prep	1 cup	87
Bournvita		
Extract	2 heaping tsp	34
Bovril		
Extract	1 heaping tsp	9
Cajun King		
Oil-Less Roux And Gravy Mix	3.5 oz	394
Durkee		
Au Jus as prep	¼ cup	5
Brown as prep	¼ cup	10
Brown Herb as prep	¼ cup	15
Brown Mushroom as prep	¼ cup	15
Brown Onion as prpe	¼ cup	15
Chicken as prep	¼ cup	20
Country as prep	¼ cup	35
Homestyle as prep	¼ cup	15
Mushroom as prep	¼ cup	15
Onion as prep	¼ cup	10
Pork as prep	¼ cup	10
Sausage as prep	¼ cup	35
Swiss Steak as prep	¼ cup	15
Turkey as prep	¼ cup	20
French's		
Au Jus as prep	¼ cup	5
Brown as prep	¼ cup	10
Chicken as prep	¼ cup	25
Herb Brown as prep	¼ cup	15
Homestyle as prep	¼ cup	10

FOOD	PORTION	CALS.
French's (CONT.)		
Mushroom as prep	¼ cup	10
Onion	¼ cup	15
Pork as prep	¼ cup	10
Sausage as prep	¼ cup	35
Turkey as prep	¼ cup	20
Hain		
Brown	¼ pkg	16
LaLoma		
Brown Gravy Quik as prep	2 tsp	45
Chicken Gravy Quik as prep	2 tsp	45
Country Quik Gravy as prep	2 tsp	10
Mushroom Quik Gravy as prep	2 tsp	10
Onion Quik Gravy as prep	2 tsp	10
Marmite		
Extract	1 heaping tsp	9
Pillsbury		
Brown	¼ cup	15
Chicken	¼ cup	25
Home Style	¼ cup	15
Weight Watchers		
Brown as prep	¼ cup	5
Brown With Mushrooms as prep	¼ cup	10
Brown With Onion as prep	¼ cup	10
Chicken as prep	¼ cup	10

GREAT NORTHERN BEANS

FOOD	PORTION	CALS.
CANNED		
great northern	1 cup	300
Allen		
Great Northern	½ cup (4.5 oz)	100
Green Giant		
Great Northern	½ cup	80
Hanover		
Great Northern	½ cup	110
Trappey		
With Sausage	½ cup (4.5 oz)	100
DRIED		
cooked	1 cup	210
Bean Cuisine		
Dried	½ cup	115

GREEN BEANS

FOOD	PORTION	CALS.
CANNED		
green beans	½ cup	13

FOOD	PORTION	CALS.
italian	½ cup	13
italian low sodium	½ cup	13
low sodium	½ cup	13
Allen		
Cut	½ cup (4.2 oz)	30
Cut No Added Salt	½ cup (4.2 oz)	15
French Style	½ cup (4.2 oz)	25
Italian	½ cup (4.2 oz)	35
Shell Outs	½ cup (4.5 oz)	30
Alma		
Cut	½ cup (4.2 oz)	30
Crest Top		
Cut	½ cup (4.2 oz)	30
Del Monte		
Cut	½ cup (4.3 oz)	20
Cut 50% Less Salt	½ cup (4.3 oz)	20
Cut Italian	½ cup (4.3 oz)	30
Cut No Salt Added	½ cup (4.3 oz)	20
French Style	½ cup (4.3 oz)	20
French Style 50% Less Salt	½ cup (4.3 oz)	20
French Style No Salt Added	½ cup (4.3 oz)	20
French Style Seasoned	½ cup (4.3 oz)	20
Whole	½ cup (4.3 oz)	20
GaBelle		
Cut	½ cup (4.2 oz)	30
Green Giant		
Almondine	½ cup	45
Cut	½ cup	16
French	½ cup	16
Kitchen Sliced	½ cup	16
Hanover		
Cut	½ cup	20
Owatonna		
Cut	½ cup	20
French	½ cup	20
S&W		
Cut Water Pack	½ cup	20
Cut Premium Blue Lake	½ cup	20
Dilled	½ cup	60
French Style Premium Blue Lake	½ cup	20
Green Beans & Wax Beans	½ cup	20
Whole Fancy Stringless	½ cup	20
Whole Vertical Pack	½ cup	20

FOOD	PORTION	CALS.
Seneca		
Cut	½ cup	20
Cuts Natural Pack	½ cup	25
French	½ cup	20
French Natural Pack	½ cup	25
Whole	½ cup	20
Sunshine		
Cut	½ cup (4.2 oz)	30
Italian	½ cup (4.2 oz)	35
FRESH		
cooked	½ cup	22
raw	½ cup	17
FROZEN		
cooked	½ cup	18
italian cooked	½ cup	18
Birds Eye		
Cut	½ cup	25
Farm Fresh Whole	¾ cup	30
French Cut	½ cup	25
In Sauce French Green Beans With Toasted Almonds	½ cup	50
Italian	½ cup	30
Polybag Cut	½ cup	25
Polybag Deluxe Whole	½ cup	20
Polybag French Cut	½ cup	25
Whole Deluxe	½ cup	45
Fresh Like		
Cut	3.5 oz	29
French	3.5 oz	29
Italian	3.5 oz	35
Whole	3.5 oz	29
Green Giant		
Cut	½ cup	16
Cut In Butter Sauce	½ cup	30
Green Beans	½ cup	14
One Serve In Butter Sauce	1 pkg	60
Hanover		
Cut	½ cup	20
French Style Blue Lake	½ cup	25
Italian Cut	½ cup	35
Whole Blue Lake	½ cup	30
Southland		
Cut Beans	3 oz	25
French	3 oz	25

FOOD	PORTION	CALS.
Stouffer's		
Green Bean Mushroom Casserole	½ cup (1.9 oz)	130
Tree Of Life		
Green Beans	⅔ cup (2.8 oz)	25
SHELF-STABLE		
Pantry Express		
Cut	½ cup	12
GREENS		
CANNED		
Allen		
Mixed	½ cup (4.2 oz)	30
Sunshine		
Mixed	½ cup (4.2 oz)	30
GROUNDCHERRIES		
fresh	½ cup	37
GROUPER		
cooked	3 oz	100
cooked	1 fillet (7.1 oz)	238
raw	3 oz	78
GUANABANA JUICE		
Libby		
Nectar	1 can (11.5 fl oz)	210
GUAVA		
fresh	1	45
guava sauce	½ cup	43
GUAVA JUICE		
Kern's		
Nectar	6 fl oz	110
Libby		
Nectar	6 oz	110
Nectar	1 can (11.5 fl oz)	220
Snapple		
Guava Mania	8 fl oz	110
GUINEA HEN		
w/ skin raw	½ hen (12.1 oz)	545
w/o skin raw	½ hen (9.3 oz)	292
HADDOCK		
FRESH		
cooked	1 fillet (5.3 oz)	168
cooked	3 oz	95

FOOD	PORTION	CALS.
raw	3 oz	74
roe raw	3½ oz	130
FROZEN		
Gorton's		
Fishmarket Fresh	5 oz	110
Microwave Entree Haddock In Lemon Butter	1 pkg	360
Mrs. Paul's		
Crunchy Batter Fillets	2 fillets	190
Light Fillets	1 fillet	220
Van De Kamp's		
Battered Fillets	2 (4 oz)	260
Breaded Fillets	2 (3.5 oz)	280
Lightly Breaded Fillets	1 (4 oz)	220
SMOKED		
smoked	1 oz	33
smoked	3 oz	99

HAKE
raw	3½ oz	84

HALIBUT
FRESH		
atlantic & pacific cooked	3 oz	119
atlantic & pacific cooked	½ fillet (5.6 oz)	223
atlantic & pacific raw	3 oz	93
greenland baked	3 oz	203
greenland baked	5.6 oz	380
FROZEN		
Van De Kamp's		
Battered Fillets	3 (4 oz)	300

HALVA
(*see* SESAME)

HAM
(*see also* HAM DISHES, PORK, TURKEY)

boneless 11% fat	3 oz	151
boneless extra lean roasted	3 oz	140
canned 13% fat	1 oz	54
canned 13% fat	3 oz	192
canned extra lean	3 oz	142
canned extra lean	1 oz	41
canned extra lean 4% fat	3 oz	116
center slice lean & fat	4 oz	229
center slice lean only	4 oz	220

FOOD	PORTION	CALS.
chopped	1 oz	65
chopped canned	1 oz	68
ham & cheese loaf	1 oz	73
ham & cheese spread	1 tbsp	37
ham & cheese spread	1 oz	69
ham salad spread	1 tbsp	32
ham salad spread	1 oz	61
minced	1 oz	75
patties uncooked	1 (2.3 oz)	206
patties grilled	1 patty (2 oz)	203
sliced extra lean 5% fat	1 oz	37
sliced regular 11% fat	1 oz	52
steak boneless extra lean	1 oz	35
whole lean & fat roasted	3 oz	207
whole lean only roasted	3 oz	133
Alpine Lace		
Boneless Cooked	2 oz	60
Armour		
Chopped Ham canned	2 oz	120
Deviled Ham canned	1 pkg (3 oz)	200
Golden Star Boneless	1 oz	33
Golden Star Canned	1 oz	32
Lower Salt 93% Fat Free	1 oz	35
Lower Salt Boneless	1 oz	34
Star Boneless	1 oz	41
Star Canned	1 oz	34
Star Speedy Cut	1 oz	44
1877 Boneless	1 oz	42
Black Label		
Chopped	2 oz	140
Carl Buddig		
Ham	1 oz	50
Honey Ham	1 oz	50
Hansel n'Gretel		
Baked Virginia	1 oz	34
Black Forest	1 oz	32
Cappy	1 oz	31
Cooked Fresh	1 oz	33
Deluxe	1 oz	31
Honey Valley	1 oz	31
Jalapeno	1 oz	25
Lessalt	1 oz	30
Lessalt Virginia	1 oz	32
Light AM	1 oz	27

FOOD	PORTION	CALS.
Hansel n'Gretel (CONT.)		
Travane	1 oz	31
Healthy Choice		
Baked Cooked	3 slices (2.2 oz)	70
Cooked	3 slices (2.2 oz)	70
Deli-Thin Baked Cooked With Natural Juices	6 slices (2 oz)	60
Deli-Thin Cooked	6 slices (2 oz)	60
Deli-Thin Honey With Natural Juices	6 slices (2 oz)	60
Deli-Thin Smoked With Natural Juices	6 slices (2 oz)	60
Fresh-Trak Cooked	1 slice (1 oz)	30
Fresh-Trak Honey	1 slice (1 oz)	30
Honey Boneless	3 oz	100
Smoked	3 slices (2.2 oz)	70
Variety Pack Regular	3 slice (2.2 oz)	70
Hillshire		
Brown Sugar	1 oz	40
Cooked Ham	1 oz	30
Deli Select Baked Ham	1 slice	10
Deli Select Brown Sugar Baked	1 slice	10
Deli Select Cajun Ham	1 slice	10
Deli Select Honey Ham	1 slice	10
Deli Select Lower Salt	1 slice	10
Deli Select Smoked Ham	1 slice	10
Flavor Pack 90-99% Fat Free Brown Sugar Baked	1 slice (0.6 oz)	20
Flavor Pack 90-99% Fat Free Honey Ham	1 slice (0.6 oz)	20
Flavor Pack 90-99% Fat Free Smoked	1 slice (0.6 oz)	20
Genuine Baked	1 oz	35
Honey Ham	1 oz	40
Lower Salt	1 oz	30
Lunch 'N Munch Cooked Ham/Swiss	1 pkg (4.5 oz)	360
Lunch 'N Munch Cooked Ham/Swiss Oreo	1 pkg (4.125 oz)	370
Lunch 'N Munch Cooked Ham/Swiss Snickers/Hi-C	1 pkg (4.25 oz + 6 fl oz)	470
Lunch 'N Munch Honey Ham/ Cheddar/ Snickers/Hi-C	1 pkg (4.25 oz + 6 fl oz)	500
Hormel		
Black Label Canned (refrigerated)	3 oz	100
Black Label Canned (self stable)	3 oz	110
Canned Chunk	2 oz	90
Cure 81 Half Ham	3 oz	100
Curemaster	3 oz	80
Deli Cooked	1 oz	29

FOOD	PORTION	CALS.
Hormel (CONT.)		
Deviled Ham	4 tbsp (2 oz)	150
Ham & Cheese Patties	1 patty (2 oz)	190
Light & Lean	3 oz	90
Light & Lean 97	3 oz	90
Light & Lean 97 Cuts	16 pieces (1 oz)	35
Light & Lean 97 Sliced	1 slice (1 oz)	25
Patties	1 patty (2 oz)	180
Primissimo Proscuitti	1 oz	70
Spread	4 tbsp (2 oz)	100
Supreme Cut Canned	1 oz	31
Jones		
Family Ham	1 slice	40
Ham Slices	1 slice	30
Krakus		
Ham	1 oz	25
Louis Rich		
Carving Board Baked With Natural Juices	2 slices (1.6 oz)	45
Carving Board Carved Thin Honey With Natural Juices	6 slices (2.1 oz)	70
Carving Board Honey With Natural Juices	2 slices (1.6 oz)	50
Carving Board Smoked Cooked With Natural Juices	1 slice (1.6 oz)	50
Dinner Slices Baked	1 slice (3.3 oz)	80
Mr. Turkey		
Deli Cuts Honey Cured	3 slices	35
Oscar Mayer		
Baked	3 slices (2.2 oz)	60
Boiled	3 slices (2.2 oz)	60
Chopped	1 slice (1 oz)	50
Deli-Thin Boiled	4 slices (1.8 oz)	50
Deli-Thin Honey Ham	4 slices (1.8 oz)	60
Deli-Thin Smoked	4 slices (1.8 oz)	50
Dinner Slice	3 oz	90
Dinner Steaks	1 (2 oz)	60
Ham & Cheese Loaf	1 slice (1 oz)	70
Healthy Favorites Baked	4 slices (1.8 oz)	50
Healthy Favorites Honey Ham	4 slices (1.8 oz)	50
Healthy Favorites Smoked Cooked	4 slices (1.8 oz)	50
Honey Ham	3 slices (2.2 oz)	70
Lower Sodium	3 slices (2.2 oz)	70
Lunchables Cookies/Ham/ Swiss	1 pkg (4.2 oz)	360
Lunchables Dessert Chocolate Pudding/ Ham/ American	1 pkg (6.2 oz)	390

FOOD	PORTION	CALS.
Oscar Mayer (CONT.)		
Lunchables Ham/Cheddar	1 pkg (4.5 oz)	340
Lunchables Ham/Garden Vegetable Cheese	1 pkg (4.5 oz)	380
Lunchables Honey Ham/Herb & Chive Cheese	1 pkg (4.5 oz)	390
Smoked Cooked	3 slices (2.2 oz)	60
Russer		
Baked	2 oz	70
Canadian Brand Maple	2 oz	70
Chopped	2 oz	130
Cooked Ham	2 oz	60
Ham & Cheese Loaf	2 oz	120
Honey & Maple Cured	2 oz	70
Honey Cured	2 oz	60
Hot	2 oz	70
Light Cooked	2 oz	60
Light Smoked	2 oz	60
Smoked Virginia	2 oz	70
Spiced	2 oz	160
Sara Lee		
Bavarian Brand Baked	2 oz	80
Bavarian Brand Baked Honey	2 oz	80
Golden Cure Smoked	2 oz	80
Honey Ham	2 oz	60
Honey Roasted	2 oz	90
Spreadables		
Ham Salad	¼ can	100
Underwood		
Deviled	2.08 oz	220
Deviled Light	2.08 oz	120
Deviled Smoked	2.08 oz	190
Weight Watchers		
Deli Thin Oven Roasted	5 slices (⅓ oz)	12
Deli Thin Oven Roasted Honey Ham	5 slices (⅓ oz)	12
Deli Thin Premium Smoked	5 slices (⅓ oz)	12
Oven Roasted Honey Ham	2 slices (¾ oz)	25
Oven Roasted Smoked	2 slices (¾ oz)	25
Premium Cooked	2 slices (¾ oz)	25

HAM DISHES
FROZEN

FOOD	PORTION	CALS.
Croissant Pocket		
Stuffed Sandwich Ham & Cheddar	1 piece (4.5 oz)	360

FOOD	PORTION	CALS.
Hot Pocket		
Stuffed Sandwich Ham & Cheese	1 (4.5 ox)	340
Ovenstuffs		
Ham/Turkey Deli Melt	1 (4.75 oz)	360
Weight Watchers		
Ham & Cheese Pocket Sandwich	1 (5 oz)	240
Hickory Smoked Ham & Cheddar Pretzel Sandwich	1 (4 oz)	260
TAKE-OUT		
croquettes	1 (3.1 oz)	217
salad	½ cup	287
sandwich w/ cheese	1	353

HAMBURGER
(*see also* BEEF)

FOOD	PORTION	CALS.
FROZEN		
Jimmy Dean		
Burger	1 (2 oz)	220
Flamed Broiled Cheeseburger	1 (6.3 oz)	540
Mini Cheeseburger	2 (3 oz)	270
Kid Cuisine		
Beef Patty Sandwich w/ Cheese	1 (8.5 oz)	410
MicroMagic		
Cheeseburger	1 pkg (4.75 oz)	450
Hamburger	1 pkg (4 oz)	350
Rudy's Farm		
Mild Burger	1 (3 oz)	360
White Castle		
Cheeseburger	2 (3.6 oz)	310
Hamburger	2 (3.2 oz)	270
TAKE-OUT		
double patty w/ bun	1 reg	544
double patty w/ catsup mayonnaise onion pickle tomato & bun	1 reg	649
double patty w/ catsup cheese mayonnaise mustard pickle tomato & bun	1 lg	706
double patty w/ catsup mustard mayonnaise onion pickle tomato & bun	1 lg	540
double patty w/ catsup mustard onion pickle & bun	1 reg	576
double patty w/ cheese & bun	1 reg	457
double patty w/ cheese & double bun	1 reg	461
double patty w/ cheese catsup mayonnaise onion pickle tomato & bun	1 reg	416

FOOD	PORTION	CALS.
single patty w/ bacon catsup cheese mustard onion pickle & bun	1 lg	609
single patty w/ bun	1 reg	275
single patty w/ bun	1 lg	400
single patty w/ catsup cheese ham mayonnaise pickle tomato & bun	1 lg	745
single patty w/ catsup mustard mayonnaise onion pickle tomato & bun	1 reg	279
single patty w/ cheese & bun	1 lg	608
single patty w/ cheese & bun	1 reg	320
triple patty w/ catsup mustard pickle & bun	1 lg	693
triple patty w/ cheese & bun	1 lg	769

HAZELNUTS

FOOD	PORTION	CALS.
dried blanched	1 oz	191
dried unblanched	1 oz	179
dry roasted unblanched	1 oz	188
oil roasted unblanched	1 oz	187
Crumpy		
Chocolate Hazelnut Spread	1 tbsp (0.5 oz)	80

HEART

FOOD	PORTION	CALS.
beef simmered	3 oz	148
chicken simmered	1 cup (5 oz)	268
lamb braised	3 oz	158
turkey simmered	1 cup (5 oz)	257
veal braised	3 oz	158

HEARTS OF PALM

FOOD	PORTION	CALS.
canned	1 (1.2 oz)	9
canned	1 cup (5.1 oz)	41

HERBAL TEA

(*see* TEA/HERBAL TEA)

HERBS/SPICES

(*see also individual names*)

FOOD	PORTION	CALS.
curry powder	1 tsp	6
poultry seasoning	1 tsp	5
pumpkin pie spice	1 tsp	6
Ac'cent		
Flavor Enhancer	½ tsp	5
Herbal All Purpose Seasoning	½ tsp	0
Golden Dipt		
All Purpose Seafood	¼ tsp	2
Blackened Redfish	¼ tsp	2

FOOD	PORTION	CALS.
Golden Dipt (CONT.)		
Broiled Fish	¼ tsp	2
Cajun Style Shrimp & Crab	¼ tsp	2
Lemon Pepper Seafood	¼ tsp	8
Ka-Me		
Five Spice Powder	¼ tsp (1 g)	0
Lawry's		
Seasoning Blend Sloppy Joe	1 pkg	126
McIlhenny		
Crab Boil	3 oz	378
Mrs. Dash		
Extra Spicy	1 tsp (3.4 g)	12
Garlic & Herb	1 tsp (3.4 g)	12
Lemon & Herb	1 tsp (3.4 g)	12
Low Pepper Blend	1 tsp (3.4 g)	12
Original	1 tsp (3.4 g)	12
Table Blend	1 tsp (3.4 g)	12
Watkins		
Apple Bake Seasoning	¼ tsp (0.5 g)	0
Barbecue Spice	¼ tsp (0.5 g)	0
Bean Soup Seasoning	¾ tsp (2 g)	5
Beef Jerky Seasoning	2 tsp (6 g)	15
Chicken Seasoning	½ tsp (1 g)	0
Cole Slaw Seasoning	½ tsp (1.5 g)	5
Egg Sensations	1 tsp (3 g)	10
Fajita Seasoning	½ tsp (3 g)	10
Grill Seasoning	¼ tsp (1 g)	0
Ground Beef Seasoning	⅛ tsp (0.5 g)	0
Italian Blend	1 tsp (3 g)	1
Meat Tenderizer	⅛ tsp (0.5 g)	0
Meatloaf Seasoning	½ tsp (5 g)	15
Mexican Blend	½ tbsp (4 g)	15
Omelet & Souffle Seasoning	¾ tsp (2 g)	5
Oriental Ginger Garlic Liquid Spice Blend	1 tbsp (0.5 oz)	120
Potato Salad Seasoning	¼ tsp (1 g)	0
Pumpkin Pie Spice	¼ tsp (0.5 g)	0
Smokehouse Liquid Blend	1 tbsp (0.5 oz)	120
Soup & Vegetable Seasoning	¼ tsp (0.5 g)	0
Spanish Seasoning Blend	¼ tsp (0.5 oz)	0
HERRING		
CANNED		
roe	3.5 oz	118
FRESH		
atlantic cooked	3 oz	172

FOOD	PORTION	CALS.
atlantic cooked	1 fillet (5 oz)	290
atlantic raw	3 oz	134
pacific baked	3 oz	213
pacific fillet baked	5.1 oz	360
roe raw	3½ oz	130
READY-TO-USE		
atlantic kippered	1 fillet (1.4 oz)	87
atlantic pickled	½ oz	39

HICKORY NUTS
dried	1 oz	187

HOMINY
CANNED

canned	½ cup	57
Allen		
Golden	½ cup (4.5 oz)	120
Mexican	½ cup (4.5 oz)	120
White	½ cup (4.5 oz)	100
Uncle William		
Golden	½ cup (4.5 oz)	120
Mexican	½ cup (4.5 oz)	120
White	½ cup (4.5 oz)	100
Van Camp's		
Golden	½ cup (4.3 oz)	80
White	½ cup (4.3 oz)	80

HONEY
honey	1 cup (11.9 oz)	1031
honey	1 tbsp (0.7 oz)	64
Burleson's		
Clover	1 tbsp	60
Creamed	1 tbsp	60
Natural	1 tbsp	60
Pure	1 tbsp	60
Raw	1 tbsp	60
Rocky Mountain Clover	1 tbsp	60
Golden Blossom		
Honey	1 tsp	20
Smucker's		
Single Serving	½ oz	45
Tree Of Life		
Alfalfa	1 tbsp (0.7 oz)	60
Avocado	1 tbsp (0.7 oz)	60
Buckwheat	1 tbsp (0.7 oz)	60

FOOD	PORTION	CALS.
Tree Of Life (CONT.)		
Clover	1 tbsp (0.7 oz)	60
Honeybear Wildflower	1 tbsp (0.7 oz)	60
Orange	1 tbsp (0.7 oz)	60
Tupelo	1 tbsp (0.7 oz)	60
Wildflower	1 tbsp (0.7 oz)	60
HONEYDEW		
FRESH		
cubed	1 cup	60
wedge	1/10	46
Chiquita		
Fresh	1 cup	70
Dole		
Honeydew	1/10	50
FROZEN		
Big Valley		
Balls	3/4 cup (4.9 oz)	45
HORSE		
roasted	3 oz	149
HORSERADISH		
Gold's		
Hot	1 tsp	4
Red	1 tsp	4
White	1 tsp	4
Hebrew National		
White	1 tbsp	7
Heluva Good Cheese		
Horseradish	1 tsp (5 g)	0
Ka-Me		
Wasabi Powder	1/4 tsp (1 g)	0
Kraft		
Cream Style	1 tsp (0.2 oz)	0
Horseradish Mustard	1 tsp (0.2 oz)	0
Prepared	1 tsp (0.2 oz)	0
Rosoff's		
Red	1 tbsp (0.5 oz)	8
White	1 tbsp (0.5 oz)	7
Sauceworks		
Horseradish	1 tsp (0.2 oz)	20
Schorr's		
Red	1 tbsp (0.5 oz)	8

FOOD	PORTION	CALS.
Schorr's (CONT.)		
White	1 tbsp (0.5 oz)	7

HOT CAKES
(*see* PANCAKES)

HOT DOG
(*see also* MEAT SUBSTITUTES, SAUSAGE, SAUSAGE SUBSTITUTES)

FOOD	PORTION	CALS.
CHICKEN		
chicken	1 (1.5 oz)	116
Empire		
Hot Dog	1 (2 oz)	100
Health Valley		
Weiners	1	96
Tyson		
Cheese	1	145
Chicken Hot Dog	1	115
Wampler Longacre		
Chicken	1 (2 oz)	130
Chicken	1 (1.6 oz)	110
MEAT		
beef	1 (2 oz)	180
beef	1 (1.5)	142
beef & pork	1 (2 oz)	183
beef & pork	1 (1.5 oz)	144
pork cheesefurter smokie	1 (1.5 oz)	141
Armour		
Lower Salt Jumbo	1	170
Lower Salt Jumbo Beef	1	170
Star Jumbo	1	190
Star Jumbo Beef	1	190
Chefwich		
Chili Dog	5 oz	380
Healthy Choice		
Beef	1 (1.8 oz)	60
Bunsize	1 (2 oz)	70
Franks	1 (1.6 oz)	50
Jumbo	1 (2 oz)	70
Hebrew National		
Beef	1 (1.7 oz)	150
Cocktail Beef	6 (1.8 oz)	160
Dinner Beef	1 (4 oz)	350
Reduced Fat Beef	1 (1.7 oz)	120
Hillshire		
Franks Bun Size Beef	2 oz	180

FOOD	PORTION	CALS.
Hillshire (CONT.)		
Light & Mild Franks Jumbo	1 link	110
Light & Mild Wieners	1 link	90
Lit'l Franks Beef	2 oz	180
Lit'l Wieners	2 oz	180
Wieners Bun Size	2 oz	180
Wieners Natural Casing	2 oz	180
Hormel		
Big 8	1 (2 oz)	170
Light & Lean 97	1 (1.6 oz)	45
Light & Lean 97 Beef	1 (1.6 oz)	45
Jimmy Dean		
Mini	1 (2 oz)	110
Nathan's		
Natural Casing Franks	1	158
Skinless Franks	1	176
Oscar Mayer		
Beef	1 (1.6 oz)	150
Big & Juicy Deli Style Beef	1 (2.7 oz)	250
Big & Juicy Hot 'N Spicy	1 (2.7 oz)	220
Big & Juicy Original	1 (2.7 oz)	240
Big & Juicy Original Beef	1 (2.7 oz)	230
Big & Juicy Quarter Pound Beef	1 (4 oz)	350
Big & Juicy Smokie Links	1 (2.7 oz)	200
Bun-Length Beef	1 (2 oz)	180
Cheese	1 (1.6 oz)	150
Free	1 (1.8 oz)	40
Healthy Favorites Turkey & Beef	1 (2 oz)	60
Light Beef	1 (2 oz)	110
Wieners Bun-Length Pork & Turkey	1 (2 oz)	180
Wieners Little	6 (2 oz)	170
Wieners Pork & Turkey	1 (1.6 oz)	150
Wieners Light Pork Turkey Beef	1 (2 oz)	110
Russer		
Lil'Salt Deli Franks	1 (2.67 oz)	160
Shofar		
Kosher Beef	1 (1.8 oz)	150
Kosher Beef Reduced Fat Reduced Sodium	1 (1.8 oz)	120
Wrangler		
Beef	1 (2 oz)	170
Cheese	1 (2 oz)	170
Smoked	1 (2 oz)	170

FOOD	PORTION	CALS.
TAKE-OUT		
corndog	1	460
w/ bun chili	1	297
w/ bun plain	1	242
TURKEY		
turkey	1 (1.5 oz)	102
Empire		
Hot Dog	1 (2 oz)	90
Health Valley		
Weiners	1	96
Louis Rich		
Bun Length	1 (2 oz)	110
Turkey	1 (1.6 oz)	90
Turkey	1 (1.5 oz)	80
Turkey Cheese	1 (1.6 oz)	90
Mr. Turkey		
Bun Size	1	130
Cheese	1	140
Hot Dog	1	110
Wampler Longacre		
Turkey	1 (2 oz)	130
Turkey	1 (1.6 oz)	110

HUMMUS

hummus	⅓ cup	140
hummus	1 cup	420
Casbah		
Mix as prep	¼ cup	120
Cedar's		
No Salt Added Hommus Tahini	2 tbsp (1 oz)	50

HYACINTH BEANS

dried cooked	1 cup	228

ICE CREAM AND FROZEN DESSERTS

(*see also* ICES AND ICE POPS, PUDDING POPS, SHERBET, YOGURT FROZEN)

chocolate	½ cup (4 fl oz)	143
dixie cup chocolate	1 (3.5 fl oz)	125
dixie cup strawberry	1 (3.5 fl oz)	112
dixie cup vanilla	1 (3.5 fl oz)	116
freeze dried ice cream chocolate strawberry & vanilla	1 pkg (0.75 oz)	158
french vanilla soft serve	½ gal	3014
french vanilla soft serve	½ cup (4 fl oz)	185
strawberry	½ cup (4 fl oz)	127

FOOD	PORTION	CALS.
vanilla	½ cup (4 fl oz)	132
vanilla light	½ cup	92
vanilla rich	½ cup	178
vanilla soft serve	½ cup	111
vanilla 10% fat	½ gal	2153
vanilla 16% fat	½ gal	2805
vanilla light	½ gal	1469
vanilla light	1 cup	184
vanilla light soft serve	½ gal	1787
vanilla light soft serve	1 cup	223
3 Musketeers		
Single Chocolate	1 (2 fl oz)	160
Single Vanilla	1 (2 fl oz)	160
Snack Chocolate	1 (0.72 fl oz)	60
Snack Vanilla	1 (0.72 fl oz)	60
Avari		
Creme Glace All Flavors	1 oz	10
Ben & Jerry's		
Banana Walnut	½ cup (3.9 oz)	290
Butter Pecan	½ cup (3.9 oz)	310
Cherry Garcia	½ cup (3.7 oz)	240
Cherry Vanilla	½ cup (3.9 oz)	240
Chocolate Chip Cookie Dough	½ cup (3.7 oz)	270
Chocolate Fudge Brownie	½ cup (3.7 oz)	250
Chunky Monkey	½ cup (3.7 oz)	280
Coconut Almond	½ cup (3.7 oz)	260
Coconut Almond Fudge Chip	½ cup (3.8 oz)	320
Coffee Almond Fudge	½ cup (3.7 oz)	290
Coffee Toffee Crunch	½ cup (3.7 oz)	280
English Toffee Crunch	½ cup (4 oz)	310
Mint Chocolate Cookie	½ cup (3.8 oz)	260
New York Super Fudge Chunk	½ cup (3.7 oz)	290
No Fat Strawberry	½ cup (3.3 oz)	140
No Fat Vanilla Fudge Swirl	½ cup (3.1 oz)	150
Peanut Butter Cup	½ cup (4.1 oz)	370
Pop Chocolate Chip Cookie Dough	1 (4.1 oz)	450
Pop English Toffee Crunch	1 (3.7 oz)	340
Pop Vanilla	1 (3.9 oz)	360
Rain Forest Crunch	½ cup (3.7 oz)	300
Smooth Aztec Harvest Coffee	½ cup (3.8 oz)	230
Smooth Deep Dark Chocolate	½ cup (3.9 oz)	260
Smooth Double Chocolate Fudge	½ cup (4.1 oz)	280
Smooth Mocho Fudge	½ cup (4 oz)	270
Smooth Vanilla	½ cup (3.8 oz)	230

FOOD	PORTION	CALS.
Ben & Jerry's (CONT.)		
Smooth Vanilla Bean	½ cup (3.8 oz)	230
Smooth Vanilla Caramel Fudge	½ cup (4.1 oz)	280
Smooth White Russian	½ cup (3.8 oz)	240
Vanilla	½ cup (3.7 oz)	230
Wavy Gravy	½ cup (4.1 oz)	330
Bon Bons		
Vanilla With Milk Chocolate Coating	5 pieces	200
Vanilla With Milk Chocolate Coating	8 pieces	330
Borden		
Buttered Pecan	½ cup	180
Chocolate Swirl	½ cup	130
Dutch Chocolate Olde Fashioned Recipe	½ cup	130
Fat Free Black Cherry	½ cup	90
Fat Free Chocolate	½ cup	100
Fat Free Peach	½ cup	90
Fat Free Strawberry	½ cup	90
Fat Free Vanilla	½ cup	90
Ice Milk Chocolate	½ cup	100
Ice Milk Strawberry	½ cup	90
Ice Milk Vanilla	½ cup	90
Strawberries 'N Cream Olde Fashioned Recipe	½ cup	130
Strawberry	½ cup	130
Sundae Cone	1	210
Vanilla Olde Fashioned Recipe	½ cup	130
Bounty		
Cherry/Dark	1 (0.84 fl oz)	70
Coconut/Dark	1 (0.84 fl oz)	70
Coconut/Milk	1 (0.84 fl oz)	70
Bresler's		
All Flavors Ice Cream	3.5 oz	230
All Flavors Royale Cremes	4 oz	260
All Flavors Royale Lites	4 oz	217
Breyers		
Bar Vanilla	1 (2.7 oz)	250
Bar Vanilla Carmel w/ Chocolate Brittle Coating	1 (2.7 oz)	260
Bar Vanilla With Chocolate Coating	1 (2.6 oz)	230
Butter Almond	½ cup	170
Butter Pecan	½ cup (2.6 oz)	180
Cherry Vanilla	½ cup	150
Chocolate	½ cup (2.6 oz)	160
Chocolate Chocolate Chip	½ cup (2.5 oz)	180

FOOD	PORTION	CALS.
Breyers (CONT.)		
Chocolate Peanut Butter Twirl	½ cup (2.6 oz)	220
Coffee	½ cup (2.6 oz)	150
Cookies n'Cream	½ cup (2.6 oz)	170
Deluxe Rocky Road	½ cup (2.5 oz)	190
French Vanilla	(2.5 oz)	170
Light Brownie Marble Fudge	½ cup (2.6 oz)	150
Light Chocolate	½ cup (2.4 oz)	130
Light Chocolate Fudge Twirl	½ cup (2.6 oz)	140
Light Heavenly Hash	½ cup (2.4 oz)	150
Light Rocky Road Deluxe	½ cup (2.4 oz)	150
Light Strawberry	½ cup (2.4 oz)	120
Light Toffee Fudge Parfait	½ cup (2.6 oz)	150
Light Vanilla	½ cup (2.4 oz)	130
Light Vanilla Chocolate Strawberry	½ cup (2.4 oz)	120
Mint Chocolate Chip	½ cup (2.6 oz)	170
Mocha Almond Fudge	½ cup (2.7 oz)	190
Peach	½ cup (2.6 oz)	130
Reduced Fat Chocolate Chocolate Chip	½ cup (2.4 oz)	150
Reduced Fat Heavenly Hash	½ cup (2.4 oz)	150
Reduced Fat Mocha Almond Fudge	½ cup (2.5 oz)	160
Reduced Fat Praline Almond Crunch	½ cup (2.4 oz)	140
Reduced Fat Swiss Almond Fudge Twirl	½ cup (2.5 oz)	160
Sandwich Vanilla	1 (2.8 oz)	250
Strawberry	½ cup (2.6 oz)	130
Toffee Bar Crunch	½ cup (2.5 oz)	180
Vanilla	½ cup (2.6 oz)	150
Vanilla Caramel Praline	½ cup (2.6 oz)	190
Vanilla Chocolate	½ cup (2.5 oz)	160
Vanilla Chocolate Strawberry	½ cup (2.5 oz)	150
Vanilla Peanut Butter Fudge Sundae	½ cup (2.5 oz)	170
Butterfinger		
Bar	1 (2.5 oz)	170
Nuggets	8	340
Carnation		
Berry Swirl Bar Raspberry	1 bar	70
Berry Swirl Bar Strawberry	1 bar	70
Cheesecake Bar Original	1 bar	120
Cheesecake Bar Strawberry	1 bar	125
Chocolate Malted Bar	1 bar	70
Creamy Lites Bar Chocolate	1 bar	50
Creamy Lites Bar Strawberry	1 bar	50
Sundae Cup Strawberry	1 (3.3 oz)	200

FOOD	PORTION	CALS.
Chiquita		
Cherry & Ice Cream Swirl	1 bar	80
Mixed Berry & Ice Cream Swirl	1 bar	80
Orange & Ice Cream Swirl	1 bar	80
Raspberry & Ice Cream Swirl	1 bar	80
Strawberry & Ice Cream Swirl	1 bar	80
Cool 'N Creamy		
Amarello With Chocolate Swirl	1 bar	62
Chocolate Vanilla	1 bar	54
Double Chocolate Fudge	1 bar	55
Orange Vanilla	1 bar	31
Cool Creations		
Cookies & Cream Sandwich	1 (3.5 oz)	240
Mini Sandwich	1 (2.3 oz)	110
Cyrk		
Chocolate	3 oz	209
Maple Walnut	3 oz	299
Mint Chocolate Chip	3 oz	258
Strawberry	3 oz	208
Vanilla	3 oz	209
DoveBar		
Almond	1 (3.67 fl oz)	335
Bite Size Almond Praline	1 (0.75 fl oz)	80
Bite Size Cherry Royale	1 (0.75 fl oz)	70
Bite Size Classic Vanilla	1 (0.75 fl oz)	70
Bite Size French Vanilla	1 (0.75 fl oz)	70
Bite Size Mint Supreme	1 (0.75 fl oz)	80
Caramel Pecan	1 (3.67 fl oz)	350
Chocolate Milk Chocolate	1 (3.8 fl oz)	340
Coffee Cashew	1 (3.67 fl oz)	335
Crunchy Cookie	1 (3.8 fl oz)	340
Peanut	1 (3.8 fl oz)	380
Single Vanilla/Dark	1 (2 fl oz)	200
Vanilla Dark Chocolate	1 (3.8 fl oz)	340
Vanilla Milk Chocolate	1 (3.8 fl oz)	340
Drumstick		
Cone Chocolate	1 (4.6 oz)	340
Cone Chocolate Dipped	1 (4.6 oz)	340
Cone Vanilla	1 (4.6 oz)	350
Cone Vanilla Caramel	1 (4.6 oz)	360
Cone Vanilla Fudge	1 (4.6 oz)	370
Eagle Brand		
Vanilla	½ cup	150

FOOD	PORTION	CALS.
Edy's		
American Dream Chocolate	3 oz	90
American Dream Chocolate Chip	3 oz	100
American Dream Cookies'N'Cream	3 oz	100
American Dream Mocha Almond Fudge	3 oz	110
American Dream Strawberry	3 oz	70
American Dream Toasted Almond	3 oz	110
American Dream Vanilla	3 oz	80
American Dream Vanilla Chocolate Strawberry	3 oz	80
Light Almond Praline	4 oz	140
Light Banana-Politan	4 oz	110
Light Butter Pecan	4 oz	140
Light Cafe Au Lait	4 oz	110
Light Candy Bar	4 oz	140
Light Chocolate Chip	4 oz	120
Light Chocolate Fudge Mousse	4 oz	130
Light Cookies'N'Cream	4 oz	120
Light Dreamy Caramel Cream	4 oz	140
Light Malt Ball 'N' Fudge	4 oz	140
Light Marble Fudge	4 oz	120
Light Mocha Almond Fudge	4 oz	140
Light Peanut Butter & Chocolate	4 oz	130
Light Raspberry Truffle	4 oz	110
Light Rocky Road	4 oz	130
Light Strawberry	4 oz	110
Light Vanilla	4 oz	100
Vanilla Chocolate Strawberry	4 oz	110
Fi-Bar		
Banana Cream	1 bar	93
Cocoa-Fudge 'N Cream	1 bar	93
Raspberries 'N Cream	1 bar	93
Wildberry Cream	1 bar	93
Flintstones		
Cool Cream	1 (2.75 oz)	90
Push-Up	1 (2.75 oz)	100
Friendly's		
Black Raspberry	½ cup	150
Chocolate Almond Chip	½ cup	170
Forbidden Chocolate	½ cup	150
Fudge Nut Brownie	½ cup	200
Heath English Toffee	½ cup (2.7 oz)	190
Purely Pistachio	½ cup	160
Vanilla	½ cup	150

FOOD	PORTION	CALS.
Friendly's (CONT.)		
Vanilla Chocolate Strawberry	½ cup	150
Vienna Mocha Chunk	½ cup	180
Frusen Gladje		
Butter Pecan	½ cup	280
Chocolate	½ cup	240
Chocolate Chocolate Chip	½ cup	270
Strawberry	½ cup	230
Swiss Chocolate Candy Almond	½ cup	270
Vanilla	½ cup	230
Vanilla Swiss Almond	½ cup	270
Good Humor		
Banana Bob	1 (3 fl oz)	155
Bar Classic Toasted Almond	1 (3.1 fl oz)	170
Bar Classic Vanilla	1 (3.1 fl oz)	190
Bar Classic Almond	1 (3.1 fl oz)	210
Bar Sidewalk Sundae	1	280
Bubble O'Bill	1 (3.6 fl oz)	170
Bubble Play	1	110
Chip Burrrger	1 (4.7 oz)	320
Chip Sandwich	1 (4.7 fl oz)	320
Choco Taco	1 (4.4 fl oz)	320
Chocolate Eclair Classic	1 (3.1 fl oz)	170
Classic Candy Center Crunch Vanilla	1	280
Colonel Crunch Chocolate	1 (3.1 oz)	160
Colonel Crunch Strawberry	1 (3.1 oz)	170
Combo Cup	1 (6.2 fl oz)	200
Cone Olde Nut Sundae	1 (3.9 oz)	230
Cone Sidewalk Sundae	1 (4.2 oz)	270
Creamee Burrrger	1 (4.7 oz)	310
Crunch Classic Candy Center	1 (3.1 fl oz)	260
Dinosaur Bar	1	110
Far Frog	1 (3.6 fl oz)	150
Fun Box Ice Cream Sandwich	1 (3.1 fl oz)	160
King Cone	1 (5.7 fl oz)	300
King Cone Classic Vanilla	1 (4.8 oz)	300
King Cone Strawberry	1 (5.7 oz)	250
Light Chocolate Chocolate Chip	½ cup (2.4 oz)	130
Light Chocolate Chip	½ cup (2.4 oz)	130
Light Coffee	½ cup (2.4 oz)	110
Light Cookies N'Cream	½ cup (2.4 oz)	140
Light Heavenly Hash	½ cup (2.4 oz)	140
Light Praline Almond Crunch	½ cup (2.4 oz)	130
Light Toffee Bar Crunch	½ cup (2.4 oz)	130

FOOD	PORTION	CALS.

Good Humor (CONT.)

FOOD	PORTION	CALS.
Light Vanilla	½ cup (2.4 oz)	110
Light Vanilla Chocolate Strawberry	½ cup (2.4 oz)	110
Light Vanilla Fudge	½ cup (2.6 oz)	120
Magmun Almond	1 (4.2 fl oz)	270
Magnum Chocolate	1 (4.2 fl oz)	260
Number One Bar	1 (4.1 fl oz)	190
Popsicle Ice Cream Sandwich	1 (3.6 fl oz)	190
Sandwich Giant Vanilla	1 (5.2 fl oz)	240
Sandwich Ice Cream	1	190
Sandwich Sidewalk Sundae	1 (3.1 fl oz)	160
Sandwich Sprinkle	1 (3.1 fl oz)	180
Strawberry Shortcake Bar Classic	1 (3.1 fl oz)	160
Sundae Twist Cup	1	160
Toffee Taco	1 (4.4 fl oz)	300
Viennetta Chocolate	1 (4.2 fl oz)	160
Viennetta Vanilla	1 (4.2 fl oz)	160
WWF Bar	1 (3.7 fl oz)	200
X-Men Bar	1 (3 fl oz)	150

Haagen-Dazs

FOOD	PORTION	CALS.
Baileys Original Irish Cream	½ cup (3.6 oz)	280
Brownies A La Mode	½ cup (3.7 oz)	280
Butter Pecan	½ cup (3.7 oz)	320
Cappuccino Commotion	½ cup (3.6 oz)	310
Caramel Cone Explosion	½ cup (3.6 oz)	310
Chocolate	½ cup (3.7 oz)	270
Chocolate Chocolate Chip	½ cup (3.7 oz)	300
Coffee	½ cup (3.7 oz)	270
Cookie Dough Dynamo	½ cup (3.6 oz)	300
Cookies & Cream	½ cup (3.6 oz)	270
DiSaronno Amaretto	½ cup (3.6 oz)	260
Macadamia Brittle	½ cup (3.7 oz)	300
Multi Pack Bars Caramel Cone Explosion	1 (3.1 oz)	330
Multi Pack Bars Chocolate & Dark Chocolate	1 (3.2 oz)	320
Multi Pack Bars Coffee & Almond Crunch	1 (3 oz)	290
Multi Pack Bars Iced Cappuccino Explosion	1 (2.9 oz)	290
Multi Pack Bars Triple Brownie Overload	1 (3 oz)	320
Multi Pack Bars Vanilla & Almonds	1 (3 oz)	300
Multi Pack Bars Vanilla & Dark Chocolate	1 (3.2 oz)	320
Multi Pack Bars Vanilla & Milk Chocolate	1 (3 oz)	280
Peanut Butter Burst	½ cup (3.6 oz)	330
Rum Raisin	½ cup (3.7 oz)	270

FOOD	PORTION	CALS.
Haagen-Dazs (CONT.)		
Single Pack Bars Caramel Cone Explosion	1 (3.3 oz)	350
Single Pack Bars Chocolate & Dark Chocolate	1 (3.9 oz)	400
Single Pack Bars Coffee & Almond Crunch	1 (3.7 oz)	360
Single Pack Bars Cookie Dough Dynamo	1 (3.5 oz)	380
Single Pack Bars Iced Cappuccino	1 (3.4 oz)	330
Single Pack Bars Triple Brownie Overload	1 (3.5 oz)	380
Single Pack Bars Vanilla & Almonds	1 (3.7 oz)	370
Single Pack Bars Vanilla & Dark Chocolate	1 (3.9 oz)	400
Single Pack Bars Vanilla & Milk Chocolate	1 (3.5 oz)	330
Strawberry	½ cup (3.7 oz)	250
Strawberry Cheesecake Craze	½ cup (3.7 oz)	290
Triple Brownie Overload	½ cup (3.5 oz)	300
Vanilla	½ cup (3.7 oz)	270
Vanilla Fudge	½ cup (3.7 oz)	280
Vanilla Swiss Almond	½ cup (3.7 oz)	310
Healthy Choice		
Black Forest	½ cup (2.5 oz)	120
Bordeaux Cherry Chocolate Chip	½ cup (2.5 oz)	110
Butter Pecan Crunch	½ cup (2.5 oz)	120
Cappuccino Chocolate Chunk	½ cup (2.5 oz)	120
Cookies 'N Cream	½ cup (2.5 oz)	120
Double Fudge Swirl	½ cup (2.5 oz)	120
Fudge Brownie	½ cup (2.5 oz)	120
Malt Caramel Cone	½ cup (2.5 oz)	120
Mint Chocolate Chip	½ cup (2.5 oz)	120
Peanut Butter Cookie Dough 'N Fudge	½ cup (2.5 oz)	120
Praline & Caramel	½ cup (2.5 oz)	130
Rocky Road	½ cup (2.5 oz)	140
Vanilla	½ cup	100
Heath		
Bar	1 (2.5 oz)	160
Nuggets	8	180
Heaven		
Sundae Bars Chocolate Fudge	1 bar	150
Sundae Bars Vanilla Fudge	1 bar	150
Vanilla Caramel Nut	1 bar	225
Vanilla Nut Fudge	1 bar	222
Hood		
Bar Orange Cream	1 bar (1.8 oz)	90
Bar Vanilla	1 bar (1.6 oz)	160
Caramel Butterscotch Blast	½ cup (2.3 oz)	160
Chocolate	½ cup (2.3 oz)	140

FOOD	PORTION	CALS.
Hood (CONT.)		
Chocolate Chip	½ cup (2.3 oz)	160
Chocolate Eclair	1 bar (1.6 oz)	150
Christmas Tree	½ cup (2.3 oz)	140
Coffee	½ cup (2.3 oz)	140
Cookie Dough Delight	½ cup (2.3 oz)	160
Cookies N Cream	½ cup (2.3 oz)	160
Cooler Cups	1 (2.1 oz)	80
Crispy Bar	1 (1.9 oz)	180
Egg Nog	½ cup (2.3 oz)	130
Fabulous Fudge & Peanut Butter Swirled Fudge Bars	1 bar (2.1 oz)	110
Fabulous Fudgies Assorted Bars	1 bar (2.1 oz)	100
Fat Free Chocolate Passion	½ cup (2.5 oz)	100
Fat Free Classic Harlequin	½ cup (2.5 oz)	100
Fat Free Double Brownie Sundae	½ cup (2.5 oz)	120
Fat Free Heavenly Hash	½ cup (2.5 oz)	120
Fat Free Mississippi Mud Pie	½ cup (2.5 oz)	130
Fat Free Praline Pecan Delight	½ cup (2.5 oz)	120
Fat Free Super Strawberry Swirl	½ cup (2.5 oz)	100
Fat Free Vanilla Fudge Twist	½ cup (2.5 oz)	120
Fat Free Very Vanilla	½ cup (2.5 oz)	100
Fudge Bars	1 bar (2.7 oz)	100
Grasshopper Pie	½ cup (2.3 oz)	160
Heavenly Hash	½ cup (2.3 oz)	140
Hendrie's Cherry Chocolate Dips	1 bar (1.3 oz)	120
Hoodsie Cup Vanilla & Chocolate	1 (1.7 oz)	100
Light Almond Praline Delight	½ cup (2.4 oz)	110
Light Brownie Nut Sundae	½ cup (2.4 oz)	140
Light Caribbean Coffee Royale	½ cup (2.4 oz)	110
Light Chocolate Chocolate Chip Cookie Dough	½ cup (2.4 oz)	140
Light Cookies N Cream	½ cup (2.4 oz)	130
Light Heath Toffee Chunk Swirl	½ cup (2.4 oz)	140
Light Heavenly Hash	½ cup (2.4 oz)	130
Light Maple Sugar Shack	⅓ cup (2.4 oz)	130
Light Massachusetts Mud Pie	½ cup (2.4 oz)	140
Light Raspberry Swirl	½ cup (2.4 oz)	120
Light Strawberry Supreme	½ cup (2.4 oz)	110
Light Triple Nut Cluster Sundae	½ cup (2.4 oz)	140
Light Vanilla	½ cup (2.4 oz)	110
Light Vanilla Chocolate Strawberry	½ cup (2.4 oz)	110
Low Fat No Sugar Added Caramel Swirl	½ cup (2.4 oz)	120
Low Fat No Sugar Added Chocolate Supreme	½ cup (2.4 oz)	120

FOOD	PORTION	CALS.
Hood (cont.)		
Low Fat No Sugar Added Mocha Fudge	½ cup (2.4 oz)	110
Low Fat No Sugar Added Raspberry Swirl	½ cup (2.4 oz)	110
Low Fat No Sugar Added Vanilla	½ cup (2.4 oz)	100
Maple Walnut	½ cup (2.3 oz)	160
Rockets	1 (2 oz)	120
Sandwich Light	1 (2.2 oz)	160
Sandwich Vanilla	1 (2.2 oz)	180
Sports Bar	1 (2.9 oz)	250
Spumoni	½ cup (2.3 oz)	140
Strawberry	½ cup (2.3 oz)	130
Super Sortment Chocolate & Banana Fudge Bar	1 bar (2.1 oz)	100
Super Sortment Root Beer Float & Orange Cream Bar	1 bar (1.5 oz)	70
Vanilla	½ cup (2.3 oz)	140
Vanilla Chocolate Patchwork	½ cup (2.3 oz)	140
Vanilla Chocolate Strawberry	½ cup (2.3 oz)	140
Vanilla Fudge	½ cup (2.3 oz)	140
Klondike		
Almond Bar	1 (5.2 fl oz)	310
Caramel Crunch	1 (5.2 fl oz)	300
Chocolate Chocolate Bar	1 (5.2 fl oz)	280
Coffee Bar	1 (5.2 fl oz)	290
Dark Chocolate Bar	1 (5.2 fl oz)	290
Gold Bar	1 (5.2 fl oz)	340
Krispy Bar	1 (5.2 fl oz)	300
Krunch	1 (3.1 fl oz)	200
Lite Bar	1 (2.3 fl oz)	110
Lite Bar Caramel	1 (2.4 fl oz)	120
Movie Bites Chocolate	8 pieces (4.6 fl oz)	340
Movie Bites Vanilla	8 pieces (4.6 fl oz)	320
Original Bar	1 (5.2 fl oz)	290
Sandwich Chocolate	1 (5.2 fl oz)	270
Sandwich Lite	1 (2.9 fl oz)	100
Sandwich Vanilla	1 (5.2 fl oz)	250
Mars		
Almond Bar	1 (1.85 fl oz)	210
Meadow Gold		
Sundae Cone	1	210
Milky Way		
Single Chocolate/Milk	1 (2 fl oz)	210
Snack Chocolate/Milk	1 (0.72 fl oz)	70
Snack Vanilla/Dark	1 (0.72 fl oz)	70

FOOD	PORTION	CALS.
Mocha Mix		
Berry Berry Berry	½ cup	140
Dutch Chocolate	½ cup (2.3 oz)	140
Mocha Almond Fudge	½ cup (2.3 oz)	150
Neapolitan	½ cup (2.3 oz)	140
Strawberry Swirl	½ cup (2.3 oz)	140
Vanilla	½ cup (2.3 oz)	140
Nestle Crunch		
Chocolate	1 bar (3 oz)	200
Cones	1 (4.6 oz)	300
Crunch King	1 (4 oz)	270
Nuggets	8 pieces	140
Reduced Fat	1 (2.5 oz)	130
Vanilla	1 bar (3 oz)	200
Rice Dream		
Bar Chocolate	1	270
Bar Chocolate Nutty	1	330
Bar Strawberry	1	260
Bar Vanilla	1	275
Bar Vanilla Nutty	1	330
Cappuccino	½ cup	130
Carob	½ cup	130
Carob Almond	½ cup	140
Carob Chip	½ cup	140
Carob Chip Mint	½ cup	140
Cocoa Marble Fudge	½ cup	140
Dream Pie Chocolate	1	380
Dream Pie Mint	1	380
Dream Pie Mocha	1	380
Dream Pie Vanilla	1	380
Lemon	½ cup	130
Peanut Butter Fudge	½ cup	160
Strawberry	½ cup	130
Vanilla	½ cup	130
Vanilla Fudge	½ cup	140
Vanilla Swiss Almond	½ cup	140
Wildberry	½ cup	130
Sealtest		
American Glory	½ cup (2.4 oz)	130
Butter Pecan	½ cup (2.4 oz)	160
Candy Cane Crunch	½ cup (2.4 oz)	150
Chocolate	½ cup (2.4 oz)	140
Chocolate Butter Pecan	½ cup (2.4 oz)	150
Chocolate Chip	½ cup (2.4 oz)	150

FOOD	PORTION	CALS.
Sealtest (CONT.)		
Coconut Chocolate	½ cup (2.4 oz)	160
Coffee	½ cup (2.4 oz)	140
Cupid's Scoops	½ cup (2.5 oz)	140
Dessert Bar Free Chocolate Fudge	1	90
Dessert Bar Free Vanilla Strawberry Swirl	1	80
Free Black Cherry	½ cup	100
Free Chocolate	½ cup	100
Free Peach	½ cup	100
Free Strawberry	½ cup	100
Free Vanilla	½ cup	100
Free Vanilla Strawberry Royale	½ cup	100
French Vanilla	½ cup (2.4 oz)	140
Fudge Royale	½ cup (2.5 oz)	150
Heavenly Hash	½ cup (2.4 oz)	150
Maple Walnut	½ cup (2.4 oz)	160
Strawberry	½ cup (2.4 oz)	130
Triple Chocolate Passion	½ cup (2.5 oz)	160
Vanilla	½ cup (2.4 oz)	140
Vanilla Chocolate Strawberry	½ cup (2.4 oz)	140
Vanilla With Orange Sherbet	½ cup (2.7 oz)	130
Simple Pleasures		
Chocolate	4 oz	140
Chocolate Caramel Sundae Light	4 oz	90
Chocolate Light	4 oz	80
Coffee	4 oz	120
Cookies n' Cream	4 oz	150
Mint Chocolate Chip	4 oz	150
Peach	4 oz	120
Pecan Praline	4 oz	140
Rum Raisin	4 oz	130
Strawberry	4 oz	120
Toffee Crunch	4 oz	130
Vanilla	4 oz	120
Vanilla Light	4 oz	80
Snickers		
Single	1 (2 fl oz)	220
Snack	1 (1 fl oz)	110
Tofu Ice Creme		
Carob	4 fl oz	190
Vanilla	4 fl oz	190
Tofutti		
Frutti Vanilla Apple Orchard	4 fl oz	100

FOOD	PORTION	CALS.
Turkey Hill		
Black Cherry	½ cup (2.3 oz)	140
Butter Pecan	½ cup (2.3 oz)	170
Choco Mint Chip	½ cup (2.3 oz)	160
Cookies 'N Cream	½ cup (2.3 oz)	160
Lite Butter Pecan	½ cup (2.3 oz)	130
Lite Choco Mint Chip	½ cup (2.3 oz)	140
Lite Cookies 'N Cream	½ cup (2.3 oz)	130
Lite Vanilla & Chocolate	½ cup (2.3 oz)	110
Lite Vanilla Bean	½ cup (2.3 oz)	110
Neapolitan	½ cup (2.3 oz)	150
Rocky Road	½ cup (2.3 oz)	170
Tin Roof Sundae	½ cup (2.3 oz)	160
Vanilla	½ cup (2.3 oz)	140
Vanilla & Chocolate	½ cup (2.3 oz)	150
Vanilla Bean	½ cup (2.3 oz)	140
Ultra Slim-Fast		
Bar Fudge	1	90
Bar Vanilla Cookie Crunch	1	90
Chocolate	4 oz	100
Chocolate Fudge	4 oz	120
Peach	4 oz	100
Pralines & Caramel	4 oz	120
Sandwich Vanilla	1	140
Sandwich Vanilla Chocolate	1	140
Sandwich Vanilla Oatmeal	1	150
Vanilla	4 oz	90
Vanilla Fudge Cookie	4 oz	110
Weight Watchers		
Artic D'Lites	1 bar	130
Berries 'n Creme Mousse	2 bars	70
Caramel Nut Bars	1 bar	130
Chocolate Chip Cookie Dough Sundae	1 (5.43 oz)	180
Chocolate Dip	1 bar	100
Chocolate Mousse Bar	2 bars	70
Chocolate Treat	1 bar	100
Crispy Pralines 'n Creme Bars	1 bar	130
English Toffee Crunch Bars	1 bar	120
Light Cookie Dough Craze	½ cup	140
Oh! So Very Vanilla!	½ cup	120
Orange Vanilla Treat	2 bars	70
Positively Praline Crunch	½ cup	140
Praline Toffee Crunch Parfait	1 (5.1 oz)	190
Reckless Rocky Road	½ cup	140

FOOD	PORTION	CALS.
Weight Watchers (CONT.)		
Triple Chocolate Tornado	½ cup	150
Vanilla Sandwich	1 bar	160
TAKE-OUT		
cone vanilla light soft serve	1 (4.6 oz)	164
gelato chocolate hazelnut	½ cup (5.3 oz)	370
gelato vanilla	½ cup (3 oz)	211
sundae caramel	1 (5.4 oz)	303
sundae hot fudge	1 (5.4 oz)	284
sundae strawberry	1 (5.4 oz)	269

ICE CREAM CONES AND CUPS

FOOD	PORTION	CALS.
sugar cone	1	40
wafer cone	1	17
Comet		
Cups	1 (5 g)	20
Sugar Cones	1 (12 g)	50
Waffle Cone	1 (17 g)	70
Dutch Mill		
Chocolate Covered Wafer Cups	1 (0.5 oz)	80
Keebler		
Sugar Cones	1	45
Vanilla Cups	1	15
Oreo		
Chocolate Cones	1 (13 g)	50
Teddy Grahams		
Cinnamon Cones	1 (0.5 oz)	60

ICE CREAM TOPPINGS
(*see also* SYRUP)

FOOD	PORTION	CALS.
butterscotch	2 tbsp (1.4 oz)	103
caramel	2 tbsp (1.4 oz)	103
marshmallow cream	1 jar (7 oz)	615
marshmallow cream	1 oz	88
pineapple	2 tbsp (1.5 oz)	106
pineapple	1 cup (11.5 oz)	861
strawberry	2 tbsp (1.5 oz)	107
strawberry	1 cup (11.5 oz)	863
walnuts in syrup	2 tbsp (1.4 oz)	167
Hershey		
Chocolate Fudge	2 tbsp	100
Chocolate Shoppe Candy Bar Sprinkles York	2 tbsp (1.1 oz)	170
Kraft		
Butterscotch	2 tbsp (1.4 oz)	130

FOOD	PORTION	CALS.
Kraft (CONT.)		
Caramel	2 tbsp (1.4 oz)	120
Chocolate	2 tbsp (1.4 oz)	110
Hot Fudge	2 tbsp (1.4 oz)	140
Pineapple	2 tbsp (1.4 oz)	110
Strawberry	2 tbsp (1.4 oz)	110
Marzetti		
Caramel Apple	2 tbsp	60
Caramel Apple Reduced Fat	2 tbsp	30
Peanut Butter Caramel	2 tbsp	60
Planters		
Nut	2 tbsp (0.5 oz)	100
Smucker's		
Butterscotch	2 tbsp	140
Butterscotch Special Recipe	2 tbsp	160
Caramel	2 tbsp	140
Chocolate	2 tbsp	130
Chocolate Fudge	2 tbsp	130
Dark Chocolate Special Recipe	2 tbsp	130
Hot Caramel	2 tbsp	150
Hot Fudge	2 tbsp	110
Hot Fudge Special Recipe	2 tbsp	150
Hot Toffee Fudge	2 tbsp	110
Magic Shell Chocolate	2 tbsp	190
Magic Shell Chocolate Fudge	2 tbsp	190
Magic Shell Chocolate Nut	2 tbsp	200
Marshmallow	2 tbsp	120
Peanut Butter Caramel	2 tbsp	150
Pecans in Syrup	2 tbsp	130
Pineapple	2 tbsp	130
Strawberry	2 tbsp	120
Swiss Milk Chocolate Fudge	2 tbsp	140
Walnuts in Syrup	2 tbsp	130

ICE TEA
(*see also* TEA/HERBAL TEA)

MIX

FOOD	PORTION	CALS.
instant artificially sweetened lemon flavored as prep w/ water	8 oz	5
instant sweetened lemon flavor as prep w/ water	9 oz	87
instant unsweetened lemon flavor as prep w/ water	8 oz	4
4C		
Instant	8 oz	90

FOOD	PORTION	CALS.
Bigelow		
Nice Over Ice	5 fl oz	1
Celestial Seasonings		
Iced Delight	8 fl oz	4
Crystal Light		
Decaffeinated Sugar Free	8 oz	2
Sugar Free	8 oz	3
Lipton		
Calorie Free Decaf as prep	1 serv	0
Calorie Free as prep	1 serv	0
Citrus as prep	1 serv	90
Decaf Lemon as prep	1 serv	90
Family Size Bags Lemon as prep	1 qt	0
Family Size Bags Lemon Lime as prep	1 qt	0
Family Size Bags Peach as prep	1 qt	0
Lemon as prep	1 serv	90
Lemon Lime as prep	1 serv	90
No Lemon as prep	1 serv	80
Sugar Free Decaf as prep	1 serv	5
Sugar Free Lemon as prep	1 serv	5
Sugar Free No Lemon as prep	1 serv	0
Sugar Free Peach as prep	1 serv	5
Sugar Free Raspberry as prep	1 serv	5
Sugar Free Tropical as prep	1 serv	5
Tea & Lemonade as prep	1 serv	90
Tea Bag Herbal Iced Refresher as prep	1 serv	0
Tropical as prep	1 serv	90
Nestea		
100% Instant Tea as prep	8 oz	2
Ice Teasers Citrus	8 oz	6
Ice Teasers Lemon	8 oz	6
Ice Teasers Orange	8 oz	6
Ice Teasers Tropical	8 oz	6
Ice Teasers Wild Cherry	8 oz	6
Lemon	8 oz	6
Peach	8 fl oz	88
Raspberry	8 fl oz	88
Sugarfree	8 oz	4
With Sugar & Lemon	1 bottle (16 fl oz)	176
With Sugar & Lemon	1 can (11.5 fl oz)	127
With Sugar & Lemon as prep	8 oz	70
READY-TO-DRINK		
Arizona		
Raspberry	8 fl oz	95

FOOD	PORTION	CALS.
Clearly Canadian		
Clearly Tea Original	8 fl oz	80
Clearly Tea Tangy Lemon	8 fl oz	80
Lipton		
Chilled Diet Lemon	8 fl oz	0
Chilled Lemon	8 fl oz	80
Chilled No Lemon	8 fl oz	90
Chilled Peach	8 fl oz	80
Chilled Raspberry	8 fl oz	80
Royal Mistic		
Diet	12 fl oz	8
Lemon	12 fl oz	144
Orange	12 fl oz	144
Wild Berry	12 fl oz	144
Schweppes		
Ice Tea	8 fl oz	90
Shasta		
Ice Tea	12 oz	124
Sipps		
Ice Tea	8.45 oz	100
Snapple		
Cranberry	8 fl oz	110
Diet	8 fl oz	0
Diet Peach	8 fl oz	0
Diet Raspberry	8 fl oz	0
Lemon	8 fl oz	110
Mango	8 fl oz	110
Mint	8 fl oz	120
Old Fashioned	8 fl oz	80
Orange	8 fl oz	110
Peach	8 fl oz	110
Raspberry	8 fl oz	120
Strawberry	8 fl oz	100
Tropicana		
Diet Lemon Fruit	8 fl oz	15
Lemon Fruit	8 fl oz	100
Peach Fruit	8 fl oz	120
Peach Fruit	1 can (11.5 fl oz)	160
Peach Fruit	1 bottle (10 fl oz)	140
Raspberry Fruit	1 can (11.5 fl oz)	160
Raspberry Fruit	8 fl oz	120
Raspberry Fruit	1 bottle (10 fl oz)	140
Tangerine Fruit	1 bottle (10 fl oz)	140
Tangerine Fruit	1 can (11.5 fl oz)	170

FOOD	PORTION	CALS.
Tropicana (CONT.)		
Tangerine Fruit	8 fl oz	110
Twister Apple Berry	8 fl oz	100
Twister Lemon Citrus	8 fl oz	110
Turkey Hill		
Diet Decaffeinated	1 cup (8 oz)	0
Raspberry Cooler	1 cup (8 oz)	110
Regular	1 cup (8 oz)	90
Veryfine		
With Lemon	8 oz	80

ICES AND ICE POPS

(*see also* ICE CREAM AND FROZEN DESSERTS, PUDDING POPS, SHERBET, YOGURT FROZEN)

FOOD	PORTION	CALS.
fruit & juice bar	1 (3 fl oz)	75
gelatin pop	1 (1.5 oz)	31
ice coconut pineapple	½ cup (4 fl oz)	109
ice fruit w/ Equal	1 bar (1.7 oz)	12
ice lime	½ cup (4 fl oz)	75
ice pop	1 (2 fl oz)	42
Ben & Jerry's		
Cherry Pop	1	330
Bresler's		
All Flavors Ice	3.5 oz	120
Chiquita		
Fruit & Cream Banana	1 bar	80
Fruit & Cream Blueberry	1 bar	80
Fruit & Cream Peach	1 bar	80
Fruit & Cream Raspberry	1 bar	80
Fruit & Cream Strawberry	1 bar	80
Fruit & Cream Strawberry Banana	1 bar	80
Fruit & Juice Bar Cherry	1 bar (2 oz)	50
Fruit & Juice Bar Raspberry	1 bar (2 oz)	50
Fruit & Juice Bar Raspberry Banana	1 bar (2 oz)	50
Fruit & Juice Bar Strawberry	1 bar (2 oz)	50
Fruit & Juice Bar Strawberry Banana	1 bar (2 oz)	50
Cool Creations		
10 Pack	1 pop (2 oz)	60
Lion King Cone	1 (4 oz)	280
Mickey Mouse Bar	1 (2.5 oz)	110
Mickey Mouse Bar	1 (4 oz)	170
Surprise Pops	1 (2 oz)	60
Crystal Light		
Berry Blend	1 bar	13

FOOD	PORTION	CALS.
Crystal Light (CONT.)		
Cherry	1 bar	13
Fruit Punch	1 bar	14
Orange	1 bar	13
Pina Colada	1 bar	14
Pineapple	1 bar	14
Pink Lemonade	1 bar	14
Raspberry	1 bar	13
Strawberry	1 bar	13
Strawberry Daiquiri	1 bar	14
Cyrk		
Ice Chocolate	4 oz	85
Ice Vanilla	4 oz	75
Sorbet Apricot	4 oz	104
Sorbet Blueberry	4 oz	77
Sorbet Cherry	4 oz	98
Sorbet Lemon	4 oz	66
Sorbet Mango	4 oz	83
Sorbet Pina Colada	4 oz	107
Sorbet Plum	4 oz	90
Sorbet Raspberry	4 oz	88
Sorbet Strawberry	4 oz	79
Sorbet Sugar Free Apricot	4 oz	36
Sorbet Sugar Free Mango	4 oz	48
Sorbet Sugar Free Pina Colada	4 oz	66
Sorbet Sugar Free Raspberry	4 oz	35
Sorbet White Peach	4 oz	96
Dole		
Fruit 'n Juice Coconut	1 bar (4 oz)	210
Fruit 'n Juice Lemonade	1 bar (4 oz)	120
Fruit 'n Juice Lime	1 bar (4 oz)	110
Fruit 'n Juice Peach Passion	1 bar (2.5 oz)	70
Fruit 'n Juice Pineapple Coconut	1 bar (4 oz)	140
Fruit 'n Juice Pineapple Orange Banana	1 bar (2.5 oz)	70
Fruit 'n Juice Pineapple Orange Banana	1 bar (4 oz)	110
Fruit 'n Juice Raspberry	1 bar (2.5 oz)	70
Fruit 'n Juice Strawberry	1 bar (4 oz)	110
Fruit 'n Juice Strawberry	1 bar (2.5 oz)	70
Fruit Juice Grape	1 bar (1.75 oz)	45
Fruit Juice No Sugar Added Grape	1 bar (1.75 oz)	25
Fruit Juice No Sugar Added Strawberry	1 bar (1.75 oz)	25
Fruit Juice Raspberry	1 bar (1.75 oz)	25
Fruit Juice Raspberry	1 bar (1.75 oz)	45
Fruit Juice Strawberry	1 bar (1.75 oz)	45

FOOD	PORTION	CALS.
Fi-Bar		
Juice Bar Lemoney-Lime	1 bar	63
Juice Bar Strawberry Nectar	1 bar	63
Juice Bar Tropical Delight	1 bar	63
Flintstones		
Rock Pops	1 (3.5 oz)	80
Frozfruit		
Strawberry	1 (4 oz)	80
Good Humor		
Big Stick Cherry Pineapple	1 (3.6 fl oz)	50
Big Stick Popsicle	1 (3.6 fl oz)	50
Calippo Cherry	1 (3.8 fl oz)	100
Calippo Grape Lemon	1 (3.9 fl oz)	90
Calippo Orange	1 (3.9 fl oz)	90
Citrus Bites	1 (1.8 fl oz)	35
Creamsicle Orange	1 (1.8 fl oz)	70
Creamsicle Orange	1 (2.8 fl oz)	110
Creamsicle Orange Raspberry	1 (2.6 fl oz)	100
Creamsicle Sugar Free	1 (1.8 fl oz)	25
Flintstones Push-Up Yabba Dabba Doo Orange	1 (2.75 fl oz)	90
Fudgsicle Pop	1 (1.8 fl oz)	60
Fudgsicle Sugar Free	1 (1.8 fl oz)	40
Fun Box Fudge Bar	1 (2.3 fl oz)	80
Fun Box Pops	1 (2 fl oz)	35
Fun Box Twin Box Cherry	1 (2.6 fl oz)	50
Fun Box Twin Pop Banana	1 (2.6 fl oz)	50
Fun Box Twin Pop Blue Raspberry	1 (2.6 fl oz)	50
Fun Box Twin Pop Cherry Lemon	1 (2.6 fl oz)	50
Fun Box Twin Pop Orange Cherry Grape	1 (2.6 oz)	50
Fun Box Twin Pop Root Beer	1 (2.6 fl oz)	50
Garfield Bar	1 (3.9 fl oz)	90
Great White	1 (3.1 fl oz)	70
Hyperstripe	1 (2.8 fl oz)	80
Ice Stripe Cherry Orange	1 (1.5 fl oz)	35
Jumbo Jet Star	1 (4.7 fl oz)	80
Laser Blazer	1 (2.6 oz)	70
Popsicle All Natural	1 (1.8 fl oz)	45
Popsicle Orange Cherry Grape	1 (1.8 fl oz)	45
Popsicle Rainbow Pops	1 (1.8 fl oz)	45
Popsicle Rootbeer Banana Lime	1 (1.8 fl oz)	45
Popsicle Strawberry Raspberry Wildberry	1 (1.8 fl oz)	45
Popsicle Supersicle Traffic Signal	1	80
Popsicle Twin Pop Cherry	1 (2.6 fl oz)	70

FOOD	PORTION	CALS.
Good Humor (CONT.)		
Popsicle Twin Pop Orange Cherry Grape Lime	1 (2.6 fl oz)	70
Snow Cone	1	60
Snowfruit Coconut Bar	1 (3.75 fl oz)	150
Snowfruit Orange Bar	1	140
Snowfruit Strawberry Bar	1	120
Snowfruit Tropical Fruit Bar	1	110
Sugar Free Pop Orange Cherry Grape	1 (1.8 fl oz)	15
Super Mario Bar	1	120
Supersicle Cherry Banana	1 (4.7 fl oz)	80
Supersicle Cherry Cola	1 (4.7 fl oz)	80
Supersicle Double Fudge	1 (4.7 fl oz)	150
Supersicle Firecracker	1 (4.7 fl oz)	90
Supersicle Firecracker Jr.	1	72
Supersicle Sour Tower	1	80
Swirl Bubble Gum	1 (2.7 fl oz)	55
Swirl Cherry Banana	1 (2.7 fl oz)	55
Torpedo Cherry	1 (1.8 fl oz)	35
Twister Blue Raspberry Cherry Cherry Cola Cherry	1 (1.8 fl oz)	45
Twister Cherry Lemon Orange Lemon	1 (1.8 fl oz)	45
Vampire's Deadly Secret	1 (2.8 fl oz)	100
Watermelon Bar	1 (3.6 fl oz)	80
Haagen-Dazs		
Sorbet Banana Strawberry	½ cup (4 oz)	140
Sorbet Chocolate	½ cup (4 oz)	130
Sorbet Manago	½ cup (4 oz)	120
Sorbet Orchard Peach	½ cup (4 oz)	140
Sorbet Raspberry	½ cup (4 oz)	120
Sorbet Strawberry	½ cup (4 oz)	130
Sorbet Zesty Lemon	½ cup (4 oz)	130
Sorbet & Cream Blueberry	4 oz	190
Sorbet & Cream Keylime	4 oz	190
Sorbet & Cream Orange	½ cup (3.7 oz)	200
Sorbet & Cream Orange	4 oz	190
Sorbet & Cream Raspberry	½ cup (3.7 oz)	190
Sorbet Bar Chocolate	1 (2.7 oz)	80
Sorbet Bar Wild Berry	1 (2.7 oz)	90
Hood		
Hendrie's Sizzle'N Sour Stix	1 bar (2 oz)	80
Hoodsie Pop	1 (3.3 oz)	60
Natural Blenders Pineapple	1 bar (1 oz)	60
Natural Blenders Raspberry	1 bar (1 oz)	60

FOOD	PORTION	CALS.
Hood (CONT.)		
Natural Blenders Strawberry	1 bar (1 oz)	60
Pop Banana	1 (3.3 oz)	60
Pop Blue Raspberry	1 (3.3 oz)	60
Pop Cherry	1 (3.3 oz)	60
Pop Grape	1 (3.3 oz)	60
Pop Orange	1 (3.3 oz)	60
Pop Root Beer	1 (3.3 oz)	60
Super Sortment Juice Bars	1 bar (1.9 oz)	40
Jell-O		
Lemon Lime	1 bar	33
Mixed Berry	1 bar	31
Orange	1 bar	31
Orange Pineapple	1 bar	31
Raspberry	1 bar	29
Raspberry Peach	1 bar	29
Side By Side Apple Cherry	1 bar	36
Side By Side Grape Lemon	1 bar	36
Strawberry	1 bar	31
Strawberry Banana	1 bar	31
Kool-Aid		
Berry Punch	1 bar	31
Cherry	1 bar	42
Grape	1 bar	42
Mountain Berry Punch	1 bar	42
Lifesavers		
Ice Pops	1	35
Ice Pops	1 (1.75 oz)	35
Sunkist		
Orange Juice Bar	1 (3.4 fl oz)	80
Wildberry	1 (3.4 fl oz)	120
Tofutti		
Frutti Apricot Mango	4 fl oz	100
Frutti Three Berry	4 fl oz	100
Vitari		
Passion-Fruit	4 oz	80
Peach	4 oz	80

ICING
(see CAKE)

INSTANT BREAKFAST
(see BREAKFAST DRINKS)

JACKFRUIT

fresh	3½ oz	70

FOOD	PORTION	CALS.
JALAPENO		
(*see* PEPPERS)		
JAM/JELLY/PRESERVES		
all flavors jam	1 tbsp (0.7 oz)	48
all flavors jam	1 pkg (0.5 oz)	34
all flavors jelly	1 pkg (0.5 oz)	38
all flavors jelly	1 tbsp (0.7 oz)	52
all flavors preserve	1 pkg (0.5 oz)	34
all flavors preserve	1 tbsp (0.7 oz)	48
apple butter	1 cup (9.9 oz)	519
apple butter	1 tbsp (0.6 oz)	33
apple jelly	3½ oz	259
apple jelly	1 pkg (0.5 oz)	38
apple jelly	1 tbsp (0.7 oz)	52
apricot jam	3½ oz	250
blackberry jam	3½ oz	237
cherry jam	3½ oz	250
linganberry jam	0.5 oz	23
orange jam	3½ oz	243
orange marmalade	1 tbsp (0.7 oz)	49
orange marmalade	1 pkg (0.5 oz)	34
plum jam	3½ oz	241
quince jam	3½ oz	236
raspberry jam	3½ oz	248
raspberry jelly	3½ oz	259
red currant jam	3½ oz	237
red currant jelly	3½ oz	265
rose hip jam	3½ oz	250
strawberry jam	1 tbsp (0.7 oz)	48
strawberry jam	1 pkg (0.5 oz)	34
strawberry preserve	1 tbsp (0.7 oz)	48
strawberry preserve	1 pkg (0.5 oz)	34
BAMA		
Apple Butter	2 tsp	25
Apple Jelly	2 tsp	30
Grape Jelly	2 tsp	30
Peach Preserves	2 tsp	30
Red Plum Jam	2 tsp	30
Strawberry Preserves	2 tsp	30
Eden		
Apple Butter	1 tbsp (0.5 fl oz)	25
Estee		
Apple Reduced Calorie	1 pkg (0.5 oz)	10

FOOD	PORTION	CALS.
Estee (CONT.)		
Apple Slice	1 tbsp (0.5 oz)	10
Apricot	1 tbsp (0.5 oz)	5
Blackberry	1 tbsp (0.5 oz)	5
Cherry	1 tbsp (0.5 oz)	5
Grape	1 tbsp (0.5 oz)	10
Orange	1 tbsp (0.5 oz)	10
Peach	1 tbsp (0.5 oz)	5
Red Raspberry	1 tbsp (0.5 oz)	5
Strawberry	1 tbsp (0.5 oz)	10
Harvest Moon		
Apricot Fruit Spread	1 tbsp (0.6 oz)	35
Blueberry Fruit Spread	1 tbsp (0.6 oz)	35
Cherry Fruit Spread	1 tbsp (0.6 oz)	35
Grape Fruit Spread	1 tbsp (0.6 oz)	35
Peach Fruit Spread	1 tbsp (0.6 oz)	35
Raspberry Fruit Spread	1 tbsp (0.6 oz)	35
Strawberry Fruit Spread	1 tbsp (0.6 oz)	35
Home Brands		
All Flavors Jelly	2 tsp	35
All Flavors Preserves	2 tsp	35
Kraft		
Apple Jelly	1 tbsp (0.7 oz)	60
Apple Strawberry Jelly	1 tbsp (0.7 oz)	50
Apricot Preserves	1 tbsp (0.7 oz)	50
Blackberry Jelly	1 tbsp (0.7 oz)	50
Blackberry Preserves	1 tbsp (0.7 oz)	50
Grape Jam	1 tbsp (0.7 oz)	60
Grape Jelly	1 tbsp (0.7 oz)	50
Grape Reduced Calorie	1 tbsp (0.6 oz)	20
Guava Jelly	1 tbsp (0.7 oz)	50
Orange Marmalade	1 tbsp (0.7 oz)	50
Peach Preserves	1 tbsp (0.7 oz)	50
Pineapple Preserves	1 tbsp (0.7 oz)	50
Red Currant Jelly	1 tbsp (0.7 oz)	50
Red Plum Jam	1 tbsp (0.7 oz)	60
Red Raspberry Preserves	1 tbsp (0.7 oz)	50
Strawberry Jam	1 tbsp (0.7 oz)	50
Strawberry Jelly	1 tbsp (0.7 oz)	60
Strawberry Preserves	1 tbsp (0.7 oz)	50
Strawberry Reduced Calorie	1 tbsp	20
Red Wing		
Apple Jelly	1 tbsp (0.7 oz)	50
Apple Blackberry Jelly	1 tbsp (0.7 oz)	50

FOOD	PORTION	CALS.
Red Wing (CONT.)		
Apple Cherry Jelly	1 tbsp (0.7 oz)	50
Apple Currant Jelly	1 tbsp (0.7 oz)	50
Apple Grape Jelly	1 tbsp (0.7 oz)	50
Apple Raspberry Jelly	1 tbsp (0.7 oz)	50
Apple Strawberry Jelly	1 tbsp (0.7 oz)	50
Black Raspberry Jelly	1 tbsp (0.7 oz)	50
Blackberry Jelly	1 tbsp (0.7 oz)	50
Cherry Jelly	1 tbsp (0.7 oz)	50
Concord Grape Jelly	1 tbsp (0.7 oz)	50
Crabapple Jelly	1 tbsp (0.7 oz)	50
Cranberry Jelly	1 tbsp (0.7 oz)	50
Cranberry Grape Jelly	1 tbsp (0.7 oz)	50
Currant Jelly	1 tbsp (0.7 oz)	50
Damson Plum Jelly	1 tbsp (0.7 oz)	50
Elderberry Jelly	1 tbsp (0.7 oz)	50
Grape Jelly	1 tbsp (0.7 oz)	50
Mint Jelly	1 tbsp (0.7 oz)	50
Mint Apple Jelly	1 tbsp (0.7 oz)	50
Mixed Fruit Jelly	1 tbsp (0.7 oz)	50
Red Plum Jelly	1 tbsp (0.7 oz)	50
Red Raspberry Jelly	1 tbsp (0.7 oz)	50
Strawberry Jelly	1 tbsp (0.7 oz)	50
Strawberry Apple Jelly	1 tbsp (0.7 oz)	50
S&W		
Apricot Pineapple Reduced Calorie Preserves	1 tsp	4
Blueberry Reduced Calorie Jam	1 tsp	4
Concord Grape Reduced Calorie Jelly	1 tsp	4
Orange Marmalade Reduced Calorie	1 tsp	4
Red Raspberry Reduced Calorie Jam	1 tsp	4
Red Tart Cherry Reduced Calorie Preserves	1 tsp	4
Strawberry Reduced Calorie Jam	1 tsp	4
Smucker's		
All Flavors Jam	1 tsp	18
All Flavors Jelly	1 tsp	18
All Flavors Low Sugar Spread	1 tsp	8
All Flavors Preserves	1 tsp	18
All Flavors Simply Fruit	1 tsp	16
All Flavors Single Serving Jelly	½ oz	38
All Flavors Single Serving Preserves	½ oz	38
All Flavors Slenderella	1 tsp	7
Apple Butter Autumn Harvest	1 tsp	12

FOOD	PORTION	CALS.
Smucker's (CONT.)		
Apple Butter Simply Fruit	1 tsp	12
Apple Butter Natural	1 tsp	12
Apple Cider Butter	1 tsp	12
Blackberry Single Serving Imitation Jelly	1 pkg (0.4 oz)	4
Cherry Singley Serving Imitation Jelly	1 pkg (0.4 oz)	4
Grape Single Serving Imitation Jelly	1 pkg (0.4 oz)	4
Orange Marmalade	1 tsp	18
Peach Butter	1 tsp	15
Pumpkin Butter Autumn Harvest	1 tsp	12
Tree Of Life		
Apricot Fruit Spread	1 tbsp (0.6 oz)	45
Blueberry Fruit Spread	1 tbsp (0.6 oz)	35
Cherry Fruit Spread	1 tbsp (0.6 oz)	40
Grape Fruit Spread	1 tbsp (0.6 oz)	35
Peach Fruit Spread	1 tbsp (0.6 oz)	45
Raspberry Fruit Spread	1 tbsp (0.6 oz)	30
Strawberry Fruit Spread	1 tbsp (0.6 oz)	35
Whistling Wings		
Blueberry Jam	1 oz	50
Raspberry Jam	1 oz	60
White House		
Apple Butter	1 oz	50

JAPANESE FOOD
(*see* ORIENTAL FOOD)

JAVA PLUM

fresh	1 cup	82
fresh	3	5

JELLY
(*see* JAM/JELLY/PRESERVE)

JERUSALEM ARTICHOKE
(*see* ARTICHOKE)

JEW'S EAR

pepeao dried	½ cup	36
pepeao raw sliced	1 cup	25

JUJUBE

fresh	3½ oz	105

KALE
FRESH

chopped cooked	½ cup	21
raw chopped	½ cup	21
scotch chopped cooked	½ cup	18

FOOD	PORTION	CALS.
Dole		
Chopped	½ cup	17
FROZEN		
chopped cooked	½ cup	20
KEFIR		
kefir	3½ oz	66
KETCHUP		
ketchup	1 tbsp	16
ketchup	1 pkg (0.2 oz)	6
low sodium	1 tbsp	16
Del Monte		
Ketchup	1 tbsp (0.5 oz)	15
Estee		
Imitation Sodium Free	1 pkg (0.5 oz)	15
Hain		
Natural	1 tbsp	16
Natural No Salt Added	1 tbsp	16
Healthy Choice		
Ketchup	1 tbsp (0.5 oz)	9
Heinz		
Hot	1 tbsp	14
Lite	1 tbsp	8
Hunt's		
Ketchup	1 tbsp (0.6 oz)	16
No Salt Added	1 tbsp (0.6 oz)	16
McIlhenny		
Ketchup	1 tbsp (0.6 oz)	23
Spicy	1 tbsp (0.6 oz)	23
Muir Glen		
Organic	1 tbsp (0.6 oz)	15
Red Wing		
Extra Fancy	1 tbsp (0.6 oz)	20
Smucker's		
Ketchup	1 tsp	8
Tree Of Life		
Ketchup	1 tbsp (0.5 oz)	10
Salsa Ketchup	1 tbsp (0.5 oz)	10
KIDNEY		
beef simmered	3 oz	122
lamb braised	3 oz	117
pork braised	3 oz	128
veal braised	3 oz	139

FOOD	PORTION	CALS.
KIDNEY BEANS		
CANNED		
kidney beans	1 cup	208
red	1 cup	216
B&M		
Red Baked Beans	½ cup (4.6 oz)	170
Eden		
Organic	½ cup (4.4 oz)	100
Friend's		
Red Baked Beans	½ cup (4.6 oz)	160
Goya		
Spanish Style	7.5 oz	140
Green Giant		
Dark Red	½ cup	90
Light Red	½ cup	90
Hanover		
Dark Red	½ cup	110
Light Red In Sauce	½ cup	120
Hunt's		
Red	4 oz	100
Luck's		
Seasoned w/ Pork	7.5 oz	220
Special Cook Red	7.5 oz	190
Progresso		
Red	½ cup (4.6 oz)	110
S&W		
Dark Red Lite 50% Less Salt	½ cup	120
Dark Red Premium	½ cup	120
Water Pack	½ cup	90
Trappey		
Dark Red	½ cup (4.5 oz)	130
Light Red	½ cup (4.5 oz)	120
Light Red New Orleans Style With Bacon	½ cup (4.5 oz)	110
Light Red With Jalapeno	½ cup (4.5 oz)	110
With Chili Gravy	½ cup (4.5 oz)	110
Van Camp's		
Dark Red	½ cup (4.6 oz)	90
Light Red	½ cup (4.6 oz)	90
DRIED		
california red cooked	1 cup	219
cooked	1 cup	225
red cooked	1 cup	225
royal red cooked	1 cup	218

FOOD	PORTION	CALS.
Arrowhead		
Red	¼ cup (1.6 oz)	160
Hurst		
Kidney Beans	1.2 oz	120
SPROUTS		
cooked	1 lb	152
raw	½ cup	27
KIWI JUICE		
After The Fall		
Kiwi Bear	1 cup (8 oz)	100
KIWIS		
fresh	1 med	46
Dole		
Kiwis	2	90
Sonoma		
Dried	7-8 pieces (1 oz)	90
KNISH		
Brand's		
Cheese 'N Blueberry	1 (7 oz)	378
Cheese 'N Cherry	1 (7 oz)	378
Everything	1 (7 oz)	221
Kashe	1 (7 oz)	270
Potato	1 (7 oz)	290
Potato w/ Broccoli & Cheese	1 (7 oz)	312
Potato w/ Spinach & Mushroom	1 (7 oz)	214
Joshua's		
Coney Island Potato	1 (4.6 oz)	280
TAKE-OUT		
cheese & blueberry	1 (7 oz)	378
cheese & cherry	1 (7 oz)	378
everything	1 (7 oz)	221
kashe	1 (7 oz)	270
potato	1 lg (7 oz)	332
potato	1 med (3.5 oz)	166
potato w/ broccoli & cheese	1 (7 oz)	312
potato w/ spinach & mushroom	1 (7 oz)	214
KOHLRABI		
raw sliced	½ cup	19
sliced cooked	½ cup	24
KUMQUATS		
fresh	1	12

FOOD	PORTION	CALS.
LAMB		
(see also LAMB DISHES*)*		
FRESH		
cubed lean only braised	3 oz	190
cubed lean only broiled	3 oz	158
ground broiled	3 oz	240
leg lean & fat Choice roasted	3 oz	219
loin chop w/ bone lean & fat Choice broiled	1 chop (2.3 oz)	201
loin chop w/ bone lean only Choice broiled	1 chop (1.6 oz)	100
rib chop lean & fat Choice broiled	3 oz	307
rib chop lean only Choice broiled	3 oz	200
shank lean & fat Choice braised	3 oz	206
shank lean & fat Choice roasted	3 oz	191
shoulder chop w/ bone lean & fat Choice braised	1 chop (2.5 oz)	244
shoulder chop w/ bone lean only Choice braised	1 chop (1.9 oz)	152
sirloin lean & fat Choice roasted	3 oz	248
FROZEN		
New Zealand lean & fat cooked	3 oz	259
New Zealand lean only cooked	3 oz	175
LAMB DISHES		
TAKE-OUT		
curry	¾ cup	345
moussaka	5.6 oz	312
stew	¾ cup	124
LAMBSQUARTERS		
chopped cooked	½ cup	29
LECITHIN		
(see SOY*)*		
LEEKS		
chopped cooked	¼ cup	8
cooked	1 (4.4 oz)	38
freeze dried	1 tbsp	1
raw	1 (4.4 oz)	76
raw chopped	¼ cup	16
LEMON		
FRESH		
lemon	1 med	22
peel	1 tbsp	0
wedge	1	5

FOOD	PORTION	CALS.
Dole		
Lemon	1	18
LEMON CURD		
lemon curd made w/ egg	2 tsp	29
lemon curd made w/ starch	2 tsp	28
LEMON EXTRACT		
Virginia Dare		
Extract	1 tsp	22
LEMON JUICE		
bottled	1 tbsp	3
fresh	1 tbsp	4
frzn	1 tbsp	3
After The Fall		
Spicy Lemon	1 can (12 oz)	150
Realemon		
Juice	1 fl oz	6
LEMONADE		
FROZEN		
as prep w/ water	1 cup	100
not prep	1 can (6 oz)	397
Bright & Early		
Lemonade	8 fl oz	120
Minute Maid		
Country Style	8 fl oz	120
Cranberry Lemonade	8 fl oz	80
Lemonade	8 fl oz	110
Pink	8 fl oz	120
Raspberry	8 fl oz	120
Seneca		
as prep	8 fl oz	110
MIX		
powder as prep w/ water	9 fl oz	113
powder w/ equal	1 pitcher (67 oz)	40
4C		
Instant as prep	8 fl oz	80
Country Time		
Mix	8 fl oz	82
Pink	8 fl oz	82
Pink Sugar Free	8 fl oz	4
Sugar Free	8 fl oz	4
Crystal Light		
Mix	8 fl oz	5

FOOD	PORTION	CALS.
Kool-Aid		
Mix	8 fl oz	99
Pink	8 fl oz	99
Sugar Free	8 fl oz	4
Sugar Sweetened Pink	8 fl oz	82
READY-TO-DRINK		
After The Fall		
Apple Raspberry	1 bottle (10 oz)	120
Crystal Geyser		
Juice Squeeze Pink	1 bottle (12 fl oz)	140
Diet Rite		
Salt/Sodium Free	8 fl oz	2
Fruitopia		
Lemonade	8 fl oz	120
Kool-Aid		
Koolers	1 pkg (8.45 fl oz)	120
Minute Maid		
Chilled	8 fl oz	110
Cranberry Chilled	8 fl oz	120
Juices To Go	1 bottle (16 fl oz)	110
Juices To Go	1 can (11.5 fl oz)	160
Juices To Go Canberry Lemonade	1 bottle (16 fl oz)	110
Juices To Go Raspberry Lemonade	1 bottle (16 fl oz)	120
Pink Chilled	8 fl oz	110
Raspberry Chilled	8 fl oz	120
Mott's		
Lemonade	10 fl oz	160
Nehi		
Lemonade	8 fl oz	130
Newman's Own		
Roadside Virginia	8 fl oz	100
Ocean Spray		
Lemonade	8 fl oz	110
With Cranberry Juice	8 fl oz	110
With Raspberry Juice	8 fl oz	110
Odwalla		
Honey	8 fl oz	70
Strawberry	8 fl oz	150
Royal Mistic		
Lemonade Limeade	16 fl oz	230
Tropical Pink	16 fl oz	230
Shasta		
Lemonade	12 fl oz	146

FOOD	PORTION	CALS.
Sipps		
Lemonade	8.45 fl oz	85
Snapple		
Diet Pink	8 fl oz	13
Lemonade	8 fl oz	110
Pink	8 fl oz	110
Strawberry	8 fl oz	110
Tropicana		
Lemonade	1 can (11.5 oz)	160
Lemonade	8 fl oz	110
Twister Orange Cranberry	8 fl oz	130
Twister Wild Berry	8 fl oz	120
Turkey Hill		
Lemonade	8 fl oz	110
Veryfine		
Lemonade	8 fl oz	120

LENTILS
CANNED
Health Valley

Fast Menu Hearty Lentils Garden Vegetables	7½ oz	150
Fast Menu Organic Lentils With Tofu Weiner	7½ oz	170
DRIED		
cooked	1 cup	231
Hurst		
Lentils	1.2 oz	120
FROZEN		
Natural Touch		
Lentil Rice Loaf	2.5 in slice (113 g)	200
MIX		
Casbah		
Pilaf as prep	1 cup	200
SPROUTS		
raw	½ cup	40

LETTUCE
(*see also* SALAD)

bibb	1 head (6 oz)	21
boston	1 head (6 oz)	21
boston	2 leaves	2
iceberg	1 leaf	3
iceberg	1 head (19 oz)	70
looseleaf shredded	½ cup	5
romaine shredded	½ cup	4

FOOD	PORTION	CALS.
Dole		
Butter	1 head	21
Iceberg	1/6 med head	20
Leaf shredded	1½ cup	12
Romaine shredded	1½ cups	18
Western Express		
Heart's Of Romaine	6 leaves (3 oz)	20

LIMA BEANS

FOOD	PORTION	CALS.
CANNED		
large	1 cup	191
lima beans	½ cup	93
Allen		
Green	½ cup (4.5 oz)	120
Green & White	½ cup (4.5 oz)	110
Del Monte		
Green	½ cup (4.4 oz)	80
Dennison's		
With Ham	7.5 oz	250
East Texas Fair		
Green	½ cup (4.5 oz)	120
Luck's		
Small Seasoned w/ Pork	7.5 oz	220
S&W		
Small Fancy	½ cup	80
Seneca		
Limas	½ cup	80
Trappey		
Baby Green With Bacon	½ cup (4.5 oz)	120
DRIED		
baby cooked	1 cup	229
cooked	½ cup	104
large cooked	1 cup	217
FROZEN		
cooked	½ cup	94
fordhook cooked	½ cup	85
Birds Eye		
Baby	½ cup	130
Fordhook	½ cup	100
Fresh Like		
Baby	3.5 oz	138
Green Giant		
Harvest Fresh	½ cup	80
In Butter Sauce	½ cup	100

FOOD	PORTION	CALS.
Hanover		
Baby	½ cup	110
Fordhook	½ cup	100
LIME		
fresh	1	20
LIME JUICE		
bottled	1 tbsp	3
fresh	1 tbsp	4
After The Fall		
Caribbean Lime	1 can (12 oz)	170
Key West	1 cup (8 oz)	100
Lifesavers		
Lime Punch	8 fl oz	140
Odwalla		
Summertime Lime	8 fl oz	90
Realime		
Juice	1 oz	6
LING		
blue raw	3½ oz	83
fresh baked	3 oz	95
fresh fillet baked	5.3 oz	168
LINGCOD		
baked	3 oz	93
fillet baked	5.3 oz	164
LIQUOR/LIQUEUR		
(*see also* BEER AND ALE, CHAMPAGNE, DRINK MIXERS, MALT, WINE, WINE COOLERS)		
anisette	⅔ oz	74
apricot brandy	⅔ oz	64
aquavit	3.5 oz	229
benedictine	⅔ oz	69
bloody mary	5 oz	116
bourbon & soda	4 oz	105
coffee liqueur	1½ oz	174
coffee w/ cream liqueur	1½ oz	154
cognac	3.5 oz	233
creme de menthe	1½ oz	186
curacao liqueur	⅔ oz	54
daiquiri	2 oz	111
gin	1½ oz	110
gin & tonic	7.5 oz	171

FOOD	PORTION	CALS.
gin ricky	4 oz	150
manhattan	2 oz	128
martini	2½ oz	156
mint julep	10 oz	210
old-fashioned	2½ oz	127
pina colada	4½ oz	262
planter's punch	3½ oz	175
rum	1½ oz	97
screwdriver	7 oz	174
sloe gin fizz	2½ oz	132
tequila sunrise	5½ oz	189
tom collins	7½ oz	121
vodka	1½ oz	97
whiskey	1½ oz	105
whiskey sour	3 oz	123
whiskey sour mix not prep	1 pkg (0.6 oz)	64

LIVER
(see also PATE*)*

beef braised	3 oz	137
beef pan-fried	3 oz	184
chicken stewed	1 cup (5 oz)	219
duck raw	1 (1.5 oz)	60
goose raw	1 (3.3 oz)	125
lamb braised	3 oz	187
lamb fried	3 oz	202
pork braised	3 oz	141
sheep raw	3½ oz	131
turkey simmered	1 cup (5 oz)	237
veal braised	3 oz	140
veal fried	3 oz	208
Dakota Lean		
Beef raw	3 oz	100

LOBSTER
(see also CRAYFISH*)*
CANNED
Progresso

Rock Lobster Sauce	½ cup (4.3 oz)	100
FRESH		
northern cooked	1 cup	142
northern cooked	3 oz	83
northern raw	1 lobster (5.3 oz)	136
northern raw	3 oz	77
spiny steamed	3 oz	122
spiny steamed	1 (5.7 oz)	233

FOOD	PORTION	CALS.
FROZEN		
Cajun Cookin'		
Crawfish Etouffee	12 oz	390
TAKE-OUT		
newburg	1 cup	485
LOGANBERRIES		
frzn	1 cup	80
LONGANS		
fresh	1	2
LOQUATS		
fresh	1	5
LOTUS		
root raw sliced	10 slices	45
root sliced cooked	10 slices	59
seeds dried	1 oz	94
LOX		
(*see* SALMON)		
LUPINES		
dried cooked	1 cup	197
LYCHEES		
fresh	1	6
Ka-Me		
Whole Pitted In Syrup	15 pieces (5 oz)	130
MACADAMIA NUTS		
dried	1 oz	199
oil roasted	1 oz	204
Mauna Loa		
Candy Glazed	1 oz	170
Chocolate Covered	1 oz	170
Honey Roasted	1 oz	200
Macadamia Nut Brittle	1 oz	150
Roasted & Salted	1 oz	210
MACARONI		
(*see* PASTA)		
MACE		
ground	1 tsp	8
MACKEREL		
CANNED		
jack	1 cup	296
jack	1 can (12.7 oz)	563

FOOD	PORTION	CALS.
Empress		
Jack	4 oz	140
FRESH		
atlantic cooked	3 oz	223
atlantic raw	3 oz	174
jack baked	3 oz	171
jack fillet baked	6.2 oz	354
king baked	3 oz	114
king fillet baked	5.4 oz	207
pacific baked	3 oz	171
pacific fillet baked	6.2 oz	354
spanish cooked	3 oz	134
spanish cooked	1 fillet (5.1 oz)	230
spanish raw	3 oz	118

MALT

nonalcoholic	12 fl oz	32
Bartles & Jaymes		
Malt Cooler Berry	12 fl oz	210
Malt Cooler Black Cherry	12 fl oz	190
Malt Cooler Light Berry	12 fl oz	140
Malt Cooler Mandarin Lemon	12 fl oz	210
Malt Cooler Margarita	12 fl oz	250
Malt Cooler Original	12 fl oz	180
Malt Cooler Peach	12 fl oz	200
Malt Cooler Pina Colada	12 fl oz	270
Malt Cooler Planter's Punch	12 fl oz	220
Malt Cooler Red Sangria	12 fl oz	190
Malt Cooler Strawberry	12 fl oz	200
Malt Cooler Strawberry Daiquiri	12 fl oz	220
Malt Cooler Tropical	12 fl oz	220
Olde English		
Malt	12 oz	163
Schaefer		
Malt	12 oz	165
Schlitz		
Malt	12 oz	177

MALTED MILK

chocolate as prep w/ milk	1 cup	229
chocolate flavor powder	3 heaping tsp (¾ oz)	79
natural flavor as prep w/ milk	1 cup	237
natural flavor powder	3 heaping tsp (¾ oz)	87
Carnation		
Chocolate	3 heaping tsp (21 g)	79

FOOD	PORTION	CALS.
Carnation (CONT.)		
Original	3 heaping tsp (21 g)	90
Kraft		
Instant Chocolate	3 tsp (0.7 oz)	80
Instant Chocolate as prep w/ 2% milk	1 serv (9.5 oz)	200
Instant Natural	3 tsp (0.7 oz)	90
Instant Natural as prep w/ 2% milk	1 serv (9.5 oz)	210

MAMMY-APPLE
fresh	1	431

MANGO
fresh	1	135
CANNED		
Ka-Me		
Mango	4 pieces (5 oz)	102
DRIED		
Sonoma		
Pieces	8 pieces (2 oz)	180

MANGO JUICE
After The Fall		
Hawaiian Mango	1 can (12 oz)	180
Mango Ginger	1 can (12 oz)	150
Kern's		
Nectar	6 fl oz	100
Libby		
Nectar	1 can (11.5 fl oz)	210
Snapple		
Diet Mango Madness	8 fl oz	13
Mango Madness Cocktail	8 fl oz	110

MARGARINE
(*see also* BUTTER BLENDS, BUTTER SUBSTITUTES)

squeeze soybean & cottonseed	1 tsp	34
stick corn	1 tsp	34
stick corn	1 stick (4 oz)	815
stick salted	1 tsp	39
stick salted	1 stick (4 oz)	815
stick unsalted	1 stick (4 oz)	809
stick unsalted	1 tsp	34
tub corn	1 tsp	34
tub corn	1 cup	1626
tub diet	1 tsp	17
tub diet	1 cup	800
tub safflower	1 tsp	34

FOOD	PORTION	CALS.
tub safflower	1 cup	1626
tub salted	1 tsp	34
tub salted	1 cup	1626
tub soybean salted	1 cup	1626
tub soybean salted	1 tsp	34
tub soybean unsalted	1 cup	1626
tub soybean unsalted	1 tsp	34
tub unsalted	1 cup	1626
tub unsalted	1 tsp	34
Blue Bonnet		
Stick	1 tbsp	100
Tub	1 tbsp	100
Whipped	1 tbsp	80
Chiffon		
Stick	1 tbsp	100
Tub	1 tbsp (0.5 oz)	100
Whipped	1 tbsp (0.3 oz)	70
Fleischmann's		
Stick	1 tbsp	100
Stick Light Corn Oil	1 tbsp	80
Stick Sweet Unsalted	1 tbsp	100
Hain		
Stick Safflower	1 tbsp	100
Stick Safflower Unsalted	1 tbsp	100
Tub Safflower	1 tbsp	100
Hollywood		
Safflower	1 tbsp	100
Safflower Unsalted Sweet	1 tbsp	100
Soft Spread	1 tbsp	90
I Can't Believe Its Not Butter		
Tub	1 tbsp	90
Krona		
Stick	1 tbsp	100
Land O'Lakes		
Stick	1 tbsp (0.5 oz)	90
Stick With Sweet Cream	1 tbsp (0.5 oz)	90
Stick With Sweet Cream Unsalted	1 tbsp (0.5 oz)	90
Tub	1 tbsp (0.5 oz)	80
Tub With Sweet Cream	1 tbsp (0.5 oz)	80
Mazola		
Stick	1 tbsp (14 g)	100
Stick	1 cup (229 g)	1650
Stick Unsalted	1 tbsp (14 g)	100
Stick Unsalted	1 cup (229 g)	1635

FOOD	PORTION	CALS.
Mazola (CONT.)		
Tub Diet	1 cup (235 g)	815
Tub Diet	1 tbsp (14 g)	50
Tub Light Corn Oil Spread	1 tbsp (14 g)	50
Mother's		
Stick Unsalted	1 tbsp	100
Sticks	1 tbsp	100
Tub Salted	1 tbsp	100
Tub Unsalted	1 tbsp	100
Nucanola		
Stick	1 tbsp (14 g)	90
Stick	1 tbsp	90
Parkay		
Squeeze	1 tbsp (0.5 oz)	80
Stick	1 tbsp (0.5 oz)	90
Stick ⅓ Less Fat	1 tbsp (0.5 oz)	70
Tub	1 tbsp (0.5 oz)	60
Tub Light	1 tbsp (0.5 oz)	50
Tub Soft	1 tbsp (0.5 oz)	100
Tub Soft Diet	1 tbsp (0.5 oz)	50
Whipped	1 tbsp (0.3 oz)	70
Promise		
Stick	1 tbsp	90
Smart Beat		
Tub	1 tbsp	25
Tub Unsalted	1 tbsp	25
Touch Of Butter		
Squeeze	1 tbsp (0.5 oz)	80
Stick	1 tbsp (0.5 oz)	90
Tree Of Life		
Canola Soft	1 tbsp (0.5 oz)	100
Stick 100% Soy	1 tbsp (0.5 oz)	100
Stick 100% Soy Salt Free	1 tbsp (0.5 oz)	100
Stick Canola Soy	1 tbsp (0.5 oz)	100
Stick Canola Soy Salt Free	1 tbsp (0.5 oz)	100
Weight Watchers		
Light	1 tbsp	45
Light Sodium Free	1 tbsp	45
Reduced Fat Stick	1 tbsp	60

MARINADE
(*see* SAUCE)

MARJORAM

dried	1 tsp	2

FOOD	PORTION	CALS.
MARSHMALLOW		
marshmallow	1 reg (0.3 oz)	23
marshmallow	1 cup (1.6 oz)	146
Campfire		
Large	2	40
Miniature	24	40
Joyva		
Twists Chocolate Covered	2 (1.5 oz)	190
Kraft		
Funmallows	4 (1.1 oz)	110
Funmallows Miniature	½ cup (1.1 oz)	100
Jet-Puffed	5 (1.2 oz)	110
Marshmallow Creme	2 tbsp (0.4 oz)	40
Miniature	½ cup (1.1 oz)	100
Teddy Bear Cocoa-Flavored	½ cup (1.1 oz)	100
MATZO		
egg	1 (1 oz)	111
egg & onion	1 (1 oz)	111
plain	1 (1 oz)	112
whole wheat	1 (1 oz)	99
Goodman's		
Matzo Ball Mix 50% Less Salt	2 tbsp (0.5 oz)	50
Matzo Ball Mix as prep	2 tbsp (0.5 oz)	60
Horowitz Margareten		
Egg Milk Chocolate Coated	1 oz	97
Manischewitz		
American Matzo	1	115
Daily Thin Tea	1	103
Dietetic Thins	1	91
Egg Dark Chocolate Coated	½ matzo (1 oz)	97
Egg n' Onion	1	112
Matzo Cracker Miniatures	10	90
Matzo Farfel	1 cup	180
Matzo Meal	1 cup	514
Passover	1	129
Passover Egg	1	132
Passover Egg Matzo Crackers	10	108
Salted Thin	1	100
Unsalted	1	110
Wheat Matzo Crackers	10	90
Whole Wheat w/ Bran	1	110
Streit's		
Dietetic	1 (1 oz)	100

FOOD	PORTION	CALS.
Streit's (CONT.)		
Lightly Salted	1 (1 oz)	110
Matzoh Meal	¼ cup (1 oz)	110
Passover	1 (1 oz)	110
Unsalted	1 (0.9 oz)	100
Whole Wheat	1 (1 oz)	110

MAYONNAISE

(*see also* MAYONNAISE TYPE SALAD DRESSING, RELISH)

FOOD	PORTION	CALS.
mayonnaise	1 cup	1577
mayonnaise	1 tbsp	99
reduced calorie	1 tbsp	34
reduced calorie	1 cup	556
sandwich spread	1 tbsp	60
BAMA		
Mayonnaise	1 tbsp	100
Bennett's		
Mayonnaise	1 tbsp	110
Best Foods		
Cholesterol Free Reduced Calorie	1 tbsp (15 g)	50
Cholesterol Free Reduced Calorie	1 cup (233 g)	760
Light	1 cup (233 g)	760
Light	1 tbsp (15 g)	50
Real	1 tbsp	100
Real	1 cup	1570
Hain		
Canola	1 tbsp	60
Canola	1 tbsp	100
Cold Processed	1 tbsp	110
Eggless No Salt Added	1 tbsp	110
Light Low Sodium	1 tbsp	60
Real No Salt Added	1 tbsp	110
Safflower	1 tbsp	110
Hellman's		
Chlesterol Free Reduced Calorie	1 tbsp (15 g)	50
Cholesterol Free Reduced Calorie	1 cup (233 g)	760
Light Reduced Calorie	1 tbsp (15 g)	50
Light Reduced Calorie	1 cup (233 g)	760
Mayonnaise	1 tbsp	100
Mayonnaise	1 cup (220 g)	1570
Hollywood		
Canola	1 tbsp	100
Mayonnaise	1 tbsp	110
Safflower	1 tbsp	100

FOOD	PORTION	CALS.
Kraft		
Free	1 tbsp (0.6 oz)	10
Light	1 tbsp (0.5 oz)	50
Real	1 tbsp (0.5 oz)	100
McIlhenny		
Spicy	1 tbsp (0.5 oz)	108
Mother's		
Mayonnaise	1 tbsp	100
Red Wing		
"H" Style	1 tbsp (0.5 oz)	110
Smart Beat		
Canola Oil	1 tbsp	40
Corn Beat	1 tbsp	40
Weight Watchers		
Fat Free	1 tbsp	10
Light	1 tbsp	25
Light Low Sodium	1 tbsp	25

MAYONNAISE TYPE SALAD DRESSING
(*see also* MAYONNAISE, RELISH)

home recipe	1 tbsp	25
home recipe	1 cup	400
mayonnaise type salad dressing	1 cup	916
mayonnaise type salad dressing	1 tbsp	57
reduced calorie w/o cholesterol	1 tbsp	68
reduced calorie w/o cholesterol	1 cup	1084
BAMA		
Dressing	1 tbsp	50
Bright Day		
Salad Dressing	1 tbsp	60
Miracle Whip		
Free	1 tbsp (0.6 oz)	15
Light	1 tbsp (0.5 oz)	40
Salad Dressing	1 tbsp (0.5 oz)	70
Smart Beat		
Dressing	1 tbsp (15 g)	12
Spin Blend		
Cholesterol Free	1 tbsp	40
Dressing	1 tbsp	60
Weight Watchers		
Fat Free Whipped Dressing	1 tbsp	15

MEAT STICKS

jerky beef	1 oz	96
jerky beef	1 lg piece (0.7 oz)	67

FOOD	PORTION	CALS.
smoked	1 (0.7 oz)	109
smoked	1 oz	156
Tombstone		
Beef Jerky	1 stick (0.5 oz)	35
Beef Sticks	1 (0.8 oz)	110
Snappy Sticks	1 (0.8 oz)	110

MEAT SUBSTITUTES

(*see also* BACON SUBSTITUTES, CHICKEN SUBSTITUTES, SAUSAGE
SUBSTITUTES, TURKEY SUBSTITUTES)

FOOD	PORTION	CALS.
simulated sausage	1 link (25 g)	64
simulated sausage	1 patty (38 g)	97
simulated meat product	1 oz	88
Boca Burgers		
Original	1 patty (2.5 oz)	110
Green Giant		
Harvest Burgers Original	1 (3 oz)	140
Harvest Direct		
TVP Beef Chunks	3.5 oz	280
TVP Beef Chunks Flavored	3.5 oz	250
TVP Beef Strips	3.5 oz	280
TVP Ground Beef	3.5 oz	280
TVP Ground Beef Flavored	3.5 oz	250
Jaclyn's		
Salisbury Steak Style Dinner	11 oz	260
Sirloin Strips Style Dinner	12 oz	290
Ken & Robert's		
Veggie Burger	1 (62 g)	110
Knox Mountain Farm		
Wheat Balls Mix	1 serv (1/10 pkg)	110
LaLoma		
Big Franks	1 (51 g)	110
Corn Dogs	1 (71 g)	190
Dinner Cuts	2 pieces (99 g)	110
Griddle Steaks	1 piece (54 g)	140
Nuteena	1/2 in slice (65 g)	160
Patty Mix	1/4 cup (16 g)	50
Redi-Burger	1/2 in slice (68 g)	130
Sandwich Spread	3 tbsp (48 g)	70
Savory Dinner Loaf Mix not prep	1/4 cup (16 g)	50
Savory Meatballs	7 (70 g)	190
Sizzle Burger	1 patty (71 g)	220
Sizzle Franks	2 (68 g)	170
Swiss Steak	1 piece (92 g)	170

FOOD	PORTION	CALS.
LaLoma (CONT.)		
Tender Bits	4 pieces (57 g)	80
Tender Rounds	6 pieces (73 g)	120
Vege-Burger	½ cup (108 g)	110
Vita-Burger Chunk	¼ cup (21 g)	70
Vita-Burger Granules	3 tbsp (21 g)	70
Lightlife		
American Grill	2.75 oz	110
Barbecue Grill	2.75 oz	130
Smart Deli Slices	2 slices (1.5 oz)	44
Smart Dogs	1 (1.5 oz)	40
Smart Dogs To Go	1 (5 oz)	115
Tofu Pups	1 (1.5 oz)	92
Vegetarian Sloppy Joe	4.3 oz	130
Midland Harvest		
Burger n' Loaf Chili w/o Beans	0.8 oz	90
Burger n' Loaf Herbs & Spice	3.2 oz	140
Burger n' Loaf Italian	3.2 oz	140
Burger n' Loaf Original	3.2 oz	140
Burger n' Loaf Sloppy Joe w/o Sauce	0.8 oz	80
Burger n' Loaf Taco	2.7 oz	90
Morningstar Farms		
Breaded Cutlet	1 patty (71 g)	230
Deli Franks	1 (35 g)	90
Sandwich Burger Pattie w/ Cheese	1 (4.75 oz)	370
Sandwich Pattie Biscuit	1 (3.5 oz)	280
Natural Touch		
Dinner Entree	1 patty (85 g)	230
Garden Pattie	1 (67 g)	120
Loaf Mix as prep	4 oz	180
Okara Pattie	1 (64 g)	160
Stroganoff Mix as prep	4 oz	90
Taco Mix as prep	2 tbsp	90
Sovex		
Better Than Burger?	½ cup (1.9 oz)	165
Spring Creek		
Soysage	1 patty (1.6 oz)	63
White Wave		
Meatless Healthy Franks	1 (1.5 oz)	90
Meatless Jumbo Franks	1 (3 oz)	170
Meatless Sandwich Slices Beef	2 slices (1.6 oz)	90
Meatless Sandwich Slices Bologna	2 slices (1.6 oz)	120
Meatless Sandwich Slices Pastrami	2 slices (1.6 oz)	90
Meatless Healthy Franks	1 (1.5 oz)	90

FOOD	PORTION	CALS.
White Wave (CONT.)		
Veggie Burger	1 patty (2.5 oz)	110
Worthington		
Beef Style Meatless	4 slices (70 g)	130
Bolono	2 slices (38 g)	60
Choplets	2 slices (92 g)	100
Corn Beef Sliced	4 slices (57 g)	120
Country Stew	9.5 oz (270 g)	220
Dinner Roast	2 oz	120
FriPats	1 (64 g)	180
Granburger not prep	6 tbsp (33 g)	110
Multigrain Cutlet	2 slices (92 g)	90
Non-Meat Balls	3 (54 g)	100
Numete	½ in slice (68 g)	150
Prime Stakes	1 piece (92 g)	160
Prosage Patties	2 (76 g)	210
Prosage Roll	2⅜ in slice (70 g)	180
Protose	½ in slice (76 g)	180
Salami Meatless	2 slices (38 g)	70
Savory Slices	2 slices (56 g)	100
Smoked Beef Slices	6 slices (56 g)	120
Stakelets	1 piece (71 g)	150
Veelets	1 patty (71 g)	230
Vegetable Skallops	½ cup (85 g)	90
Vegetable Skallops No Added Salt	½ cup (85 g)	80
Vegetable Steaks	2.5 pieces (90 g)	110
Vegetarian Burger	½ cup (113 g)	150
Vegetarian Burger No Added Salt	½ cup (113 g)	150
Vegetarian Beef Pie	1 (227 g)	360
Wham	3 slices (68 g)	120
Zoglo's		
Crispy Vegetarian Cutlets	1 (3.5 oz)	200
Savory Vegetarian Kebabs	1 serv (2.8 oz)	135
Tender Vegetarian Burgers	1 (2.6 oz)	150
Vegetable Patties	1 (2.6 oz)	130
Vegetarian Franks	1 (2.6 oz)	125
MELON		
(*see also individual names*)		
FRESH		
Chiquita		
Cantalene	1 cup	60
Honey Mist	1 cup	80
FROZEN		
melon balls	1 cup	55

FOOD	PORTION	CALS.
Big Valley		
Mixed	¾ cup (4.9 oz)	40

MEXICAN FOOD
(*see also* SALSA, SAUCE, SPANISH FOODS, TORTILLA)

MILK
(*see also* CHOCOLATE, COCOA, MILK DRINKS)

FOOD	PORTION	CALS.
CANNED		
condensed sweetened	1 oz	123
condensed sweetened	1 cup	982
evaporated	½ cup	169
evaporated skim	½ cup	99
Carnation		
Evaporated	2 tbsp	40
Evaporated Lowfat	2 tbsp	25
Lite Evaporated Skimmed	½ cup (4 fl oz)	100
Sweetened Condensed	2 tbsp	130
Eagle		
Sweetened Condensed	⅓ cup	320
Pet		
Evaporated	½ cup	170
Evaporated Filled	½ cup	150
Evaporated Light Skimmed	½ cup	100
DRIED		
buttermilk	1 tbsp	25
nonfat instantized	1 pkg (3.2 oz)	244
Carnation		
Nonfat	⅓ cup dry	80
Nutra/Balance		
Lactose Reduced as prep	8 oz	80
Sanalac		
As Prep	8 oz	80
REFRIGERATED		
1%	1 cup	102
1%	1 qt	409
1% protein fortified	1 qt	477
1% protein fortified	1 cup	119
2%	1 cup	121
2%	1 qt	485
buffalo	3½ oz	112
buttermilk	1 cup	99
buttermilk	1 qt	396
camel	3½ oz	80
donkey	3½ oz	43

FOOD	PORTION	CALS.
goat	1 cup	168
goat	1 qt	672
human	1 cup	171
indian buffalo	1 cup	236
low sodium	1 cup	149
mare	3½ oz	49
sheep	1 cup	264
skim	1 cup	86
skim	1 qt	342
skim protein fortified	1 qt	400
skim protein fortified	1 cup	100
whole	1 cup	150
BodyWise		
Nonfat	8 fl oz	100
Borden		
Acidophilus 1%	8 fl oz	100
Buttermilk Lowfat Golden Churn	8 fl oz	120
Hi-Calcium	8 fl oz	150
Hi-Protein 2%	8 fl oz	140
Milk	8 fl oz	150
Skim	8 fl oz	90
Skim-line	8 fl oz	100
CaliMilk		
CalciMilk	8 fl oz	102
Farmland		
1%	8 fl oz	100
2%	8 fl oz	130
Cholesterol Reduced	8 oz	150
Easylac 1%	8 fl oz	100
Easylac Nonfat	8 fl oz	90
Skim	8 fl oz	80
Skim Plus	8 fl oz	100
Friendship		
Buttermilk	8 fl oz	120
Hood		
1%	1 cup (8 oz)	110
Better Taste 2%	1 cup (8 oz)	130
Buttermilk	1 cup (8 oz)	90
Whole	1 cup (8 oz)	150
Lactaid		
1%	8 fl oz	102
Nonfat	8 fl oz	86
Nuform		
1%	1 cup (8 oz)	120

FOOD	PORTION	CALS.
Nuform (CONT.)		
Skim	1 cup (8 oz)	100
Silovet		
Skim	1 cup (8 oz)	90
Viva		
2%	8 fl oz	120
Skim	8 fl oz	100
Weight Watchers		
Skim	1 cup	90
SHELF-STABLE		
Parmalat		
1%	1 cup (8 oz)	110
2%	1 cup (8 oz)	130
Skim	1 cup (8 oz)	90
Whole	1 cup (8 oz)	160

MILK DRINKS

(*see also* BREAKFAST DRINKS, CHOCOLATE, COCOA)

FOOD	PORTION	CALS.
chocolate milk	1 cup	208
chocolate milk	1 qt	833
chocolate milk 1%	1 cup	158
chocolate milk 1%	1 qt	630
chocolate milk 2%	1 cup	179
strawberry flavor mix as prep w/ whole milk	9 oz	234
Body Wise		
Chocolate Nonfat Milk	1 cup (8 fl oz)	180
Borden		
Chocolate Lowfat Dutch Brand	8 fl oz	180
Bosco		
Chocolate Milk	1 cup (8 fl oz)	230
Hershey		
Chocolate Milk 2%	1 cup	190
Whole Chocolate Milk	8 oz	210
Hood		
Chocolate Lowfat	1 cup (8 oz)	150
Lactaid		
Chocolate Milk 1%	8 fl oz	158
Meadow Gold		
Chocolate Milk	8 fl oz	210
Parmalat		
Chocolate 2%	1 box (8 oz)	180
Quik		
Banana Lowfat Milk	8 oz	190
Chocolate	2½ tsp (0.75 oz)	90

FOOD	PORTION	CALS.
Quik (CONT.)		
Chocolate Lowfat Milk	8 oz	200
Chocolate as prep w/ 2% milk	8 oz	210
Chocolate as prep w/ skim milk	8 oz	170
Chocolate as prep w/ whole milk	8 oz	230
Ready To Drink Chocolate	8 oz	230
Ready To Drink Lite Chocolate Lowfat	8 oz	130
Ready To Drink Strawberry	8 oz	230
Strawberry	2½ tsp (0.75 oz)	80
Strawberry Lowfat Milk	8 oz	200
Strawberry as prep w/ 2% milk	8 oz	200
Strawberry as prep w/ skim milk	8 oz	160
Strawberry as prep w/ whole milk	8 oz	220
Sugar Free Chocolate	1 heaping tsp (5.8 g)	18
Sugar Free Chocolate as prep w/ 2% milk	8 oz	140
Syrup Chocolate as prep w/ 2% milk	8 oz	220
Syrup Chocolate as prep w/ skim milk	8 oz	220
Syrup Chocolate as prep w/ whole milk	8 oz	240
Syrup Strawberry as prep w/ 2% milk	8 oz	220
Syrup Strawberry as prep w/ skim milk	8 oz	180
Syrup Strawberry as prep w/ whole milk	8 oz	240
Vanilla Lowfat Milk	8 oz	200

MILK SUBSTITUTES

(*see also* COFFEE WHITENERS)

FOOD	PORTION	CALS.
imitation milk	1 cup	150
imitation milk	1 qt	600
Better Than Milk		
Carob	8 fl oz	130
Chocolate	8 fl oz	125
Light	8 fl oz	80
Natural	8 fl oz	90
Eden		
Original	1 pkg (8.8 oz)	135
Original	8 fl oz	130
EdenBlend		
Original	8 fl oz	120
EdenRice		
Milk	8 fl oz	110
Edensoy		
Carob	8 fl oz	150
Extra Original	8 fl oz	130
Extra Original	1 pkg (8.8 oz)	140
Extra Vanilla	1 pkg (8.8 fl oz)	150

FOOD	PORTION	CALS.
Edensoy (CONT.)		
Extra Vanilla	8 fl oz	140
Vanilla	8 fl oz	150
Vanilla	1 pkg (8.8 fl oz)	150
Health Valley		
Soo Moo	1 cup	120
Rice Dream		
Carob Lite	8 fl oz	150
Chocolate	8 fl oz	190
Chocolate	8 fl oz	190
Lite Organic Original	8 fl oz	130
Lite Vanilla	8 fl oz	130
Spring Creek		
!Honey Vanilla	1 oz	23
Original	1 oz	21
Plain	1 oz	15
Vegelicious		
Milk	8 fl oz	100
Vitamite		
Milk	8 fl oz	100
Vitasoy		
Carob Supreme	8 fl oz	150
Cocoa Light	8 fl oz	140
Cocoa Rich	8 fl oz	160
Original Creamy	8 fl oz	100
Original Light	8 fl oz	90
Vanilla Delite	8 fl oz	150
Vanilla Light	8 fl oz	110
Westsoy		
Cocoa Lite	8 fl oz	140
Plain Lite	8 fl oz	100
Vanilla Lite	8 fl oz	110

MILKFISH

baked	3 oz	162

MILKSHAKE

chocolate	10 oz	360
strawberry	10 oz	319
thick shake chocolate	10.6 oz	356
thick shake vanilla	11 oz	350
vanilla	10 oz	314
Frostee		
Chocolate	8 fl oz	200
Strawberry	8 fl oz	180

FOOD	PORTION	CALS.
Hood		
Shake Up Chocolate	1 cup (8 oz)	240
Shake Up Strawberry	1 cup (8 oz)	220
Shake Up Vanilla	1 cup (8 oz)	220
MicroMagic		
Chocolate	1 (10.5 oz)	290
Milky Way		
Shake	1 (10 fl oz)	390
Parmalat		
Shake A Shake Chocolate	1 box (6 oz)	180
Shake A Shake Orange Vanilla	1 box (6 oz)	110
Shake A Shake Vanilla	1 box (6 oz)	170
Weight Watchers		
Chocolate Fudge Shake Mix as prep	1 pkg	80

MILLET

cooked	½ cup	143

MINERAL/BOTTLED WATER

FOOD	PORTION	CALS.
Artesia		
Almund	7 oz	0
Cranberi	7 oz	0
Lemin	7 oz	0
Orange	7 oz	0
Plain	7 oz	0
Canada Dry		
Sparkling Water	8 fl oz	0
Crystal Geyser		
Sparking Natural Wild Cherry	1 bottle 12 fl oz	0
Sparkling Lemon	1 bottle (12 fl oz)	0
Sparkling Mineral	1 bottle (12 fl oz)	0
Sparkling Natural Cola Berry	1 bottle (12 fl oz)	0
Sparkling Orange	1 bottle (12 fl oz)	0
Diamond Spring		
Water	1 qt	0
Evian		
Water	1 liter	0
Glennpatrick		
Irish Spring Pure	8 oz	0
LaCroix		
Sparkling Berry	12 fl oz	0
Sparkling Lemon	12 fl oz	0
Sparkling Lime	12 fl oz	0
Sparkling Orange	12 fl oz	0
Sparkling Regular	12 fl oz	0

FOOD	PORTION	CALS.
Mountain Valley		
Mineral Water	1 qt	0
San Pellegrino		
Mineral Water	1 liter (33.8 oz)	0
Saratoga		
Sparkling	1 liter	0
MISO		
miso	½ cup	284
Eden		
Genmai Miso Organic	1 tbsp (0.5 oz)	25
Hacho Miso Organic	1 tbsp (0.5 oz)	35
Kome Miso Organic	1 tbsp (0.6 oz)	25
Mugi Miso Organic	1 tbsp (0.6 oz)	25
Shiro Miso Organic	1 tbsp (0.6 oz)	35
MOLASSES		
blackstrap	1 tbsp (0.7 oz)	47
blackstrap	1 cup (11.5 oz)	771
molasses	1 tbsp (0.7 oz)	53
molasses	1 cup (11.5 oz)	873
Brer Rabbit		
Dark	2 tbsp	110
Light	2 tbsp	110
McIlhenny		
Molasses	1 tbsp (0.7 oz)	66
Tree Of Life		
Blackstrap	1 tbsp (0.5 oz)	45
MONKFISH		
baked	3 oz	82
MOOSE		
roasted	3 oz	114
MOTH BEANS		
dried cooked	1 cup	207
MOUSSE		
FROZEN		
Pepperidge Farm		
San Francisco Chocolate Mousse	1	490
Sara Lee		
Chocolate	1 slice (2.7 oz)	260
Chocolate Light	1 (3 oz)	170
Light Classics Strawberry	1 slice (53.8 g)	180

FOOD	PORTION	CALS.
Weight Watchers		
Chocolate Mousse	1 (2.75 oz)	190
Praline Pecan	1 (2.71 oz)	170
Triple Chocolate Caramel Mousse	1 (2.75 oz)	200
HOME RECIPE		
chocolate	½ cup (7.1 oz)	447
crab	¼ cup	364
orange	½ cup	87
MIX		
Jell-O		
Rich & Luscious Chocolate	½ cup	145
Rich & Luscious Chocolate Fudge	½ cup	143
Knorr		
Dark Chocolate as prep	½ cup	90
Milk Chocolate as prep	½ cup	90
Unflavored as prep	½ cup	80
White Chocolate as prep	½ cup	80
Royal		
Chocolate Mousse No-Bake	⅛ pie	130
TAKE-OUT		
chocolate	½ cup (7.1 oz)	447

MUFFIN
FROZEN
Health Valley

FOOD	PORTION	CALS.
Almond & Date Oat Bran Fancy Fruit	1	180
Fat Free Apple Spice	1	140
Fat Free Banana	1	130
Fat Free Raisin Spice	1	140
Oat Bran Fancy Fruit Blueberry	1	140
Oat Bran Fancy Fruit Raisin	1	180
Rice Bran Fancy Fruit Raisin	1	210
Pepperidge Farm		
Banana Nut	1	170
Blueberry	1	170
Cholesterol Free Multi Grain Muesli	1	200
Cholesterol Free Oatbran With Apple	1	190
Cholesterol Free Raisin Bran	1	170
Cinnamon Swirl	1	190
Corn	1	180
Sara Lee		
Apple Oat Bran	1	190
Apple Spice	1	220
Blueberry	1	200

FOOD	PORTION	CALS.
Sara Lee (CONT.)		
Blueberry Free & Light	1	120
Cheese Streusel	1	220
Chocolate Chunk	1	220
Golden Corn	1	240
Oat Bran	1	210
Raisin Bran	1	220
Weight Watchers		
Banana Nut	1 (2.5 oz)	190
Blueberry	1 (2.5 oz)	250
Chocolate Chocolate Chip	1 (2.5 oz)	200
Harvest Honey Bran	1 (2.5 oz)	220
HOME RECIPE		
blueberry as prep w/ 2% milk	1 (2 oz)	163
blueberry as prep w/ whole milk	1 (2 oz)	165
corn as prep w/ 2% milk	1 (2 oz)	180
corn as prep w/ whole milk	1 (2 oz)	183
plain as prep w/ 2% milk	1 (2 oz)	169
plain as prep w/ whole milk	1 (2 oz)	172
wheat bran as prep w/ 2% milk	1 (2 oz)	161
wheat bran as prep w/ whole milk	1 (2 oz)	164
MIX		
blueberry	1 (1¾ oz)	149
corn	1 (1.75 oz)	160
wheat bran as prep	1 (1¾ oz)	138
Arrowhead		
Bran	⅓ cup (1.4 oz)	150
Oat Bran Wheat Free	⅓ cup (1.5 oz)	160
Betty Crocker		
Apple Cinnamon	1	120
Apple Cinnamon No Cholesterol Recipe	1	110
Banana Nut	1	120
Banana Nut No Cholesterol Recipe	1	110
Blueberry Streusel Bake Shop	1	210
Cinnamon Streusel	1	200
Oat Bran	1	190
Oat Bran No Cholesterol Recipe	1	180
Twice The Blueberries	1	120
Twice The Blueberries No Cholesterol Recipe	1	110
Wild Blueberry	1	120
Wild Blueberry Light	1	70
Wild Blueberry Light No Cholesterol Recipe	1	70

FOOD	PORTION	CALS.
Betty Crocker (CONT.)		
Wild Blueberry No Cholesterol Recipe	1	110
Dromedary		
Corn Muffin	1	120
Flako		
Corn	⅓ cup (1.4 oz)	160
Hain		
Oat Bran Apple Cinnamon	1	140
Oat Bran Banana Nut	1	140
Oat Bran Raspberry Spice	1	140
Jiffy		
Apple Cinnamon as prep	1	190
Banana Nut as prep	1	180
Blueberry as prep	1	190
Bran Date	1	110
Bran With Dates as prep	1	170
Corn as prep	1	180
Honey Date as prep	1	170
Oatmeal as prep	1	180
Wanda's		
Blue Corn	¼ cup mix per serv (1.2 oz)	130
READY-TO-EAT		
blueberry	1 (2 oz)	158
corn	1 (2 oz)	174
oat bran wheat free	1 (2 oz)	154
toaster type blueberry	1	103
toaster type corn	1	114
toaster type wheat bran w/ raisins	1 (36 g)	106
Arnold		
Bran'nola	1 (2.3 oz)	160
Raisin	1 (2.3 oz)	160
Dutch Mill		
Apple Oat Bran	1 (2 oz)	180
Banana Walnut	1 (2 oz)	220
Carrot	1 (2 oz)	190
Corn	1 (2 oz)	190
Cranberry Orange	1 (2 oz)	170
Raisin Bran	1 (2 oz)	230
Entenmann's		
Blueberry	1 (2 oz)	200
Freihofer's		
Corn Toasters	1 (1.3 oz)	130

FOOD	PORTION	CALS.
Hostess		
Mini Apple Cinnamon	5 (2 oz)	260
Mini Banana Nut	5 (2 oz)	260
Mini Blueberry	5 (2 oz)	240
Mini Chocolate Chip	5 (2 oz)	260
Muffin Loaf Blueberry	1 (3.8 oz)	440
Oat Bran	1 (1.5 oz)	160
Oat Bran Banana Nut	1 (1.5 oz)	150

MULBERRIES
fresh	1 cup	61

MULLET
striped cooked	3 oz	127
striped raw	3 oz	99

MUNG BEANS
DRIED		
cooked	1 cup	213
SPROUTS		
canned	½ cup	8
cooked	½ cup	13
raw	½ cup	16
stir fried	½ cup	31

MUNGO BEANS
dried cooked	1 cup	190

MUSHROOMS
CANNED		
chanterelle	3½ oz	12
pieces	½ cup	19
whole	1 (0.4 oz)	3
B In B		
Mushrooms	¼ cup	12
With Garlic	¼ cup	12
Empress		
Button	2 oz	14
Button Sliced	2 oz	14
Pieces & Stems	2 oz	14
Straw Broken	2 oz	10
Green Giant		
Oriental Straw	¼ cup	12
Pieces And Stems	¼ cup	12
Sliced	¼ cup	12
Whole	¼ cup	12

FOOD	PORTION	CALS.
Ka-Me		
Stir Fry	½ cup (4.5 oz)	20
Straw Whole Peeled	½ cup (4.5 oz)	20
Seneca		
Mushrooms	½ cup	25
DRIED		
chanterelle	3½ oz	89
shitake	4 (½ oz)	44
FRESH		
chanterelle	3½ oz	11
enoki raw	1 (4 in)	2
morel	3½ oz	9
oyster	3.5 oz	11
raw	1 (½ oz)	5
raw sliced	½ cup	9
shitake cooked	4 (2.5 oz)	40
sliced cooked	½ cup	21
whole cooked	1 (0.4 oz)	3
FROZEN		
Empire		
Breaded	7 (2.8 oz)	90
Fresh Like		
Mushrooms	3.5 oz	28

MUSKRAT
roasted	3 oz	199

MUSSELS
blue raw	3 oz	73
blue raw	1 cup	129
fresh blue cooked	3 oz	147

MUSTARD
dry mustard seed yellow	1 tsp	15
yellow ready-to-use	1 tsp	5
Blanchard & Blanchard		
Mustard	1 tsp (5 g)	0
Eden		
Hot Organic	1 tsp (5 g)	0
Estee		
Sodium Free	1 pkg (0.5 oz)	5
Grey Poupon		
Country Dijon	1 tsp	6
Dijon	1 tsp	6
Parisian	1 tsp	6

FOOD	PORTION	CALS.
Gulden's		
Diablo	1 tsp	8
Mild	1 tsp	6
Spicy Brown	1 tsp	8
Hain		
Stone Ground	1 tbsp	14
Stone Ground No Salt Added	1 tbsp	14
Heinz		
Mild Yellow	1 tbsp	8
Spicy Brown	1 tbsp	14
Ka-Me		
Hot Mustard Powder Chinese Style	¼ tsp (1 g)	5
Kosciuszko		
Spicy Brown	1 tsp	5
Kraft		
Mustard	1 tsp (0.2 oz)	0
McIlhenny		
Coarse Ground	1 tsp (0.2 oz)	4
Spicy	1 tsp (0.2 oz)	6
Plochman		
Dijon	1 tsp (5 g)	7
Spoonable Salad	1 tsp (5 g)	4
Squeeze Salad	1 tsp (5 g)	4
Stone Ground	1 tsp (5 g)	6
Russer		
Deli	1 tsp (5 g)	4
Tree Of Life		
Dijon	1 tsp (5 g)	0
Dijon Imported	1 tsp (5 g)	5
Low Sodium	1 tsp (5 g)	3
Stone Ground	1 tsp (5 g)	0
Yellow	1 tsp (5 g)	0
Watkins		
Country Mill	1 tsp (7 oz)	15
Dusseldorf	1 tsp (7 oz)	10
Horseradish	1 tsp (7 oz)	10
Jalapeno	1 tsp (7 oz)	10
Onion	1 tsp (7 oz)	10
Parisienne	1 tsp (7 oz)	10

MUSTARD GREENS
CANNED
Allen

Mustard Greens	½ cup (4.1 oz)	30

FOOD	PORTION	CALS.
Sunshine		
Mustard Greens	½ cup (4.1 oz)	30
FRESH		
chopped cooked	½ cup	11
raw chopped	½ cup	7
FROZEN		
chopped cooked	½ cup	14

NATTO
natto	½ cup	187

NAVY BEANS
CANNED		
navy	1 cup	296
Allen		
Navy Beans	½ cup (4.5 oz)	110
Eden		
Organic	½ cup (4.3 oz)	100
Hanover		
Navy	½ cup	100
Luck's		
Seasoned w/ Pork	7.5 oz	230
Trappey		
With Bacon	½ cup (4.5 oz)	110
With Bacon & Jalapeno	½ cup (4.5 oz)	110
DRIED		
cooked	1 cup	259
SPROUTS		
cooked	3½ oz	78
raw	½ cup	35

NECTARINE
fresh	1	67
Dole		
Nectarine	1	70

NEUFCHATEL
neufchatel	1 oz	74
neufchatel	1 pkg (3 oz)	221
Philadelphia		
Neufchatel	1 oz	70
Spreadery		
Classic Ranch	2 tbsp (1 oz)	60
Garden Vegetable	2 tbsp (1 oz)	70
Garlic & Herb	2 tbsp (1 oz)	80
With Strawberry	1 oz	70

FOOD	PORTION	CALS.
WisPride		
Garden Vegetable Cup	2 tbsp (1.1 oz)	60
Garlic & Herb Cup	2 tbsp (1.1 oz)	60

NON-DAIRY CREAMERS
(*see* COFFEE WHITENERS)

NON-DAIRY WHIPPED TOPPINGS
(*see* WHIPPED TOPPINGS)

NOODLE DISHES
(*see also* NOODLES, PASTA DINNERS)

CANNED

FOOD	PORTION	CALS.
Dinty Moore		
Noodles & Chicken	1 can (7.5 oz)	180
Micro Cup Meals		
Noodles & Chicken	1 cup (10.4 oz)	250
Van Camp's		
Noodlee Weenee	1 can (8 oz)	230

FROZEN

FOOD	PORTION	CALS.
Luigino's		
Stroganoff	1 pkg (8 oz)	310

MIX

FOOD	PORTION	CALS.
Kraft		
Chicken Egg Noodle	1 cup	330
La Choy		
Ramen Noodles Beef as prep	1 cup	200
Ramen Noodles Chicken as prep	1 cup	200
Lipton		
Noodles & Sauce Alfredo	⅔ cup (2.2 oz)	250
Noodles & Sauce Alfredo Broccoli as prep	⅔ cup (2.2 oz)	260
Noodles & Sauce Beef	⅔ cup (2.1 oz)	220
Noodles & Sauce Butter	⅔ cup (2.2 oz)	260
Noodles & Sauce Butter & Herb	⅔ cup (2.2 oz)	250
Noodles & Sauce Cheddar & Bacon	⅔ cup (2.1 oz)	230
Noodles & Sauce Cheese	⅔ cup (2.3 oz)	250
Noodles & Sauce Chicken	⅔ cup (2.1 oz)	230
Noodles & Sauce Chicken Tetrazzini	⅔ cup (2 oz)	220
Noodles & Sauce Creamy Chicken	⅔ cup (2.1 oz)	230
Noodles & Sauce Parmesan	⅔ cup (2.1 oz)	250
Noodles & Sauce Romanoff	⅔ cup (2.3 oz)	260
Noodles & Sauce Sour Cream & Chive	⅔ cup (2.2 oz)	260
Noodles & Sauce Stroganoff	⅔ cup (2 oz)	210
Minute		
Microwave Chicken Flavored	½ cup	157

FOOD	PORTION	CALS.
Minute (CONT.)		
Microwave Parmesan	½ cup	178
Noodle Roni		
Chicken & Mushroom	½ cup	160
Fettuccini	½ cup	300
Herb & Butter	½ cup	160
Parmesano	½ cup	240
Romanoff	½ cup	240
Stroganoff	½ cup	350
Noodles By Leonardo		
Macaroni & Cheese as prep	1 cup (2.5 oz)	250
Ultra Slim-Fast		
Noodles & Alfredo Sauce	2.3 oz	240
Noodles & Beef	2.3 oz	230
Noodles & Cheese	2.3 oz	230
Noodles & Chicken Sauce	2.3 oz	220
Noodles & Tomato Herb Sauce	2.3 oz	220
TAKE-OUT		
noodle pudding	½ cup	132
NOODLES		
cellophane	1 cup	492
chow mein	1 cup	237
egg	1 cup (38 g)	145
egg cooked	1 cup	212
japanese soba cooked	½ cup	56
japanese soba not prep	2 oz	192
japanese somen cooked	½ cup	115
japanese somen not prep	2 oz	203
spinach/egg cooked	1 cup	211
spinach/egg not prep	1 cup	145
Azumaya		
Chinese	4 oz	293
Japanese	4 oz	289
Creamette		
Egg	2 oz	221
Egg	2 oz	220
Golden Grain		
Egg	2 oz	210
Herb's		
Egg Fine	2 oz	220
Egg Medium	2 oz	220
Kluski Medium	2 oz	220
Kluski Wide	2 oz	220

FOOD	PORTION	CALS.
Hodgson Mill		
Veggie Egg	2 oz	200
Whole Wheat Spinach Egg	2 oz	190
Ka-Me		
Chinese Egg	½ cup (2 oz)	210
Chinese Plain	½ cup (2 oz)	200
Chuka Soba Curly Noodles	2 oz	200
Lo Mein Wide Chinese	½ cup (2 oz)	200
Py Mai Fun Rice Sticks	2 oz	193
Sai Fun Bean Thread	1 cup (2 oz)	190
Soba Shin Shu Japanese Buckwheat	2 oz	200
Tomoshiraga Somen Noodles	2 oz	190
Udon Japanese Thick	2 oz	190
La Choy		
Chow Mein Narrow	½ cup	150
Chow Mein Wide	½ cup	150
Rice	½ cup	130
Mueller's		
Egg	2 oz (57 g)	220
Noodle Trio	2 oz (57 g)	220
Noodles By Leonardo		
Egg Fine	2 oz	210
Egg Medium	2 oz	210
Egg Wide	2 oz	210
San Giorgio		
Egg	2 oz	210
Shofar		
No Yolks	2 oz	210

NOPALES

cooked	1 cup (5.2 oz)	23
raw sliced	½ cup (1.5 oz)	7
raw sliced	1 cup (3 oz)	14

NUTMEG

ground	1 tsp	12
Watkins		
Ground	¼ tsp (0.5 g)	0

NUTRITIONAL SUPPLEMENTS

(*see also* BREAKFAST BAR, BREAKFAST DRINKS)

DIET

Dynatrim		
Dutch Chocolate as prep w/ 1% milk	8 oz	220
Strawberry Royale as prep w/ 1% milk	8 oz	220

FOOD	PORTION	CALS.
Dynatrim (CONT.)		
Vanilla as prep w/ 1% milk	8 oz	220
Figurines		
Chocolate	1 bar	100
Chocolate Caramel	1 bar	100
Chocolate Peanut Butter	1 bar	100
S'Mores	1 bar	100
Vanilla	1 bar	100
Sego		
Lite Chocolate	10 fl oz	150
Lite Dutch Chocolate	10 fl oz	150
Lite French Vanilla	10 fl oz	150
Lite Strawberry	10 fl oz	150
Lite Vanilla	10 fl oz	150
Very Chocolate	10 fl oz	225
Very Chocolate Malt	10 fl oz	225
Very Strawberry	10 fl oz	225
Very Vanilla	10 fl oz	225
Slim-Fast		
Powder Chocolate as prep w/ skim milk	8 oz	190
Powder Chocolate Malt as prep w/ skim milk	8 oz	190
Powder Strawberry as prep w/ skim milk	8 oz	190
Powder Vanilla as prep w/ skim milk	8 oz	190
Sweet Success		
Chewy Bar Chocolate Brownie	1 (1.6 oz)	120
Chewy Bar Chocolate Peanut Butter	1 (1.6 oz)	120
Chewy Bar Chocolate Raspberry	1 (1.6 oz)	120
Chewy Bar Chocolate Chip	1 (1.6 oz)	120
Chewy Bar Oatmeal Raisin	1 (1.6 oz)	120
Chocolate Raspberry Truffle	1 can (10 fl oz)	200
Chocolate Raspberry as prep w/ skim milk	9 fl oz	180
Chocolate Mocha Supreme	1 can (10 fl oz)	200
Chocolate Mocha Supreme as prep w/ skim milk	9 fl oz	180
Classic Chocolate Chip as prep w/ skim milk	9 fl oz	180
Creamy Milk Chocolate	1 can (10 fl oz)	200
Creamy Milk Chocolate	1 carton (12 fl oz)	220
Creamy Milk Chocolate as prep w/ skim milk	9 fl oz	180
Creamy Vanilla Delight as prep w/ skim milk	9 fl oz	180
Dark Chocolate Fudge	1 can (10 fl oz)	200

FOOD	PORTION	CALS.
Sweet Success (CONT.)		
Dark Chocolate Fudge	1 carton (12 fl oz)	220
Dark Chocolate Fudge as prep w/ skim milk	9 fl oz	180
Rich Chocolate Almond	1 can (10 fl oz)	200
Rich Chocolate Almond	1 carton (12 fl oz)	220
Rich Chocolate Almond as prep w/ skim milk	9 fl oz	180
Smooth Vanilla Creme	1 can (10 fl oz)	200
Ultra Slim-Fast		
Cafe Mocha as prep w/ skim milk	8 oz	200
Chocolate Royale as prep w/ skim milk	8 oz	200
Crunch Bar Cocoa Almond	1	110
Crunch Bar Cocoa Raspberry	1	100
Crunch Bar Vanilla Almond	1	110
Dutch Chocolate as prep w/ water	8 oz	220
French Vanilla as prep w/ skim milk	8 oz	190
French Vanilla as prep w/ water	8 oz	220
Fruit Juice Mix as prep w/ fruit juice	8 oz	200
Nutrition Bar Dutch Chocolate	1	130
Pina Colada as prep w/ skim milk	8 oz	180
Ready-To-Drink Chocolate Royale	11 oz	230
Ready-To-Drink Chocolate Royale	12 oz	250
Ready-To-Drink French Vanilla	11 oz	230
Ready-To-Drink French Vanilla	12 oz	220
Ready-To-Drink Strawberry Supreme	12 oz	220
Strawberry Supreme as prep w/ water	8 oz	220
Strawberry as prep w/ skim milk	8 oz	190
REGULAR		
BeneFit		
Chocolate	1 serv	120
Nutrition Bar	1 (2 oz)	240
Vanilla	1 serv	120
Boost		
Chocolate	1 can (8 oz)	240
Vanilla	8 oz	240
Fi-Bar		
Apple	1 (1 oz)	90
Cocoa Almond	1	130
Cocoa Peanut	1	130
Cranberry & Wild Berries	1 (1 oz)	100
Lemon	1 (1 oz)	90
Mandarin Orange	1 (1 oz)	99
Nuggets Almond Cappuccino Crunch	1 pkg	136

FOOD	PORTION	CALS.
Fi-Bar (CONT.)		
Nuggets Almond Butter Crunch	1 pkg	163
Nuggets Coconut Almond Crunch	1 pkg	136
Nuggets Peanut Butter Crunch	1 pkg	160
Raspberry	1 (1 oz)	100
Strawberry	1 (1 oz)	100
Treat Yourself Right Almond	1	152
Treat Yourself Right Peanutty Butter	1	152
Vanilla Almond	1	130
Vanilla Peanut	1	130
Gatorade		
GatorBar	1 (1.17 oz)	110
GatorLode	1 can (11.6 fl oz)	280
GatorPro	1 can (11 fl oz)	360
ReLode	1 pkt (0.75 oz)	80
Gookinaid		
Lemonade	1 cup (8 fl oz)	45
Malsovit		
Mealwafers	2	152
Meal On The Go		
Apple	1 bar (3 oz)	294
Banana w/ Pecans	1 bar (3 oz)	289
Original	1 bar (3 oz)	286
Nutra/Balance		
Frozen Pudding Chocolate	4 oz	225
Frozen Pudding Tapioca	4 oz	225
Frozen Pudding Vanilla	4 oz	225
NutraShake		
Chocolate	4 oz	200
Strawberry	4 oz	200
Vanilla	4 oz	200
With Fiber Vanilla	6 oz	300
Power Bar		
Malt-Nut	1 bar (2.3 oz)	230
Resource		
Fructose Sweetened	1 pkg (8 oz)	250
Fruit Beverage	1 pkg (8 oz)	180
Liquid Food	1 pkg (8 oz)	250
Plus Liquid Food	1 pkg (8 oz)	355
Sustacal		
Vanilla	8 oz	240
Vita-J		
Apple Juice	11.5 fl oz	8
Fruit Punch	11.5 fl oz	8

FOOD	PORTION	CALS.
Vita-J (CONT.)		
Grapefruit Cocktail w/ Raspberry	11.5 fl oz	8
Orange Juice	11.5 fl oz	8

NUTS MIXED
(*see also individual names*)

FOOD	PORTION	CALS.
dry roasted w/ peanuts	1 oz	169
dry roasted w/ peanuts salted	1 oz	169
oil roasted w/ peanuts	1 oz	175
oil roasted w/ peanuts salted	1 oz	175
oil roasted w/o peanuts	1 oz	175
oil roasted w/o peanuts salted	1 oz	175
Fisher		
Mixed Deluxe Lightly Salted	1 oz	180
Mixed Deluxe Salted	1 oz	180
Mixed Oil Roasted 25% More Cashews Lightly Salted	1 oz	180
Mixed Oil Roasted 25% More Cashews Salted	1 oz	180
Nut & Fruit Pina Colada	1 oz	150
Nut & Fruit Raisin Cranberry	1 oz	150
Nut & Fruit Tropical Fruit	1 oz	140
Nut Toppings Oil Roasted With Peanuts	1 oz	190
Peanuts Cashews	1 oz	170
Guy's		
Mixed With Peanuts	1 oz	180
Tasty Mix	1 oz	130
Planters		
Cashews & Peanuts Honey Roasted	1 oz	150
Deluxe Oil Roasted	1 oz	170
Dry Roasted	1 oz	170
Honey Roasted	1 oz	140
Lightly Salted Oil Roasted	1 oz	170
No Brazils Lightly Salted Oil Roasted	1 oz	170
No Brazils Oil Roasted	1 oz	170
Oil Roasted	1 oz	170
Select Mix Cashews Almonds & Macadamias Oil Roasted	1 oz	170
Select Mix Cashews Almonds & Pecans Oil Roasted	1 oz	170
Unsalted Oil Roasted	1 oz	170

OCTOBER BEANS

FOOD	PORTION	CALS.
Luck's		
Seasoned w/ Pork	7.25 oz	230

FOOD	PORTION	CALS.
OCTOPUS		
fresh steamed	3 oz	140
OHELOBERRIES		
fresh	1 cup	39
OIL		
(see also FAT)		
almond	1 cup	1927
almond	1 tbsp	120
apricot kernel	1 cup	1927
apricot kernel	1 tbsp	120
avocado	1 tbsp	124
avocado	1 cup	1927
babassu palm	1 tbsp	120
butter oil	1 cup	1795
butter oil	1 tbsp	112
canola	1 cup	1927
canola	1 tbsp	124
coconut	1 tbsp	117
corn	1 cup	1927
corn	1 tbsp	120
cottonseed	1 cup	1927
cottonseed	1 tbsp	120
cupu assu	1 tbsp	120
grapeseed	1 tbsp	120
hazelnut	1 cup	1927
hazelnut	1 tbsp	120
mustard	1 cup	1927
mustard	1 tbsp	124
oat	1 tbsp	120
olive	1 tbsp	119
olive	1 cup	1909
palm	1 tbsp	120
palm	1 cup	1927
palm kernel	1 tbsp	117
palm kernel	1 cup	1879
peanut	1 cup	1909
peanut	1 tbsp	119
poppyseed	1 tbsp	120
poppyseed	3.5 fl oz	900
pumpkin seed	3½ oz	925
rice bran	1 tbsp	120
safflower	1 cup	1927
safflower	1 tbsp	120

FOOD	PORTION	CALS.
sesame	1 tbsp	120
sheanut	1 tbsp	120
soybean	1 tbsp	120
soybean	1 cup	1927
sunflower	1 tbsp	120
sunflower	1 cup	1927
teaseed	1 tbsp	120
tomatoseed	1 tbsp	120
vegetable soybean & cottonseed	1 tbsp	120
vegetable soybean & cottonseed	1 cup	1927
walnut	1 tbsp	120
walnut	1 cup	1927
wheat germ	1 tbsp	120
Arrowhead		
Flax Seed	1 tbsp (0.5 fl oz)	120
Hazelnut	1 tbsp (0.5 fl oz)	120
Bertolli		
Classico	1 tbsp	120
Extra Light	1 tbsp	120
Extra Virgin	1 tbsp	120
Crisco		
Corn Canola	1 tbsp (0.5 fl oz)	120
Oil	1 tbsp (0.5 fl oz)	120
Puritan Canola	1 tbsp (0.5 fl oz)	120
Eden		
Hot Pepper Sesame	1 tbsp (0.5 oz)	130
Toasted Sesame	1 tbsp (0.5 oz)	130
Hain		
All Blend	1 tbsp	120
Almond	1 tbsp	120
Apricot Kernel	1 tbsp	120
Avocado	1 tbsp	120
Canola	1 tbsp	120
Canola Organic	1 tbsp	120
Coconut	1 tbsp	120
Corn	1 tbsp	120
Garlic & Oil	1 tbsp	120
Olive	1 tbsp	120
Peanut	1 tbsp	120
Rice Bran	1 tbsp	120
Safflower	1 tbsp	120
Safflower Hi-Oleic	1 tbsp	120
Safflower Organic	1 tbsp	120
Sesame	1 tbsp	120

FOOD	PORTION	CALS.
Hain (CONT.)		
Soy	1 tbsp	120
Sunflower	1 tbsp	120
Sunflower Organic	1 tbsp	120
Walnut	1 tbsp	120
Hollywood		
Canola	1 tbsp	120
Peanut	1 tbsp	120
Safflower	1 tbsp	120
Soy	1 tbsp	120
Sunflower	1 tbsp	120
House Of Tsang		
Hot Chili Sesame	1 tsp (5 g)	45
Mongolian Fire	1 tsp (5 g)	45
Pure Sesame	1 tsp (5 g)	45
Singapore Curry	1 tsp (5 g)	45
Wok Oil	1 tbsp (0.5 oz)	130
Italica		
Olive Oil	1 tbsp	120
Ka-Me		
Chili Hot	1 tbsp (0.5 fl oz)	130
Sesame	1 tbsp (0.5 fl oz)	130
Sesame Tempura	1 tbsp (0.5 fl oz)	130
Mazola		
No Stick	2.5 second spray (0.2 g)	2
Oil	1 tbsp (14 g)	120
Oil	1 cup (221 g)	1955
Orville Redenbacher's		
Oil	1 tbsp	120
Pam		
Butter	1 sec spray (0.266 g)	2
Cooking Spray	1 sec spray (0.266 g)	2
Olive Oil	1 sec spray (0.266 g)	2
Pump	1 spray (0.43 g)	4
Planters		
Peanut	1 tbsp (0.5 oz)	120
Popcorn	1 tbsp (0.5 oz)	120
Pompeian		
Olive	1 tbsp	130
Progresso		
Olive Extra Light	1 tbsp	119
Olive Extra Mild	1 tbsp (0.5 oz)	120
Olive Extra Virgin	1 tbsp (0.5 oz)	120
Olive Riviera Blend	1 tbsp (0.5 oz)	120

FOOD	PORTION	CALS.
Smart Beat		
Canola	1 tbsp (14 g)	120
Oil	1 tbsp	120
Tree Of Life		
Almond	1 tbsp (0.5 g)	130
Apricot Kernel	1 tbsp (0.5 g)	130
Avocado	1 tbsp (0.5 g)	130
Macadamia Nut	1 tbsp (0.5 g)	130
Olive Extra Virgin Organic	1 tbsp (0.5 g)	130
Sesame	1 tbsp (0.5 g)	130
Toasted Sesame	1 tbsp (0.5 oz)	130
Weight Watchers		
Butter Spray	⅓ second spray	0
Cooking Spray	⅓ second spray	0
Wesson		
Canola	1 tbsp	120
Cooking Spray Lite	0.5 sec spray	0
Corn	1 tbsp	120
Olive	1 tbsp	120
Sunflower	1 tbsp	120
Vegetable	1 tbsp	120
FISH OIL		
cod liver	1 tbsp	123
herring	1 tbsp	123
menhaden	1 tbsp	123
salmon	1 tbsp	123
sardine	1 tbsp	123
shark	3½ oz	945
whale	3½ oz	945
Hain		
Cod Liver	1 tbsp	120
Cod Liver Cherry	1 tbsp	120
Cod Liver Mint	1 tbsp	120
OKRA		
CANNED		
Allen		
Cut	½ cup (4.4 oz)	25
McIlhenny		
Pickled	2 pieces (1 oz)	7
Trappey		
Cocktail Hot	2 pieces (1 oz)	8
Cocktail Mild	1 piece (1 oz)	9
Creole Gumbo	½ cup (4.2 oz)	35

FOOD	PORTION	CALS.
Trappey (CONT.)		
Cut	½ cup (4.4 oz)	25
FRESH		
raw	8 pods	36
raw sliced	½ cup	19
sliced cooked	½ cup	25
sliced cooked	8 pods	27
FROZEN		
sliced cooked	1 pkg (10 oz)	94
sliced cooked	½ cup	34
Fresh Like		
Cut	3.5 oz	26
Whole	3.5 oz	32
Hanover		
Cut	½ cup	25
Whole	½ cup	35
OLIVES		
green	3 extra lg	15
green	4 med	15
ripe	1 sm	4
ripe	1 lg	5
ripe	1 jumbo	7
ripe	1 colossal	12
California		
Ripe	3 sm	4
Ripe	2 jumbo	188
Progresso		
Oil Cured	6 (0.5 oz)	80
Olive Salad (drained)	2 tbsp (0.8 oz)	25
S&W		
Ripe Extra Large	3.5 oz	163
Ripe Pitted Large	3.5 oz	163
Tee Pee		
Spanish Green	2 oz	98
ONION		
CANNED		
chopped	½ cup	21
whole	1 (2.2 oz)	12
S&W		
Whole Small	½ cup	35
Vlasic		
Lightly Spiced Cocktail Onions	1 oz	4

FOOD	PORTION	CALS.
Watkins		
Liquid Spice	1 tbsp (0.5 oz)	120
DRIED		
flakes	1 tbsp	16
powder	1 tsp	7
Watkins		
Flakes	¼ tsp (1 g)	0
FRESH		
chopped cooked	½ cup	47
raw chopped	1 tbsp	4
raw chopped	½ cup	30
scallions raw chopped	1 tbsp	2
scallions raw sliced	½ cup	16
welsh raw	3½ oz	34
Antioch Farms		
Vidalia	1 med	60
Dole		
Green Chopped	1 tbsp	2
Medium	1	60
FROZEN		
chopped cooked	½ cup	30
chopped cooked	1 tbsp	4
rings	7 (2.5 oz)	285
rings cooked	2 (0.7 oz)	81
whole cooked	3½ oz	28
Birds Eye		
Polybag Whole Small	½ cup	30
Small With Cream Sauce	½ cup	100
Fresh Like		
Diced	3.5 oz	29
Whole	3.5 oz	37
Kineret		
Rings	6 (3 oz)	200
Mrs. Paul's		
Crispy Onion Rings	2½ oz	190
Ore Ida		
Chopped	¾ cup (3 oz)	25
Onion Ringers	6 pieces (3 oz)	240
Southland		
Chopped	2 oz	15
TAKE-OUT		
fried	½ cup (7.5 oz)	176
rings breaded & fried	8 to 9	275

FOOD	PORTION	CALS.
OPOSSUM		
roasted	3 oz	188
ORANGE		
CANNED		
Del Monte		
Mandarin In Heavy Syrup	½ cup (4.4 oz)	80
Dole		
Mandarin Segments	½ cup	70
Pineapple Mandarin Segments	½ cup	80
Empress		
Mandarin	5.5 oz	100
Mandarin From Japan	5.5 oz	35
S&W		
Mandarin Natural Style	½ cup	60
Mandarin Selected Sections in Heavy Syrup	½ cup	76
Mandarin Unsweetened	½ cup	28
FRESH		
california valencia	1	59
florida	1	69
peel	1 tbsp	6
sections	1 cup	85
Dole		
Orange	1	50
ORANGE EXTRACT		
Virginia Dare	1 tsp	22
ORANGE JUICE		
canned	1 cup	104
chilled	1 cup	110
fresh	1 cup	111
frzn as prep	1 cup	112
frzn not prep	6 oz	339
mandarin orange	3½ oz	47
orange drink	6 oz	94
After The Fall		
Juice	1 bottle (10 oz)	110
Bright & Early		
Chilled	8 fl oz	120
Frozen	8 fl oz	120
Del Monte		
Juice	8 fl oz	110
Hawaiian Punch		
Drink	6 oz	100

FOOD	PORTION	CALS.
Hi-C		
Box	8.45 fl oz	130
Drink	8 fl oz	130
Drink	1 can (11.5 oz)	180
Hood		
From Concentrate	1 cup (8 oz)	120
Select	1 cup (8 oz)	120
With Calcium	1 cup (8 oz)	120
Juice Works		
Drink	6 oz	90
Kool-Aid		
Drink	8 oz	98
Koolers	1 (8.45 oz)	115
Sugar Sweetened	8 oz	79
Libby		
Juice	6 fl oz	80
Minute Maid		
Box	8.45 fl oz	120
Calcium Rich Chilled	8 fl oz	120
Calcium Rich frzn	8 fl oz	120
Chilled	8 fl oz	110
Country Style Chilled	8 fl oz	110
Country Style frzn	8 fl oz	110
Juices To Go	1 can (11.5 fl oz)	160
Juices To Go	1 bottle (16 fl oz)	110
Juices To Go	1 bottle (10 fl oz)	140
Orange Punch Box	8.45 fl oz	130
Premium Choice Chilled	8 fl oz	110
Pulp Free Chilled	8 fl oz	110
Pulp Free frzn	8 fl oz	110
Reduced Acid frzn	8 fl oz	110
Mott's		
From Concentrate	10 fl oz	130
Ocean Spray		
Juice	8 fl oz	120
Odwalla		
Juice	8 fl oz	110
S&W		
100% Unsweetened	6 oz	83
Sippin' Pak		
100% Pure	8.45 fl oz	110
Snapple		
Juice	10 fl oz	130
Orangeade	8 fl oz	120

FOOD	PORTION	CALS.
Tang		
Breakfast Crystals Sugar Free as prep	6 oz	5
Breakfast Crystals as prep	6 oz	86
Fruit Box	8.45 oz	127
Tropical Orange	8.45 fl oz	146
Tree Of Life		
Juice	8 fl oz	110
Tree Top		
Juice	6 oz	90
Tropicana		
Frozen as prep	6 fl oz	110
Juice	1 container (8 fl oz)	110
Juice	1 container (6 fl oz)	80
Juice	1 container (10 fl oz)	130
Juice	8 fl oz	110
Season's Best	1 bottle (7 fl oz)	90
Season's Best	1 can (11.5 fl oz)	140
Season's Best	8 fl oz	110
Season's Best	1 bottle (10 fl oz)	130
Season's Best Calcium	8 fl oz	110
Season's Best Homestyle	8 fl oz	110
Season's Best Vitamin	8 fl oz	110
Veryfine		
100%	8 oz	121
Orange Drink	8 oz	140

OREGANO

ground	1 tsp	5
Watkins		
Liquid Spice	1 tbsp (0.5 oz)	120

ORGAN MEATS

(*see* BRAINS, GIBLETS, GIZZARD, HEART, KIDNEY, LIVER, SWEETBREADS)

ORIENTAL FOOD

(*see also* EGG ROLLS, DINNER, NOODLES, RICE)

CANNED

chow mein chicken	1 cup	95
La Choy		
Bi-Pack Beef Pepper	¾ cup	80
Bi-Pack Chow Mein Chicken	¾ cup	80
Bi-Pack Chow Mein Pork	¾ cup	80
Bi-Pack Chow Mein Shrimp	¾ cup	70
Bi-Pack Sweet & Sour Chicken	¾ cup	120
Bi-Pack Teriyaki Chicken	¾ cup	85

FOOD	PORTION	CALS.
La Choy (CONT.)		
Dinner Chow Mein Chicken	¾ pkg	300
Entree Beef Pepper Oriental	¾ cup	100
Entree Chow Mein Beef	¾ cup	40
Entree Chow Mein Chicken	¾ cup	70
Entree Chow Mein Meatless	¾ cup	25
Entree Chow Mein Shrimp	¾ cup	35
Entree Sweet & Sour Chicken	¾ cup	240
Entree Sweet & Sour Pork	¾ cup	250
FRESH		
wonton wrappers	1	23
Azumaya		
Won Ton Wraps	1 (8 g)	23
FROZEN		
Banquet		
Chow Mein Chicken	1 pkg (9 oz)	400
Birds Eye		
Easy Recipe Chicken Teriyaki not prep	½ pkg	160
Easy Recipe Oriental Beef not prep	½ pkg	100
Internationals Chinese Stir Fry not prep	3.3 oz	35
Japanese Stir Fry International not prep	3.3 oz	30
Chun King		
Beef Pepper Steak	1 pkg (13 oz)	300
Chow Mein Chicken	1 pkg (13 oz)	370
Imperial Chicken	1 pkg (13 oz)	460
Sweet & Sour Pork	1 pkg (13 oz)	450
Walnut Chicken	1 pkg (13 oz)	460
Lean Cuisine		
Chicken Chow Mein With Rice	1 meal (9 oz)	210
Luigino's		
Chicken & Almonds With Rice	1 pkg (8 oz)	250
Chop Suey Pork With Rice	1 pkg (8.5 oz)	210
Lo Mein Chicken	1 pkg (8 oz)	320
Lo Mein Shrimp	1 pkg (8 oz)	190
Oriental Beef & Peppers With Rice	1 pkg (8 oz)	230
Pasta Favorites		
Chicken Lo Mein	1 pkg (10.5 oz)	270
Rice Gourmet		
Chicken Teriyaki Rice Bowl	1 bowl (10.9 oz)	430
Stouffer's		
Chicken Chow Mein With Rice	1 pkg (10.6 oz)	260
Chicken Oriental	1 pkg (9.75 oz)	320
Stir-Fry Teriyaki	1 pkg (9 oz)	260

FOOD	PORTION	CALS.
Tyson		
Stir Fry Kit With Yoshida Oriental Sauce	10.6 oz	330
Sweet & Sour Kit With Sweet & Sour Sauce	14.85 oz	440
Weight Watchers		
Chicken Chow Mein	1 pkg (9 oz)	200
MIX		
Kikkoman		
Chow Mein Seasoning	1⅛ oz pkg	98
Teriyaki Baste & Glaze	1 tbsp	24
La Choy		
Dinner Classics Egg Foo Young	2 patties + 3 oz sauce	170
Dinner Classics Sweet & Sour	¾ cup	310
TAKE-OUT		
chicken teriyaki	¾ cup	399
chicken teriyaki w/ rice	1 serv (11 oz)	430
chop suey w/ beef & pork	1 cup	300
chop suey w/ pork	1 cup	375
chow mein chicken	1 cup	255
chow mein pork	1 cup	425
chow mein shrimp	1 cup	221
chow mein vegetable	1 serv (8 oz)	90
fried rice	6.6 oz	249
fried rice w/ egg	6.7 oz	395
oriental pepper & beef	1 serv (8 oz)	90
spring roll deep fried	3.5 oz	202
sweet & sour pork	1 serv (8 oz)	250
wonton fried	½ cup (1 oz)	111
wonton soup	1 cup	205

OYSTERS

CANNED		
eastern	3 oz	58
eastern	1 cup	170
Bumble Bee		
Whole	½ cup (3.5 oz)	100
Empress		
Whole	4 oz	100
S&W		
Fancy Whole	2 oz	95
FRESH		
eastern cooked	3 oz	117
eastern cooked	6 med	58
eastern raw	1 cup	170

FOOD	PORTION	CALS.
eastern raw	6 med	58
pacific raw	3 oz	69
pacific raw	1 med	41
steamed	3 oz	138
steamed	1 med	41
TAKE-OUT		
battered & fried	6 (4.9 oz)	368
breaded & fried	6 (4.9 oz)	368
eastern breaded & fried	6 med (88 g)	173
eastern breaded & fried	3 oz	167
oysters rockefeller	3 oysters	66
stew	1 cup	278

PANCAKE/WAFFLE SYRUP
(see also SYRUP)

FOOD	PORTION	CALS.
low calorie	1 tbsp	12
maple	2 tbsp	122
maple	1 cup (11.1 oz)	824
maple	1 tbsp (0.8 oz)	52
pancake syrup	1 tbsp (0.7 oz)	57
pancake syrup	1 cup (11 oz)	903
pancake syrup light	1 oz	46
pancake syrup w/ butter	1 tbsp (0.7 oz)	59
pancake syrup w/ butter	1 cup (11 oz)	933
Alaga		
Breakfast	2 tbsp	108
Butter Lite	2 tbsp	54
Honey Flavored	2 tbsp	124
Lite	2 tbsp	54
Aunt Jemima		
Butter Rich	¼ cup (2.8 oz)	210
Butterlite	¼ cup (2.5 oz)	100
Lite	¼ cup (2.5 oz)	100
Syrup	¼ cup (2.8 oz)	210
Brer Rabbit		
Dark	2 tbsp	120
Light	2 Tbsp	120
Estee		
Lite Maple	¼ cup (2.4 oz)	80
Golden Griddle		
Syrup	1 tbsp (20 g)	50
Syrup	1 cup (321 g)	885
Karo		
Syrup	1 tbsp (21 g)	60

FOOD	PORTION	CALS.
Log Cabin		
Country Kitchen	1 oz	103
Lite	1 oz	49
Mrs.Richardson's		
Lite	¼ cup (2.5 oz)	100
Original Recipe	¼ cup (2.8 oz)	210
Red Wing		
Lite	¼ cup (2 oz)	100
Syrup	¼ cup (2 oz)	210
Tastee		
Maple	2 tbsp	113
Syrup	2 tbsp	121
Tree Of Life		
Maple	¼ cup (2.1 oz)	200
Whitfield		
White Label	2 tbsp	121
Yellow Label	2 tbsp	125
Yellow Label Butter Flavor	2 tbsp	117
Yellow Label Maple Flavor	2 tbsp	117

PANCAKES

FROZEN

FOOD	PORTION	CALS.
buttermilk	1, 4 in diam (1.3 oz)	83
plain	1, 4 in diam (1.3 oz)	83
Aunt Jemima		
Blueberry	3 (3.4 oz)	210
Buttermilk	3 (3 oz)	180
Lowfat	3 (3.4 oz)	130
Original	3 (3.4 oz)	200
Downyflake		
Blueberry	3	290
Buttermilk	3	280
Pancakes And Sausages	1 pkg (5.5 oz)	430
Regular	3	280
Great Starts		
Pancakes And Sausages	6 oz	460
Pancakes With Bacon	4½ oz	400
Silver Dollar Pancakes And Sausage	3¾ oz	310
Whole Wheat Pancakes With Lite Links	5½ oz	350
Healthy Starts		
Pancakes w/ LeanLinks	6 oz	360
Jimmy Dean		
Flapstick	1 (2.5 oz)	240
Flapstick Blueberry	1 (2.5 oz)	260

FOOD	PORTION	CALS.
Morningstar Farms		
Pancakes/Links	1 pkg (4 oz)	240
Pillsbury		
Buttermilk Microwave	3	260
Harvest Wheat Microwave	3	240
Microwave	3	250
Original Microwave	3	240
Quaker		
Lite Pancakes & Lite Links	1 pkg (6 oz)	310
Lite Pancakes & Lite Syrup	1 pkg (6 oz)	260
Pancakes & Sausages	1 pkg (6 oz)	420
Weight Watchers		
Buttermilk	2 (2.5 oz)	140
HOME RECIPE		
blueberry	1 (4 in diam)	84
plain	1 (4 in diam)	86
MIX		
buckwheat	1 (4 in diam)	62
buttermilk	1, 4 in diam (1.3 oz)	74
plain	1, 4 in diam (1.3 oz)	74
sugar free low sodium	1 (3 in diam)	44
whole wheat	1 (4 in diam)	92
Arrowhead		
Multigrain Pancake & Waffle Mix	¼ cup (1.2 oz)	120
Aunt Jemima		
Buckwheat Pancake & Waffle Mix	¼ cup (1.4 oz)	120
Buttermilk Pancake & Waffle Mix	⅓ cup (1.9 oz)	190
Original Pancake & Waffle Mix	⅓ cup (1.6 oz)	150
Pancake & Waffle Mix Regular	⅓ cup (1.9 oz)	190
Pancake & Waffle Mix Whole Wheat	¼ cup (1.4 oz)	130
Betty Crocker		
Buttermilk	3 (4 in diam)	280
Bisquick		
Apple Cinnamon Shake 'N Pour	3 (4 in diam)	240
Blueberry Shake 'N Pour	3 (4 in diam)	270
Buttermilk Shake 'N Pour	3 (4 in diam)	250
Original Shake 'N Pour	3 (4 in diam)	250
Estee		
Pancake Mix Fat Free as prep	4 (4 in diam)	180
Fast Shake		
Blueberry	1 serv (2.5 oz)	251
Buttermilk	1 serv (2.5 oz)	258
Original	1 serv (2.5 oz)	266

FOOD	PORTION	CALS.
Health Valley		
Pancake Mix not prep	1 oz	100
Hodgson Mill		
Buckwheat	⅓ cup (1.8 oz)	160
Hungry Jack		
Bluberry	3 (4 in diam)	320
Buttermilk	3 (4 in diam)	240
Buttermilk Complete	3 (4 in diam)	180
Buttermilk Complete Packets	3 (4 in diam)	180
Extra Lights	3 (4 in diam)	210
Extra Lights Complete	3 (4 in diam)	190
Panshakes	3 (4 in diam)	250
Stone-Buhr		
Buckwheat	¼ cup (1.4 oz)	130
Oat Bran	¼ cup (1.4 oz)	130
Whole Wheat	¼ cup (1.4 oz)	120
Wanda's		
Blue Corn	⅓ cup mix per serv (1.7 oz)	170
TAKE-OUT		
buckwheat	1 (4 in diam)	55
potato	1 (4 in diam)	78
w/ butter & syrup	3	519

PANCREAS
(*see* SWEETBREADS)

PAPAYA
CANNED
Ka-Me

Papaya	¾ cup	120
DRIED		
Sonoma		
Pieces	2 pieces (2 oz)	200
FRESH		
cubed	1 cup	54
papaya	1	117

PAPAYA JUICE

nectar	1 cup	142
Goya		
Nectar	6 oz	110
Kern's		
Nectar	6 fl oz	110
Libby		
Nectar	1 can (11.5 fl oz)	210

FOOD	PORTION	CALS.
PAPRIKA		
paprika	1 tsp	6
Watkins		
Ground	¼ tsp (0.5 oz)	0
PARSLEY		
dry	1 tsp	1
dry	1 tbsp	1
fresh chopped	½ cup	11
Dole		
Chopped	1 tbsp	10
PARSNIPS		
fresh cooked	1 (5.6 oz)	130
fresh sliced cooked	½ cup	63
raw sliced	½ cup	50
PASSION FRUIT		
purple fresh	1	18
PASSION FRUIT JUICE		
purple	1 cup	126
yellow	1 cup	149
Snapple		
Passion Supreme	10 fl oz	160
PASTA		
(*see also* NOODLES, PASTA DINNERS, PASTA SALAD)		
DRY		
corn cooked	1 cup	176
elbows	1 cup	389
elbows cooked	1 cup	197
protein fortified cooked	1 cup	188
shells	1 cup	389
shells cooked	1 cup	197
spaghetti	2 oz	211
spaghetti cooked	1 cup	197
spaghetti protein fortified cooked	1 cup	229
spinach spaghetti	2 oz	212
spinach spaghetti cooked	1 cup	183
spirals	1 cup	389
spirals cooked	1 cup	197
vegetable	1 cup	308
vegetable cooked	1 cup	171
whole wheat	1 cup	365
whole wheat cooked	1 cup (4.9 oz)	174

FOOD	PORTION	CALS.
whole wheat spaghetti	2 oz	198
whole wheat spaghetti cooked	1 cup	174
Anthony		
Pasta	2 oz	210
Bella Via		
Angel Hair	2 oz	200
Artichoke Angel Hair as prep	⅝ cup	200
Artichoke Spaghetti as prep	⅝ cup	200
Elbows	2 oz	200
Fettucini as prep	⅝ cup	200
Linguini	2 oz	200
Penne as prep	⅝ cup	200
Rotelli	2 oz	200
Shells	2 oz	200
Spaghetti	2 oz	200
Ziti	2 oz	200
Classico		
Gnocchi Di Toscana	1 cup (2 oz)	210
Creamette		
Elbow Macaroni not prep	2 oz	210
Linguini Egg	2 oz	221
Rotelle	2 oz	210
Rotini Rainbow	2 oz	210
Spaghetti Egg	2 oz	221
Spaghetti Thin	2 oz	210
Spaghetti not prep	2 oz	210
Spinach Ribbons not prep	2 oz	210
Ziti	2 oz	210
De Bole's		
Whole Wheat Organic Elbows	2 oz	210
DeFino		
Lasagna No Boil	1 oz	102
Ribbons No Boil	2 oz	204
Delverde		
Spaghetti Whole Wheat	2 oz	206
Eden		
Elbows Whole Wheat Organic	2 oz	210
Elbows Whole Wheat Vegetable Organic	2 oz	210
Kudzu And Sweet Potato Pasta	2 oz	190
Kudzu Kiri Pasta	2 oz	190
Mung Bean Pasta Harusame	2 oz	190
Ribbons Durum Wheat Curry Organic	2 oz	220
Ribbons Durum Wheat Organic	2 oz	220
Ribbons Durum Wheat Paella Organic	2 oz	220

FOOD	PORTION	CALS.
Eden (CONT.)		
Ribbons Durum Wheat Parsley Garlic Organic	2 oz	220
Ribbons Durum Wheat Pesto Organic	2 oz	220
Ribbons Whole Wheat Spinach Organic	2 oz	200
Rice Pasta Bifun	2 oz	200
Shells Durum Wheat Vegetable Organic	2 oz	210
Soba 100% Buckwheat	2 oz	200
Soba 40% Buckwheat	2 oz	190
Soba Lotus Root	2 oz	190
Soba Mugwort	2 oz	190
Soba Wild Yam Jinenjo	2 oz	190
Spaghetti Durum Wheat Organic	2 oz	210
Spaghetti Kamut Organic	2 oz	210
Spaghetti Pasley Garlic Organic	2 oz	210
Spaghetti Whole Wheat Organic	2 oz	210
Spirals Durum Wheat Vegetable Organic	2 oz	210
Spirals Kamut Organic	2 oz	210
Spirals Sesame Rice Organic	2 oz	200
Spirals Whole Wheat Vegetable Organic	2 oz	210
Udon	2 oz	190
Udon Brown Rice	2 oz	190
Gioia		
Pasta	2 oz	210
Golden Grain		
Pasta	2 oz	203
Hanover		
Spaghetti Wheels	½ cup	90
Health Valley		
Lasagna Whole Wheat	2 oz	170
Lasagna Spinach Whole Wheat	2 oz	170
Spagehetti Amaranth	2 oz	170
Spaghetti Oat Bran	2 oz	120
Spaghetti Spinach Whole Wheat	2 oz	170
Spaghetti Whole Wheat	2 oz	170
Hodgson Mill		
Spaghetti Whole Wheat Spinach not prep	2 oz	190
Veggie Bows not prep	2 oz	200
Veggie Rotini not prep	2 oz	200
Veggie Wagon Wheels not prep	2 oz	200
Whole Wheat Spirals not prep	2 oz	190
La Molisana		
Radiatori	2 oz	230

FOOD	PORTION	CALS.
Lupini		
Elbow uncooked	½ cup (2 oz)	190
Spaghetti Light uncooked	½ cup (2 oz)	190
Spaghetti With Triticale	1/7 pkg (2 oz)	190
Luxury		
Pasta	2 oz	210
Merlino's		
Pasta	2 oz	210
Mueller's		
Dinosaurs	2 oz (57 g)	210
Jungle Animals	2 oz (57 g)	210
Lasagne	2 oz (57 g)	210
Monsters	2 oz (57 g)	210
Outer Space	2 oz	210
Spaghetti	2 oz (57 g)	210
Teddy Bears	2 oz (57 g)	210
Twists Tri Color	2 oz (57 g)	210
Noodles By Leonardo		
Capellini	2 oz	200
Elbows not prep	½ cup (2 oz)	200
Fettucini	2 oz	200
Linguine not prep	½ cup (2 oz)	200
Rigatoni	2 oz	200
Rotini	2 oz	200
Shells not prep	½ cup (2 oz)	200
Spaghetti not prep	½ cup (2 oz)	200
Spaghettini	2 oz	200
Vermicelli not prep	½ cup (2 oz)	200
Penn Dutch		
Pasta	2 oz	210
Pomi		
Capellini	2 oz	210
Prince		
Egg	2 oz	221
Pasta	2 oz	210
Rainbow	2 oz	210
Spinach Egg	2 oz	220
Pritikin		
Spaghetti Whole Wheat	⅛ box (2 oz)	190
Spiral	⅔ cup (2 oz)	190
Red Cross		
Pasta	2 oz	210
Ronco		
Pasta	2 oz	210

FOOD	PORTION	CALS.
Ronzoni		
Elbows	¾ cup (2 oz)	210
Fettucini	¾ cup (2 oz)	210
Fusilli	¾ cup (2 oz)	210
Lasagne	¾ cup (2 oz)	210
Manicotti	¾ cup (2 oz)	210
Mostaccioli	¾ cup (2 oz)	210
Rigatoni	¾ cup (2 oz)	210
Rotelle uncooked	¾ cup (2 oz)	210
Rotini uncooked	¾ cup (2 oz)	210
Shells uncooked	¾ cup (2 oz)	210
Shells Jumbo	¾ cup (2 oz)	210
Spaghetti not prep	¾ cup (2 oz)	210
Tubettini	¾ cup (2 oz)	210
San Giorgio		
Bowties Egg	2 oz	210
Capellini	2 oz	210
Elbow Macaroni	2 oz	210
Fettuccine Egg	2 oz	210
Fettuccini Florentine	2 oz	210
Lasagne	2 oz	210
Linguini	2 oz	210
Manicotti	2 oz	210
Mostaccioli Rigati	2 oz	210
Rigatoni	2 oz	210
Rotini	2 oz	210
Shells	2 oz	210
Spaghetti	2 oz	210
Spaghetti Thin	2 oz	210
Vermicelli	2 oz	210
Ziti Cut	2 oz	210
Tree Of Life		
Cajun as prep	⅝ cup (4.9 oz)	200
Confetti as prep	⅝ cup (4.9 oz)	200
Garlic & Parsley as prep	⅝ cup (4.9 oz)	200
Jamaican Spice as prep	⅝ cup (4.9 oz)	200
Lemon Pepper as prep	⅝ cup (4.9 oz)	200
Spinach as prep	⅝ cup (4.9 oz)	200
Tex Mex as prep	⅝ cup (4.9 oz)	200
Thai as prep	⅝ cup (4.9 oz)	200
Tomato Basil as prep	⅝ cup (4.9 oz)	200
Vimco		
Pasta	2 oz	210

FOOD	PORTION	CALS.
FRESH		
plain made w/ egg cooked	2 oz	75
spinach made w/ egg cooked	2 oz	74
Contadina		
Angel's Hair	1¼ cup (2.8 oz)	240
Fettuccine	1¼ cup (2.9 oz)	250
Fettuccine Cholesterol Free	1 cup (2.9 oz)	240
Light Ravioli Cheese	1 cup (3.1 oz)	240
Light Ravioli Garden Vegetable	1¼ cup (3.8 oz)	290
Light Tortellini Garlic & Cheese	1 cup (3.6 oz)	280
Linguine	1¼ cup (3 oz)	260
Linguine Cholesterol Free	1¼ cup (3.1 oz)	250
Ravioli Beef And Garlic	1¼ cup (4 oz)	350
Ravioli Cheese	1 cup (3.1 oz)	280
Ravioli Chicken And Rosemary	1¼ cup (4 oz)	330
Tagliatelli Spinach	1¼ cup (3.1 oz)	270
Tortelloni Cheese	¾ cup (3 oz)	260
Tortelloni Cheese And Basil	1 cup (4 oz)	360
Tortelloni Chicken And Prosciutto	1 cup (3.8 oz)	360
Tortelloni Chicken And Vegetable	¾ cup (2.9 oz)	260
Tortelloni Spicy Italian Sausage And Bell Pepper	1 cup (3.6 oz)	330
Di Giorno		
Angel's Hair	2 oz	160
Fettuccine	2.5 oz	190
Fettuccine Spinach	2.5 oz	190
Linguine	2.5 oz	190
Linguine Herb	2.5 oz	190
Ravioli Italian Herb Cheese	1 cup (3.8 oz)	350
Ravioli Light Cheese & Garlic	1 cup (3.7 oz)	270
Ravioli Light Tomato & Cheese	1 cup (3.7 oz)	280
Ravioli With Italian Sausage	¾ cup (3.6 oz)	340
Tortellini Cheese	¾ cup (2.8 oz)	260
Tortellini Mozzarella Garlic	1 cup (3.5 oz)	300
Tortellini Mushroom	1 cup (3.4 oz)	290
Tortellini Red Hot Pepper Cheese	1 cup (3.4 oz)	310
Tortellini With Chicken And Herbs	1 cup (3.2 oz)	260
Tortellini With Meat	¾ cup (3.1 oz)	290
Herb's		
Fettucine Bell Pepper Basil	2 oz	220
Fettucine Parsley Garlic	2 oz	220
Fettucine Spinach	2 oz	220
Ribbons Vegetable	2 oz	220
Ribbons Whole Wheat	2 oz	200

FOOD	PORTION	CALS.
Herb's (CONT.)		
Rotini Mixed Vegetable	2 oz	210
Shells Mixed Vegetable	2 oz	210
Trios		
Ravioli Cracked Pepper Garlic Cheese	1 cup (4.3 oz)	340
HOME RECIPE		
made w/ egg cooked	2 oz	74
made w/o egg cooked	2 oz	71

PASTA DINNERS
(*see also* DINNER, PASTA SALAD)
CANNED
Chef Boyardee		
ABC's & 1,2,3's In Cheese Flavor Sauce	7.5 oz	180
ABC's & 1,2,3's w/ Mini Meatballs	7.5 oz	260
Beef Ravioli	7.5 oz	190
Beefaroni	7.5 oz	220
Cheese Ravioli In Meat Sauce	7.5 oz	200
Dinosaurs In Cheese Flavor Sauce	7.5 oz	180
Dinosaurs w/ Meatballs	7.5 oz	240
Elbows In Beef Sauce	7.5 oz	210
Lasagna	7.5 oz	230
Lasagna In Garden Vegetable Sauce	7.5 oz	170
Macaroni & Cheese	7.5 oz	180
Pasta Rings & Meatballs	7.5 oz	220
Rigatoni	7.5 oz	210
Rings & Franks	7.5 oz	190
Shells In Mushroom Sauce	7.5 oz	170
Spaghetti & Meat Balls	7.5 oz	230
Tic Tac Toes In Cheese Flavor Sauce	7.5 oz	170
Tic Tac Toes w/ Mini Meatballs	7.5 oz	250
Turtles In Sauce	7.5 oz	160
Turtles w/ Meatballs	7.5 oz	210
Franco-American		
Beef RavioliO's In Meat Sauce	½ can (7½ oz)	250
CircusO's Pasta In Tomato & Cheese Sauce	½ can (7⅜ oz)	170
CircusO's Pasta With Meatballs In Tomato Sauce	½ can (7⅜ oz)	210
Macaroni & Cheese	½ can (7⅜ oz)	170
Spaghetti In Tomato Sauce w/ Cheese	½ can (7⅜ oz)	180
Spaghetti w/ Meatballs In Tomato Sauce	½ can (7⅜ oz)	220
SpaghettiO's With Meatballs	½ can (7⅜ oz)	220
SpaghettiO's In Tomato & Cheese Sauce	½ can (7⅜ oz)	170

FOOD	PORTION	CALS.
Franco-American (CONT.)		
SportyO's In Tomato & Cheese Sauce	½ can (7½ oz)	170
SportyO's Pasta With Meatballs In Tomato Sauce	½ can (7⅜ oz)	210
TeddyO's In Tomato & Cheese Sauce	½ can (7½ oz)	170
TeddyO's Pasta With Meatballs	½ can (7⅜ oz)	210
Hormel		
Lasagna	1 can (7.5 oz)	250
Spaghetti & Meatballs	1 can (7.5 oz)	210
Kid's Kitchen		
Cheezy Mac & Beef	1 cup (7.5 oz)	250
Noodle Rings & Chicken	1 cup (7.5 oz)	150
Spaghetti Rings & Franks	1 cup (7.5 oz)	230
Progresso		
Beef Ravioli	1 cup (9.1 oz)	260
Cheese Ravioli	1 cup (9.1 oz)	220
Van Camp's		
Spaghetti Weenee	1 can (8 oz)	230
FROZEN		
Armour		
Classics Chicken Fettucini	1 meal (10 oz)	230
Banquet		
Family Entree Lasagna w/ Meat Sauce	1 serv (8 oz)	240
Family Entree Macaroni & Cheese	1 serv (8 oz)	300
Family Entree Noodles & Beef	1 serv (7.47 oz)	140
Birds Eye		
Easy Recipe Chicken Primavera not prep	½ pkg	80
Budget Gourmet		
Cheese Ravioli	1 meal (9.5 oz)	290
Lasagna Italian Sausage	1 meal (10 oz)	430
Lasagna Vegetable	1 meal (10.5 oz)	390
Lasagne Three Cheese	1 meal (10 oz)	390
Lasagne With Meat Sauce	1 meal (9.4 oz)	290
Linguini With Shrimp & Clams	1 meal (9.5 oz)	280
Linguini With Shrimp And Clams	1 meal (10 oz)	270
Macaroni & Cheese With Cheddar & Parmesan	1 meal (10.5 oz)	330
Mainicotti Cheese	1 meal (10 oz)	440
Pasta Alfredo With Broccoli	1 meal (5.5 oz)	210
Penne Pasta With Chunky Tomato Sauce & Italian Sausage	1 meal (10 oz)	320
Rigatoni In Cream Sauce With Broccoli & Chicken	1 meal (10.8 oz)	290
Spaghetti With Chunky Tomato & Meat Sauce	1 meal (10 oz)	300

FOOD	PORTION	CALS.
Budget Gourmet (CONT.)		
Tortellini Cheese	1 meal (5.5 oz)	200
Ziti In Marinara Sauce	1 meal (6.25 oz)	200
Dining Light		
Cheese Cannelloni	9 oz	310
Formagg		
Penne Pasta Alfredo	⅔ cup (5 oz)	190
Penne Pasta Primavera	⅔ cup (5 oz)	190
Vegetable Pasta & Caesar Italian Garden	⅔ cup (5 oz)	190
Green Giant		
Garden Gourmet Creamy Mushroom	1 pkg	220
Garden Gourmet Pasta Dijon	1 pkg	260
Garden Gourmet Pasta Florentine	1 pkg	230
Garden Gourmet Rotini Cheddar	1 pkg	230
One Serve Cheese Tortellini	1 pkg	260
One Serve Macaroni & Cheese	1 pkg	230
One Serve Pasta Marinara	1 pkg	180
One Serve Pasta Parmesan With Green Peas	1 pkg	170
Pasta Accents Creamy Cheddar	½ cup	100
Pasta Accents Garden Herb	½ cup	80
Pasta Accents Garlic Seasoning	½ cup	110
Pasta Accents Pasta Primavera	½ cup	110
Healthy Choice		
Beef Macaroni Casserole	1 meal (8.5 oz)	200
Cheese Ravioli Parmigiana	1 meal (9 oz)	250
Chicken Fettucini Alfredo	1 meal (8.5 oz)	250
Classics Pasta Shells Marinara	1 meal (12 oz)	360
Classics Turkey Fettuccine Alla Crema	1 meal (12.5 oz)	350
Fettucini Alfredo	1 meal (8 oz)	240
Lasagna Roma	1 meal (13.5 oz)	390
Macaroni & Cheese	1 meal (9 oz)	290
Spaghetti Bolognese	1 meal (10 oz)	260
Three Cheese Manicotti	1 meal (11 oz)	310
Vegetable Pasta Italiano	1 meal (10 oz)	220
Zucchini Lasagna	1 meal (14 oz)	330
Kid Cuisine		
Macaroni & Cheese	1 pkg (10.6 oz)	420
Mini Cheese Ravioli	1 pkg (9.82 oz)	320
Le Menu		
Entree LightStyle Garden Vegetables Lasagna	10½ oz	260
Entree LightStyle Lasagna With Meat Sauce	10 oz	290

FOOD	PORTION	CALS.
Le Menu (CONT.)		
Entree LightStyle Meat Sauce & Cheese Tortellini	8 oz	250
Entree LightStyle Spaghetti With Beef Sauce And Mushrooms	9 oz	280
LightStyle 3-Cheese Stuffed Shells	10 oz	280
Manicotto With Three Cheeses	11¾ oz	390
Lean Cuisine		
Angel Hair Pasta	1 meal (10 oz)	210
Cannelloni Cheese	1 meal (9.1 oz)	270
Cheddar Bake With Pasta	1 meal (9 oz)	220
Chicken Fettucini	1 pkg (9 oz)	270
Fettucini Alfredo	1 meal (9 oz)	270
Fettucini Primavera	1 meal (10 oz)	260
Lasagna Classic Cheese	1 meal (11.5 oz)	290
Lasagna Tuna	1 meal (9.75 oz)	230
Lasagna Zucchini	1 meal (11 oz)	240
Lasagne With Meat Sauce	1 pkg (10.25 oz)	270
Macaroni & Cheese	1 pkg (9 oz)	270
Marinara Twist	1 pkg (10 oz)	240
Ravioli Cheese	1 meal (8.5 oz)	250
Rigatoni	1 pkg (9 oz)	180
Spaghetti With Meat Sauce	1 meal (11.5 oz)	290
Life Choice		
Linguini Roma	1 meal (13.2 oz)	230
Sun Dried Tomato Manicotti	1 meal (11.65 oz)	220
Vegetable Lasagna Primavera	1 meal (11.2 oz)	170
Luigino's		
& Pomodoro Sauce With Meatballs	1 pkg (9 oz)	320
& Pomodoro Sauce With Meatballs	1 cup (6.3 oz)	270
Cheese Ravioli & Alfredo With Broccoli Sauce	1 pkg (8.5 oz)	420
Fettuccine Alfredo	1 cup (7.5 oz)	330
Fettuccine Alfredo	1 pkg (9.4 oz)	390
Fettuccine Alfredo With Broccoli	1 pkg (9.2 oz)	360
Fettuccine Carbonara	1 pkg (9 oz)	360
Lasagna Alfredo	1 pkg (9 oz)	360
Lasagna Alfredo	1 cup (6.3 oz)	300
Lasagna Pollo	1 pkg (9 oz)	320
Lasagna With Meat Sauce	1 cup (7.2 oz)	240
Lasagna With Meat Sauce	1 pkg (9 oz)	290
Lasagna With Vegetables	1 pkg (9 oz)	290
Linguini With Clams & Sauce	1 pkg (9 oz)	270
Linguini With Seafood	1 pkg (9 oz)	290

FOOD	PORTION	CALS.
Luigino's (CONT.)		
Macaroni & Cheese	1 cup (7.2 oz)	310
Macaroni & Cheese	1 pkg (9 oz)	370
Marinara Sauce Penne Pasta Italian Sausage & Peppers	1 pkg (9 oz)	350
Marinara Sauce Penne Pasta Italian Sausage & Peppers	1 cup (7.4 oz)	290
Meat Ravioli & Pomodoro Sauce	1 pkg (8.5 oz)	320
Minestrone With Penne Pasta	1 cup (6.3 oz)	180
Penne Pollo	1 pkg (9 oz)	330
Penne Primavera	1 pkg (9 oz)	350
Rigatoni Pomodoro Italiano	1 pkg (9 oz)	290
Shells & Cheese With Jalapenos	1 pkg (8.5 oz)	360
Spaghetti Bolognese	1 pkg (9 oz)	270
Spaghetti Marinara	1 pkg (10 oz)	250
Spinach Ravioli & Primavera Sauce	1 pkg (8.5 oz)	360
Morton		
Macaroni & Cheese	1 serv (8 oz)	220
Mrs. Paul's		
Entrees Light Seafood Lasagne	9½ oz	290
Entrees Light Seafood Rotini	9 oz	240
Seafood Rotini	9 oz	240
Palmazone		
Macaroni 'n Cheese	½ pkg (6 oz)	260
Pasta Favorites		
Chicken Pasta Primavera	1 pkg (10.5 oz)	330
Fettuccini Alfredo	1 pkg (10.5 oz)	370
Italian Sausage & Peppers	1 pkg (10.5 oz)	340
Lasagna	1 pkg (10.5 oz)	290
Macaroni & Cheese	1 pkg (10.5 oz)	350
Pasta Primavera	1 pkg (10.5 oz)	320
Spaghetti w/ Meatballs	1 pkg (10.5 oz)	370
Vegetable Lasagna	1 pkg (10.5 oz)	260
White Cheddar & Rotini	1 pkg (10.5 oz)	350
Senor Felix's		
Lasagna Southwestern	1 serv (6 oz)	160
Stouffer's		
Beef Ravioli	1 pkg (9.5 oz)	370
Cheese Manicotti	1 pkg (9 oz)	340
Cheese Ravioli With Tomato Sauce	1 pkg (9.5 oz)	360
Cheese Shells With Tomato Sauce	1 pkg (9.25 oz)	340
Cheese Tortellini With Tomato Sauce	1 pkg (9.25 oz)	290
Fettucini Alfredo	1 pkg (10 oz)	480
Four Cheese Lasagna	1 pkg (10.75 oz)	410

FOOD	PORTION	CALS.
Stouffer's (CONT.)		
Homestyle Chicken Fettucini	1 pkg (10.5 oz)	380
Lasagna With Meat Sauce	1 cup (7 oz)	260
Lasagna With Meat Sauce	1 pkg (10.5 oz)	360
Lunch Express Cheese Lasagna Casserole	1 pkg (9.5 oz)	270
Lunch Express Cheese Ravioli	1 pkg (8.5 oz)	310
Lunch Express Chicken Fettucini	1 pkg (10.25 oz)	250
Lunch Express Macaroni & Cheese & Broccoli	1 pkg (9.5 oz)	240
Lunch Express Macaroni & Cheese With Broccoli	1 pkg (10.4 oz)	360
Lunch Express Pasta & Chicken Marinara	1 pkg (9.1 oz)	270
Lunch Express Pasta & Tuna Casserole	1 pkg (9.6 oz)	280
Lunch Express Pasta & Turkey Dijon	1 pkg (9.9 oz)	270
Lunch Express Rigatoni With Meat Sauce	1 pkg (10.75 oz)	340
Lunch Express Spaghetti With Meat Sauce	1 pkg (9.6 oz)	320
Macaroni & Cheese	1 cup (6 oz)	330
Noodles Romanoff	1 pkg (12 oz)	460
Spaghetti With Meat Sauce	1 pkg (12.9 oz)	430
Spaghetti With Meatballs	1 pkg (12.6 oz)	420
Tuna Noodle Casserole	1 pkg (10 oz)	330
Turkey Tettrazini	1 pkg (10 oz)	360
Vegetable Lasagna	1 cup (8 oz)	280
Vegetable Lasagna	1 pkg (10.5 oz)	370
Swanson		
Homestyle Lasagne With Meat Sauce	10½ oz	400
Homestyle Macaroni & Cheese	10 oz	390
Homestyle Spaghetti With Italian Style Meatballs	13 oz	490
Macaroni & Cheese	12¼ oz	370
Macaroni & Cheese	7 oz	200
Spaghetti & Meatballs	12½ oz	390
Tabatchnick		
Macaroni & Cheese	7.5 oz	280
Tyson		
Parmigiana	1 pkg (11.25 oz)	380
Ultra Slim-Fast		
Pasta Primavera	12 oz	340
Spaghetti With Beef & Mushroom Sauce	12 oz	370
Weight Watchers		
Angel Hair Pasta	1 pkg (9 oz)	180
Cheese Manicotti	1 pkg (9.25 oz)	290
Chicken Fettucini	1 pkg (8.25 oz)	280
Fettucini Alfredo With Broccoli	1 pkg (8.5 oz)	220

FOOD	PORTION	CALS.
Weight Watchers (CONT.)		
Garden Lasagne	1 pkg (11 oz)	230
Italian Cheese Lasagna	1 pkg (11 oz)	300
Lasagna Florentine	1 pkg (10 oz)	210
Lasagna With Meat Sauce	1 pkg (10.25 oz)	290
Macaroni & Beef	1 pkg (8.5 oz)	220
Penne Pasta With Sun-Dried Tomatoes	1 pkg (10 oz)	290
Ravioli Florentine	1 pkg (8.5 oz)	200
Spaghetti With Meat Sauce	1 pkg (10 oz)	250
Tuna Noodle Casserole	1 pkg (9.5 oz)	240
HOME RECIPE		
macaroni & cheese	1 cup	430
spaghetti w/ meatballs & tomato sauce	1 cup	330
MIX		
Casbah		
Pasta Fasul	1 pkg (1.6 oz)	150
Golden Grain		
Macaroni & Cheese	½ cup	310
Hain		
Pasta & Sauce Creamy Parmesan	¼ pkg	150
Pasta & Sauce Creamy Swiss	¼ pkg	170
Pasta & Sauce Fettuccine Alfredo	¼ pkg	180
Pasta & Sauce Italian Herb	¼ pkg	110
Pasta & Sauce Primavera	¼ pkg	140
Pasta & Sauce Tangy Cheddar	¼ pkg	180
Kraft		
Cheddar Cheese Egg Noodle	1 cup (8 oz)	430
Macaroni & Cheese Deluxe Original	1 cup (6.1 oz)	320
Macaroni & Cheese Dinosaurs	1 cup (6.8 oz)	390
Macaroni & Cheese Flintstones	1 cup (6.8 oz)	390
Macaroni & Cheese Milk White Cheddar	1 cup (6.8 oz)	390
Macaroni & Cheese Original	1 cup (6.9 oz)	390
Macaroni & Cheese Santa Mac	1 cup	390
Macaroni & Cheese Spirals	1 cup (6.8 oz)	390
Macaroni & Cheese Super Mario Bros	1 cup (6.8 oz)	390
Macaroni & Cheese Teddy Bears	1 cup (6.8 oz)	390
Macaroni & Cheese Thick 'N Creamy	1 cup (6.1 oz)	320
Spaghetti Mild American	1 cup (8.1 oz)	270
Spaghetti Tangy Italian	1 cup (7.9 oz)	270
Spaghetti With Meat Sauce	1 cup (8.2 oz)	330
Lipton		
Golden Saute Angel Hair Chicken	⅓ cup (2.1 oz)	210
Golden Saute Angel Hair Parmesan	⅓ cup (2.2 oz)	240
Golden Saute Chicken Herb Parmesan	½ cup (2.2 oz)	230

FOOD	PORTION	CALS.
Lipton (CONT.)		
Golden Saute Chicken Herb Parmesan	½ cup (2.2 oz)	230
Golden Saute Chicken Stir Fry	½ cup (2.2 oz)	220
Golden Saute Garlic Butter	½ cup (2.1 oz)	230
Golden Saute Penne Herb & Garlic	⅓ cup (2.1 oz)	230
Pasta & Sauce Cheddar Broccoli as prep	½ cup (2.4 oz)	260
Pasta & Sauce Cheese Bow Ties	½ cup (2 oz)	230
Pasta & Sauce Chicken Primavera as prep	½ cup (2 oz)	220
Pasta & Sauce Creamy Garlic as prep	½ cup (2.4 oz)	260
Pasta & Sauce Herb Tomato as prep	½ cup (2.3 oz)	240
Pasta & Sauce Primavera as prep	½ cup (2.2 oz)	240
Pasta & Sauce Three Cheese as prep	½ cup (2.2 oz)	240
Minute		
Microwave Cheddar Cheese Broccoli And Pasta as prep	½ cup	160
Nile Spice		
Pasta'n Sauce Mediterranean	1 pkg	210
Pasta'n Sauce Parmesan	1 pkg	200
Pasta'n Sauce Primavera	1 pkg	200
Terrazza		
Pasta E Fagioli as prep	½ cup	150
Ultra Slim-Fast		
Macaroni & Cheese	2.3 oz	230
Uncle Ben		
Country Inn Pasta & Sauce Angel Hair Parmesan	1 serv (2.2 oz)	245
Country Inn Pasta & Sauce Broccoli & White Cheddar	1 serv (2.2 oz)	240
Country Inn Pasta & Sauce Butter & Herb	1 serv (2 oz)	230
Country Inn Pasta & Sauce Creamy Garlic	1 serv (2.4 oz)	261
Country Inn Pasta & Sauce Fettuccine Alfredo	1 serv (2.2 oz)	310
Country Inn Pasta & Sauce Herb Linguine	1 serv (2.2 oz)	240
Country Inn Pasta & Sauce Mushroom Fettuccine	1 serv (2.2 oz)	250
Country Inn Pasta & Sauce Vegetable Alfredo	1 serv (2.2 oz)	240
Velveeta		
Rotini & Cheese Broccoli	1 cup (7.2 oz)	400
Shells & Cheese Bacon	1 cup (6.8 oz)	360
Shells & Cheese Original	1 cup (6.6 oz)	360
Shells & Cheese Salsa	1 cup (7.5 oz)	380
SHELF-STABLE		
Chef Boyardee		
Microwave Main Meal Beans & Pasta	10.5 oz	200

FOOD	PORTION	CALS.
Chef Boyardee (CONT.)		
Microwave Main Meal Beef Ravioli Suprema	10.5 oz	290
Microwave Main Meal Cheese Ravioli Suprema	10.5 oz	290
Microwave Main Meal Fettuccine	10.5 oz	290
Microwave Main Meal Lasagna	10.5 oz	290
Microwave Main Meal Meat Tortellini	10.5 oz	220
Microwave Main Meal Noodles w/ Chicken	10.5 oz	170
Microwave Main Meal Peas & Pasta	10.5 oz	190
Microwave Main Meal Zesty Macaroni	10.5 oz	290
Microwave Main Meal Ziti In Sauce	10.5 oz	210
Dinty Moore		
American Classics Lasagna With Meat & Sauce	1 bowl (10 oz)	260
Kid's Kitchen		
Microwave Meals Beefy Macaroni	1 cup (7.5 oz)	190
Microwave Meals Macaroni & Cheese	1 cup (7.5 oz)	260
Microwave Meals Mini Ravioli	1 cup (7.5 oz)	240
Microwave Meals Spaghetti Ring & Meatballs	1 cup (7.5 oz)	250
Lunch Bucket		
Elbows In Tomato Sauce	1 pkg (7.5 oz)	190
Lasagna With Meatsauce	1 pkg (7.5 oz)	220
Light'n Healthy Italian Style Pasta	1 pkg (7.5 oz)	130
Light'n Healthy Pasta In Wine Sauce	1 pkg (7.5 oz)	130
Light'n Healthy Pasta'n Garden Vegetables	1 pkg (7.5 oz)	150
Macaroni'n Cheese	1 pkg (7.5 oz)	210
Pasta'n Chicken	1 pkg (7.5 oz)	180
Spaghetti'n Meatsauce	1 pkg (7.5 oz)	240
Micro Cup Meals		
Lasagna	1 cup (7.5 oz)	230
Lasagna & Beef Tomato Sauce	1 cup	359
Macaroni & Cheese	1 cup (7.5 oz)	260
Ravioli Tomato Sauce	1 cup (7.5 oz)	260
Spaghetti & Meat Sauce	1 cup (7.5 oz)	220
My Own Meal		
Cheese Tortellini	1 pkg (10 oz)	340
Top Shelf		
Italian Lasagna	1 bowl (10 oz)	350
Spaghetti With Meat Sauce	1 bowl (10 oz)	240
TAKE-OUT		
lasagna	1 piece (2.5 in x 2.5 in)	374
macaroni & cheese	1 cup	230

FOOD	PORTION	CALS.
manicotti	¾ cup (6.4 oz)	273
rigatoni w/ sausage sauce	¾ cup	260
spaghetti w/ meatballs & cheese	1 cup	407

PASTA MACHINE MIX
Wanda's

Dried Tomato	⅓ cup mix per serv (1.9 oz)	202
Durum & Semolina	⅓ cup mix per serv (1.9 oz)	199
Semolina Blend	⅓ cup mix per serv (1.9 oz)	202
Spinach	⅓ cup mix per serv (1.9 oz)	202
Whole Wheat & Semolina	⅓ cup mix per serv (1.9 oz)	198

PASTA SALAD
MIX
Kraft

Pasta Salad Classic Ranch With Bacon	¾ cup (4.7 oz)	360
Pasta Salad Creamy Ceasar	¾ cup (4.8 oz)	350
Pasta Salad Garden Primavera	¾ cup (5 oz)	280
Pasta Salad Light Italian	¾ cup (5 oz)	190
Pasta Salad Parmesan Peppercorn	¾ cup (4.9 oz)	360

Suddenly Salad

Classic Pasta as prep	½ cup	160
Creamy Macaroni as prep	½ cup	200
Creamy Macaroni as prep low fat recipe	½ cup	140
Italian Pasta as prep	½ cup	160
Pasta Primavera as prep	½ cup	190
Pasta Primavera as prep low fat recipe	½ cup	150
Tortellini Italiano as prep	½ cup	160

TAKE-OUT

elbow macaroni salad	3.5 oz	160
italian style pasta salad	3.5 oz	140
mustard macaroni salad	3.5 oz	190
pasta salad w/ vegetables	3.5 oz	140

PASTRY
(see BROWNIE, CAKE, DANISH PASTRY)

PATE
CANNED

chicken liver	1 tbsp (13 g)	109
chicken liver	1 oz	238

FOOD	PORTION	CALS.
goose liver smoked	1 tbsp (13 g)	60
goose liver smoked	1 oz	131
liver	1 tbsp (13 g)	41
liver	1 oz	90
Sells		
Liver	2.08 oz	190

PEACH
CANNED

FOOD	PORTION	CALS.
halves in heavy sirup	1 half	60
halves in light syrup	1 half	44
halves juice pack	1 half	34
halves water pack	1 half	18
spiced in heavy sirup	1 fruit	66
spiced in heavy sirup	1 cup	180
Del Monte		
Halves Cling In Heavy Syrup	½ cup (4.5 oz)	100
Halves Cling Lite	½ cup (4.4 oz)	60
Halves Cling Melba In Heavy Syrup	½ cup (4.5 oz)	100
Halves Freestone In Heavy Syrup	½ cup (4.5 oz)	100
Sliced Cling Fruit Naturals	½ cup (4.4 oz)	60
Sliced Cling In Heavy Syrup	½ cup (4.5 oz)	100
Sliced Cling Lite	½ cup (4.4 oz)	60
Sliced Freestone In Heavy Syrup	½ cup (4.5 oz)	100
Sliced Freestone Lite	½ cup (4.4 oz)	60
Snack Cups Diced Fruit Naturals	1 serv (4.5 oz)	60
Snack Cups Diced Fruit Naturals EZ-Open Lid	1 serv (4.2 oz)	60
Snack Cups Diced In Heavy Syrup	1 serv (4.5 oz)	100
Snack Cups Diced In Heavy Syrup EZ-Open Lid	1 serv (4.2 oz)	90
Snack Cups Diced Lite	1 serv (4.5 oz)	60
Snack Cups Diced Lite EZ-Open Lid	1 serv (4.2 oz)	60
Whole Cling In Heavy Syrup	½ cup (4.2 oz)	100
Hunt's		
Halves	4 oz	90
Slices	4 oz	90
Libby		
Halves Yellow Cling Lite	½ cup (4.4 oz)	60
Sliced Yellow Cling Lite	½ cup (4.4 oz)	60
S&W		
Halves Clingstone	½ cup	100
Halves Clingstone Diet	½ cup	30
Halves Clingstone Unsweetened	½ cup	30

FOOD	PORTION	CALS.
S&W (CONT.)		
Halves Freestone Diet	½ cup	30
Halves Freestone In Heavy Syrup	½ cup	100
Sliced Clingstone Diet	½ cup	30
Sliced Clingstone Unsweetened	½ cup	30
Sliced Freestone In Heavy Syrup	½ cup	100
Sliced Yellow Cling Natural Style	½ cup	90
Sliced Yellow Cling Premium In Heavy Syrup	½ cup	100
Whole Yellow Cling Spiced In Heavy Syrup	½ cup	90
Yellow Cling Natural Lite	½ cup	50
DRIED		
halves	10	311
halves	1 cup	383
halves cooked w/ sugar	½ cup	139
halves cooked w/o sugar	½ cup	99
Del Monte		
Sun Dried	⅓ cup (1.4 oz)	90
Mariani		
Peaches	¼ cup	140
Sonoma		
Pieces	3-5 pieces (1.4 oz)	120
FRESH		
peach	1	37
sliced	1 cup	73
Dole		
Peach	2	70
FROZEN		
slices sweetened	1 cup	235
Big Valley		
Freestone	⅔ cup (4.9 oz)	50
PEACH JUICE		
nectar	1 cup	134
Goya		
Nectar	6 oz	110
Kern's		
Nectar	6 fl oz	110
Libby		
Nectar	1 can (11.5 fl oz)	210
Mott's		
Fruit Basket Orchard Peach Juice Cocktail as prep	8 fl oz	130
Smucker's		
Juice	8 oz	120

FOOD	PORTION	CALS.
Snapple		
Dixie Peach	10 fl oz	140
PEANUT BUTTER		
chunky	1 cup	1520
chunky	2 tbsp	188
chunky w/o salt	1 cup	1520
chunky w/o salt	2 tbsp	188
smooth	1 cup	1517
smooth	2 tbsp	188
smooth w/o salt	2 tbsp	188
smooth w/o salt	1 cup	1517
Arrowhead		
Creamy	2 tbsp (1.1 oz)	200
Crunchy	2 tbsp (1.1 oz)	200
BAMA		
Creamy	2 tbsp	200
Crunchy	2 tbsp	200
Jelly & Peanut Butter	2 tbsp	150
Crazy Richard's		
Natural Creamy	2 tbsp (1.1 oz)	190
Erewhon		
Chunky	2 tbsp (32 g)	190
Chunky Unsalted	2 tbsp (32 g)	190
Creamy	2 tbsp (32 g)	190
Creamy Unsalted	2 tbsp (32 g)	190
Estee		
Chunky Sodium Free	2 tbsp (1 oz)	190
Chunky Sodium Free Sorbitol Sweetened	2 tbsp (1 oz)	190
Creamy Sodium Free	2 tbsp (1 oz)	190
Creamy Sodium Free Sorbitol Sweetened	2 tbsp (1 oz)	190
Health Valley		
Chunky No Salt	2 tbsp	170
Creamy No Salt	2 tbsp	170
Hollywood		
Creamy	1 tbsp	35
Crunchy	1 tbsp	35
Unsalted	1 tbsp	35
Home Brand		
Natural Lightly Salted	2 tbsp	210
Natural Unsalted	2 tbsp	210
No-Sugar Added	2 tbsp	180
Peanut Butter	2 tbsp	210
Jif		
Creamy	2 tbsp (1.1 oz)	190

FOOD	PORTION	CALS.
Jif (CONT.)		
Extra Crunchy	2 tbsp (1.1 oz)	190
Reduced Fat	2 tbsp (1.3 oz)	190
Simply Creamy	2 tbsp (1.1 oz)	190
Simply Extra Crunchy	2 tbsp (1.1 oz)	190
Peter Pan		
Creamy	2 tbsp	190
Creamy Salt Free	2 tbsp	190
Crunchy	2 tbsp	190
Crunchy Salt Free	2 tbsp	190
Red Wing		
Creamy	2 tbsp (1.1 oz)	200
Crunchy	2 tbsp (1.1 oz)	200
Reese's		
Peanut Butter Chips	¼ cup (1.5 oz)	230
Skippy		
Creamy	1 cup (263 g)	1540
Creamy w/ 2 slices white bread	1 sandwich	340
Reduced Fat Creamy	2 tbsp	190
Super Chunk	2 tbsp (32 g)	190
Super Chunk	1 cup (260 g)	1540
Super Chunk w/ slices white bread	1 sandwich	340
Smucker's		
Goober Grape	2 tbsp	180
Honey Sweetened	2 tbsp	200
Natural	2 tbsp	200
Natural No-Salt Added	2 tbsp	200
Tree Of Life		
Creamy	2 tbsp (1 oz)	190
Creamy No Salt	2 tbsp (1 oz)	190
Creamy Organic	2 tbsp (1 oz)	190
Creamy Organic No Salt	2 tbsp (1 oz)	190
Crunchy	2 tbsp (1 oz)	190
Crunchy No Salt	2 tbsp (1 oz)	190
Crunchy Organic	2 tbsp (1 oz)	190
Crunchy Organic No Salt	2 tbsp (1 oz)	190
Peanut Wonder 78% Less Fat	2 tbsp (1 oz)	100

PEANUTS

chocolate coated	10 (1.4 oz)	208
chocolate coated	1 cup (5.2 oz)	773
cooked	½ cup	102
dry roasted	1 oz	164
dry roasted	1 cup	855

FOOD	PORTION	CALS.
oil roasted	1 oz	163
oil roasted	1 cup	837
oil roasted w/o salt	1 oz	163
oil roasted w/o salt	1 cup	837
spanish oil roasted	1 oz	162
spanish oil roasted w/o salt	1 oz	162
unroasted	1 oz	159
valencia oil roasted	1 oz	165
valencia oil roasted	1 cup	848
valencia oil roasted w/o salt	1 oz	165
valencia oil roasted w/o salt	1 cup	848
virginia oil roasted	1 cup	826
virginia oil roasted	1 oz	161
Beer Nuts		
Peanuts	1 pkg (1 oz)	180
Fisher		
Party Peanuts	1 oz	160
Salted-In-Shell shelled	1 oz	170
Spanish Roasted	1 oz	180
Frito Lay		
Dry Roasted	1.2 oz	190
Salted	1 oz	170
Guy's		
Dry Roasted	1 oz	170
Spanish Salted	1 oz	170
Lance		
Honey Toasted	1 pkg (39 g)	230
Roasted w/ Shell	1 pkg (50 g)	190
Salted	1 pkg (32 g)	190
Salted Tube	1 pkg (42 g)	240
Little Debbie		
Salted	1 pkg (1.2 oz)	230
Pennant		
Oil Roasted	1 oz	170
Planters		
Cocktail Lightly Salted Oil Roasted	1 oz	170
Cocktail Oil Roasted	1 oz	170
Cocktail Unsalted Oil Roasted	1 oz	170
Dry Roasted	1 oz	160
Fun Size! Oil Roasted	2 pkg (1 oz)	170
Heat Hot Spicy Oil Roasted	1 pkg (1.7 oz)	290
Heat Hot Spicy Oil Roasted	1 oz	160
Heat Hot Spicy Oil Roasted	1 pkg (2 oz)	330
Heat Mild Spicy Oil Roasted	1 oz	160

FOOD	PORTION	CALS.
Planters (CONT.)		
Honey Roasted	1 oz	160
Honey Roasted Dry Roasted	1 pkg (1.7 oz)	260
Lightly Salted Dry Roasted	1 oz	160
Lightly Salted Dry Roasted	1 pkg (1.75 oz)	290
Lightly Salted Oil Roasted	1 pkg (1.8 oz)	300
Munch'N Go Singles Heat Hot Spicy Oil Roasted	1 pkg (2.5 oz)	410
Reduced Fat Honey Roasted	⅓ cup (1 oz)	130
Salted Oil Roasted	1 pkg (1 oz)	170
Spanish Oil Roasted	1 oz	170
Spanish Raw	1 oz	150
Sweet N Crunchy	1 oz	140
Unsalted Dry Roasted	1 oz	160
Weight Watchers		
Honey Roasted	1 pkg (0.7 oz)	100

PEAR
CANNED

FOOD	PORTION	CALS.
halves in heavy sirup	1 cup	188
halves in heavy syrup	1 half	68
halves in light syrup	1 half	45
halves juice pack	1 cup	123
halves water pack	1 half	22
Del Monte		
Halves Fruit Naturals	½ cup (4.4 oz)	60
Halves In Heavy Syrup	½ cup (4.5 oz)	100
Halves Lite	½ cup (4.4 oz)	60
Sliced In Heavy Syrup	½ cup (4.5 oz)	100
Sliced Lite	½ cup (4.4 oz)	60
Snack Cups Diced In Heavy Syrup	1 serv (4.5 oz)	100
Snack Cups Diced In Heavy Syrup EZ-Open Lid	1 serv (4.2 oz)	90
Snack Cups Diced Lite	1 serv (4.5 oz)	60
Snack Cups Diced Lite EZ-Open Lid	1 serv (4.2 oz)	60
Hunt's		
Halves	4 oz	90
Libby		
Halves Lite	½ cup (4.3 oz)	60
Sliced Lite	½ cup (4.3 oz)	60
S&W		
Halves Bartlett In Heavy Syrup	½ cup	100
Halves Bartlett Peeled Unsweetened	½ cup	35
Halves Peeled Diet	½ cup	35

FOOD	PORTION	CALS.
S&W (CONT.)		
Quartered Peeled Diet	½ cup	35
Sliced Natural Light Bartlett	½ cup	60
Sliced Natural Style	½ cup	80
DRIED		
halves	10	459
halves	1 cup	472
halves cooked w/ sugar	½ cup	196
halves cooked w/o sugar	½ cup	163
Mariani		
Pears	¼ cup	150
Sonoma		
Pieces	3-4 pieces (1.4 oz)	120
FRESH		
asian	1 (4.3 oz)	51
pear	1	98
sliced w/ skin	1 cup	97
Dole		
Pear	1	100
PEAR JUICE		
nectar	1 cup	149
Goya		
Nectar	6 oz	120
Kern's		
Nectar	6 fl oz	120
Libby		
Nectar	1 can (11.5 fl oz)	220
PEAS		
CANNED		
green	½ cup	59
green low sodium	½ cup	59
Allen		
Crowder	½ cup (4.5 oz)	110
Purple Hull	½ cup (4.4 oz)	120
Crest Top		
Early June	½ cup (4.5 oz)	100
Del Monte		
Sweet	½ cup (4.4 oz)	60
Sweet 50% Less Salt	½ cup (4.4 oz)	60
Sweet No Salt Added	½ cup (4.4 oz)	60
Sweet Very Young	½ cup (4.4 oz)	60
East Texas Fair		
Cream Peas	½ cup (4.4 oz)	120

FOOD	PORTION	CALS.
East Texas Fair (CONT.)		
Crowder	½ cup (4.5 oz)	110
Lady Peas With Snaps	½ cup (4.3 oz)	100
Peas 'n Pork	½ cup (4.5 oz)	110
Pepper Peas	½ cup (4.5 oz)	120
Purple Hull	½ cup (4.4 oz)	120
White Acre	½ cup (4.3 oz)	100
Green Giant		
Sweet	½ cup	50
Homefolks		
Crowder	½ cup (4.5 oz)	110
Purple Hull	½ cup (4.4 oz)	120
Luck's		
Crowder Peas Seasoned w/Pork	7.5 oz	200
Owatonna		
Early June or Sweet	½ cup	70
S&W		
Petit Pois	½ cup	70
Sweet	½ cup	70
Sweet Water Pack	½ cup	40
Veri-Green Sweet	½ cup	70
Seneca		
Natural Pack	½ cup	60
Peas	½ cup	50
Sunshine		
Field Peas	½ cup (4.4 oz)	120
Lady Peas	½ cup (4.3 oz)	100
Trappey		
Field Peas With Bacon	½ cup (4.5 oz)	90
Field Peas With Snaps And Bacon	½ cup (4.5 oz)	110
DRIED		
split cooked	1 cup	231
FRESH		
edible-pod cooked	½ cup	34
edible-pod raw	½ cup	30
green cooked	½ cup	67
green raw	½ cup	58
Dole		
Sugar Peas	½ cup	30
FROZEN		
edible-pod cooked	1 pkg (10 oz)	132
edible-pod cooked	½ cup	42
green cooked	½ cup	63

FOOD	PORTION	CALS.
Birds Eye		
Green	½ cup	80
In Butter Sauce	½ cup	80
Polybag Deluxe Tender Tiny	½ cup	60
Polybag Green	½ cup	70
Sugar Snap Deluxe	½ cup	45
Tender Tiny Deluxe	½ cup	60
Chun King		
Snow Pea Pods	½ pkg (3 oz)	35
Fresh Like		
Green	3.5 oz	85
Tiny Green	3.5 oz	63
Green Giant		
Harvest Fresh Early June	½ cup	60
Harvest Fresh Sugar Snap	½ cup	30
Harvest Fresh Sweet	½ cup	50
In Butter Sauce	½ cup	80
One Serve In Butter Sauce	1 pkg	90
Sugar Snap Sweet Select	½ cup	30
Sweet	½ cup	50
Hanover		
Petite	½ cup	70
Snow Peas	½ cup	35
Sweet	½ cup	70
Le Seur		
Early In Butter Sauce	½ cup	80
Early Select	½ cup	60
Tree Of Life		
Peas	⅔ cup (3.1 oz)	70
SHELF-STABLE		
Green Giant		
Mini Sweet	½ cup	60
SPROUTS		
raw	½ cup	77
TAKE-OUT		
pea & potato curry	1 serv (7 oz)	284
pea curry	1 serv (4.4 oz)	438

PECANS

dried	1 oz	190
dry roasted	1 oz	187
dry roasted salted	1 oz	187
halves dried	1 cup	721
oil roasted	1 oz	195
oil roasted salted	1 oz	195

FOOD	PORTION	CALS.
Planters		
Chips	1 pkg (2 oz)	390
Gold Measure Halves	1 pkg (2 oz)	390
Halves	1 oz	190
Honey Roasted	1 oz	180
Pieces	1 oz	190
Pieces	1 pkg (2 oz)	390
PECTIN		
powder	1 pkg (1.75 oz)	163
powder	¼ pkg (0.4 oz)	39
Certo		
Liquid	1 tbsp	2
Slim Set		
Packet	1 pkg	208
Powder	1 tbsp	3
Sure-Jell		
Light	¼ pkg	33
Powder	¼ pkg	38
PEPPER		
black	1 tsp	5
cayenne	1 tsp	6
red	1 tsp	6
white	1 tsp	7
Ac'cent		
Lemon	½ tsp	0
Seasoned	½ tsp	0
Lawry's		
Lemon	1 tsp	6
Watkins		
Black	¼ tbsp (0.5 g)	0
Cajun	¼ tbsp (0.5 g)	0
Cracked Black	¼ tbsp (0.5 g)	0
Dijon	¼ tbsp (0.5 g)	0
Garlic Peppercorn Blend	¼ tbsp (1 g)	0
Herb	¼ tbsp (0.5 g)	0
Italian	¼ tbsp (0.5 g)	0
Lemon	¼ tbsp (1 g)	0
Mexican	¼ tbsp (0.5 g)	0
Red Pepper Flakes	¼ tsp (0.5 oz)	0
Royal Pepper Blend	¼ tbsp (0.5 g)	0
PEPPERS		
CANNED		
chili green hot	1 (2.6 oz)	18

FOOD	PORTION	CALS.
chili green hot chopped	½ cup	17
chili red hot	1 (2.6 oz)	18
chili red hot chopped	½ cup	17
green halves	½ cup	13
jalapeno chopped	½ cup	17
red halves	½ cup	13
Chi-Chi's		
Chilies Diced Green	2 tbsp (1.2 oz)	10
Chilies Green Whole	¾ pepper (1 oz)	10
Jalapenos Green Wheels	1 oz	10
Jalapenos Green Whole	1 oz	10
Jalapenos Red Wheels	1 oz	10
Jalapenos Red Whole	1 oz	15
Del Monte		
Chilpotie In Spice Sauce	2 tbsp (1.1 oz)	20
Hot Chili	4 (1 oz)	10
Jalapeno Pickled Sliced	2 tbsp (1.1 oz)	5
Jalapeno Pickled Whole	2 tbsp (1.1 oz)	5
Jalapeno Whole	1 (0.7 oz)	3
Hebrew National		
Filet	¼ pepper (1 oz)	9
Hot Cherry	⅓ pepper (1 oz)	11
Red Filet	¼ pepper (1 oz)	9
McIlhenny		
Jalapeno Nacho Slices	12 slices (1.1 oz)	7
Old El Paso		
Green Chilies Chopped	2 tbsp (1 oz)	5
Green Chilies Whole	1 (1.2 oz)	10
Jalapenos Peeled	3 (1 oz)	10
Jalapenos Pickled	2 (0.9 oz)	5
Jalapenos Slices	2 tbsp (1.1 oz)	15
Progresso		
Cherry (drained)	2 tbsp (0.9 oz)	30
Fried (drained)	2 tbsp (0.9 oz)	60
Hot Cherry	1 (1 oz)	15
Pepper Salad (drained)	2 tbsp (0.9 oz)	25
Roasted	½ piece (1 oz)	10
Tuscan (drained)	3 (1 oz)	10
Rosoff's		
Sweet	¼ pepper (1 oz)	9
Schorr's		
Filet Peppers	1 oz	9
Trappey		
Banana Mild	3 peppers (1 oz)	6

FOOD	PORTION	CALS.
Trappey (CONT.)		
Banana Sliced Rings	21 slices (1 oz)	6
Cherry Hot	2 peppers (1 oz)	7
Cherry Mild	2 peppers (1 oz)	10
Dulcito Italian Pepperoncini	4 peppers (1 oz)	8
In Vinegar Hot	15 peppers (1 oz)	9
Jalapeno Hot Sliced	21 slices (1 oz)	4
Jalapeno Whole	2 peppers (1 oz)	11
Serano	7 peppers (1 oz)	7
Tempero Golden Greek Pepperoncini	4 peppers (1 oz)	7
Torrido Santa Fe Grande	3 peppers (1 oz)	10
Vlasic		
Hot Banana Pepper Rings	1 oz	4
Hot Cherry	1 oz	10
Jalapeno Mexican Hot	1 oz	8
Mexican Tiny Hot	1 oz	6
Mild Cherry	1 oz	8
Mild Greek Pepperoncini Salad Peppers	1 oz	4
DRIED		
green	1 tbsp	1
red	1 tbsp	1
FRESH		
chili green hot raw	1	18
chili green hot raw chopped	½ cup	30
chili red hot raw	1 (1.6 oz)	18
chili red raw chopped	½ cup	30
green chopped cooked	½ cup	19
green cooked	1 (2.6 oz)	20
green raw	1 (2.6 oz)	20
green raw chopped	½ cup	13
red chopped cooked	½ cup	19
red cooked	1 (2.6 oz)	20
red raw	1 (2.6 oz)	20
red raw chopped	½ cup	13
yellow raw	1 (6.5 oz)	50
yellow raw	10 strips	14
Dole		
Medium	1	25
FROZEN		
green chopped not prep	1 oz	6
red chopped	1 oz	6
Southland		
Green Diced	2 oz	10

FOOD	PORTION	CALS.
Southland (CONT.)		
Sweet Red & Green Cut	2 oz	15
PERCH		
FRESH		
cooked	1 fillet (1.6 oz)	54
cooked	3 oz	99
ocean perch atlantic cooked	1 fillet (1.8 oz)	60
ocean perch atlantic cooked	3 oz	103
ocean perch atlantic raw	3 oz	80
raw	3 oz	77
red raw	3½ oz	114
FROZEN		
Gorton's		
Fishmarket Fresh Ocean Perch	5 oz	140
Van De Kamp's		
Battered Fillets	2 (4 oz)	300
PERSIMMONS		
dried japanese	1	93
fresh	1	32
fresh japanese	1	118
Sonoma		
Dried	6-8 pieces (1.4 oz)	140
PHEASANT		
breast w/o skin raw	½ breast (6.4 oz)	243
leg w/o skin raw	1 (3.6 oz)	143
w/ skin raw	½ pheasant (14 oz)	723
w/o skin raw	½ pheasant (12.4 oz)	470
PHYLLO DOUGH		
phyllo dough	1 oz	85
sheet	1	57
Ekizian		
Sheets	½ lb	865
PICANTE		
(*see* SALSA)		
PICKLES		
dill	1 (2.3 oz)	12
dill low sodium	1 (2.3 oz)	12
dill low sodium sliced	1 slice	1
dill sliced	1 slice	1
gerkins	3½ oz	21
kosher dill	1 (2.3 oz)	12

FOOD	PORTION	CALS.
polish dill	1 (2.3 oz)	12
quick sour	1 (1.2 oz)	4
quick sour low sodium	1 (1.2 oz)	4
quick sour sliced	1 slice	1
sweet	1 (1.2 oz)	41
sweet gherkin	1 sm (½ oz)	20
sweet low sodium	1 (1.2 oz)	41
sweet sliced	1 slice	7
Claussen		
Bread 'N Butter Slices	1 slice	7
Dill Spears	1 spear	4
Kosher Halves	1 half	9
Kosher Slices	1 slice	1
Kosher Whole	1	9
No Garlic Dills	1	17
Del Monte		
Dill Halves	¼ pickle (1 oz)	5
Dill Hamburger Chips	5 pieces (1 oz)	5
Dill Sweet Chips	5 pieces (1 oz)	40
Dill Sweet Gherkin	2 pickles (1 oz)	40
Dill Sweet Midgets	3 pickles (1 oz)	40
Dill Sweet Whole	2 pickles (1 oz)	40
Dill Tiny Kosher	1½ pickle (1 oz)	5
Dill Whole Pickles	1½ pickle (1 oz)	5
Hebrew National		
Half Sour	½ pickle (1 oz)	4
Kosher	⅓ pickle (1 oz)	4
Kosher Barrel Cured Dill	1 pkg	23
Kosher Barrel Cured Hot Dill	1 pkg	23
Kosher Chips	3 slices (1 oz)	4
Kosher Halves	⅓ pickle (1 oz)	4
Kosher Large	⅕ pickle (1 oz)	4
Kosher Spears	½ spear (1 oz)	4
Sour Garlic	⅓ pickle (1 oz)	3
McIlhenny		
Hot N' Sweet	4 (1 oz)	42
Rosoff's		
Half Sour	⅓ pickle (1 oz)	4
Half Sour Spears	½ spear (1 oz)	4
Kosher	⅓ pickle (1 oz)	4
Kosher Halves	⅓ pickle (1 oz)	4
Schorr's		
Garlic	⅓ pickle (1 oz)	3
Half Sour	½ spear (1 oz)	4

FOOD	PORTION	CALS.
Schorr's (CONT.)		
Half Sour	⅓ pickle (1 oz)	4
Kosher Deli	½ pickle (1 oz)	4
Kosher Halves	⅓ pickle (1 oz)	4
Kosher Spears	½ spear (1 oz)	4
Kosher Whole	⅓ pickle (1 oz)	4
Vlasic		
Bread & Butter Chips	1 oz	30
Bread & Butter Chunks	1 oz	25
Bread & Butter Stixs	1 oz	18
Deli Bread & Butter	1 oz	25
Deli Dill Halves	1 oz	4
Half-The-Salt Hamburger Dill Chips	1 oz	2
Half-The-Salt Kosher Crunchy Dills	1 oz	4
Half-The-Salt Kosher Dill Spears	1 oz	4
Half-The-Salt Sweet Butter Chips	1 oz	30
Hot & Spicy Garden Mix	1 oz	4
Kosher Baby Dills	1 oz	4
Kosher Crunchy Dills	1 oz	4
Kosher Dill Gherkins	1 oz	4
Kosher Dill Spears	1 oz	4
Kosher Snack Chunks	1 oz	4
No Garlic Dill Spears	1 oz	4
Original Dills	1 oz	2
Polish Snack Chunk Dills	1 oz	4
Zesty Crunchy Dills	1 oz	4
Zesty Dill Snack Chunks	1 oz	4
Zesty Dill Spears	1 oz	4

PIE
(*see also* PIE CRUST)

CANNED FILLING

FOOD	PORTION	CALS.
apple	1 can (21 oz)	599
apple	⅛ can (2.6 oz)	74
cherry	⅛ can (2.6 oz)	85
cherry	1 can (21 oz)	683
pumpkin pie mix	1 cup	282
Libby		
Pumpkin Pie Mix	½ cup	100
None Such		
Mincemeat Condensed	¼ pkg	220
Mincemeat Ready-to-Use	⅓ cup	200
Mincemeat Ready-to-Use With Brandy & Rum	⅓ cup	220

FOOD	PORTION	CALS.
S&W		
Mincemeat Old Fashioned	½ cup	206
FROZEN		
apple	⅛ of 9 in pie (4.4 oz)	297
blueberry	⅛ of 9 in pie (4.4 oz)	289
cherry	⅛ of 9 in pie (4.4 oz)	325
chocolate creme	⅙ of 8 in pie (4 oz)	344
coconut creme	⅙ of 7 in pie (2.2 oz)	191
lemon meringue	⅙ of 8 in pie (4.5 oz)	303
peach	⅙ of 8 in pie (4.1 oz)	261
Banquet		
Apple	⅕ pie (4 oz)	300
Banana Cream	⅓ pie (4.7 oz)	350
Cherry	⅕ pie (4 oz)	290
Chocolate Cream	⅓ pie (4.7 oz)	360
Coconut Cream	⅓ pie (4.7 oz)	350
Lemon Cream	⅓ pie (4.7 oz)	360
Mincemeat	⅕ pie (4 oz)	310
Peach	⅕ pie (4 oz)	260
Pumpkin	⅙ pie (4 oz)	250
Kineret		
Apple Homestyle	⅙ pie (4 oz)	313
McMillin's		
Apple	4 oz	430
Berry	4 oz	430
Cherry	4 oz	430
Chocolate Pudding	4 oz	420
Coconut Pudding	4 oz	450
Lemon	4 oz	450
Peach	4 oz	430
Strawberry	4 oz	400
Mrs. Smith's		
Apple	⅒ of 10 in pie (4.6 oz)	280
Apple	⅛ of 9 in pie (4.6 oz)	370
Apple	⅙ of 8 in pie (4.3 oz)	270
Apple Cranberry	⅙ of 8 in pie (4.3 oz)	280
Apple Lattice Ready To Serve	⅕ of 8 in pie (4.6 oz)	310
Banana Cream	¼ of 8 in pie (3.4 oz)	250
Berry	⅙ of 8 in pie (4.3 oz)	280
Blackberry	⅙ of 8 in pie (4.3 oz)	280
Blueberry	⅙ of 8 in pie	260
Boston Cream	⅛ of 8 in pie (2.4 oz)	170
Cherry	⅙ of 8 in pie	270
Cherry	⅒ of 10 in pie (4.6 oz)	410

FOOD	PORTION	CALS.
Mrs. Smith's (CONT.)		
Cherry	1/8 of 9 in pie (4.6 oz)	320
Cherry Lattice Ready To Serve	1/5 of 8 in pie (4.6 oz)	320
Chocolate Cream	1/4 of 8 in pie (3.4 oz)	290
Coconut Cream	1/4 of 8 in pie (3.4 oz)	280
Coconut Custard	1/5 of 8 in pie (5 oz)	280
Dutch Apple	1/6 of 8 in pie	310
Dutch Apple	1/10 of 10 in pie (4.6 oz)	320
Dutch Apple	1/9 of 9 in pie (4.5 oz)	300
French Silk Cream	1/5 of 8 in pie (4.8 oz)	410
Hearty Pumpkin	1/5 of 8 in pie (5.2 oz)	280
Lemon Cream	1/4 of 8 in pie (3.4 oz)	270
Lemon Meringue	1/5 of 8 in pie (4.8 oz)	300
Mince	1/6 of 8 in pie (4.3 oz)	300
Peach	1/6 of 8 in pie	260
Peach	1/8 of 9 in pie (4.6 oz)	310
Pecan	1/8 of 10 in pie (4.5 oz)	500
Pumpkin	1/9 of 10 in pie (5.1 oz)	250
Pumpkin	1/5 of 8 in pie (5.2 oz)	270
Red Raspberry	1/6 of 8 in pie (4.3 oz)	280
Strawberry Rhubarb	1/5 of 8 in pie (4.8 oz)	520
Strawberry Rhubarb	1/6 of 8 in pie (4.3 oz)	280
Pepperidge Farm		
Hyannis Boston Cream Pie	1	230
Mississippi Mud	1	310
Pet-Ritz		
Apple	1/6 pie (4.33 oz)	330
Banana Cream	1/6 pie (2.33 oz)	170
Blueberry	1/6 pie (4.33 oz)	370
Cherry	1/6 pie (4.33 oz)	300
Chocolate Cream	1/6 pie (2.33 oz)	190
Coconut Cream	1/6 pie (2.33 oz)	190
Egg Custard	1/6 pie (4.0 oz)	200
Lemon Cream	1/6 pie (2.33 oz)	190
Mince	1/6 pie (4.33 oz)	280
Neapolitan Cream	1/6 pie (2.33 oz)	180
Peach	1/6 pie (4.33 oz)	320
Pumpkin Custard	1/6 pie (4.33 oz)	250
Strawberry Cream	1/6 pie (2.33 oz)	170
Sweet Potato	1/6 pie (3.33 oz)	150
Sara Lee		
Apple Homestyle	1 slice (4 oz)	280
Apple Homestyle High	1 slice (4.9 oz)	400
Apple Streusel Free & Light	1 slice (2.9 oz)	170

FOOD	PORTION	CALS.
Sara Lee (CONT.)		
Blueberry Homestyle	1 slice (4 oz)	300
Cherry Homestyle	1 slice (4 oz)	270
Cherry Streusel Free & Light	1 slice (3.6 oz)	160
Dutch Apple Homestyle	1 slice (4 oz)	300
Mince Homestyle	1 slice (4 oz)	300
Peach Homestyle	1 slice (3.4 oz)	280
Pecan Homestyle	1 slice (3.4 oz)	400
Pumpkin Homestyle	1 slice (4 oz)	240
Raspberry Homestyle	1 slice (4 oz)	280
Weight Watchers		
Chocolate Mocha	1 (2.75 oz)	170
Mississippi Mud	1 (5.04 oz)	180
HOME RECIPE		
apple	⅛ of 9 in pie (5.4 oz)	411
banana cream	⅛ of 9 in pie (5.2 oz)	398
blueberry	⅛ of 9 in pie (5.2 oz)	360
butterscotch	⅛ of 9 in pie (4.5 oz)	355
cherry	⅛ of 9 in pie (6.3 oz)	486
coconut creme	⅛ of 9 in pie (4.7 oz)	396
custard	⅛ of 9 in pie (4.5 oz)	262
lemon meringue	⅛ of 9 in pie (4.5 oz)	362
mince	⅛ of 9 in pie (5.8 oz)	477
pecan	⅛ of 9 in pie (4.3 oz)	502
pumpkin	⅛ of 9 in pie (5.4 oz)	316
vanilla cream	⅛ of 9 in pie (4.4 oz)	350
MIX		
banana cream no-bake	⅛ of 9 in pie (3.2 oz)	231
chocolate mousse no-bake	⅛ of 9 in pie (3.3 oz)	247
coconut creme no-bake	⅛ of 9 in pie (3.3 oz)	259
Betty Crocker		
Boston Cream Classic Dessert	⅛ pie	270
Jell-O		
Banana Cream as prep w/ whole milk	⅙ of 8 in pie	103
Chocolate Cream Pie No Bake Dessert	⅛ pie	260
Chocolate Mousse	⅛ pie	259
Coconut Cream	⅛ pie	258
Coconut Cream as prep w/ whole milk	⅙ of 8 in pie	111
Lemon	⅙ of 8 in pie	175
Pumpkin	⅛ pie	253
Royal		
Key Lime Pie Filling	mix for 1 serv	50
Lemon Pie Filling	mix for 1 serv	50

FOOD	PORTION	CALS.
Royal (CONT.)		
Lemon Meringue No-Bake	⅛ pie	210
READY-TO-EAT		
Entenmann's		
Apple Homestyle	1 serv (2.1 oz)	140
Coconut Custard	1 serv (1.8 oz)	140
SNACK		
apple	1 (3 oz)	266
apple fried	1 (6.4 oz)	404
blueberry fried	1 (6.4 oz)	404
cherry	1 (3 oz)	266
cherry fried	1 (6.4 oz)	404
lemon	1 (3 oz)	266
lemon fried	1 (6.4 oz)	404
peach fried	1 (6.4 oz)	404
strawberry fried	1 (6.4 oz)	404
Drake's		
Apple	1 (2 oz)	210
Blueberry	1 (2 oz)	210
Cherry	1 (2 oz)	220
Lemon	1 (2 oz)	210
Lance		
Pecan	1 (38 g)	350
Little Debbie		
Marshmallow Banana	1 pkg (1.4 oz)	160
Marshmallow Banana	1 pkg (2.7 oz)	320
Marshmallow Banana	1 pkg (2 oz)	240
Marshmallow Chocolate	1 pkg (1.4 oz)	160
Marshmallow Chocolate	1 pkg (2.7 oz)	320
Marshmallow Chocolate	1 pkg (2 oz)	240
Oatmeal Creme	1 pkg (1.3 oz)	170
Oatmeal Creme	1 pkg (3 oz)	360
Oatmeal Creme	1 pkg (2.5 oz)	300
Raisin Creme	1 pkg (1.2 oz)	140
Raisin Creme	1 pkg (2.5 oz)	290
Tastykake		
Apple	1 pkg (113 g)	300
Banana Creme	1 pkg (120 g)	380
Blueberry	1 pkg (113 g)	310
Cherry	1 pkg (113 g)	300
Coconut Creme	1 pkg (113 g)	380
French Apple	1 pkg (120 g)	350
Lemon	1 pkg (113 g)	320
Lemon Lime	1 pkg (113 g)	320

FOOD	PORTION	CALS.
Tastykake (CONT.)		
Peach	1 pkg (113 g)	300
Pineapple Cheese	1 pkg (120 g)	340
Pumpkin	1 pkg (4 oz)	320
Strawberry	1 pkg (113 g)	340
Tasty Klair	1 pkg (113 g)	400
TAKE-OUT		
coconut custard	1/6 of 8 in pie (3.6 oz)	271
custard	1/6 pie 9 in	330
pecan	1/6 of 8 in pie (4 oz)	452
pumpkin	1/6 of 8 in pie (3.8 oz)	229

PIE CRUST
(*see also* PIE)

FOOD	PORTION	CALS.
FROZEN		
baked	9 in shell (4.4 oz)	647
baked	1/8 of 9 in pie (0.6 oz)	82
puff pastry baked	1 shell (1.4 oz)	223
Oronoque		
Deep Dish	1/6 pie (1.41 oz)	200
Pie Crust	1/6 pie (1.23 oz)	170
Pepperidge Farm		
Patty Shells	1	210
Puff Pastry Sheets	1/4 sheet	260
Pet-Ritz		
Deep Dish	1/6 pie (1 oz)	130
Graham Cracker	1/6 pie (0.83 oz)	110
Regular	1/6 pie (0.83 oz)	110
Tart Shells	1	150
HOME RECIPE		
9-inch crust	1	900
baked	9 in shell (6.3 oz)	949
baked	1/8 of 9 in crust (0.8 oz)	119
MIX		
as prep	9 in crust (5.6 oz)	801
as prep	1/8 of 9 in pie (0.7 oz)	100
Betty Crocker		
Pie Crust	1/16 pkg	120
Sticks	1/16 pkg	120
Flako		
Mix	1/4 cup (0.9 oz)	130
Jiffy		
As prep	1/7 crust	180
Pillsbury		
Mix	1/6 of 2 crust pie	270

FOOD	PORTION	CALS.
Pillsbury (CONT.)		
Stick	1/6 of a 2 crust pie	270
READY-TO-EAT		
chocolate cookie crumb baked	1/8 of 9 in pie (1 oz)	139
chocolate cookie crumb baked	9 in crust (7.7 oz)	1130
chocolate cookie crumb chilled	9 in crust (7.8 oz)	1127
chocolate cookie crumb chilled	1/8 of 9 in pie (1 oz)	142
graham cracker baked	9 in crust (8.4 oz)	1181
graham cracker baked	1/8 of 9 in pie (1 oz)	148
graham cracker chilled	9 in crust (8.6 oz)	1182
graham cracker chilled	1/8 of 9 in pie (1 oz)	150
vanilla wafer cracker crumbs baked	9 in crust (6.1 oz)	937
vanilla wafer cracker crumbs baked	1/8 of 9 in pie (0.8 oz)	119
vanilla wafer cracker crumbs chilled	9 in crust (6.2 oz)	934
vanilla wafer cracker crumbs chilled	1/8 of 9 in pie (0.8 oz)	117
Generic Label		
Graham	1/8 pie (0.7 oz)	110
Honey Maid		
Graham	1/6 crust (1 oz)	140
Nabisco		
Nilla	1/6 crust (1 oz)	140
Oreo		
Crumb Crust	1/6 crust (1 oz)	140
Ready Crust		
Chocolate	1/8 pie 9 in	100
Chocolate	1 (3 in diam)	110
Graham	1 (3 in diam)	110
Graham	1/8 pie 9 in	100
REFRIGERATED		
Pillsbury		
All Ready	1/8 of 2 crust pie	240

PIEROGI

FOOD	PORTION	CALS.
FROZEN		
Empire		
Potato Cheese	3 (4.6 oz)	260
Potato Onion	3 (4.6 oz)	250
Golden		
Potato Cheese	3 (4 oz)	250
Potato Onion	3 (4 oz)	210
Mrs. T's		
Potato And Cheddar Cheese	1 (1.3 oz)	60
Potato And Onion	1 (1.3 oz)	50
Sauerkraut	1	60

FOOD	PORTION	CALS.
TAKE-OUT		
pierogi	¾ cup (4.4 oz)	307
PIGNOLIA		
(*see* PINE NUTS)		
PIG'S EARS AND FEET		
ears frzn simmered	1 ear (3.7 oz)	183
feet pickled	1 oz	58
feet pickled	1 lb	923
feet simmered	2.5 oz	138
Hormel		
Pickled Feet	2 oz	80
Pickled Hocks	2 oz	110
PIGEON		
w/ skin & bone	3.5 oz	169
PIGEON PEAS		
dried cooked	½ cup	102
dried cooked	1 cup	204
PIKE		
northern cooked	½ fillet (5.4 oz)	176
northern cooked	3 oz	96
northern raw	3 oz	75
roe raw	3½ oz	130
walleye baked	3 oz	101
walleye fillet baked	4.4 oz	147
PILLNUTS		
pillnuts- canarytree dried	1 oz	204
PIMIENTOS		
canned	1 tbsp	3
canned	1 slice	0
Dromedary		
Pimientos	1 oz	10
PINE NUTS		
pignolia dried	1 oz	146
pignolia dried	1 tbsp	51
pinyon dried	1 oz	161
Progresso		
Pignoli	1 jar (1 oz)	170
PINEAPPLE		
CANNED		
chunks in heavy sirup	1 cup	199

FOOD	PORTION	CALS.
chunks juice pack	1 cup	150
crushed in heavy syrup	1 cup	199
slices in heavy syrup	1 slice	45
slices in light syrup	1 slice	30
slices juice pack	1 slice	35
slices water pack	1 slice	19
tidbits in heavy syrup	1 cup	199
tidbits in juice	1 cup	150
tidbits in water	1 cup	79
Del Monte		
Chunks In Heavy Syrup	½ cup (4.3 oz)	90
Chunks In Its Own Juice	½ cup (4.4 oz)	70
Crushed In Heavy Syrup	½ cup (4.4 oz)	90
Crushed In Its Own Juice	½ cup (4.3 oz)	70
Sliced In Heavy Syrup	½ cup (4.1 oz)	90
Sliced In Its Own Juice	½ cup (4 oz)	60
Snack Cups Tidbits In Juice	1 serv (4.5 oz)	70
Snack Cups Tidbits In Juice EZ-Open Lid	1 serv (4.2 oz)	60
Spears In Its Own Juice	½ cup (4.3 oz)	70
Tidbits In Its Own Juice	½ cup (4.3 oz)	70
Wedges In Its Own Juice	½ cup (4.3 oz)	70
Dole		
All Cuts Juice Pack	½ cup	70
All Cuts Syrup Pack	½ cup	90
Empress		
Chunk	4 oz	70
Crushed	4 oz	70
Sliced	4 oz	70
Libby		
Crushed	1 cup with juice	140
Sliced In Unsweetened Juice	1 cup with juice	140
S&W		
Hawaiian Slice In Heavy Syrup	½ cup	90
Hawaiian Slice Juice Pack	½ cup	70
Sliced Unsweetened	½ cup	60
DRIED		
Sonoma		
Pieces	2 pieces (1.4 oz)	140
FRESH		
diced	1 cup	77
slice	1 slice	42
Chiquita		
Fresh	1 cup	90

FOOD	PORTION	CALS.
Dole		
Pineapple	2 slices	90
FROZEN		
chunks sweetened	½ cup	104

PINEAPPLE JUICE

canned	1 cup	139
frzn as prep	1 cup	129
frzn not prep	6 oz	387
After The Fall		
Mandarin Pineapple	1 can (12 oz)	150
Bright & Early		
Frozen	8 fl oz	120
Del Monte		
Juice	8 fl oz	110
Juice	6 fl oz	80
Juice	1 serv (11.5 oz)	190
Dole		
100% frzn as prep	8 fl oz	130
Chilled	6 fl oz	90
Minute Maid		
Box	8.45 fl oz	130
Frozen	8 fl oz	130
S&W		
Unsweetened	6 oz	100
Tree Top		
Juice	6 oz	100
Veryfine		
100%	8 oz	125

PINK BEANS

CANNED		
Goya		
Spanish Style	7.5 oz	140
DRIED		
cooked	1 cup	252

PINTO BEANS

CANNED		
pinto	1 cup	186
Allen		
Pinto Beans	½ cup (4.5 oz)	110
Brown Beauty		
Pinto Beans	½ cup (4.5 oz)	110
East Texas Fair		
Pinto Beans	½ cup (4.5 oz)	110

FOOD	PORTION	CALS.
Eden		
Organic	½ cup (4.4 oz)	90
Gebhardt		
Pinto Beans	4 oz	100
Goya		
Spanish Style	7.5 oz	140
Green Giant		
Picante	½ cup	100
Pinto Beans	½ cup	90
Luck's		
Seasoned w/ Pork w/ Onions	7.5 oz	220
Old El Paso		
Pinto Beans	½ cup (4.6 oz)	110
Progresso		
Pinto Beans	½ cup (4.6 oz)	110
Trappey		
Jalapinto With Bacon	½ cup (4.5 oz)	120
With Bacon	½ cup (4.5 oz)	120
DRIED		
cooked	1 cup	235
Arrowhead		
Dried	¼ cup (1.5 oz)	150
Bean Cuisine		
Dried	½ cup	115
Hurst		
Pinto Beans	1.2 oz	120
With Spanish Seasoning	1.3 oz	120
FROZEN		
cooked	3 oz	152
SPROUTS		
cooked	3½ oz	22
raw	3½ oz	62
PISTACHIOS		
dried	1 oz	164
dried	1 cup	739
dry roasted	1 oz	172
dry roasted salted	1 oz	172
dry roasted salted	1 cup	776
Dole		
Shelled	1 oz	163
Shells On	1 oz	90
Fisher		
Red Tint	1 oz	170

FOOD	PORTION	CALS.
Lance		
Pistachios	1 pkg (32 g)	100
Planters		
Munch'N Go Singles Shelled Dry Roasted	1 pkg (2 oz)	330
Red Salted Dry Roasted	1 pkg	160
Uncolored Dry Roasted	½ cup	160
Sonoma		
Salted Shelled	¼ cup (1 oz)	190

PINYON
(*see* PINE NUTS)

PITANGA
fresh	1 cup	57
fresh	1	2

PIZZA
DOUGH
Boboli		
Shell + Sauce	⅛ lg shell (2.6 oz)	170
Shell + Sauce	⅙ sm shell (2.6 oz)	170
House of Pasta		
Frozen	⅛ of 14 in pie (1.9 oz)	140
Jiffy		
As prep	¼ crust	180
Sassafras		
Cornmeal Pizza Crust	1 slice (1.4 oz)	140
Italian Pizza Crust Mix	1 slice (1.4 oz)	140
Wanda's		
Crust Mix Oregano & Basil	⅒ pie (1.4 oz)	149
Crust Mix Oregano & Basil Whole Wheat	⅒ pie (1.4 oz)	141
Watkins		
Crust Mix	⅛ pkg (1.8 oz)	180

FROZEN
Celeste		
Italian Bread Deluxe	1 (5.1 oz)	290
Italian Bread Garlic & Herb Zesty Chicken	1 (5 oz)	260
Italian Bread Pepperoni	1 (5 oz)	320
Italian Bread Zesty Four Cheese	1 (4.6 oz)	300
Large Cheese	¼ pie (4.4 oz)	320
Large Deluxe	¼ pie (5.5 oz)	350
Large Pepperoni	¼ pie (4.7 oz)	350
Large Suprema With Meat	⅕ pie (4.6 oz)	290
Large Zesty Four Cheese	¼ pie (4.4 oz)	330
Small Cheese	1 (7.5 oz)	540

FOOD	PORTION	CALS.
Celeste (CONT.)		
Small Deluxe	1 (8.2 oz)	540
Small Hot & Zesty Four Cheese	1 (7 oz)	530
Small Original Four Cheese	1 (7 oz)	540
Small Pepperoni	1 (6.7 oz)	520
Small Sausage	1 (7.5 oz)	530
Small Suprema Vegetable	1 (7.5 oz)	480
Small Suprema With Meat	1 (9 oz)	580
Small Zesty Four Cheese	1 (7 oz)	530
Croissant Pocket		
Stuffed Sandwich Pepperoni Pizza	1 piece (4.5 oz)	350
Empire		
3 Pack	1 (3 oz)	210
Bagel	1 (2 oz)	150
English Muffin	1 (2 oz)	130
Pizza	½ pie (5 oz)	340
Fox		
Deluxe Golden Topping	½ pizza	240
Deluxe Hamburger	½ pizza	260
Deluxe Pepperoni	½ pizza	250
Deluxe Sausage	½ pizza	260
Deluxe Sausage & Pepperoni	½ pizza	260
Healthy Choice		
French Bread Cheese	1 (5.6 oz)	310
French Bread Pepperoni	1 (6 oz)	360
French Bread Sausage	1 (6 oz)	330
French Bread Supreme	1 (6.35 oz)	340
Hot Pocket		
Stuffed Sandwich Pepperoni & Sausage Pizza	1 (4.5 oz)	340
Stuffed Sandwich Pepperoni Pizza	1 (4.5 oz)	350
Jeno's		
4-Pack Cheese	1 pizza	160
4-Pack Combination	1 pizza	180
4-Pack Hamburger	1 pizza	180
4-Pack Pepperoni	1 pizza	170
4-Pack Sausage	1 pizza	180
Crisp 'n Tasty Canadian Bacon	½ pizza	250
Crisp 'n Tasty Cheese	½ pizza	270
Crisp 'n Tasty Hamburger	½ pizza	290
Crisp 'n Tasty Pepperoni	½ pizza	280
Crisp 'n Tasty Sausage	½ pizza	300
Crisp 'n Tasty Sausage & Pepperoni	½ pizza	300
Microwave Pizza Rolls Pepperoni & Cheese	6	240

FOOD	PORTION	CALS.
Jeno's (CONT.)		
Microwave Pizza Rolls Sausage & Cheese	6	250
Pizza Rolls Cheese	6	240
Pizza Rolls Hamburger	6	240
Pizza Rolls Pepperoni & Cheese	6	230
Pizza Rolls Sausage & Pepperoni	6	230
Kid Cuisine		
Cheese	1 (8 oz)	430
Hamburger	1 (8.30 oz)	400
Kineret		
Bagel Pizza	2 (4 oz)	300
Slice	1 (4.9 oz)	490
Lean Cuisine		
French Bread Cheese	1 pkg (6 oz)	350
French Bread Deluxe	1 pkg (6.1 oz)	350
French Bread Pepperoni	1 pkg (5.25 oz)	330
Lean Pockets		
Stuffed Sandwich Pizza Deluxe	1 (4.5 oz)	270
MicroMagic		
Deep Dish Combination	1 (6.5 oz)	605
Deep Dish Pepperoni	1 (6.5 oz)	615
Deep Dish Sausage	1 (6.5 oz)	590
Mrs. P's		
Combination	½ pizza	260
Golden Topping	½ pizza	240
Hamburger	½ pizza	260
Pepperoni	½ pizza	250
Sausage	½ pizza	260
Old El Paso		
Pizza Burrito Cheese	1 (3.5 oz)	320
Pizza Burrito Pepperoni	1 (3.5 oz)	260
Pizza Burrito Sausage	1 (3.5 oz)	260
Pappalo's		
French Bread Cheese	1 pizza	360
French Bread Combination	1 pizza	430
French Bread Pepperoni	1 pizza	410
French Bread Sausage	1 pizza	410
Pan Combination	⅙ pizza	340
Pan Hamburger	⅙ pizza	310
Pan Pepperoni	⅙ pizza	330
Pan Sausage	⅙ pizza	360
Thin Crust Combination	⅙ pizza	260
Thin Crust Hamburger	⅙ pizza	240
Thin Crust Pepperoni	⅙ pizza	270

FOOD	PORTION	CALS.
Pappalo's (CONT.)		
Thin Crust Sausage	1/6 pizza	250
Pepperidge Farm		
Croissant Pastry Cheese	1	430
Croissant Pastry Deluxe	1	440
Croissant Pastry Pepperoni	1	420
Pillsbury		
Microwave Cheese	1/2 pizza	240
Microwave Combination	1/2 pizza	310
Microwave French Bread	1 pizza	370
Microwave French Bread Pepperoni	1 pizza	430
Microwave French Bread Sausage	1 pizza	410
Microwave French Bread Sausage & Pepperoni	1 pizza	450
Microwave Pepperoni	1/2 pizza	300
Microwave Sausage	1/2 pizza	280
Small World		
Four Cheese	1 (4 oz)	240
Special Delivery		
Organic	1/3 pizza (5.3 oz)	320
Organic Soy Kaas	1/3 pizza (5.3 oz)	320
Stouffer's		
French Bread Bacon Cheddar	1 piece (5.8 oz)	440
French Bread Cheese	1 piece (5.2 oz)	350
French Bread Cheeseburger	1 piece (6 oz)	440
French Bread Deluxe	1 piece (6.2 oz)	440
French Bread Double Cheese	1 piece (5.9 oz)	420
French Bread Garden Vegetable	1 piece (5.8 oz)	340
French Bread Pepperoni	1 piece (5.6 oz)	420
French Bread Pepperoni & Mushroom	1 piece (6.1 oz)	430
French Bread Sausage	1 piece (6 oz)	420
French Bread Sausage & Pepperoni	1 piece (6.25 oz)	460
French Bread Vegetable Deluxe	1 piece (6.4 oz)	380
French Bread White Pizza	1 piece (5.1 oz)	460
Lunch Express Deluxe	1 pkg (6.6 oz)	460
Lunch Express Double Cheese	1 pkg (5.9 oz)	420
Lunch Express Pepperoni	1 pkg (5.75 oz)	440
Lunch Express Sausage	1 pkg (6.5 oz)	460
Lunch Express Sausage & Pepperoni	1 pkg (6.4 oz)	500
Tombstone		
12 in Canadian Bacon	1/5 pie (5.5 oz)	360
12 in Cheese & Hamburger	1/5 pie (4.4 oz)	320
12 in Cheese & Pepperoni	1/5 pie (4.4 oz)	340
12 in Cheese & Sausage	1/5 pie (4.4 oz)	320

FOOD	PORTION	CALS.
Tombstone (CONT.)		
12 in Cheese Sausage & Mushroom	⅕ pie (4.5 oz)	320
12 in Deluxe	⅕ pie (4.7 oz)	320
12 in Extra Cheese	⅕ pie (5.1 oz)	370
12 in Sausage & Pepperoni	⅕ pie (4.4 oz)	340
12 in Special Order Four Cheese	⅕ pie (5.2 oz)	400
12 in Special Order Four Meat	⅙ pie (4.7 oz)	350
12 in Special Order Pepperoni	⅙ pie (4.5 oz)	360
12 in Special Order Super Supreme	⅙ pie (4.8 oz)	350
12 in Special Order Three Sausage	⅙ pie (4.6 oz)	340
12 in Supreme	⅕ pie (4.6 oz)	330
12 in ThinCrust Italian Style Three Cheese	¼ pie (4.8 oz)	380
9 in Cheese & Hamburger	⅓ pie (4.1 oz)	310
9 in Cheese & Pepperoni	⅓ pie (4.1 oz)	340
9 in Cheese & Sausage	⅓ pie (4.1 oz)	310
9 in Deluxe	⅓ pie (4.5 oz)	320
9 in Extra Cheese	⅓ pie (5.6 oz)	420
9 in Pepperoni & Sausage	⅓ pie (4.4 oz)	360
9 in Special Order Four Meat	⅓ pie (5.3 oz)	400
9 in Special Order Pepperoni	⅓ pie (5.1 oz)	400
9 in Special Order Super Supreme	⅓ pie (5.5 oz)	400
9 in Special Order Three Sausage	⅓ pie (5.2 oz)	390
Double Top Pepperoni With Double Cheese	⅙ pie (4.5 oz)	350
Double Top Sausage & Pepperoni With Double Cheese	⅙ pie (4.7 oz)	360
Double Top Sausage With Double Cheese	⅙ pie (4.7 oz)	350
For One ½ Less Fat Cheese	1 pie (6.5 oz)	360
For One ½ Less Fat Pepperoni	1 pie (6.7 oz)	400
For One ½ Less Fat Supreme	1 pie (7.7 oz)	400
For One ½ Less Fat Vegetable	1 pie (7.2 oz)	360
For One Cheese & Pepperoni	1 pie (7 oz)	580
For One Extra Cheese	1 pie (7 oz)	540
For One Italian Sausage	1 pie (7 oz)	560
For One Sausage & Pepperoni	1 pie (7 oz)	590
For One Supreme	1 pie (7.5 oz)	570
Light Supreme	⅕ pie (4.8 oz)	270
Light Vegetable	⅕ pie (4.6 oz)	240
ThinCrust Italian Style Four Meat Combo	¼ pie (5.1 oz)	410
ThinCrust Italian Style Pepperoni	¼ pie (5 oz)	420
ThinCrust Italian Style Sausage	¼ pie (5.1 oz)	400
ThinCrust Italian Style Supreme	¼ pie (5.3 oz)	400
ThinCrust Mexican Style Supreme Taco	¼ pie (5.1 oz)	380

FOOD	PORTION	CALS.
Totino's		
Microwave Cheese	1 pizza	250
Microwave Pepperoni	1 pizza	280
Microwave Sausage	1 pizza	320
Microwave Sausage Pepperoni Combination	1 pizza	310
My Classic Deluxe Cheese	⅙ pizza	210
My Classic Deluxe Combination	⅙ pizza	270
My Classic Deluxe Pepperoni	⅙ pizza	260
Pan Pepperoni	⅙ pizza	330
Pan Sausage	⅙ pizza	320
Pan Sausage & Pepperoni Combination	⅙ pizza	340
Pan Three Cheese	⅙ pizza	290
Party Bacon	½ pizza	370
Party Canadian Bacon	½ pizza	310
Party Cheese	½ pizza	340
Party Combination	½ pizza	380
Party Hamburger	½ pizza	370
Party Mexican Style	½ pizza	380
Party Pepperoni	½ pizza	370
Party Sausage	½ pizza	390
Party Vegetable	½ pizza	300
Slices Cheese	1	170
Slices Combination	1	200
Slices Pepperoni	1	190
Slices Sausage	1	200
Weight Watchers		
Deluxe Combo	1 (6.57 oz)	380
Deluxe Pocket Pizza Sandwich	1 (5 oz)	300
Extra Cheese	1 (5.74 oz)	390
Pepperoni	1 (5.56 oz)	390
SAUCE		
Boboli		
Sauce	1 pkg (1.2 oz)	20
Sauce	¼ cup (2.5 oz)	40
Contadina		
Flavored With Pepperoni	¼ cup	40
Pizza Sauce	¼ cup	35
Squeeze	¼ cup	35
With Italian Cheeses	¼ cup	40
Eden		
Pizza Pasta Sauce	½ cup (4.4 oz)	80
Muir Glen		
Organic	¼ cup (2.2 oz)	40

FOOD	PORTION	CALS.
Progresso		
Pizza Sauce	¼ cup (2.2 oz)	35
Ragu		
Quick Traditional	3 tbsp (1.7 oz)	35
Tree Of Life		
Sauce	¼ cup (1.9 oz)	30
TAKE-OUT		
cheese	12 in pie	1121
cheese	⅛ of 12 in pie	140
cheese deep dish individual	1 (5.5 oz)	460
cheese meat & vegetables	12 in pie	1472
cheese meat & vegetables	⅛ of 12 in pie	184
pepperoni	⅛ of 12 in pie	181
pepperoni	12 in pie	1445

PLANTAINS

FOOD	PORTION	CALS.
fresh uncooked	1 (6.3 oz)	218
sliced cooked	½ cup	89
Top Banana		
All Natural Plantain Chips	1 oz	150
TAKE-OUT		
ripe fried	2.8 oz	214

PLUMS
CANNED

FOOD	PORTION	CALS.
purple in heavy sirup	3	119
purple in heavy syrup	1 cup	320
purple in light syrup	3	83
purple in light syrup	1 cup	158
purple juice pack	3	55
purple juice pack	1 cup	146
purple water pack	1 cup	102
purple water pack	3	39
S&W		
Halves Purple Fancy Unpeeled In Extra Heavy Syrup	½ cup	135
Whole Purple Fancy Unpeeled In Extra Heavy Syrup	½ cup	135
Whole Unpeeled Diet	½ cup	52
FRESH		
plum	1	36
sliced	1 cup	91
Dole		
Plums	2	70

FOOD	PORTION	CALS.
POI		
poi	½ cup	134
POKEBERRY SHOOTS		
cooked	½ cup	16
raw	½ cup	18
Allen		
Pokeberry Shoots	½ cup (4.1 oz)	35
POLLACK		
altantic fillet baked	5.3 oz	178
FROZEN		
Mrs. Paul's		
Fillets Light	1 fillet (4.5 oz)	240
POMEGRANATES		
pomegranate	1	104
POMPANO		
florida cooked	3 oz	179
florida raw	3 oz	140
POLENTA		
(*see* CORNMEAL)		
POPCORN		
(*see also* CHIPS, POPCORN CAKES, PRETZELS, SNACKS)		
air-popped	1 cup (0.3 oz)	31
air-popped	1 oz	108
caramel coated	1 oz	122
caramel coated	1 cup (1.2 oz)	152
carmel coated w/ peanuts	⅔ cup (1 oz)	114
cheese	1 oz	149
cheese	1 cup (0.4 oz)	58
oil popped	1 oz	142
oil popped	1 cup (0.4 oz)	55
Barrel O' Fun		
Baked Curl	1 oz	150
Caramel Corn	1 oz	115
Corn Pop	1 oz	190
Popcorn	1 oz	160
White Cheddar Pops	1 oz	170
Cheetos		
Cheddar Cheese	0.5 oz	80
Chesters		
Cheddar Cheese	0.5 oz	80
Microwave	3 cups	110

FOOD	PORTION	CALS.
Chesters (CONT.)		
Microwave Butter	3 cups	120
Microwave Cheese	3 cups	110
Popcorn	0.5 oz	70
Cracker Jack		
Original	1 oz	120
Estee		
No Sugar Added Caramel	1 cup (1 oz)	120
General Mills		
Popcorn Bars Caramel	1 (0.6 oz)	70
Greenfield		
Caramel	1 cup (1 oz)	120
Jiffy Pop		
Bag Butter	3 cups	90
Bag Lite	3 cups	70
Bag Regular	3 cups	100
Glazed Popcorn Clusters	1 oz	120
Microwave Butter	4 cup	140
Microwave Regular	4 cup	140
Pan Butter	4 cup	130
Pan Regular	4 cup	130
Lance		
Cheese	1 pkg (25 g)	130
Plain	1 pkg (25 g)	140
White Cheddar Cheese	1 pkg (25 g)	140
Louise's		
Fat-Free Apple Cinnamon	1 oz	100
Fat-Free Buttery Toffee	1 oz	100
Fat-Free Caramel	1 oz	100
Newman's Own		
Oldstyle Picture Show	3 ⅓ cups	80
Oldstyle Picture Show Microwave Natural Butter	3 cups	150
Oldstyle Picture Show Microwave No Salt	3 cups	150
Oldstyle Picture Show Microwave Light Butter	3 cups	90
Oldstyle Picture Show Microwave Light Natural	3 cups	90
Orville Redenbacher's		
Gourmet Hot Air	3 cups	40
Gourmet Original	3 cups	80
Gourmet White	3 cups	80
Microwave Gourmet	3 cups	100
Microwave Gourmet Butter Toffee	2½ cups	210

FOOD	PORTION	CALS.
Orville Redenbacher's (CONT.)		
Microwave Gourmet Caramel	2½ cups	240
Microwave Gourmet Cheddar Cheese	3 cups	130
Microwave Gourmet Salt Free	3 cups	100
Microwave Gourmet Salt Free Butter	3 cups	100
Microwave Gourmet Sour Cream 'n Onion	3 cups	160
Pillsbury		
Microwave Butter	3 cups	210
Microwave Original	3 cups	210
Microwave Salt Free	3 cups	170
Pop Secret		
Butter Flavor	3 cups	100
Butter Flavor Singles	6 cups	250
Light Butter Flavor	3 cups	70
Light Butter Flavor Singles	6 cups	140
Light Natural Flavor	3 cups	70
Light Natural Flavor Singles	6 cups	150
Natural Flavor	3 cups	100
Natural Flavor Salt Free	3 cups	100
Pop Chips	1½ cups (1 oz)	130
Pop Qwiz Butter Flavor	3 cups	100
Pop Qwiz Natural Flavor	3 cups	100
Smartfood		
Cheddar Cheese	0.5 oz	80
Light Butter	0.5 oz	70
Snyder's		
Butter	1 oz	140
Ultra Slim-Fast		
Lite N' Tasty	½ oz	60
Weight Watchers		
Butter	1 pkg (0.66 oz)	90
Butter Toffee	1 pkg (0.9 oz)	110
Caramel	1 pkg (0.9 oz)	100
Microwave	1 pkg (1 oz)	90
White Cheddar Cheese	1 pkg (0.66 oz)	90
Wise		
Tender Eating	0.5 oz	70
With Real Premium White Cheddar Cheese	0.5 oz	70

POPCORN CAKES

FOOD	PORTION	CALS.
popcorn cake	1 (0.3 oz)	38
Lundberg		
Organic Lightly Salted	1	60
Organic Unsalted	1	60

FOOD	PORTION	CALS.
Lundberg (CONT.)		
Rye With Caraway Lightly Salted	1	59
Mother's		
Butter Flavor	1 (0.3 oz)	35
Unsalted	1 (0.3 oz)	35
Quaker		
Blueberry Crunch	1 (0.5 oz)	50
Butter Mini	6 (0.5 oz)	50
Butter Popped	1 (0.3 oz)	35
Caramel	1 (0.5 oz)	50
Caramel Mini	5 (0.5 oz)	50
Cheddar Cheese Mini	6 (0.5 oz)	50
Lightly Salted Mini	7 (0.5 oz)	50
Monterey Jack	1 (0.4 oz)	40
Strawberry Crunch	1 (0.5 oz)	50
White Cheddar	1 (0.4 oz)	40

POPOVER

FOOD	PORTION	CALS.
home recipe as prep w/ 2% milk	1 (1.4 oz)	87
home recipe as prep w/ whole milk	1 (1.4 oz)	90
mix as prep	1 (1.2 oz)	67

POPPY SEEDS

FOOD	PORTION	CALS.
poppy seeds	1 tsp	15

PORK

(*see also* BACON, BACON SUBSTITUTES, CANADIAN BACON, HAM, DELI MEATS/COLD CUTS, SAUSAGE)

The values for cooked pork may differ slightly from values for raw pork. When meat is cooked some moisture and fat is lost, changing the nutritive value slightly. As a rule of thumb, it can be assumed that a 4 oz raw portion will equal a 3 oz cooked portion of meat.

FOOD	PORTION	CALS.
CANNED		
Hormel		
Pickled Tidbits	2 oz	100
FRESH		
blade chop roasted	1 (3.1 oz)	321
center loin chop broiled	1 (3.1 oz)	275
center loin chop lean & fat braised	1 chop (2.6 oz)	266
center loin chop lean & fat broiled	1 chop (3.1 oz)	275
center loin chop lean & fat panfried	1 chop (3.1 oz)	333
center loin chop lean & fat roasted	1 chop (3.1 oz)	268
center loin chop lean only braised	1 chop (2.1 oz)	166
center loin chop lean only broiled	1 chop (2.5 oz)	166

FOOD	PORTION	CALS.
center loin chop lean only panfried	1 chop (2.4 oz)	178
center loin chop lean only roasted	1 chop (2.4 oz)	180
center loin lean & fat braised	3 oz	301
center loin lean & fat panfried	3 oz	318
center loin lean only broiled	3 oz	196
center loin lean only panfried	3 oz	226
center loin lean only roasted	3 oz	204
center loin roasted	3 oz	259
ham fresh rump half lean & fat roasted	3 oz	233
ham fresh rump half lean only roasted	3 oz	187
ham fresh shank half lean & fat roasted	3 oz	258
ham fresh shank half lean only roasted	3 oz	183
ham fresh whole lean & fat roasted	3 oz	250
ham fresh whole lean only roasted	3 oz	187
leg loin & shoulder lean only roasted	3 oz	198
loin blade chop lean & fat braised	1 chop (3.1 oz)	321
loin blade chop lean & fat braised	1 chop (2.4 oz)	275
loin blade chop lean & fat panfried	1 chop (3.1 oz)	368
loin blade chop lean only braised	1 chop (1.8 oz)	156
loin blade chop lean only broiled	1 chop (2.1 oz)	177
loin blade chop lean only panfried	1 chop (2.2 oz)	175
loin blade chop lean only roasted	1 chop (2.5 oz)	198
loin blade lean & fat braised	3 oz	348
loin blade lean & fat broiled	3 oz	334
loin blade lean & fat panfried	3 oz	352
loin blade lean & fat roasted	3 oz	310
loin blade lean only broiled	3 oz	255
loin blade lean only panfried	3 oz	240
loin blade lean only roasted	3 oz	238
loin chop lean & fat braised	1 chop (2.5 oz)	261
loin chop lean & fat roasted	1 chop (2.9 oz)	262
loin chop lean & fat braised	1 chop (2.3 oz)	267
loin chop lean & fat broiled	1 chop (2.7 oz)	295
loin chop lean & fat panfried	1 chop (2.9 oz)	337
loin chop lean & fat roasted	1 chop (2.8 oz)	274
loin chop lean only braised	1 chop (1.8 oz)	147
loin chop lean only broiled	1 chop (2.1 oz)	165
loin chop lean only panfried	1 chop (2 oz)	157
loin chop lean only roasted	1 chop (2.3 oz)	167
loin lean & fat braised	3 oz	312
loin lean & fat broiled	3 oz	294
loin lean only braised	3 oz	232
loin lean only broiled	3 oz	218
loin lean only roasted	3 oz	204
loin w/ fat roasted	3 oz	271

FOOD	PORTION	CALS.
lungs braised	3 oz	84
pancreas braised	3 oz	186
rib chop lean only braised	1 chop (1.8 oz)	147
rib chop lean only broiled	1 chop (2.1 oz)	162
rib chop lean only panfried	1 chop (2 oz)	160
rib chop lean only roasted	1 chop (2.2 oz)	162
rib chop lean & fat braised	1 chop (2.2 oz)	246
rib chop lean & fat broiled	1 chop (2.6 oz)	264
rib chop lean & fat panfried	1 chop (2.9 oz)	343
rib chop lean & fat roasted	1 chop (2.6 oz)	252
shoulder arm picnic cured lean & fat roasted	3 oz	238
shoulder arm picnic cured lean only roasted	3 oz	145
shoulder arm picnic lean only braised	3 oz	211
shoulder arm picnic lean only roasted	3 oz	194
shoulder arm picnic lean & fat braised	3 oz	293
shoulder arm picnic lean & fat roasted	3 oz	281
shoulder blade boston steak lean & fat braised	1 steak (5.6 oz)	594
shoulder blade boston steak lean & fat broiled	1 steak (6.5 oz)	647
shoulder blade boston steak lean & fat roasted	1 steak (6.5 oz)	594
shoulder blade boston steak lean only braised	1 steak (4.6 oz)	382
shoulder blade boston steak lean only broiled	1 steak (5.3 oz)	413
shoulder blade boston steak lean only roasted	1 steak (5.5 oz)	404
shoulder blade roll cured lean & fat	3 oz	304
shoulder boston blade lean & fat braised	3 oz	316
shoulder boston blade lean & fat broiled	3 oz	297
shoulder boston blade lean & fat roasted	3 oz	273
shoulder boston blade lean only braised	3 oz	250
shoulder boston blade lean only broiled	3 oz	233
shoulder boston blade lean only roasted	3 oz	218
shoulder whole lean only roated	3 oz	207
shoulder whole roasted	3 oz	277
sirloin chop lean & fat braised	1 chop (2.4 oz)	250
sirloin chop lean & fat broiled	1 chop (2.8 oz)	278
sirloin chop lean & fat roasted	1 chop (2.8 oz)	244
sirloin chop lean only braised	1 chop (1.9 oz)	149
sirloin chop lean only broiled	1 chop (2.3 oz)	165
sirloin chop lean only roasted	1 chop (2.5 oz)	175
spareribs braised	3 oz	338
spleen braised	3 oz	127

FOOD	PORTION	CALS.
tail simmered	3 oz	336
tenderloin lean only roasted	3 oz	141
Oscar Mayer		
Sweet Morsel Smoked Boneless Pork Shoulder	3 oz	180
TAKE-OUT		
pork roast	2 oz	70

PORK DISHES
FROZEN
Jimmy Dean

BBQ Pork Rib Sandwich	1 (5.4 oz)	440
TAKE-OUT		
tourtiere	1 piece (4.9 oz)	451

POSOLE
(*see* HOMINY)

POT PIE
FROZEN
Award Brand

Beef	1 (7 oz)	350
Chicken	1 (7 oz)	350
Banquet		
Family Entree Chicken Pie	1 serv (8 oz)	450
Macaroni & Cheese	1 pkg (6.5 oz)	200
Vegetable & Cheese	1 (7 oz)	390
Vegetable Pie w/ Beef	1 (7 oz)	330
Vegetable Pie w/ Chicken	1 (7 oz)	350
Vegetable Pie w/ Turkey	1 (7 oz)	370
Empire		
Chicken	1 (8.1 oz)	440
Turkey	1 (8.1 oz)	470
Great Value		
Beef	1 (7 oz)	390
Chicken	1 (7 oz)	380
Turkey	1 (7 oz)	400
Morton		
Beef	1 (7 oz)	310
Chicken	1 (7 oz)	320
Macaroni & Cheese	1 (6 oz)	160
Turkey	1 (7 oz)	300
Ozark Valley		
Chicken	1 (7 oz)	330
Macaroni & Cheese	1 (6.5 oz)	160

FOOD	PORTION	CALS.
Ozark Valley (CONT.)		
Turkey	1 (7 oz)	280
Stouffer's		
Beef Pie	1 pkg (10 oz)	450
Chicken Pie	1 pkg (10 oz)	520
Chicken Pie	½ pkg (8 oz)	460
Turkey	1 cup (8 oz)	500
Turkey	1 pkg (10 oz)	530
Swanson		
Beef	7 oz	370
Beef Hungry Man	16 oz	610
Chicken	7 oz	380
Chicken Homestyle	8 oz	410
Hungry Man Chicken	16 oz	630
Hungry Man Turkey	16 oz	650
Turkey	7 oz	380
TAKE-OUT		
beef	⅓ of 9 in pie (7.4 oz)	515
chicken	⅓ of 9 in pie (8.1 oz)	545

POTATO
(*see also* CHIPS, KNISH)

FOOD	PORTION	CALS.
CANNED		
potatoes	½ cup	54
Allen		
Refried Potatoes	½ cup (4.5 oz)	150
Butterfield		
Diced	⅔ cup (5.7 oz)	100
Sliced	½ cup (5.7 oz)	100
Whole	2½ pieces (5.6 oz)	90
Del Monte		
New Sliced	⅔ cup (5.4 oz)	60
New Whole	⅔ cup (5.5 oz)	60
Hormel		
Au Gratin & Bacon	1 can (7.5 oz)	250
Scalloped & Ham	1 can (7.5 oz)	260
Hunt's		
Whole New	4 oz	70
S&W		
New Potatoes Extra Small	½ cup	45
Seneca		
Potatoes	½ cup	80
Sunshine		
Whole	2½ pieces (5.6 oz)	90

FOOD	PORTION	CALS.
FRESH		
baked skin only	1 skin (2 oz)	115
baked w/ skin	1 (6½ oz)	220
baked w/o skin	1 (5 oz)	145
baked w/o skin	½ cup	57
boiled	½ cup	68
microwaved	1 (7 oz)	212
microwaved w/o skin	½ cup	78
raw w/o skin	1 (3.9 oz)	88
Yukon Gold		
Fresh	1 (5.3 oz)	110
FROZEN		
french fries	10 strips	111
french fries thick cut	10 strips	109
hashed brown	½ cup	170
potato puffs	½ cup	138
potato puffs as prep	1	16
Budget Gourmet		
Baked With Broccoli And Cheese	1 pkg (10.5 oz)	300
Cheddared Potatoes	1 pkg (5.5 oz)	260
Cheddared Potatoes With Broccoli	1 pkg (5 oz)	150
Three Cheese Potatoes	1 pkg (5.75 oz)	220
Empire		
Crinkle Cut French Fries	½ cup (3 oz)	90
Latkes Potato Pancakes	1 (2 oz)	80
Latkes Mini Potato Pancakes	2 (2 oz)	90
Golden		
Potato Pancakes	1 (1.33 oz)	71
Green Giant		
One Serve Au Gratin	1 pkg	200
One Serve Potatoes & Broccoli In Cheese Sauce	1 pkg	130
Healthy Choice		
Cheddar Broccoli Potatoes	1 meal (10.5 oz)	310
Garden Potato Casserole	1 meal (9.25 oz)	200
Kineret		
Crinkle Cut	18 pieces (3 oz)	120
Kugel	1 piece (2.5 oz)	150
Latkes	1 (1.5 oz)	90
Latkes Mini	10 (3 oz)	160
Lean Cuisine		
Deluxe Cheddar	1 pkg (10.4 oz)	270
MicroMagic		
French Fries	1 pkg (3 oz)	290

FOOD	PORTION	CALS.
MicroMagic (CONT.)		
Skinny Fries	1 pkg (3 oz)	350
Oh Boy!		
Stuffed With Cheddar Cheese	1 (6 oz)	130
Stuffed With Real Bacon	1 (6 oz)	120
Ore Ida		
Cheddar Browns	1 patty (3 oz)	90
Cottage Fries	14 pieces (3 oz)	130
Crispers!	17 pieces (3 oz)	220
Crispers! Nacho	10 pieces (3 oz)	170
Crispers! Texas	3 oz	170
Crispy Crowns!	12 pieces (3 oz)	100
Crispy Crunchies	12 pieces (3 oz)	160
Deep Fries Crinkle Cuts	18 pieces (3 oz)	160
Deep Fries French Fries	22 pieces (3 oz)	160
Dinner Fries Country Style	8 pieces (3 oz)	110
Fast Fries	23 pieces (3 oz)	140
Fast Fries Ranch	22 pieces (3 oz)	150
Golden Crinkles	16 pieces (3 oz)	120
Golden Fries	16 pieces (3 oz)	120
Golden Patties	1 (2.5 oz)	140
Golden Twirls	28 pieces (3 oz)	160
Hash Browns Country Style	1 cup (2.6 oz)	60
Hash Browns Shredded	1 patty (3 oz)	70
Hash Browns Southern Style	¾ cup (3 oz)	70
Hot Tots	9 pieces (3 oz)	150
Mashed Natural Butter	½ cup (2.1 oz)	80
Microwave Crinkle Cuts	1 pkg (3.5 oz)	180
Microwave Hash Browns	1 patty (2 oz)	110
Microwave Tater Tots	1 pkg (3.75 oz)	190
O'Brien Potatoes	¾ cup (3 oz)	60
Pixie Crinkles	33 pieces (3 oz)	140
Shoestrings	38 pieces (3 oz)	150
Snackin' Fries	1 pkg (5 oz)	180
Snackin' Fries Extra Zesty	1 pkg (5 oz)	180
Tater ABC's	10 pieces (3 oz)	190
Tater Tots	9 pieces (3 oz)	160
Tater Tots Bacon	9 pieces (3 oz)	150
Tater Tots Onion	9 pieces (3 oz)	150
Toaster Hash Browns	2 patties (3.5 oz)	190
Topped Broccoli & Cheese	½ (6 oz)	150
Topped Salsa & Cheese	½ (5.5 oz)	160
Topped Vegetable Primavera	1 (6.13 oz)	160
Twice Baked Butter	1 (5 oz)	200

FOOD	PORTION	CALS.
Ore Ida (CONT.)		
Twice Baked Cheddar Cheese	1 (5 oz)	190
Twice Baked Ranch	1 (5 oz)	180
Twice Bakes Sour Cream & Chives	1 (5 oz)	180
Waffle Fries	15 pieces (3 oz)	140
Wedges With Skin	9 pieces (3 oz)	110
Zesties!	12 pieces (3 oz)	160
Stouffer's		
Au Gratin	½ cup (2.25 oz)	130
Baked Broccoli & Cheese	1 pkg (10.1 oz)	320
Baked Cheddar Cheese & Bacon	1 pkg (9.4 oz)	380
Lunch Express Baked Broccoli & Cheese	1 pkg (10.25 oz)	250
Scalloped	½ cup (2.25 oz)	130
Weight Watchers		
Baked Broccoli & Cheese	1 pkg (10 oz)	230
HOME RECIPE		
au gratin	½ cup	160
mashed	½ cup	111
scalloped	½ cup	105
MIX		
au gratin as prep	4½ oz	127
instant mashed flakes as prep w/ whole milk & butter	½ cup	118
instant mashed flakes not prep	½ cup	78
instant mashed granules as prep w/ whole milk & butter	½ cup	114
instant mashed granules not prep	½ cup	372
scalloped as prep	4½ oz	127
Betty Crocker		
Au Gratin as prep	½ cup	140
Cheddar 'N Bacon as prep	½ cup	140
Cheesy Scalloped as prep	½ cup	140
Hash Browns as prep	½ cup	160
Hash Browns as prep w/o salt	½ cup	160
Homestyle American Cheese as prep	½ cup	140
Homestyle Broccoli Au Gratin as prep	½ cup	130
Homestyle Cheddar Cheese as prep	½ cup	140
Homestyle Cheesy Scalloped as prep	½ cup	140
Julienne as prep	½ cup	130
Potato Buds as prep	½ cup	130
Potato Buds as prep w/o salt	½ cup	130
Scalloped as prep	½ cup	140
Scalloped & Ham as prep	½ cup	160
Smokey Cheddar as prep	½ cup	140

FOOD	PORTION	CALS.
Betty Crocker (CONT.)		
Sour Cream 'N Chive as prep	½ cup	140
Twice Baked Bacon & Cheddar as prep	½ cup	210
Twice Baked Cheddar With Mild Onion as prep	½ cup	190
Twice Baked Herbed Butter as prep	½ cup	220
Twice Baked Sour Cream & Chive as prep	½ cup	200
Country Store		
Mashed not prep	⅓ cup	70
French's		
Cheddar & Bacon Casserole	½ cup	130
Creamy Stroganoff	½ cup	130
Crispy Top Scalloped With Savory Onion	½ cup	140
Real Cheese Scalloped	½ cup	140
Real Sour Cream & Chives	½ cup	150
Spuds Mashed	½ cup	140
Tangy Au Gratin	½ cup	130
Hungry Jack		
Mashed Flakes	½ cup	40
Kraft		
Potatoes & Cheese Au Gratin	½ cup	130
Potatoes & Cheese Broccoli Au Gratin	½ cup	120
Potatoes & Cheese Scalloped	½ cup	140
Potatoes & Cheese Scalloped With Ham	½ cup	150
REFRIGERATED		
Simply Potatoes		
Au Gratin	¼ pkg (3 oz)	130
Hash Browns	⅕ pkg (4 oz)	100
Hash Browns Onion	⅕ pkg (4 oz)	120
Hash Browns Southwest Style	⅕ pkg (4 oz)	100
Mashed	⅕ pkg (4 oz)	90
Scalloped	¼ pkg (3 oz)	100
SHELF-STABLE		
Lunch Bucket		
Scalloped	1 pkg (7.5 oz)	160
Micro Cup Meals		
Scalloped Potatoes & Ham	1 cup (10.4 oz)	360
Scalloped Potatoes With Ham	1 cup (7.5 oz)	260
Pantry Express		
Augratin	½ cup	120
TAKE-OUT		
au gratin w/ cheese	½ cup	178
baked topped w/ cheese sauce	1	475
baked topped w/ cheese sauce & bacon	1	451

FOOD	PORTION	CALS.
baked topped w/ cheese sauce & broccoli	1	402
baked topped w/ cheese sauce & chili	1	481
baked topped w/ sour cream & chives	1	394
curry	1 serving (6 oz)	292
french fried in beef tallow	1 lg	358
french fried in beef tallow	1 reg	237
french fried in vegetable oil	1 reg	235
french fried in vegetable oil	1 lg	355
hash brown	½ cup	163
mashed w/ whole milk & margarine	⅓ cup	66
mustard potato salad	3.5 oz	120
o'brien	1 cup	157
potato dumpling	3½ oz	334
potato pancakes	1 (1.3 oz)	101
potato salad	½ cup	179
potato salad	⅓ cup	108
potato salad w/ vegetables	3.5 oz	120
scalloped	½ cup	127

POTATO STARCH

potato starch	3½ oz	335
Manischewitz		
Potato Starch	1 cup	570

POUT

ocean baked	3 oz	86
ocean fillet baked	4.8 oz	139

PRESERVE
(*see* JAM/JELLY/PRESERVE)

PRETZELS
(*see also* CHIPS, POPCORN, SNACKS)

chocolate covered	1 (0.4 oz)	50
chocolate covered	1 oz	130
dutch twist	4 (2.1 oz)	229
pretzels	1 oz	108
rods	4 (2 oz)	229
sticks	10	10
sticks	120 (2 oz)	229
twist	1 (½ oz)	65
twists	10 (2.1 oz)	229
whole wheat	2 sm (1 oz)	103
whole wheat	2 med (2 oz)	205
Barrel O' Fun		
Mini	1 oz	110

FOOD	PORTION	CALS.
Barrel O' Fun (CONT.)		
Sticks	1 oz	110
Twists	1 oz	110
Estee		
Dutch Unsalted	2 (1.1 oz)	130
Nuggets Ranch Reduced Sodium	23 (1 oz)	130
Nuggets Reduced Sodium	30 (1 oz)	120
Unsalted	23 (1 oz)	120
Formagg		
Pretzel Nuts	1 oz	120
J&J		
Soft	1 (2.25 oz)	170
Soft Bites	5 bites	110
Lance		
Twist	1 pkg (42 g)	150
Manischewitz		
Bagel Pretzels Original	4 (1 oz)	110
Mister Salty		
Chips	16 (1 oz)	110
Dutch	2 (1.1 oz)	120
Fat Free Chips	16 (1 oz)	100
Mini	22 (1 oz)	110
Sticks Fat Free	47 (1 oz)	110
Twist Fat Free	9 (1 oz)	110
Mr. Phipps		
Chips Lower Sodium	16 (1 oz)	120
Chips Original Fat Free	16 (1 oz)	100
Planters		
Twists	1 oz	100
Twists	1 pkg (1.5 oz)	160
Quinlan		
Beers	1 oz	110
Hard Sourdough	1 oz	110
Logs	1 oz	110
Nuggets	1 oz	110
Rods	1 oz	110
Sticks	1 oz	110
Thins	1 oz	110
Rold Gold		
Bavarian	3 pieces (1 oz)	120
Pretzel Chips	1 oz	110
Pretzel Chips Cheese	1 oz	120
Rods	3 pieces (1 oz)	110
Snack Mix	½ cup (1 oz)	140

FOOD	PORTION	CALS.
Rold Gold (CONT.)		
Sour Dough	1½ pieces (1 oz)	110
Sticks	50 pieces (1 oz)	110
Thin Twist	10 pieces (1 oz)	110
Tiny Twist	15 pieces (1 oz)	110
Seyfart's		
Butter Rods	1 oz	110
Snyder's		
Logs	1 oz	310
Minis	1 oz	310
Minis Unsalted	1 oz	310
Nibblers	1 oz	310
Oat Bran	1 oz	120
Old Fashioned Hard	1 oz	111
Old Fashioned Hard Unsalted	1 oz	100
Old Tyme	1 oz	310
Old Tyme Unsalted	1 oz	110
Rods	1 oz	310
Sourdough Hard Buttermilk Ranch	1 oz	130
Sourdough Hard Cheddar Cheese	1 oz	160
Sourdough Hard Honey Mustard & Onion	1 oz	130
Stix	1 oz	310
Very Thins	1 oz	310
Sunshine		
California Pretzels	1 oz	110
Ultra Slim-Fast		
Lite N' Tasty	1 oz	100
Wege		
Sourdough	1 oz	102
Unsalted	1 oz	102
Whole Wheat	1 oz	109
Weight Watchers		
Oat Bran Nuggets	1 pkg (1.5 oz)	170
PRICKLYPEAR		
fresh	1	42
PRUNE JUICE		
canned	1 cup	181
Del Monte		
Juice	8 fl oz	170
S&W		
Unsweetened	6 oz	120

FOOD	PORTION	CALS.
PRUNES		
CANNED		
in heavy syrup	5	90
in heavy syrup	1 cup	245
DRIED		
cooked w/ sugar	½ cup	147
cooked w/o sugar	½ cup	113
dried	10	201
dried	1 cup	385
Del Monte		
Pitted	¼ cup (1.4 oz)	120
Unpitted	⅓ cup (1.4 oz)	110
Mariani		
Pitted	¼ cup	140
Whole	¼ cup	140
Sonoma		
Pitted	¼ cup (1.4 oz)	120
Sunsweet		
Orange Essence Pitted Prunes	6 (1.4 oz)	100
PUDDING		
(*see also* CUSTARD, PUDDING POPS)		
HOME RECIPE		
bread pudding	½ cup (4.4 oz)	212
bread pudding	1 recipe 6 serv (26.4 oz)	1266
chocolate as prep w/ whole milk	½ cup (5.5 oz)	221
corn	⅔ cup	181
cornstarch	½ cup (4.4 oz)	137
rice	½ cup (5.3 oz)	217
yorkshire as prep w/ skim milk	3.5 oz	93
yorkshire as prep w/ whole milk	3.5 oz	104
MIX		
lemon	½ cup (5.1 oz)	163
Knorr		
Creme Caramel Flan & Sauce as prep	½ cup + 1 tbsp sauce	190
My*T*Fine		
Butterscotch	mix for 1 serv	90
Chocolate	mix for 1 serv	100
Chocolate Almond	mix for 1 serv	100
Chocolate Fudge	mix for 1 serv	100
Lemon	mix for 1 serv	90
Vanilla	mix for 1 serv	90
Vanilla Tapioca	mix for 1 serv	80
Royal		
Banana Cream	mix for 1 serv	80

FOOD	PORTION	CALS.
Royal (CONT.)		
Banana Cream Instant	mix for 1 serv	90
Butterscotch	mix for 1 serv	90
Butterscotch Instant	mix for 1 serv	90
Cherry Vanilla Instant	mix for 1 serv	90
Chocolate	mix for 1 serv	90
Chocolate Chocolate Chip Instant	mix for 1 serv	110
Chocolate Instant	mix for 1 serv	110
Chocolate Sugar Free Instant	mix for 1 serv	50
Dark 'n Sweet Chocolate	mix for 1 serv	90
Dark 'N Sweet Instant	mix for 1 serv	110
Lemon Instant	mix for 1 serv	90
Pistachio Instant	mix for 1 serv	90
Strawberry Instant	mix for 1 serv	100
Toasted Coconut Instant	mix for 1 serv	100
Vanilla	mix for 1 serv	80
Vanilla Chocolate Chip Instant	mix for 1 serv	90
Vanilla Instant	mix for 1 serv	90
MIX WITH 2% MILK		
banana	½ cup (4.9 oz)	142
banana instant	½ cup (5.2 oz)	152
chocolate	½ cup (5 oz)	150
chocolate instant	½ cup (5.2 oz)	149
coconut cream	½ cup (4.9 oz)	148
coconut cream instant	½ cup (5.2 oz)	157
lemon instant	½ cup (5.2 oz)	155
rice	½ cup (5.1 oz)	161
tapioca	½ cup (5 oz)	147
vanilla	½ cup (4.9 oz)	141
vanilla instant	½ cup (5 oz)	147
Jell-O		
Banana Instant Sugar Free	½ cup	84
Chocolate Instant Sugar Free	½ cup	92
Chocolate Sugar Free	½ cup	91
Pistachio Instant Sugar Free	½ cup	94
Vanilla Instant Sugar Free	½ cup	82
MIX WITH SKIM MILK		
D-Zerta		
Butterscotch	½ cup	68
Chocolate	½ cup	65
Vanilla	½ cup	69
Emes		
Dietetic	½ cup (4 fl oz)	71

FOOD	PORTION	CALS.
MIX WITH WHOLE MILK		
banana	½ cup (4.9 oz)	157
banana instant	½ cup (5.2 oz)	167
chocolate	½ cup (5 oz)	158
chocolate instant	½ cup (5.2 oz)	164
coconut cream	½ cup (4.9 oz)	160
coconut cream instant	½ cup (5.2 oz)	172
lemon instant	½ cup (5.2 oz)	169
rice	½ cup (5.1 oz)	175
tapioca	½ cup (5 oz)	161
vanilla	½ cup (4.9 oz)	155
vanilla instant	½ cup (5 oz)	181
Jell-O		
Banana Cream Instant	½ cup	165
Butter Pecan Instant	½ cup	170
Butterscotch	½ cup	169
Butterscotch Instant	½ cup	164
Chocolate Instant	½ cup	176
Chocolate Tapioca Americana	½ cup	169
Coconut Cream Instant	½ cup	178
French Vanilla	½ cup	169
French Vanilla Instant	½ cup	165
Golden Egg Custard Americana	½ cup	167
Lemon Instant	½ cup	168
Milk Chocolate Instant	½ cup	179
Pineapple Cream Instant	½ cup	165
Pistachio Instant	½ cup	170
Rice Americana	½ cup	175
Vanilla	½ cup	156
Vanilla Instant	½ cup	168
Vanilla Tapioca Americana	½ cup	160
READY-TO-USE		
banana	1 pkg (5 oz)	180
chocolate	1 pkg (5 oz)	189
lemon	1 pkg (5 oz)	177
rice	1 pkg (5 oz)	231
tapioca	1 pkg (5 oz)	169
vanilla	1 pkg (4 oz)	146
Del Monte		
Snack Cups Butterscotch	1 serv (4 oz)	140
Snack Cups Chocolate	1 serv (4 oz)	160
Snack Cups Chocolate Peanut Butter	1 serv (4 oz)	160
Snack Cups Lite Chocolate	1 serv (4 oz)	100
Snack Cups Lite Vanilla	1 serv (4 oz)	90

FOOD	PORTION	CALS.
Del Monte (CONT.)		
Snack Cups Tapioca	1 serv (4 oz)	140
Snack Cups Vanilla	1 serv (4 oz)	150
Imagine Foods		
Lemon Dream	1 (4 oz)	120
Jell-O		
Chocolate	1 (4 oz)	171
Chocolate Caramel Swirl	1 (4 oz)	175
Chocolate Vanilla Swirl	1 (4 oz)	175
Chocolate Vanilla Swirl	1 (5.5 oz)	240
Light Chocolate	1 (4 oz)	104
Light Chocolate Vanilla	1 (4 oz)	104
Light Vanilla	1 (4 oz)	104
Milk Chocolate	1 (4 oz)	173
Tapioca	1 (5.5 oz)	229
Tapioca	1 (4 oz)	167
Vanilla	1 (4 oz)	182
Vanilla	1 (5.5 oz)	250
Vanilla Chocolate Swirl	1 (4 oz)	178
Matthew Walker		
Plum	3.5 oz	290
Snack Pack		
Banana	4.25 oz	145
Butterscotch	4.25 oz	170
Chocolate	4.25 oz	170
Chocolate Marshmallow	4.25 oz	165
Lemon	4.25 oz	150
Light Chocolate	4.25 oz	100
Light Tapioca	4.25 oz	100
Tapioca	4.25 oz	150
Vanilla	4.25 oz	170
Swiss Miss		
Butterscotch	4 oz	180
Chocolate	4 oz	180
Chocolate Fudge	4 oz	220
Chocolate Sundae	4 oz	220
Light Chocolate	4 oz	100
Light Chocolate Fudge	4 oz	100
Light Vanilla	4 oz	100
Light Vanilla Chocolate Parfait	4 oz	100
Tapioca	4 oz	160
Vanilla	4 oz	190
Vanilla Parfait	4 oz	180
Vanilla Sundae	4 oz	200

FOOD	PORTION	CALS.
Ultra Slim-Fast		
Butterscotch	4 oz	100
Chocolate	4 oz	100
Vanilla	4 oz	100
TAKE-OUT		
blancmange	1 serv (4.7 oz)	154
bread pudding	1 serv (6.7 oz)	564
bread pudding	½ cup (4.4 oz)	212
bread w/ raisins	½ cup	180
chocolate	½ cup (5.5 oz)	206
queen of puddings	1 serv (4.4 oz)	266
rice pudding	1 serv (3 oz)	110
rice w/ raisins	½ cup	246
tapioca	½ cup (5.3 oz)	189
vanilla	½ cup (4.3 oz)	130

PUDDING POPS

  (*see also* ICE CREAM AND FROZEN DESSERTS, PUDDING)

chocolate	1 (1.6 oz)	72
vanilla	1 (1.6 oz)	75
Jell-O		
Chocolate	1 pop	79
Chocolate Fudge	1 pop	79
Chocolate Peanut Butter Swirl	1 bar	78
Chocolate Swirl	1 pop	80
Deluxe Chocolate Covered	1 pop	201
Deluxe Peanuts And Chocolate	1 bar	185
Milk Chocolate	1 pop	80
Vanilla	1 pop	77

PUMMELO

fresh	1	228
sections	1 cup	71

PUMPKIN

CANNED		
pumpkin	½ cup	41
Libby		
Solid Pack	½ cup	60
Owatonna		
Pumpkin	½ cup	40
FRESH		
cooked mashed	½ cup	24
flowers cooked	½ cup	10
flowers raw	1	0

FOOD	PORTION	CALS.
leaves cooked	½ cup	7
leaves raw	½ cup	4
raw cubed	½ cup	15
SEEDS		
dried	1 oz	154
roasted	1 cup	1184
roasted	1 oz	148
salted & roasted	1 oz	148
salted & roasted	1 cup	1184
whole roasted	1 oz	127
whole roasted	1 cup	285
whole salted roasted	1 cup	285
whole salted roasted	1 oz	127

PURSLANE

cooked	1 cup	21
raw	1 cup	7

QUAHOGS
(see CLAM)

QUAIL

breast w/o skin raw	1 (2 oz)	69
w/ skin raw	1 quail (3.8 oz)	210
w/o skin raw	1 quail (3.2 oz)	123

QUICHE
HOME RECIPE

lorraine	⅛ of 8 in pie	600
TAKE-OUT		
cheese	1 slice (3 oz)	283
lorraine	1 slice (3 oz)	352
mushroom	1 slice (3 oz)	256

QUINCE

fresh	1	53

QUINOA

quinoa	½ cup	318
Arrowhead		
Quinoa	¼ cup (1.4 oz)	140
Eden		
Not Prep	¼ cup (1.6 oz)	170

RABBIT

domestic w/o bone roasted	3 oz	167
wild w/o bone stewed	3 oz	147

FOOD	PORTION	CALS.
RACCOON		
roasted	3 oz	217
RADICCHIO		
leaf	3.5 oz	18
raw shredded	½ cup	5
RADISHES		
DRIED		
chinese	½ cup	157
daikon	½ cup	157
FRESH		
chinese raw	1 (12 oz)	62
chinese raw sliced	½ cup	8
chinese sliced cooked	½ cup	13
daikon raw	1 (12 oz)	62
daikon raw sliced	½ cup	8
daikon sliced cooked	½ cup	13
red raw	10	7
red sliced	½ cup	10
white icicle raw	1 (½ oz)	2
white icicle raw sliced	½ cup	7
Dole		
Radishes	7	20
SPROUTS		
raw	½ cup	8
RAISINS		
chocolate coated	10 (0.4 oz)	39
chocolate coated	1 cup (6.7 oz)	741
golden seedless	1 cup	437
seedless	1 cup	434
seedless	1 tbsp	27
sultanas	1 oz	88
Cinderella		
Seedless	½ cup	250
Del Monte		
Golden	¼ cup (1.4 oz)	130
Raisins	1 box (1.5 oz)	140
Raisins	¼ cup (1.4 oz)	130
Raisins	1 box (1 oz)	90
Raisins	1 box (0.5 oz)	45
Yogurt Raisins Strawberry	1 pkg (0.9 oz)	110
Yogurt Raisins Vanilla	1 pkg (0.9 oz)	110
Yogurt Raisins Vanilla	1 pkg (1 oz)	120

FOOD	PORTION	CALS.
Del Monte (CONT.)		
Yogurt Raisins Vanilla	3 tbsp (1 oz)	130
Dole		
Golden	½ cup	250
Seedless	½ cup	250
Sonoma		
Monukka Thompson	¼ cup (1.4 oz)	130
Tree Of Life		
Organic	¼ cup (1.4 oz)	130

RASPBERRIES
CANNED
in heavy syrup	½ cup	117
FRESH		
raspberries	1 cup	61
raspberries	1 pint	154
Dole		
Raspberries	1 cup	45
FROZEN		
sweetened	1 cup	256
sweetened	1 pkg (10 oz)	291
Big Valley		
Raspberries	⅔ cup (4.9 oz)	80
Birds Eye		
Whole In Lite Syrup	½ cup	100

RASPBERRY JUICE
Crystal Geyser		
Juice Squeeze Mountain Raspberry	1 bottle (12 fl oz)	135
Kool-Aid		
Raspberry	8 oz	98
Sugar Free	8 oz	2
Smucker's		
Juice	8 oz	120
Juice Sparkler	10 oz	130

RED BEANS
CANNED
Allen		
Red Beans	½ cup (4.5 oz)	160
Green Giant		
Red Beans	½ cup	90
Hunt's		
Small	4 oz	90

FOOD	PORTION	CALS.
Van Camp's		
Red Beans	½ cup (4.6 oz)	90
DRIED		
Bean Cuisine		
Dried	½ cup	115
MIX		
Bean Cuisine		
Pasta & Beans Barcelona Red With Radiatore	½ cup	170
Mahatma		
Red Beans & Rice	1 cup	190

RELISH

FOOD	PORTION	CALS.
cranberry orange	½ cup	246
hamburger	1 tbsp	19
hamburger	½ cup	158
hot dog	1 tbsp	14
hot dog	½ cup	111
piccalilli	1.4 oz	13
sweet	1 tbsp	19
sweet	½ cup	159
Claussen		
Pickle Relish	1 tbsp	14
Del Monte		
Hamburger	1 tbsp (0.5 oz)	20
Hot Dog	1 tbsp (0.5 oz)	15
Sweet Pickle	1 tbsp (0.5 oz)	20
Hellman's		
Sandwich Spread	1 tbsp (15 g)	55
Old El Paso		
Jalapeno	1 tbsp (0.5 oz)	5
Vlasic		
Dill	1 oz	2
Hamburger	1 oz	40
Hot Dog	1 oz	40
Hot Piccalilli	1 oz	35
India	1 oz	30
Sweet	1 oz	30

RENNIN

FOOD	PORTION	CALS.
tablet	1 (0.9 g)	1

RHUBARB

FOOD	PORTION	CALS.
fresh	½ cup	13
frzn	½ cup	60
frzn as prep w/ sugar	½ cup	139

FOOD	PORTION	CALS.

RICE
(see also BRAN, CEREAL, FLOUR, RICE CAKES, WILD RICE)

BROWN

long-grain cooked	½ cup	109
medium-grain cooked	½ cup	109
Arrowhead		
Basmati	¼ cup (1.5 oz)	150
Quick Regular	⅓ cup (1.5 oz)	150
Quick Spanish Style	¼ pkg (1.4 oz)	150
Quick Vegetable Herb	¼ pkg (1.4 oz)	150
Quick Wild Rice & Herb	¼ pkg (1.3 oz)	140
Minute		
Precooked as prep	½ cup	121
Near East		
Pilaf as prep	1 cup	220
S&W		
Quick Natural Long Grain	3.5 oz	110
Quick Natural Long Grain cooked	3.5 oz	119
Uncle Ben		
Brown Rice	1 serv (1.6 oz)	158

CANNED

Old El Paso		
Mexican	½ cup (4 oz)	410
Spanish	1 cup (8.6 oz)	130
Van Camp's		
Spanish	1 cup (9 oz)	180

FROZEN

Birds Eye		
Rice & Broccoli Au Gratin	½ pkg	150
Budget Gourmet		
Oriental Rice With Vegetables	1 pkg (5.75 oz)	230
Rice Pilaf With Green Beans	1 pkg (5.5 oz)	230
Chun King		
Fried Rice	1 pkg (8 oz)	290
Fried Rice With Chicken	1 pkg (8 oz)	270
Green Giant		
Garden Gourmet Asparagus Pilaf	1 pkg	190
Garden Gourmet Sherry Wild Rice	1 pkg	210
One Serve Rice 'N Broccoli In Cheese Sauce	1 pkg	180
One Serve Rice Peas & Mushrooms With Sauce	1 pkg	130
Rice Originals Italian Rice s Spinach In Cheese Sauce	½ cup	140

FOOD	PORTION	CALS.
Green Giant (CONT.)		
Rice Originals Pilaf	½ cup	110
Rice Originals Rice 'N Broccoli In Cheese Sauce	½ cup	120
Rice Originals Rice Medley	½ cup	100
Rice Originals White & Wild	½ cup	130
Luigino's		
Fried Rice Chicken	1 pkg (8 oz)	250
Fried Rice Pork	1 pkg (8 oz)	250
Fried Rice Pork & Shrimp	1 pkg (8 oz)	250
Fried Rice Shrimp	1 pkg (8 oz)	220
Risotto Parmesano	1 pkg (8 oz)	360
MIX		
Casbah		
Jambalaya	1 pkg (1.4 oz)	130
La Fiesta	1 pkg (1.59 oz)	170
Nutted Pilaf as prep	1 cup	220
Pilaf as prep	1 cup	200
Spanish Pilaf as prep	1 cup	200
Thai Yum	1 pkg (1.7 oz)	180
Goodman's		
Rice & Vermicelli For Beef	¾ cup	160
Rice & Vermicelli For Chicken	¾ cup	160
Hain		
Rice Almondine	½ cup	130
Rice Oriental 3-Grain Goodness	½ cup	120
Kikkoman		
Fried Rice Seasoning Mix	1 oz pkg	91
Kitchen Del Sol		
Mediterranean Paella Costa Brave as prep	½ cup (1.2 oz)	130
Mediterranean Sunny Lemon Pilaf as prep	½ cup (1.2 oz)	110
Mediterranean Tomato & Basil With Pine Nuts	½ cup (1 oz)	110
Knorr		
Risotto Milanese With Saffron	½ cup	130
Risotto Tomato	½ cup	110
Risotto With Mushrooms	½ cup	110
Risotto With Onion	½ cup	110
Risotto With Peas And Corn	½ cup	110
La Choy		
Chinese Fried Rice	¾ cup	190
Lipton		
Golden Saute Beef	½ cup (2.1 oz)	230
Golden Saute Chicken	1 cup (2.2 oz)	240

FOOD	PORTION	CALS.
Lipton (CONT.)		
Golden Saute Chicken Broccoli	½ cup (2.3 oz)	260
Golden Saute Fried Rice	½ cup (2.1 oz)	240
Golden Saute Herb & Butter	½ cup (2.1 oz)	240
Golden Saute Onion Mushroom	½ cup (2.1 oz)	240
Golden Saute Oriental	½ cup (2.1 oz)	240
Golden Saute Savory Herb	½ cup (2.1 oz)	240
Golden Saute Spanish	½ cup (2.3 oz)	250
Rice & Beans Cajun as prep	½ cup (2.5 oz)	260
Rice & Sauce Alfredo Broccoli as prep	½ cup (2.2 oz)	250
Rice & Sauce Beef Broccoli as prep	½ cup (2.1 oz)	230
Rice & Sauce Beef Flavor as prep	½ cup (2.2 oz)	230
Rice & Sauce Cajun as prep	½ cup (2.2 oz)	230
Rice & Sauce Cheddar Broccoli as prep	½ cup (2.2 oz)	250
Rice & Sauce Chicken Broccoli as prep	½ cup (2.2 oz)	250
Rice & Sauce Chicken Flavor as prep	½ cup (2.2 oz)	240
Rice & Sauce Chicken Risotto	½ cup (2.1 oz)	230
Rice & Sauce Creamy Chicken as prep	½ cup (2.2 oz)	260
Rice & Sauce Herb & Butter as prep	½ cup (2.1 oz)	240
Rice & Sauce Long Grain Mushroom	½ cup (2.2 oz)	250
Rice & Sauce Medley as prep	½ cup (2.1 oz)	240
Rice & Sauce Mushroom as prep	½ cup (2.1 oz)	220
Rice & Sauce Oriental as prep	½ cup (2.1 oz)	230
Rice & Sauce Original Long Grain as prep	½ cup (2.2 oz)	250
Rice & Sauce Pilaf as prep	½ cup (2.1 oz)	230
Rice & Sauce Spanish as prep	½ cup (2.2 oz)	230
Mahatma		
Broccoli & Cheese	1 cup	200
Jambalaya	1 cup (2 oz)	190
Long Grain & Wild	1 cup (2 oz)	190
Pilaf	1 cup (2 oz)	190
Spanish	1 cup (2 oz)	180
Yellow Rice Mix	1 cup	190
Minute		
Fried Rice With Vermicelli as prep	½ cup	158
Microwave Broccoli Almondin	½ cup	143
Microwave Cheddar Cheese Broccoli	½ cup	164
Microwave French Pilaf	½ cup	133
Microwave Long Grain Brown And Wild	½ cup	140
Microwave Rice With Savory Cheese Sauce as prep	½ cup	162
Rice Drumstick With Vermicelli as prep	½ cup	153
Rice Rib Roast With Vermicelli as prep	½ cup	151

FOOD	PORTION	CALS.
Near East		
Barley Pilaf as prep	1 cup	220
Beef Pilaf as prep	1 cup	220
Curry Rice as prep	1 cup	220
Lentil Pilaf as prep	1 cup	210
Long Grain & Wild as prep	1 cup	220
Pilaf Chicken as prep	1 cup	220
Pilaf Kosher as prep	1 cup	220
Spanish Pilaf as prep	1 cup	230
Pritikin		
Mexican	⅓ cup (2 oz)	200
Oriental	⅓ cup (2 oz)	190
Rice-A-Roni		
Beef	½ cup	140
Beef & Mushroom	½ cup	150
Chicken	½ cup	150
Chicken & Broccoli	½ cup	150
Chicken & Mushroom	½ cup	180
Chicken & Vegetables	½ cup	140
Fried Rice	½ cup	110
Herb & Butter	½ cup	130
Long Grain & Wild Chicken w/ Almonds	½ cup	140
Long Grain & Wild Original	½ cup	130
Long Grain & Wild Pilaf	½ cup	130
Pilaf	½ cup	150
Risotto	½ cup	200
Spanish	½ cup	150
Stroganoff	½ cup	200
Yellow Rice	½ cup	140
Success		
Beef Oriental	½ cup	190
Broccoli & Cheese	½ cup	200
Brown & Wild	½ cup	190
Classic Chicken	½ cup	150
Long Grain & Wild	½ cup	190
Pilaf	½ cup	200
Spanish	½ cup	190
Ultra Slim-Fast		
Oriental Style	2.3 oz	240
Rice & Chicken Sauce	2.3 oz	240
Uncle Ben		
Brown & Wild Fast Cooking	1 serv (1.3 oz)	120
Country Inn Broccoli Almondine	1 serv (1.2 oz)	124
Country Inn Broccoli & White Cheddar	1 serv (1.2 oz)	131

FOOD	PORTION	CALS.
Uncle Ben (CONT.)		
Country Inn Broccoli Au Gratin	1 serv (1.1 oz)	116
Country Inn Chicken With Wild Rice	1 serv (1.1 oz)	108
Country Inn Creamy Chicken & Mushroom	1 serv (1.3 oz)	138
Country Inn Creamy Chicken & Wild Rice	1 serv (1.3 oz)	135
Country Inn Green Bean Almondine	1 serv (1.2 oz)	128
Country Inn Herbed Au Gratin	1 serv (1.2 oz)	119
Country Inn Homestyle Chicken & Vegetables	1 serv (1.3 oz)	139
Country Inn Rice Florentine	1 serv (1.2 oz)	212
Country Inn Vegetable Pilaf	1 serv (1.2 oz)	115
Long Grain & Wild Chicken Stock Sauce	1 serv (1.3 oz)	133
Long Grain & Wild Fast Cooking	1 serv (1 oz)	101
Long Grain & Wild Garden Vegetable Blend	1 serv (1.3 oz)	128
Long Grain & Wild Original	1 serv (1 oz)	96
Watkins		
Brown & Wild	¼ cup (1.6 oz)	160
Calico Medley	¼ cup (1.6 oz)	160
East/West Medley	¼ cup (1.6 oz)	160
Heartland Medley	¼ cup (1.6 oz)	160
Minnesota Medley	¼ cup (1.6 oz)	160
White & Wild	¼ cup (1.6 oz)	160
TAKE-OUT		
pilaf	½ cup	84
risotto	6.6 oz	426
spanish	¾ cup	363
WHITE		
glutinous cooked	½ cup	116
long-grain cooked	½ cup	131
long-grain instant cooked	½ cup	80
long-grain parboiled cooked	½ cup	100
medium-grain cooked	½ cup	132
short-grain cooked	½ cup	133
starch	3½ oz	343
Arrowhead		
Basmati	¼ cup (1.5 oz)	150
Casbah		
Basmati as prep	1 cup	158
Minute		
Boil In Bag Long Grain as prep	½ cup	94
Long Grain as prep	⅔ cup	150
Rice as prep	⅔ cup	141
Rice Long Grain & Wild as prep	½ cup	149

FOOD	PORTION	CALS.
S&W		
Long Grain cooked	3.5 oz	106
Superfino		
Arborio Rice	½ cup	100
Uncle Ben		
Boil-In-Bag	1 serv (0.9 oz)	94
Converted	1 serv (1.2 oz)	123
In An Instant	1 serv (1.1 oz)	111

RICE CAKES
(see also POPCORN CAKES)

FOOD	PORTION	CALS.
brown rice	1 (0.3 oz)	35
brown rice & buckwheat	1 (0.3 oz)	34
brown rice & buckwheat unsalted	1 (0.3 oz)	34
brown rice & corn	1 (0.3 oz)	35
brown rice & rye	1 (0.3 oz)	35
brown rice & sesame seed	1 (0.3 oz)	35
brown rice multigrain	1 (0.3 oz)	35
brown rice multigrain unsalted	1 (0.3 oz)	35
brown rice unsalted	1 (0.3 oz)	35
Hain		
5-Grain	1	40
Mini Apple Cinnamon	½ oz	60
Mini Barbeque	½ oz	70
Mini Cheese	½ oz	60
Mini Honey Nut	½ oz	60
Mini Nacho Cheese	½ oz	70
Mini Plain	½ oz	60
Mini Plain No Salt Added	½ oz	60
Mini Ranch	½ oz	70
Mini Teriyaki	½ oz	50
Plain	1	40
Plain No Salt Added	1	40
Sesame	1	40
Sesame No Salt	1	40
Ka-Me		
Cheese	16 pieces (1 oz)	120
Onion	16 pieces (1 oz)	120
Plain	16 pieces (1 oz)	120
Seaweed	16 pieces (1 oz)	120
Sesame	16 pieces (1 oz)	120
Unsalted	16 pieces (1 oz)	120
Lundberg		
Organic Lightly Salted	1	60

FOOD	PORTION	CALS.
Lundberg (CONT.)		
Organic Unsalted	1	60
Premium Lightly Salted	1	60
Premium Unsalted	1	60
Sesame Lightly Salted	1	59
Mother's		
Mini Apple	5 (0.5 oz)	50
Mini Caramel	5 (0.5 oz)	50
Mini Cinnamon	5 (0.5 oz)	50
Mini Plain Unsalted	7 (0.5 oz)	60
Multigrain Lightly Salted	1 (0.3 oz)	35
Rye Unsalted	1 (0.3 oz)	35
Wheat Unsalted	1 (0.3 oz)	35
Pritikin		
Mini Apple Crisp	5 (0.5 oz)	50
Multigrain	1 (0.3 oz)	35
Multigrain Unsalted	1 (0.3 oz)	35
Plain	1 (0.3 oz)	35
Plain Unsalted	1 (0.3 oz)	35
Sesame Low Sodium	1 (0.3 oz)	35
Sesame Unsalted	1 (0.3 oz)	35
Quaker		
Apple Cinnamon	1 (0.5 oz)	50
Banana Crunch	1 (0.5 oz)	50
Cinnamon Crunch	1 (0.5 oz)	50
Mini Apple Cinnamon	5 (0.5 oz)	50
Mini Banana Nut	5 (0.5 oz)	50
Mini Butter Popped Corn	6 (0.5 oz)	50
Mini Caramel Corn	5 (0.5 oz)	50
Mini Chocolate Crunch	5 (0.5 oz)	50
Mini Cinnamon Crunch	5 (0.5 oz)	50
Mini Honey Nut	5 (0.5 oz)	50
Mini Monterey Jack	6 (0.5 oz)	50
Mini White Cheddar	6 (0.5 oz)	50
Salt-Free	1 (0.3 oz)	35
Salted	1 (0.3 oz)	35
Tree Of Life		
Fat Free Mini Apple Cinnamon	15	60
Fat Free Mini Caramel	15	60
Fat Free Mini Honey Nut	15	60
Fat Free Mini Jalapeno	15	60
Fat Free Mini Plain	15	50
ROCKFISH		
pacific cooked	1 fillet (5.2 oz)	180

FOOD	PORTION	CALS.
pacific cooked	3 oz	103
pacific raw	3 oz	80

ROE
(see individual fish names)

FOOD	PORTION	CALS.
fish	3.5 oz	39
fresh baked	1 oz	58
fresh baked	3 oz	173

ROLL
(see also BISCUIT, CROISSANT, ENGLISH MUFFIN, MUFFIN, POPOVER, SCONE)

FROZEN
Pepperidge Farm

FOOD	PORTION	CALS.
Cinnamon Roll	1 (2¼ oz)	220
Sara Lee		
All Butter Cinnamon Roll w/ Icing	1	280
All Butter Cinnamon Roll w/o Icing	1	230
Weight Watchers		
Glazed Cinnamon Rolls	1 (2.1 oz)	200
HOME RECIPE		
dinner as prep w/ 2% milk	1 (2½ in)	111
dinner as prep w/ whole milk	1 (2½ in)	112
raisin & nut	1 (2 oz)	196
MIX		
Dromedary		
Hot Roll Mix	2	239
Natural Ovens		
German Hard	1 (2.1 oz)	138
Gourmet Dinner	1 (1 oz)	50
Hearty Sandwich	1 (1.8 oz)	110
Pillsbury		
Hot Roll Mix	2	240
READY-TO-EAT		
brown & serve	1 (1 oz)	85
cheese	1 (2.3 oz)	238
cinnamon raisin	1 (2¾ in)	223
dinner	1 (1 oz)	85
egg	1 (2½ in)	107
french	1 (1.3 oz)	105
hamburger	1 (1½ oz)	123
hamburger multi-grain	1 (1½ oz)	113
hamburger reduced calorie	1 (1½ oz)	84
hard	1 (3½ in)	167
hot cross bun	1	202

FOOD	PORTION	CALS.
hotdog	1 (1½ oz)	123
hotdog multi-grain	1 (1½ oz)	113
hotdog reduced calorie	1 (1½ oz)	84
kaiser	1 (3½ in)	167
oat bran	1 (1.2 oz)	78
rye	1 (1 oz)	81
submarine	1 (4.7 oz)	155
wheat	1 (1 oz)	77
whole wheat	1 (1 oz)	75
Alvarado St. Bakery		
Burger Buns	1 (2.2 oz)	140
Hot Dog Buns	1 (2.2 oz)	140
Arnold		
8-inch Francisco	1 (2.5 oz)	210
Augusto Pan Cubano	1	230
Bakery Light	1 (1.5 oz)	80
Bran'nola Buns	1 (1.5 oz)	100
Deli Kaiser	1	170
Deli Onion	1	170
Dinner Plain	1 (0.7 oz)	50
Dinner Sesame	1 (0.7 oz)	50
Dutch Egg	1	130
French Francisco	1 (2.5 oz)	210
French Mini Francisco	1	130
Hamburger	1	120
Hot Dog	1 (1.5 oz)	110
Hot Dog Bran'nola	1 (1.5 oz)	110
Hot Dog New England Style	1	110
Italian 8-inch Savoni	1	210
Kaiser Francisco	1 (2 oz)	180
Onion Premium	1 (2.6 oz)	180
Onion Soft	1	140
Party Petite	2	70
Potato	1	140
Sandwich Soft Sesame	1	130
Sourdough Brown N' Serve	1 (1 oz)	100
Sourdough Francisco	1 (1 oz)	100
Wheat Old Fashioned	2	80
August Bros.		
Dinner	1	90
Kaiser	1	170
Onion	1	160
Sesame Cubano	1	170

FOOD	PORTION	CALS.
Bread Du Jour		
Bavarian Cracked Wheat	1 (1.2 oz)	90
Crusty Italian	1 (1.2 oz)	80
French Petite	1 (3.5 oz)	230
Rye	1 (1.2 oz)	90
Sourdough	1 (2.2 oz)	140
Country Kitchen		
Frankfurt	1	120
Dicarlo's		
Extra Sourdough	1 (1.6 oz)	100
French	1 (1 oz)	70
Hollywood		
Dark Bread	1	40
Dinner Light Pan Special Formula	1	60
Sliced Light Special Formula	1	80
Home Pride		
Dinner Wheat	1 (1.9 oz)	160
Hamburger Potato Bun	1 (1.9 oz)	130
Hot Dog Potato Bun	1 (1.9 oz)	130
Sandwich Roll Wheat	1 (1.9 oz)	160
White	2 (1.6 oz)	130
Levy		
Sub Old Country	1	180
Martin's		
Big Marty Poppy	1	170
Big Marty Sesame	1	170
Hoagie	1	240
Hoagie Sesame	1	240
Potato Dinner	1	100
Potato Long	1	140
Potato Party	1	50
Potato Sandwich	1	140
Sandwich Whole Wheat 100% Stoneground	1	160
Matthew's		
Salad Roll	1	110
Sandwich	1	110
Pepperidge Farm		
Brown 'N Serve Club	1	100
Brown 'N Serve French	½ roll	180
Brown 'N Serve Hearth	1	50
Dinner	1	60
Dinner Country Style Classic	1	50
Finger Poppy Seed	1	50

FOOD	PORTION	CALS.
Pepperidge Farm (CONT.)		
Finger Sesame Seed	1	60
Frankfurter Dijon	1	160
Frankfurter Side Sliced	1	140
Frankfurter w/ Poppy Seeds	1	130
French Style	1	100
Hamburger	1	130
Hamburger	1	130
Heat & Serve Butter Crescent	1	110
Heat & Serve Golden Twist	1	110
Hoagie Soft	1	210
Old Fashioned	1	50
Parker House	1	60
Party	1	30
Potato Sandwich	1	160
Sandwich Onion w/ Poppy Seeds	1	150
Sandwich Salad	1	110
Sandwich w/ Sesame Seeds	1	140
Soft Family	1	100
Sourdough French	1	100
Roman Meal		
Brown & Serve	2 (2 oz)	140
Dinner	2 (2 oz)	136
Hamburger	1 (1.6 oz)	111
Hotdog	1 (1.5 oz)	103
Sandwich	1 (2.7 oz)	181
Sandwich	1 (2.7 oz)	181
San Francisco		
Sourdough	1 (1.8 oz)	180
The Baker		
Honey Cinnamon Raisin	1 (2 oz)	150
Wonder		
Brown 'N Serve Wheat	1 (1 oz)	70
Brown 'N Serve White	1 (1 oz)	70
Dinner White Light	1 (1 oz)	60
Hamburger	1 (1.5 oz)	110
Hamburger Light	1 (1.5 oz)	80
Hamburger Wheat	1 (2.2 oz)	170
Hot Dog	1 (1.5 oz)	110
Hot Dog Light	1 (1.5 oz)	80
Tea Dinner Rolls	1 (1.5 oz)	80
REFRIGERATED		
cinnamon w/ frosting	1	109
crescent	1 (1 oz)	98

FOOD	PORTION	CALS.
Pillsbury		
Best Quick Cinnamon Rolls w/ Icing	1	110
Butterflake	1	140
Crescent	1	100
ROSE APPLE		
fresh	3½ oz	32
ROSE HIP		
fresh	3½ oz	91
ROSELLE		
fresh	1 cup	28
ROSEMARY		
dried	1 tsp	4
ROUGHY		
orange baked	3 oz	75
RUTABAGA		
CANNED		
Sunshine		
Diced	½ cup (4.2 oz)	30
FRESH		
cooked mashed	½ cup	41
raw cubed	½ cup	25
SABLEFISH		
baked	3 oz	213
fillet baked	5.3 oz	378
smoked	1 oz	72
smoked	3 oz	218
SAFFLOWER		
seeds dried	1 oz	147
SAFFRON		
saffron	1 tsp	2
SAGE		
ground	1 tsp	2
Watkins		
Sage	¼ tsp (0.5 g)	0
SALAD		
(*see also* LETTUCE, PASTA SALAD)		
MIX		
Dole		
Caesar Salad	⅓ pkg (3.5 oz)	170

FOOD	PORTION	CALS.
Dole (CONT.)		
Classic Blend	3.5 oz	25
Coleslaw Blend	3.5 oz	30
French Blend	3.5 oz	25
Italian Blend	3.5 oz	25
Salad-In-A- Minute Oriental	3.5 oz	110
Salad-In-A- Minute Spinach	3.5 oz	180
Fresh Express		
American Salad	1½ cups (3 oz)	20
Caesar Salad	1½ cups (3 oz)	140
European Salad	1½ cups (3 oz)	20
Garden Salad	1½ cups (3 oz)	20
Italian Salad	1½ cups (3 oz)	20
Oriental Salad	1½ cups (3 oz)	120
Riviera Salad	1½ cups (3 oz)	10
Spinach Salad	1½ cups (3 oz)	130
Suddenly Salad		
Caesar as prep	½ cup	170
Ranch & Bacon as prep	½ cup	210
Ranch & Bacon as prep low fat recipe	½ cup	160
TAKE-OUT		
chef w/o dressing	1½ cups	386
tossed w/o dressing	¾ cup	16
tossed w/o dressing	1½ cups	32
tossed w/o dressing w/ cheese & egg	1½ cups	102
tossed w/o dressing w/ chicken	1½ cups	105
tossed w/o dressing w/ pasta & seafood	1½ cups (14.6 oz)	380
tossed w/o dressing w/ shrimp	1½ cups	107
waldorf	½ cup	79

SALAD DRESSING

HOME RECIPE		
french	1 tbsp	88
vinegar & oil	1 tbsp	72
MIX		
Good Seasons		
Blue Cheese & Herbs as prep	1 tbsp	72
Buttermilk Farm as prep	1 tbsp	58
Cheese Garlic as prep	1 tbsp	72
Cheese Italian as prep	1 tbsp	72
Classic Dill	1 pkg	28
Garlic & Herbs as prep	1 tbsp	71
Italian as prep	1 tbsp	71
Italian Lite as prep	1 tbsp	27

FOOD	PORTION	CALS.
Good Seasons (CONT.)		
Italian No Oil as prep	1 tbsp	7
Lemon & Herbs as prep	1 tbsp	71
Lite Cheese Italian as prep	1 tbsp	27
Lite Ranch as prep	1 tbsp	29
Lite Zesty Italian as prep	1 tbsp	26
Mild Italian as prep	1 tbsp	73
Ranch as prep	1 tbsp	57
Zesty Italian as prep	1 tbsp	71
Hain		
No Oil 1000 Island	1 tbsp	12
No Oil Bleu Cheese	1 tbsp	14
No Oil Buttermilk	1 tbsp	11
No Oil Caesar	1 tbsp	6
No Oil French	1 tbsp	12
No Oil Garlic & Cheese	1 tbsp	6
No Oil Herb	1 tbsp	2
No Oil Italian	1 tbsp	2
READY-TO-USE		
blue cheese	1 tbsp	77
french	1 tbsp	67
french reduced calorie	1 tbsp	22
italian	1 tbsp	69
italian reduced calorie	1 tbsp	16
russian	1 tbsp	76
russian reduced calorie	1 tbsp	23
sesame seed	1 tbsp	68
thousand island	1 tbsp	59
thousand island reduced calorie	1 tbsp	24
Estee		
Blue Cheese	2 tbsp (1 oz)	15
Creamy French	2 tbsp (1 oz)	10
Creamy French Fat Free	1 pkg (0.5 oz)	5
Creamy Garlic	2 tbsp (1 oz)	60
Creamy Garlic Fat Free	1 pkg (0.5 oz)	5
Creamy Italian	2 tbsp (1 oz)	15
Italian	2 tbsp (1 oz)	5
Italian Fat Free	1 pkg (0.5 oz)	0
Low Fat Blue Cheese	1 pkg (0.5 oz)	5
Thousand Island	2 tbsp (1 oz)	10
Hain		
1000 Island	1 tbsp	50
Canola Garden Tomato	1 tbsp	60
Canola Italian	1 tbsp	50

FOOD	PORTION	CALS.
Hain (CONT.)		
Canola Spicy French Mustard	1 tbsp	50
Canola Tangy Citrus	1 tbsp	50
Creamy Caesar	1 tbsp	60
Creamy Caesar Low Salt	1 tbsp	60
Creamy French	1 tbsp	60
Creamy Italian	1 tbsp	80
Creamy Italian No Salt Added	1 tbsp	80
Cucumber Dill	1 tbsp	80
Dijon Vinaigrette	1 tbsp	50
Garlic & Sour Cream	1 tbsp	70
Honey & Sesame	1 tbsp	60
Italian Cheese Vinaigrette	1 tbsp	55
Old Fashioned Buttermilk	1 tbsp	70
Poppyseed Rancher's	1 tbsp	60
Savory Herb No Salt Added	1 tbsp	90
Swiss Cheese Vinaigrette	1 tbsp	60
Traditional Italian	1 tbsp	80
Hollywood		
Caesar	1 tbsp	70
Creamy French	1 tbsp	70
Creamy Italian	1 tbsp	90
Dijon Vinaigrette	1 tbsp	60
Italian	1 tbsp	90
Old Fashion Buttermilk	1 tbsp	75
Poppy Seed Rancher's	1 tbsp	75
Thousand Island	1 tbsp	60
Kraft		
Bacon & Tomato	2 tbsp (1.1 oz)	140
Buttermilk Ranch	2 tbsp (1 oz)	150
Caesar Ranch	2 tbsp (1 oz)	140
Catalina With Honey	2 tbsp (1.2 oz)	140
Chunky Blue Cheese	2 tbsp (1.2 oz)	90
Coleslaw	2 tbsp (1.2 oz)	150
Creamy Caesar	2 tbsp (1 oz)	140
Creamy Garlic	2 tbsp (1.1 oz)	110
Creamy Italian	2 tbsp (1.1 oz)	110
Cucumber Ranch	2 tbsp (1.1 oz)	150
Deliciously Right Bacon & Tomato	2 tbsp (1.1 oz)	60
Deliciously Right Caesar	2 tbsp (1.1 oz)	50
Deliciously Right Catalina French	2 tbsp (1.2 oz)	80
Deliciously Right Creamy Italian	2 tbsp (1.1 oz)	50
Deliciously Right Cucumber Ranch	2 tbsp (1.1 oz)	60
Deliciously Right French	2 tbsp (1.2 oz)	50

FOOD	PORTION	CALS.
Kraft (CONT.)		
Deliciously Right Italian	2 tbsp (1.1 oz)	70
Deliciously Right Ranch	2 tbsp (1.1 oz)	110
Deliciously Right Thousand Island	2 tbsp (1.2 oz)	70
Free Blue Cheese	2 tbsp (1.2 oz)	50
Free Catalina	2 tbsp (1.2 oz)	45
Free French	2 tbsp (1.2 oz)	50
Free Honey Dijon	2 tbsp (1.2 oz)	50
Free Italian	2 tbsp (1.1 oz)	10
Free Peppercorn Ranch	2 tbsp (1.2 oz)	50
Free Ranch	1 tbsp (1.2 oz)	50
Free Red Wine Vinegar	2 tbsp (1.1 oz)	15
Free Thousand Island	2 tbsp (1.2 oz)	45
French	2 tbsp (1.1 oz)	120
Honey Dijon	2 tbsp (1.1 oz)	150
House Italian	2 tbsp (1.1 oz)	120
Oil-Free Italian	2 tbsp (1.1 oz)	5
Peppercorn Ranch	2 tbsp (1 oz)	170
Pesto Italian	2 tbsp (1 oz)	140
Ranch	2 tbsp (1 oz)	170
Roka Blue Cheese	2 tbsp (1.2 oz)	90
Russian	2 tbsp (1.2 oz)	130
Salsa Ranch	2 tbsp (1 oz)	130
Salsa Zesty Garden	2 tbsp (1.1 oz)	70
Sour Cream & Onion Ranch	2 tbsp (1 oz)	170
Thousand Island	2 tbsp (1.1 oz)	110
Thousand Island With Bacon	2 tbsp (1 oz)	120
Zesty Italian	2 tbsp (1.1 oz)	110
Marzetti		
Bacon Spinach Salad	2 tbsp	80
Blue Cheese	2 tbsp	160
Buttermilk Parmesan Pepper	2 tbsp	170
Buttermilk Parmesan Ranch	2 tbsp	160
Buttermilk Veggie Dip	2 tbsp	170
Caesar	2 tbsp	150
Caesar Ranch	2 tbsp	190
California French	2 tbsp	160
Celery Seed	2 tbsp	160
Chunky Blue Cheese	2 tbsp	150
Classic Caesar Ranch	2 tbsp	190
Country French	2 tbsp	150
Cracked Peppercorn	2 tbsp	140
Creamy Garlic Italian	2 tbsp	160
Creamy Italian	2 tbsp	150

FOOD	PORTION	CALS.
Marzetti (CONT.)		
Crispy Celery Seed	2 tbsp	160
Dijon Honey Mustard	2 tbsp	140
Dijon Ranch	2 tbsp	170
Dutch Sweet'N Sour	2 tbsp	160
Fat Free California French	2 tbsp	45
Fat Free Honey Dijon	2 tbsp	60
Fat Free Honey French	2 tbsp	45
Fat Free Italian	2 tbsp	15
Fat Free Peppercorn Ranch	2 tbsp	30
Fat Free Ranch	2 tbsp	30
Fat Free Raspberry	2 tbsp	70
Fat Free Slaw	2 tbsp	45
Fat Free Sweet & Sour	2 tbsp	45
Fat Free Thousand Island	2 tbsp	35
Garden Ranch	2 tbsp	180
Gusto Italian	2 tbsp	120
Honey Dijon	2 tbsp	140
Honey Dijon Ranch	2 tbsp	150
Honey French	2 tbsp	160
Honey French Blue Cheese	2 tbsp	160
House Caesar	2 tbsp	150
Italian With Olive Oil	2 tbsp	120
Light Blue Cheese	2 tbsp	60
Light Buttermilk Ranch	2 tbsp	90
Light California French	2 tbsp	80
Light Chunky Blue Cheese	2 tbsp	80
Light French	2 tbsp	40
Light French	2 tbsp	40
Light Honey French	2 tbsp	80
Light Italian	2 tbsp	60
Light Ranch	2 tbsp	90
Light Red Wine Vinegar & Oil	2 tbsp	20
Light Sweet & Sour	2 tbsp	100
Light Thousand Island	2 tbsp	70
Old Fashioned Poppyseed	2 tbsp	140
Olde Venice Italain	2 tbsp	130
Olde World Caesar	2 tbsp	150
Parmesan Pepper	2 tbsp	160
Peppercorn Ranch	2 tbsp	180
Poppyseed	2 tbsp	160
Potato Salad Dressing	2 tbsp	120
Ranch	2 tbsp	180
Red Wine Vinegar & Oil	2 tbsp	130

FOOD	PORTION	CALS.
Marzetti (CONT.)		
Romano Cheese Caesar	2 tbsp	150
Romano Italian	2 tbsp	160
Savory Italian	2 tbsp	110
Slaw	2 tbsp	170
Southern Slaw	2 tbsp	100
Sweet & Saucy	2 tbsp	140
Sweet & Sour	2 tbsp	160
Thousand Island	2 tbsp	150
Vintage Champagne	2 tbsp	150
Wilde Raspberry	2 tbsp	150
Newman's Own		
Italian Light	1 tbsp (0.5 fl oz)	10
Olive Oil & Vinegar	1 tbsp (0.5 fl oz)	80
Ranch	1 tbsp (0.5 fl oz)	90
Pfeiffer		
1000 Island	2 tbsp	140
California French	2 tbsp	140
French	2 tbsp	150
Honey Dijon	2 tbsp	140
Lite Italian	2 tbsp	50
Ranch	2 tbsp	180
Savory Italian	2 tbsp	110
Pritikin		
Dijon Balsamic Vinaigrette	2 tbsp (1 oz)	3
French	2 tbsp (1 oz)	35
Honey Dijon	2 tbsp (1 oz)	45
Honey French	2 tbsp (1 oz)	40
Italian	2 tbsp (1 oz)	20
Raspberry Vinaigrette	2 tbsp (1 oz)	45
Red Wing		
"K" Dressing	1 tbsp (0.5 oz)	70
Chunky Blue Cheese	2 tbsp (1 oz)	130
Creamy Ranch	2 tbsp (1 oz)	150
French Traditional	2 tbsp (1 oz)	130
Italian Traditional	2 tbsp (1 oz)	100
Spicy Sweet French	2 tbsp (1 oz)	130
Thousand Island Thick & Rich	2 tbsp (1 oz)	110
S&W		
Blue Cheese Low Calorie	1 tbsp	25
Creamy Cucumber Low Calorie	1 tbsp	25
Creamy Italian Low Calorie	1 tbsp	10
French Low Calorie	1 tbsp	18
Italian No-Oil	1 tbsp	2

FOOD	PORTION	CALS.
S&W (CONT.)		
Russian Low Calorie	1 tbsp	25
Thousand Island Low Calorie	1 tbsp	25
Seven Seas		
Creamy Italian	2 tbsp (1.1 oz)	110
Free Italian	2 tbsp (1.1 oz)	10
Free Ranch	2 tbsp (1.2 oz)	50
Free Red Wine Vinegar	2 tbsp (1.1 oz)	15
Green Goddess	2 tbsp (1 oz)	120
Herbs & Spices	2 tbsp (1.1 oz)	120
Ranch	2 tbsp (1 oz)	150
Red Wine Vinegar & Oil	2 tbsp (1.1 oz)	110
Reduced Calorie Creamy Italian	2 tbsp (1.1 oz)	60
Reduced Calorie Italian With Olive Oil	2 tbsp (1.1 oz)	50
Reduced Calorie Ranch	2 tbsp (1.1 oz)	100
Reduced Calorie Red Wine Vinegar & Oil	2 tbsp (1.1 oz)	60
Two Cheese Italian	2 tbsp (1.1 oz)	70
Viva Buttermilk	2 tbsp (1.1)	150
Viva Caesar	2 tbsp (1.1 oz)	120
Viva Italian	2 tbsp (1.1 oz)	110
Viva Reduced Calorie Italian	2 tbsp (1.1 oz)	45
Tree Of Life		
Cafe Venice	2 tbsp (1 oz)	100
Fat Free Blue Cheese	2 tbsp (1 oz)	15
Fat Free Honey French	2 tbsp (1 oz)	35
Fat Free Italian Garlic	2 tbsp (1 oz)	20
Fat Free Oriental Ginger	2 tbsp (1 oz)	15
Frisco's Raspberry	2 tbsp (1 oz)	120
Maison Caesar	2 tbsp (1 oz)	70
Shanghai Palace	2 tbsp (1 oz)	80
Ultra Slim-Fast		
French	1 tbsp	20
Italian	1 tbsp	6
W.J. Clark		
Ginger Orange Vinaigrette	1 tbsp	73
Herbs & Romano	1 tbsp	67
Lemon Peppercorn	1 tbsp	72
Lime Cilantro Vinaigrette	1 tbsp	73
Poppy Seed	1 tbsp	75
Sweet Pepper Basil	1 tbsp	69
Tarragon Honey Mustard	1 tbsp	66
Walden Farms		
Bleu Cheese Fat Free	2 tbsp (1 oz)	25
Creamy Italian With Parmesan Fat Free	1 tbsp (1 oz)	25

FOOD	PORTION	CALS.
Walden Farms (CONT.)		
French Style Fat Free	2 tbsp (1 oz)	25
Honey Dijon Fat Free	2 tbsp (1 oz)	25
Italian Sodium Free Fat Free	2 tbsp (1 oz)	10
Italian Sugar Free Fat Free	2 tbsp (1 oz)	0
Italian With Sun Dried Tomato	2 tbsp (1 oz)	15
Ranch Fat Free	2 tbsp (1 oz)	25
Ranch With Sun Dried Tomato	2 tbsp (1 oz)	25
Thousand Island Fat Free	2 tbsp (1 oz)	35
Weight Watchers		
Fat Free Caesar	2 tbsp	10
Fat Free Caesar	1 pkg (0.75 oz)	6
Fat Free Creamy Italian	2 tbsp	30
Fat Free French Style	2 tbsp	40
Fat Free Honey Dijon	2 tbsp	45
Fat Free Italian	2 tbsp	10
Fat Free Ranch	2 tbsp	35
Fat Free Ranch	1 pkg (0.75 oz)	25
Salad Celebrations 3 Cheese Ceasar	2 tbsp	40
Salad Celebrations Russian	2 tbsp	45
Salad Celebrations Thousand Island	2 tbsp	45
Wishbone		
Caesar Olive Oil	2 tbsp (1 oz)	90
Chunky Blue Cheese	2 tbsp (1 oz)	170
Classic House Italian	2 tbsp (1 oz)	140
Classic Olive Oil Italian	2 tbsp (1 oz)	70
Creamy Italian	2 tbsp (1 oz)	100
Creamy Roasted Garlic	2 tbsp (1 oz)	140
Deluxe French	2 tbsp (1 oz)	120
Fat Free Chunky Blue Cheese	2 tbsp (1 oz)	35
Fat Free Creamy Roasted Garlic	2 tbsp (1 oz)	40
Fat Free Honey Dijon	2 tbsp (1 oz)	45
Fat Free Italian	2 tbsp (1 oz)	15
Fat Free Ranch	2 tbsp (1 oz)	40
Fat Free Sweet & Spicy French	2 tbsp (1 oz)	30
Fat Free Thousand Island	2 tbsp (1 oz)	35
Honey Dijon	2 tbsp (1 oz)	130
Italian	2 tbsp (1 oz)	80
Lite Caesar With Olive Oil	2 tbsp	60
Lite Chunky Blue Cheese	2 tbsp (1 oz)	80
Lite Classic Dijon Vinaigrette	2 tbsp (1 oz)	60
Lite Creamy Italian	2 tbsp (1 oz)	60
Lite French	2 tbsp	50
Lite Italian	2 tbsp (1 oz)	24

FOOD	PORTION	CALS.
Wishbone (CONT.)		
Lite Ranch	2 tbsp (1 oz)	100
Lite Thousand Island	2 tbsp (1 oz)	80
Olive Oil Vinaigrette	2 tbsp (1 oz)	60
Ranch	2 tbsp (1 oz)	160
Robusto Italian	2 tbsp (1 oz)	100
Russian	2 tbsp (1 oz)	110
Santa Fe	2 tbsp (1 oz)	150
Sierra	2 tbsp	150
Sweet 'N Spicy French	2 tbsp (1 oz)	130
Thousand Island	2 tbsp (1 oz)	130

SALMON
CANNED		
chum w/ bone	1 can (13.9 oz)	521
chum w/ bone	3 oz	120
pink w/ bone	3 oz	118
pink w/ bone	1 can (15.9 oz)	631
sockeye w/ bone	3 oz	130
sockeye w/ bone	1 can (12.9 oz)	566
Bumble Bee		
Keta	3.5 oz	160
Pink	3.5 oz	160
Pink Skinless & Boneless	3.25 oz	120
Red	3.5 oz	180
Red Skinless & Boneless	3.25 oz	130
Deming's		
Alaska Keta	½ cup	140
Alaska Pink	½ cup	140
Alaska Red Sockeye	½ cup	170
Double Q		
Alaska Pink	½ cup	140
Humpty Dumpty		
Alaska Chum	½ cup	140
Libby		
Keta	½ can (3.8 oz)	140
Pink	½ can (3.8 oz)	150
S&W		
Bluepack Fancy Diet	½ cup	188
Red Fancy Sockeye Bluepack	½ cup	190
FRESH		
atlantic baked	3 oz	155
chinook baked	3 oz	196
chum baked	3 oz	131

FOOD	PORTION	CALS.
coho cooked	3 oz	157
coho cooked	½ fillet (5.4 oz)	286
coho raw	3 oz	124
pink baked	3 oz	127
roe raw	3.5 oz	207
sockeye cooked	3 oz	183
sockeye cooked	½ fillet (5.4 oz)	334
sockeye raw	3 oz	143
SMOKED		
chinook	1 oz	33
chinook	3 oz	99
Nathan's		
Nova	2 oz	80
TAKE-OUT		
salmon cake	1 (3 oz)	241

SALSA

(*see also* KETCHUP, SAUCE, SPANISH FOODS)

FOOD	PORTION	CALS.
Casa Fiesta		
Chili Salsa	1 oz	9
Picante Mild	1 oz	9
Chi-Chi's		
Hot	2 tbsp (1 oz)	10
Medium	1 tbsp (1 oz)	10
Mild	2 tbsp (1 oz)	10
Verde Medium	2 tbsp (1.2 oz)	15
Verde Mild	2 tbsp (1.2 oz)	15
Del Monte		
Mexicana	2 tbsp (1.1 oz)	5
Taquera	2 tbsp (1.1 oz)	5
Verde	2 tbsp (1.1 oz)	10
Frito Lay		
Hot	1 oz	12
Medium	1 oz	12
Mild	1 oz	12
Guiltless Gourmet		
Picante Hot	1 oz	6
Picante Medium	1 oz	6
Hain		
Hot	¼ cup	22
Mild	¼ cup	20
Heluva Good Cheese		
Cheese & Salsa	2 tbsp (1.1 oz)	80
Thick & Chunky Hot	2 tbsp (1.2 oz)	10

FOOD	PORTION	CALS.
Heluva Good Cheese (CONT.)		
Thick & Chunky Mild	2 tbsp (1.2 oz)	10
Hot Cha Cha		
Medium	2 tbsp (1 oz)	5
Louise's		
Fat Free BBQ Black Bean	1 oz	10
Fat Free Black Bean	1 oz	10
Fat Free Medium	1 oz	10
Fat Free Mild	1 oz	10
Fat Free Nacho Queso	1 oz	15
Muir Glen		
Organic Fat Free Hot	2 tbsp (1.1 oz)	10
Organic Fat Free Medium	2 tbsp (1.1 oz)	10
Organic Fat Free Mild	2 tbsp (1.1 oz)	10
Newman's Own		
Bandito Hot	1 tbsp (0.7 oz)	6
Bandito Medium	1 tbsp (0.7 oz)	6
Bandito Mild	1 tbsp (0.7 oz)	6
Old El Paso		
Green Chili Medium	2 tbsp (1 oz)	10
Homestyle	2 tbsp (1 oz)	5
Homestyle Mild	2 tbsp (1 oz)	5
Picante Hot	2 tbsp (1 oz)	10
Picante Medium	2 tbsp (1 oz)	10
Picante Mild	2 tbsp (1 oz)	10
Picante Thick'n Chunky Hot	2 tbsp (1 oz)	10
Picante Thick'n Chunky Medium	2 tbsp (1 oz)	10
Picante Thick'n Chunky Mild	2 tbsp (1 oz)	10
Pico De Gallo Hot	2 tbsp (1 oz)	5
Pico De Gallo Medium	1 tbsp (1 oz)	5
Salsa Verde	2 tbsp (1 oz)	10
Thick'n Chunky Hot	2 tbsp (1 oz)	10
Thick'n Chunky Medium	2 tbsp (1 oz)	10
Thick'n Chunky Mild	2 tbsp (1 oz)	10
Ortega		
Hot Green Chili	1 tbsp	6
Medium Green Chili	1 tbsp	6
Mild Green Chili	1 tbsp	8
Pace		
Picante	2 tbsp (1 fl oz)	7
Thick & Chunky	2 tbsp (1 fl oz)	12
Progresso		
Italian Hot	2 tbsp (1 oz)	30
Italian Medium	2 tbsp (1 oz)	10

FOOD	PORTION	CALS.
Progresso (CONT.)		
Italian Mild	2 tbsp (1 oz)	10
Roserita		
Chunky Hot	3 tbsp (1.5 oz)	25
Chunky Medium	3 tbsp (1.5 oz)	25
Chunky Mild	3 tbsp (1.5 oz)	25
Taco Salsa Chunky Medium	3 tbsp (1.5 oz)	25
Taco Salsa Chunky Mild	3 tbsp (1.5 oz)	25
Tabasco		
Picante	2 tbsp (1.5 oz)	17
Tree Of Life		
Hot	2 tbsp (1 oz)	10
Medium	2 tbsp (1 oz)	10
Mild	2 tbsp (1 oz)	10
No Salt	2 tbsp (1 oz)	10
Watkins		
Salsa Seasoning Blend	⅛ tsp (0.5 g)	0
Tropical	2 tbsp (1 oz)	60
Wise		
Picante	2 tbsp	12

SALSIFY

fresh sliced cooked	½ cup	46
raw sliced	½ cup	55

SALT SUBSTITUTES

Morton		
Salt Substitute	1 tsp	2
Papa Dash		
Lite Lite Lite Salt	¼ tsp (0.5 g)	1
Salt Lover's Blend	¼ tsp (0.7 g)	tr

SALT/SEASONED SALT
(*see also* SALT SUBSTITUTES)

salt	1 tbsp (18 g)	0
salt	1 tsp (6 g)	0
Hain		
Sea Salt	1 tsp	0
Sea Salt Iodized	1 tsp	0
Morton		
Garlic	1 tsp	3
Iodized	1 tsp	tr
Kosher	1 tsp	0
Lite	1 tsp	tr
Nature's Season Seasoning Blend	1 tsp	3

FOOD	PORTION	CALS.
Morton (CONT.)		
Non-Iodized	1 tsp	0
Seasoned	1 tsp	4
Watkins		
Bacon Cheese Salt	¼ tbsp (1 g)	0
Butter Salt	¼ tbsp (1 g)	0
Cheese Salt	¼ tbsp (1 g)	0
Garlic Salt	¼ tsp (1 g)	0
Salt & Vinegar Seasoning	¼ tsp (1 g)	0
Seasoning Salt	¼ tsp (1 g)	0
Sour Cream & Onion Salt	¼ tbsp (1 g)	0

SAPODILLA

FOOD	PORTION	CALS.
fresh	1	140
fresh cut up	1 cup	199

SAPOTES

FOOD	PORTION	CALS.
fresh	1	301

SARDINES

FOOD	PORTION	CALS.
CANNED		
atlantic in oil w/ bone	2	50
atlantic in oil w/ bone	1 can (3.2 oz)	192
pacific in tomato sauce w/ bone	1 can (13 oz)	658
pacific in tomato sauce w/ bone	1	68
Del Monte		
In Tomato Sauce	1 fish (1.4 oz)	50
Empress		
Skinless & Boneless Olive Oil	1 can (3.8 oz)	420
Skinless & Boneless Soy Oil	1 can (4.4 oz)	500
Port Clyde		
In Louisiana Hot Sauce	1 can (3.75 oz)	170
In Mustard Sauce	1 can (3.75 oz)	150
In Soybean Oil Select Small	1 can (3.3 oz)	220
In Soybean Oil With Hot Chilies	1 can (3.3 oz)	155
In Soybean Oil drained	1 can (3.3 oz)	220
In Spring Water	1 can (3.3 oz)	170
In Tomato Sauce	1 can (3.75 oz)	150
S&W		
Norwegian Brisling	1.5 oz	130
Underwood		
Brisling In Olive Oil	3.75 oz	260
In Mustard Sauce	3.75 oz	220
In Sild Oil drained	3.75 oz	460
In Soya Oil drained	3 oz	230

FOOD	PORTION	CALS.
Underwood (CONT.)		
In Tomato Sauce	3.75 oz	220
With Tabasco Pepper Sauce drained	3 oz	220
Viking's Delight		
Brisling In Olive Oil	1 can (3.75 oz)	460
Brisling In Olive Oil drained	1 can (3.75 oz)	260
FRESH		
raw	3½ oz	135

SAUCE

(*see also* BARBECUE SAUCE, GRAVY, PIZZA, SALSA, SPAGHETTI SAUCE, TOMATO)

FOOD	PORTION	CALS.
JARRED		
teriyaki	1 tbsp	15
teriyaki	1 oz	30
Armour		
Chili Hot Dog	¼ cup (2.2 oz)	120
Meatless Sloppy Joe Sauce	¼ cup (2.2 oz)	30
Best Foods		
Tartar	1 tbsp (14 g)	70
Bright Day		
Tartar	1 tbsp	50
Casa Fiesta		
Taco Mild	1 oz	9
Chi-Chi's		
Taco Thick & Chunky	1 tbsp (0.5 oz)	10
Contadina		
Sweet 'n Sour	2 tbsp	40
Del Monte		
Cocktail	¼ cup (2.7 oz)	100
Sloppy Joe Hickory Flavor	¼ cup (2.4 oz)	70
Sloppy Joe Italian Style	¼ cup (2.4 oz)	70
Sloppy Joe Original	¼ cup (2.4 oz)	70
El Molino		
Taco Red Mild	2 tbsp	10
Escoffier		
Diable	1 tbsp	20
Gebhardt		
Enchilada Sauce	3 tbsp (1.5 oz)	25
Hot Dog Chili Sauce	2 tbsp	30
Hot Sauce	½ tsp	tr
Gold's		
Rib	1 oz	60
Golden Dipt		
Cajun Style	1 oz	90

FOOD	PORTION	CALS.
Golden Dipt (CONT.)		
Creole	1 oz	20
Dijonaisse	1 oz	52
French White	1 oz	55
Ginger Teriyaki Marinade	1 oz	120
Lemon Butter Dill	1 oz	100
Lemon Herb Marinade	1 oz	130
Seafood Cocktail	1 tbsp	20
Seafood Cocktail Extra Hot	1 tbsp	20
Tartar	1 tbsp	70
Tartar Lite	1 tbsp	50
Heinz		
Worcestershire	1 tbsp	6
Hellman's		
Tartar	1 tbsp (14 g)	70
Heluva Good Cheese		
Cocktail	¼ cup (1.6 oz)	40
Hormel		
Not-So-Sloppy- Joe Sauce	¼ cup (2.2 oz)	70
House Of Tsang		
Bangkok Padang	1 tbsp (0.6 oz)	45
Hoisin	1 tsp (6 g)	15
Mandarin Marinade	1 tbsp (0.6 oz)	25
Saigon Sizzle	1 tbsp (0.6 oz)	40
Spicy Brown Bean	1 tsp (6 g)	15
Stir Fry Sweet & Sour	1 tbsp (0.6 oz)	35
Stir Fry Szechuan Spicy	1 tbsp (0.6 oz)	20
Sweet & Sour Concentrate	1 tsp (6 g)	10
Teriyaki Korean	1 tbsp (0.6 oz)	30
Hunt's		
Barbeque	¼ cup (2.2 oz)	57
Just Rite		
Hot Dog	2 oz	60
Ka-Me		
Black Bean Sauce	1 tbsp (0.5 oz)	10
Chili Sauce Hot Garlic	1 tbsp (0.5 oz)	15
Duck Sauce	2 tbsp (1 oz)	80
Fish Sauce	1 tbsp (0.5 fl oz)	10
Hoisin Sauce	2 tbsp (1 oz)	45
Hot Sauce	1 tsp (5 g)	0
Lemon Sauce	1 tbsp (0.5 oz)	45
Mandarin Orange Sauce	2 tbsp (1 oz)	80
Oyster Sauce	1 tbsp (0.5 fl oz)	10
Plum	2 tbsp (1 fl oz)	80

FOOD	PORTION	CALS.
Ka-Me (CONT.)		
Stir Fry Sauce	1 tbsp	10
Sweet & Sour	2 tbsp (1 fl oz)	50
Szechuan	1 tbsp (0.5 oz)	20
Tamari	1 tbsp (0.5 fl oz)	10
Tempura Sauce	2 tbsp (1 fl oz)	15
Teriyaki Sauce	1 tbsp (0.5 fl oz)	10
Kikkoman		
Stir-Fry	1 tbsp	16
Sweet & Sour	1 tbsp	19
Teriyaki	1 tbsp	15
Knorr		
Grilling And Broiling Chardonnay	1.6 oz	50
Grilling And Broiling Tequilla Lime	1.6 oz	50
Grilling And Broiling Tuscan Herb	1.6 oz	50
Microwave Hollandaise	1 oz	50
Microwave Mandarin Ginger	1.6 oz	50
Microwave Parmesano	1.6 oz	50
Microwave Vera Cruz	3.3 oz	70
Kraft		
Sandwich Spread & Burger Sauce	1 tbsp (0.5 oz)	50
Sweet'n Sour	2 tbsp (1.3 oz)	80
Tartar Sauce Nonfat	2 tbsp (1.1 oz)	25
La Choy		
Duck Sauce Sweet & Sour	1 tbsp	25
Sweet & Sour	1 tbsp	25
Lawry's		
Marinade Lemon Pepper	1 tbsp (0.5 oz)	10
Teriyaki Marinade	2 tbsp	72
Lea & Perrins		
Steak	1 oz	40
Worcestershire	1 tsp	5
Worcestershire White Wine	1 tsp	4
Manwich		
Bold	¼ cup (2.2 oz)	62
Burrito	¼ cup (2.2 oz)	25
Mexican	¼ cup (2.2 oz)	27
Original	¼ cup (2.2 oz)	32
Taco	¼ cup (2.2 oz)	31
Thick & Chunky	¼ cup (2.3 oz)	44
Marzetti		
Teriyaki Stir-Fry	2 tbsp	80
McIlhenny		
7 Spice Chili	2 tbsp (1.1 fl oz)	16

FOOD	PORTION	CALS.
McIlhenny (CONT.)		
Sauce	2 tbsp (1.1 oz)	48
Tabasco	1 tsp	1
Mrs. Dash		
Steak	1 tbsp	17
Newman's Own		
Bandito Diavalo Spicy	4 oz	70
Old El Paso		
Enchilada Hot	¼ cup (2 oz)	30
Enchilada Mild	¼ cup (2 oz)	25
Green Chili Enchilada Sauce	¼ cup (2.1 oz)	30
Taco Hot	1 tbsp (0.5 oz)	5
Taco Medium	1 tbsp (0.5 oz)	5
Taco Mild	1 tbsp (0.5 oz)	5
Taco Sauce	1 tbsp (0.5 oz)	5
Taco Sauce Extra Chunky Medium	1 tbsp (0.5 oz)	5
Taco Sauce Extra Chunky Mild	1 tbsp (0.5 oz)	5
Ortega		
Taco Thick & Smooth Hot	1 tbsp	8
Taco Thick & Smooth Mild	1 tbsp	8
Taco Western Style	1 oz	8
Progresso		
Alfredo	½ cup (4.4 oz)	310
Red Wing		
Chili Sauce	1 tbsp (0.6 oz)	20
Seafood Cocktail	¼ cup (2 oz)	90
Sauce Arturo		
Original	¼ cup (2.2 fl oz)	50
Sauceworks		
Cocktail	¼ cup (2.3 oz)	60
Sweet'n Sour	2 tbsp (1.2 oz)	60
Tartar	2 tbsp (1.1 oz)	100
Tartar Natural Lemon & Herb	2 tbsp (1 oz)	150
Simmer Chef		
Golden Honey Mustard	½ cup (4 fl oz)	150
Hearty Onion & Mushroom	½ cup (4 fl oz)	50
Snow's		
Newburg With Sherry	⅓ cup	120
Welsh Rarebit Cheese	½ cup	170
Trappey		
Indi-Pep West Indian Style Pepper Sauce	1 tsp (0.1 oz)	1
Mexi Pep Louisiana Hot Sauce	1 tsp (0.1 oz)	tr
Pepper Sauce	1 tsp (0.2 oz)	1
Red Devil Buffalo Style Hot Sauce	1 tsp (0.1 oz)	1

FOOD	PORTION	CALS.
Trappey (CONT.)		
Red Devil Cayenne Pepper Sauce	1 tsp (0.1 oz)	1
Worcestershire Chef Magic	1 tsp (0.1 oz)	3
Watkins		
Beef Marinade	¼ tbsp (2 g)	5
Calypso Hot Pepper Sauce	1 tsp (5 g)	10
Caribbean Red Pepper Sauce	1 tsp (5 g)	10
Chicken & Pork Marinade	¼ tbsp (2 g)	5
Fish & Seafood Marinade	¼ tbsp (2 g)	10
Inferno Hot Pepper Sauce	2 tbsp (1 oz)	35
Meat Magic	1 tsp (6 g)	10
Steak Sauce	1 tbsp (0.5 oz)	20
Wolf Brand		
Hot Dog	1.25 oz	44
MIX		
bearnaise as prep w/ milk & butter	1 cup	701
cheese as prep w/ milk	1 cup	307
curry as prep w/ milk	1 cup	270
mushroom as prep w/ milk	1 cup	228
sourcream as prep w/ milk	1 cup	509
stroganoff as prep	1 cup	271
sweet & sour as prep	1 cup	294
teriyaki as prep	1 cup	131
white as prep w/ milk	1 cup	241
Cajun King		
Etoufee Seasoning Mix	3.5 oz	383
Jambalaya Seasoning Mix	3.5 oz	375
Durkee		
A La King as prep	1 cup	60
Cheese as prep	¼ cup	25
Hollandaise as prep	2 tbsp	10
Nacho Cheese as prep	2 tbsp	25
White as prep	¼ cup	20
French's		
Cheese as prep	¼ cup	25
Hollandaise as prep	2 tbsp	10
Kikkoman		
Marinade For Meat	1 oz pkg	64
Sweet & Sour	2⅛ oz pkg	228
Teriyaki	1½ oz pkg	125
Knorr		
Au Jus as prep	2 oz	8
Bearnaise as prep	2 oz	170
Classic Brown Gravy as prep	2 oz	25

FOOD	PORTION	CALS.
Knorr (CONT.)		
Demi-Glace as prep	2 oz	30
Hollandaise as prep	2 oz	170
Hunter as prep	2 oz	25
Lyonnaise as prep	2 oz	20
Mushroom as prep	2 oz	60
Napoli as prep	4 oz	100
Pepper as prep	2 oz	20
Weight Watchers		
Lemon Butter as prep	¼ cup	5
SHELF-STABLE		
Cheez Whiz		
Cheese Sauce With Mild Salsa Zap-A-Pack	2 tbsp (1.2 oz)	90
Zap-A-Pack	2 tbsp (1.2 oz)	90
Fresh Gourmet		
Stir 'n Sauce Italian	1 tbsp (0.5 oz)	30
SAUERKRAUT		
canned	½ cup	22
Claussen		
Canned	½ cup	17
Del Monte	½ cup (4.2 oz)	15
Eden		
Organic	½ cup (3.9 oz)	25
Hebrew National		
Gallon Kraut	½ cup	25
New Kraut	½ cup (3.1 oz)	50
Rosoff's		
Sauerkraut	½ cup (3.2 oz)	50
S&W		
Canned	½ cup	25
Schorr's		
New Kraut	½ cup (3.2 oz)	50
Seneca		
Canned	2 tbsp	5
SnowFloss		
Kraut	4 oz	28
Kraut Bavarian Style	4 oz	64
Vlasic		
Old Fashioned	1 oz	4
SAUERKRAUT JUICE		
S&W		
Juice	4 oz	14
SAUSAGE		
(*see also* HOT DOG, SAUSAGE SUBSTITUTES)		
bierschinken	3.5 oz	174

FOOD	PORTION	CALS.
bierwurst	3.5 oz	258
blutwurst uncooked	3½ oz	424
bockwurst	3.5 oz	276
bockwurst pork & veal raw	1 link (2.3 oz)	200
bratwurst pork cooked	1 link (3 oz)	256
brotwurst pork	1 oz	92
brotwurst pork & beef	1 link (2.5 oz)	226
country-style pork cooked	1 link (½ oz)	48
country-style pork cooked	1 patty (1 oz)	100
fleischwurst	3.5 oz	305
gelbwurst uncooked	3½ oz	363
italian pork cooked	1 (2.4 oz)	216
italian pork cooked	1 (3 oz)	268
jagdwurst	3.5 oz	211
kielbasa pork	1 oz	88
knockwurst pork & beef	1 (2.4 oz)	209
knockwurst pork & beef	1 oz	87
mettwurst uncooked	3½ oz	483
plockwurst uncooked	3½ oz	312
polish pork	1 (8 oz)	739
polish pork	1 oz	92
pork & beef cooked	1 link (½ oz)	52
pork & beef cooked	1 patty (1 oz)	107
pork cooked	1 patty (1 oz)	100
pork cooked	1 link (½ oz)	48
regensburger uncooked	3½ oz	354
smoked beef cooked	1 sausage (1.4 oz)	134
smoked pork	1 link (2.4 oz)	265
smoked pork	1 sm link (½ oz)	62
smoked pork & beef	1 link (2.4 oz)	229
smoked pork & beef	1 sm link (½ oz)	54
vienna canned	1 (½ oz)	45
vienna canned	7 (4 oz)	315
weisswurst uncooked	3½ oz	305
zungenwurst (tongue)	3.5 oz	285
Aidells		
Andouille Cajun Cooked	1 (3.5 oz)	220
Burmese Curry Cooked	1 (3.5 oz)	220
Chicken & Apple Fresh	1 (1.9 oz)	110
Chicken & Apple Smoked	1 (3.5 oz)	220
Chicken & Turkey New Mexico Smoked	1 (3.5 oz)	220
Chicken & Turkey Thai Fresh	1 (3.5 oz)	200
Chicken & Turkey Thai Smoked	1 (3.5 oz)	220
Chicken & Turkey With Sun-Dried Tomatoes & Basil Fresh	1 (3.5 oz)	200

FOOD	PORTION	CALS.
Aidells (CONT.)		
Chicken & Turkey With Sun-Dried Tomatoes & Basil Smoked	1 (3.5 oz)	200
Creole Hot Cooked	1 (3.5 oz)	220
Duck & Turkey Smoked	1 (3.5 oz)	220
Hunter's Cooked	1 (3.5 oz)	240
Italian Hot Fresh	1 (3.5 oz)	230
Lamb & Beef With Rosemary Fresh	1 (3.5 oz)	220
Lemon Chicken Cooked	1 (3.5 oz)	220
Mexican Chorizo Beef Fresh	1 (3.5 oz)	400
Whiskey Fennel Cooked	1 (3.5 oz)	230
Armour		
Country Sausage Lower Salt	1 oz	110
Country Sausage Lower Salt Links	1 oz	110
Pork	1 oz	110
Pork Links	1 oz	110
Pork Patties	1.5 oz	160
Vienna Sausage 25% Less Fat	3 (1.9 oz)	130
Vienna Sausage In BBQ Sauce	3 (2.1 oz)	160
Vienna Sausage In Beef Stock	3 (1.9 oz)	170
Vienna Sausage In Hot Sauce	3 (2.1 oz)	170
Vienna Sausage Smoked	3 (1.9 oz)	170
Banner		
Sausage Tripe	2 oz	90
Bilinski's		
Chicken & Vegetable	1 (3 oz)	80
Chicken Italian With Peppers & Onions	1 (3 oz)	120
Golden Brown		
Beef	1	80
Mild	1	100
Spicy	1	100
Healthy Choice		
Low Fat Smoked	2 oz	70
Low Fat Smoked Polska Kielbasa	2 oz	70
Hebrew National		
Beef Knocks	1 (3 oz)	260
Polish Beef	1 link	240
Hillshire		
Beer Bratwurst	1 (2 oz)	190
Bratwurst Fresh	1 (2 oz)	190
Bratwurst Light Fresh	1 (2 oz)	150
Bratwurst Spicy	1 (2 oz)	180
Flavorseal Kielbasa Polska	2 oz	190
Flavorseal Kielbasa Polska Beef	2 oz	190

FOOD	PORTION	CALS.
Hillshire (CONT.)		
Flavorseal Kielbasa Polska Lite	2 oz	130
Flavorseal Kielbasa Polska Mild	2 oz	190
Flavorseal Kielbasa Polska Turkey	2 oz	90
Flavorseal Smoked	2 oz	190
Flavorseal Smoked Beef	2 oz	180
Flavorseal Smoked Beef & Cheddar	2 oz	190
Flavorseal Smoked Country Recipe	2 oz	180
Flavorseal Smoked Hot	2 oz	180
Flavorseal Smoked Lite	2 oz	130
Flavorseal Smoked Turkey	2 oz	90
Flavorseal Smoked w/ Italian Seasoning	2 oz	200
Italian Mild	1 (2 oz)	190
Italian Mild Light	1 (2 oz)	150
Italian Hot	1 (2 oz)	180
Italian Hot Light	1 (2 oz)	150
Kielbasa Fresh Polska	1 (2 oz)	190
Kielbasa Fresh Polska Lower Fat	1 (2 oz)	150
Links 80% Fat Free Cheddar Hots	2 oz	150
Links 80% Fat Free Kielbasa	2 oz	130
Links Brats Fully Cooked	2 oz	170
Links Bratwurst Smoked	2 oz	190
Links Bun Size Cheddarwurst	2 oz	200
Links Bun Size Kielbasa	2 oz	180
Links Bun Size Smoked	2 oz	180
Links Bun Size Smoked Beef	2 oz	180
Links Cheddarwurst	2 oz	190
Links Cheddarwurst Lite	1 link (2.7 oz)	190
Links Hot	2 oz	190
Links Hot Beef	2 oz	190
Links Hot Lite	1 link (2.7 oz)	190
Links Keilbasa Polska	2 oz	190
Links Keilbasa Polska Lite	1 link (2.7 oz)	190
Links Knockwurst Lite	2 oz	180
Links Lit'l Polskas	2 oz	180
Links Lit'l Smokies	2 oz	180
Links Lit'l Smokies Beef	2 oz	180
Links Lit'l Smokies Cheddar	2 oz	180
Links Lit'l Smokies Light	2 oz	120
Links Polish	2 oz	190
Links Smoked	2 oz	190
Mexican Style	1 (2 oz)	190
Mexican Style Lower Fat	1 (2 oz)	150

FOOD	PORTION	CALS.
Hormel		
Light & Lean 97 Dinner Smoked	2 oz	60
Pickled Hot	6 (2 oz)	140
Pickled Smoked	6 (2 oz)	140
Vienna	2 oz	140
Vienna Chicken	2 oz	90
Jimmy Dean		
Brick Sausage	2.5 oz	270
Bulk	2.5 oz	300
Hickory Smoked Dinner Sausage	2 oz	170
Pattie Pre-Cooked	1 (1.9 oz)	230
Polska Kielbaska	2 oz	170
Sage Pattie	1 (2 oz)	200
Sausage Pattie Raw	1 (2 oz)	200
Skinless Link	4 (2 oz)	200
Skinless Link	2 (2 oz)	200
Jones		
Brown & Serve Bacon	1	90
Brown & Serve Beef	1	90
Brown & Serve Light	1	60
Brown & Serve Regular	1	100
Cello Beef	1 slice (1 oz)	130
Cello Hot Country	1 slice (1 oz)	110
Cello Original	1 slice (1 oz)	100
Dinner Link	1	280
Golden Brown Light Links	1	60
Golden Brown Mild Pattie	1	150
Italian	1	160
Light Link	1	70
Little Link	1	140
Patties	1	150
Scrapple	1 slice	90
Scrapple	1 slice (1½ oz)	90
Little Sizzlers		
Brown & Serve	2 patties (1.4 oz)	190
Brown & Serve	3 links (2.1 oz)	190
Cooked	3 links (1.4 oz)	210
Cooked	2 patties (2 oz)	250
Heat & Serve Pork cooked	3 links (1.4 oz)	210
Louis Rich		
Polska Kielbasa	2 oz	80
Smoked Sausage With Cheese cooked	1 (1 oz)	47
Turkey	2.5 oz	110
Turkey & Cheese Smoked	2 oz	90

FOOD	PORTION	CALS.
Louis Rich (CONT.)		
Turkey Links	2 (2 oz)	90
Turkey Smoked	2 oz	90
Mr. Turkey		
Breakfast	2.5 oz	130
Hearty Blend Polish Kielbasa	1 oz	70
Hearty Blend Smoked	1 oz	70
Hot Smoked	1 oz	45
Italian Smoked	1 oz	45
Polish Kielbasa	1 oz	45
Smoked	1 oz	45
Old Smokehouse		
Summer Sausage	1 oz	110
Oscar Mayer		
Pork cooked	2 links (1.7 oz)	170
Smokies Beef	1 (1.5 oz)	120
Smokies Cheese	1 (1.5 oz)	130
Smokies Links	1 (1.5 oz)	130
Smokies Little	6 (2 oz)	170
Perdue		
Breakfast Links Turkey Cooked	2 links (2 oz)	100
Hot Italian Turkey Cooked	1 link (2.4 oz)	110
Sweet Italian Turkey Cooked	1 link (2.4 oz)	110
Rudy's Farm		
Italian Hot	2.5 oz	240
Italian Mild Natural Casing	1 (2 oz)	190
Morning Right Link	3 (2.9 oz)	150
Morning Right Pattie	2 (2.9 oz)	150
Pattie Pre-Cooked	1 (1.4 oz)	100
Smoked	4 (2.1 oz)	200
Sweet Link	1 (3.9 oz)	380
Shofar		
Knockwurst Beef	1 (3 oz)	260
Tyson		
Country Pork	3.5 oz	320
Wampler Longacre		
Breakfast Links	1 (2.8 oz)	170
Italian Links	1 (2.8 oz)	170
Tinderlings Garlic & Pepper	1 (3.5 oz)	143
Turkey	1 pattie (2 oz)	120
Turkey	1 link (1 oz)	60
TAKE-OUT		
pork	1 link (.5 oz)	48
pork	1 patty (1 oz)	100

FOOD	PORTION	CALS.
SAUSAGE DISHES		
FROZEN		
Jimmy Dean		
Italian Sausage & Mozzarella Sandwich	1 (4.5 oz)	380
Ovenstuffs		
French Roll Italian Sausage	1 (4.75 oz)	390
French Roll Pepperoni	1 (4.75 oz)	370
TAKE-OUT		
sausage roll	1 (2.3 oz)	311
SAUSAGE SUBSTITUTES		
Knox Mountain Farm		
No-So-Sausage	1 serv (¹/₁₀ pkg)	120
LaLoma		
Linketts	2 (71 g)	140
Little Links	2 (46 g)	90
Lightlife		
Lean Links Breakfast	1.25 oz	69
Lean Links Italian	1.5 oz	83
Morningstar Farms		
Breakfast Patties	2 (76 g)	190
Country Crisp Patties	1 (71 g)	220
Grillers	1 (64 g)	180
White Wave		
Meatless Healthy Links	2 (1.6 oz)	140
Worthington		
Leanies	1 link (40 g)	100
Prosage Links	2 (45 g)	130
Saucettes	2 links (67 g)	150
Super-Links	1 (48 g)	100
Veja-Links	2 (62 g)	140
SAVORY		
ground	1 tsp	4
SCALLOP		
FRESH		
raw	3 oz	75
FROZEN		
Mrs. Paul's		
Fried	2 oz	160
HOME RECIPE		
breaded & fried	2 lg	67
TAKE-OUT		
breaded & fried	6 (5 oz)	386

FOOD	PORTION	CALS.
SCONE		
Finnegan's		
Irish Raisin	1 (2.7 oz)	90
HOME RECIPE		
apricot scone	1	232
TAKE-OUT		
cheese	1 (1.75 oz)	182
fruit	1 (1.75 oz)	158
plain	1 (1.75 oz)	181
SCROD		
FROZEN		
Gorton's		
Microwave Entree Baked	1 pkg	320
SCUP		
fresh baked	3 oz	115
SEA BASS		
(*see* BASS)		
SEA TROUT		
(*see* TROUT)		
SEAWEED		
agar dried	1 oz	87
agar fresh	1 oz	tr
irishmoss fresh	1 oz	14
kelp fresh	1 oz	12
kombu fresh	1 oz	12
laver fresh	1 oz	10
nori fresh	1 oz	10
spirulina dried	1 oz	83
spirulina fresh	1 oz	7
tangle fresh	1 oz	12
wakame fresh	1 oz	13
Eden		
Agar Agar Bars	1 tbsp (2.5 oz)	10
Agar Agar Flakes	1 tbsp (2.5 oz)	10
Arame	½ cup (0.3 oz)	30
Hiziki	½ cup (0.3 oz)	30
Kombu	3.5 in piece (3.3 g)	10
Nori	1 sheet (2.5 g)	10
Sushi Nori	1 sheet (2.5 g)	10
Wakame	½ cup (0.3 oz)	25
Wakame Flakes	½ cup (0.3 oz)	25

FOOD	PORTION	CALS.
Maine Coast		
Alaria	⅓ cup (7 g)	18
Dulse	⅓ cup (7 g)	18
Dulse Flakes	1 oz	75
Kelp	⅓ cup (7 g)	17
Kelp Crunch	1 bar (1 oz)	129
Kelp Crunch Peanut-Raisin	1 bar (1 oz)	129
Laver	⅓ cup (7 g)	22
Sea Seasoning Dulse	1 g	3
Sea Seasoning Dulse With Celery	1 g	3
Sea Seasoning Dulse With Garlic	1 g	3
Sea Seasoning Dulse With Sesame	1 g	3
Sea Seasoning Kelp	1 g	3
Sea Seasoning Kelp With Cayenne	1 g	3
Sea Seasoning Nori	1 g	3
Sea Seasoning Nori With Ginger	1 g	3

SEITAN
(*see* WHEAT)

SEMOLINA
dry	½ cup	303

SESAME
seeds	1 tsp	16
seeds dried	1 tbsp	52
seeds dried	1 cup	825
seeds roasted & toasted	1 oz	161
sesame butter	1 tbsp	95
sesame crunch candy	1 oz	146
sesame crunch candy	20 pieces (1.2 oz)	181
sesame sticks	1 oz	153
sesame sticks unsalted	1 oz	153
tahini from roasted & toasted kernels	1 tbsp	89
tahini from stone ground kernels	1 tbsp	86
tahini from unroasted kernels	1 tbsp	85
Arrowhead		
Sesame Tahini	1 oz	170
Casbah		
Tahini Sauce Mix as prep	¼ cup	160
Eden		
Sesame Shake	½ tsp (1.5 g)	10
Sesame Shake Garlic	½ tsp (1.5 g)	10
Sesame Shake Organic Seaweed	½ tsp (1.5 g)	10
Erewhon		
Sesame Butter	2 tbsp (32 g)	190

FOOD	PORTION	CALS.
Erewhon (CONT.)		
Sesame Tahini	2 tbsp (32 g)	200
Joyva		
Tahini	2 tbsp (1 oz)	200
Planters		
Nut Mix	1 oz	150
Stone-Buhr		
Seeds Raw	4 tsp (1 oz)	180

SESBANIA
flower	1	1
flowers	1 cup	5
flowers cooked	1 cup	23

SHAD
american baked	3 oz	214
roe baked w/ butter & lemon	3.5 oz	126
roe raw	3½ oz	130

SHALLOTS
dried	1 tbsp	3
raw chopped	1 tbsp	7

SHARK
batter-dipped & fried	3 oz	194
raw	3 oz	111

SHEEPSHEAD FISH
cooked	1 fillet (6.5 oz)	234
cooked	3 oz	107
raw	3 oz	92

SHELLFISH
(see individual names, SHELLFISH SUBSTITUTES*)*

SHELLFISH SUBSTITUTES
crab imitation	3 oz	87
scallop imitation	3 oz	84
shrimp imitation	3 oz	86
surimi	1 oz	28
surimi	3 oz	84
Louis Kemp		
Crab Delights Chunk Style	2 oz	54
Lobster Delights	2 oz	60
Maryland Style Cakes	2.5 oz	154
Ocean Magic		
Imitation King Crab	3 oz	80

FOOD	PORTION	CALS.
SHELLIE BEANS		
canned	½ cup	37
SHERBET		
(*see also* ICES AND ICE POPS)		
orange	½ cup (4 fl oz)	132
orange	½ gal	2158
orange	1 bar (2.75 fl oz)	91
orange home recipe	½ cup	120
Borden		
Orange	½ cup	110
Bresler's		
All Flavors	3.5 oz	140
Hood		
Lime Orange Lemon	½ cup (3.1 oz)	120
Orange	½ cup (3.1 oz)	120
Rainbow Swirl	½ cup (3.1 oz)	120
Raspberry Orange Lime	½ cup (3.1 oz)	120
Sealtest		
Lime	½ cup (3 oz)	130
Orange	½ cup (3 oz)	130
Rainbow Orange Red Raspberry Lime	½ cup (3 oz)	130
Red Raspberry	½ cup (3 oz)	130
SHRIMP		
CANNED		
canned	3 oz	102
canned	1 cup	154
Robinson		
Canned Shrimp	2 oz	58
S&W		
Deveined Medium Whole Shrimp	2 oz	65
FRESH		
cooked	3 oz	84
cooked	4 large	22
raw	4 large	30
raw	3 oz	90
FROZEN		
Cajun Cookin'		
Shrimp Creole	12 oz	390
Shrimp Etouffee	17 oz	360
Shrimp Jambalaya	12 oz	450
Gorton's		
Butterfly Shrimp	4 oz	160
Microwave Crunchy Shrimp	5 oz	380

FOOD	PORTION	CALS.
Gorton's (CONT.)		
Microwave Entree Shrimp Scampi	1 pkg	390
Shrimp Crisps	4 oz	280
Mrs. Paul's		
Entrees Light Seafood & Clams With Linguini	10 oz	240
Van De Kamp's		
Breaded Butterfly	7 (4 oz)	280
Breaded Popcorn	20 (4 oz)	270
Breaded Whole	7 (4 oz)	240
READY-TO-USE		
American Original		
Fried	4 oz	253
TAKE-OUT		
breaded & fried	3 oz	206
breaded & fried	6 to 8 (6 oz)	454
jambalaya	¾ cup	188

SMELT

rainbow cooked	3 oz	106
rainbow raw	3 oz	83

SNACKS

(*see also* CHIPS, FRUIT SNACKS, NUTS MIXED, POPCORN, PRETZELS)

oriental mix	1 oz	155
pork skins	½ oz	77
pork skins	1 oz	154
pork skins barbecue	1 oz	152
pork skins barbecue	½ oz	76
trail mix	1 oz	131
trail mix	1 cup (5.3 oz)	693
trail mix tropical	1 oz	115
trail mix w/ chocolate chips	1 cup (5.1 oz)	707
trail mix w/ chocolate chips	1 oz	137
Bakem-ets		
Hot'N Spicy	21 pieces (1 oz)	150
Snacks	21 pieces (1 oz)	160
Bugles		
Nacho Cheese	1 oz	160
Ranch	1 oz	150
Snacks	1 oz	150
Cheetos		
Cheddar Valley	26 pieces (1 oz)	160
Crunchy	26 pieces (1 oz)	150
Curls	15 pieces (1 oz)	150

FOOD	PORTION	CALS.
Cheetos (CONT.)		
Flamin' Hot	26 pieces (1 oz)	150
Light	38 pieces (1 oz)	140
Paws	16 pieces (1 oz)	160
Puffed Ball	38 pieces (1 oz)	160
Puffs	33 pieces (1 oz)	160
Cheez Doodles		
Crunchy	1 oz	160
Puffed	1 oz	150
Cheez Waffies		
Snacks	1 oz	140
Chex		
Snack Mix Barbeque	½ cup (1.1 oz)	130
Snack Mix Cool Sour Cream And Onion	½ cup (1 oz)	130
Snack Mix Golden Cheddar	½ cup (1 oz)	130
Snack Mix Traditional	⅔ cup (1.2 oz)	150
Combos		
Cheddar Cheese Cracker	1 pkg (1.7 oz)	250
Cheddar Cheese Cracker	1 oz	140
Cheddar Cheese Pretzel	1 pkg (1.8 oz)	240
Cheddar Cheese Pretzel	1 oz	130
Chili Cheese w/ Corn Shell	1 oz	140
Chili Cheese w/ Corn Shell	1 pkg (1.7 oz)	230
Mustard Pretzel	1 pkg (1.8 oz)	230
Mustard Pretzel	1 oz	130
Nacho Cheese Pretzel	1 pkg (1.7 oz)	230
Nacho Cheese Pretzel	1 oz	130
Nacho Cheese w/ Tortilla Shell	1 oz	140
Nacho Cheese w/ Tortilla Shell	1 pkg (1.7 oz)	230
Peanut Butter Cracker	1 oz	140
Pepperoni & Cheese Pizza	1 oz	140
Pepperoni & Cheese Pizza	1 pkg (1.7 oz)	240
Pizzeria Pretzel	1 pkg (1.8 oz)	230
Pizzeria Pretzel	1 oz	130
Tortilla Ranch	1 bag (1.7 oz)	240
Tortilla Ranch	1 oz	140
Cornnuts		
Barbecue	1 oz	120
Nacho Cheese	1 oz	120
Original	1 oz	120
Original	1 pkg (2 oz)	260
Picante	1 oz	120
Ranch	1 oz	120

FOOD	PORTION	CALS.
Doo Dads		
Sancks	1 oz	130
Energy Food Factory		
Poprice Cheddar Cheese	½ oz	60
Poprice Herb & Garlic	½ oz	50
Poprice Lite	½ oz	50
Poprice Original No Salt	½ oz	45
Estee		
Snack Crisps Apple Cinnamon	1 pkg (0.66 oz)	90
Snack Crisps Apple Cinnamon	27 crisps (1 oz)	130
Snack Crisps Chocolate	30 crisps (1 oz)	130
Snack Crisps Chocolate	1 pkg (0.66 oz)	90
Snack Crisps Lemon	1 pkg (0.66 oz)	90
Snack Crisps Lemon	30 (1 oz)	130
Snack Crisps Ranch	30 (1 oz)	130
Snack Crisps Ranch	1 pkg (0.6 oz)	90
Snack Crisps White Cheddar	1 pkg (0.6 oz)	90
Snack Crisps With Cheddar	27 crisps (1 oz)	130
Frito Lay		
Corn Nuggets Toasted	1.38 oz	170
Funyums		
Onion Rings	11 pieces (1 oz)	140
Handi-Snacks		
Peanut Butter'n Crackers	1 pkg (1.1 oz)	180
Peanut Butter'n Grahamsticks	1 pkg (1.1 oz)	170
Hapi		
Chili Bits	½ cup (1 oz)	110
Health Valley		
Cheddar Lites	0.75 oz	40
Cheddar Lites With Green Onion	0.75 oz	40
Lance		
Cheese Balls	1 pkg (32 g)	190
Crunchy Cheese Twists	1 pkg (42 g)	260
Gold-N-Chees	1 pkg (39 g)	180
Pork Skins	1 pkg (14 g)	80
Pork Skins BBQ	1 pkg (14 g)	80
Mr. Peanut		
Peanut Butter Crisps Graham	12 pieces (1.1 oz)	150
Munchos		
Snack	16 pieces (1 oz)	160
Planters		
Cheez Balls	1 oz	150
Cheez Balls	1 pkg (1 oz)	150
Cheez Curls	1 oz	150

FOOD	PORTION	CALS.
Planters (CONT.)		
Cheez Curls	1 pkg (1.2 oz)	190
Heat Snack Mix	1 oz	140
Snyder's		
Cheddar Cheese Twists	1 oz	150
Kruncheez	1 oz	160
Onion Toasters	1 oz	150
Snack Mix	1 oz	170
Sopaipillas Apple & Cinnamon	1 oz	150
Splurge		
Snack Mix Fat Free Original	⅔ cup (1 oz)	100
Ultra Slim-Fast		
Lite N' Tasty Cheese Curls	1 oz	110
Weight Watchers		
Cheese Curls	1 pkg (0.5 oz)	70
Pizza Curls	1 pkg (0.5 oz)	60
Ranch Curls	1 pkg (0.5 oz)	60

SNAIL
cooked	3 oz	233
raw	3 oz	117

SNAPPER
cooked	3 oz	109
cooked	1 fillet (6 oz)	217
raw	3 oz	85

SODA
(*see also* DRINK MIXERS, MINERAL/BOTTLED WATER)

club	12 oz	0
cola	12 oz	151
cream	12 oz	191
diet cola	12 oz	2
diet cola w/ equal	12 oz	2
diet cola w/ saccharin	12 oz	2
ginger ale	12 oz can	124
grape	12 oz	161
lemon lime	12 oz	149
orange	12 oz	177
pepper type	12 oz	151
quinine	12 oz	125
root beer	12 oz	152
tonic water	12 oz	125
7 Up		
Cherry	1 oz	13

FOOD	PORTION	CALS.
7 Up (CONT.)		
Cherry Diet	1 oz	tr
Diet	1 oz	tr
Gold	1 oz	13
Gold Diet	1 oz	tr
Orignal	1 oz	12
After The Fall		
Raspberry Ginger Ale	1 can (12 oz)	150
Barrelhead		
Root Beer	8 fl oz	110
Burst		
Cola Strawberry	8 fl oz	117
Canada Dry		
Birch Beer Brown	8 fl oz	110
Birch Beer Clear	8 fl oz	110
Black Cherry Wishniak	8 fl oz	130
Cactus Cooler	8 fl oz	110
California Strawberry	8 fl oz	110
Club	8 fl oz	0
Club Sodium Free	8 fl oz	0
Concord Grape	8 fl oz	120
Diet Ginger Ale	8 fl oz	0
Diet Ginger Ale Cherry	8 fl oz	0
Diet Ginger Ale Cranberry	8 fl oz	0
Diet Ginger Ale Lemon	8 fl oz	5
Diet Tonic Water	8 fl oz	0
Diet Tonic Water Twist Of Lime	8 fl oz	0
Ginger Ale	8 fl oz	100
Ginger Ale Cherry	8 fl oz	110
Ginger Ale Cranberry	8 fl oz	100
Ginger Ale Golden	8 fl oz	100
Ginger Ale Lemon	8 fl oz	100
Half & Half	8 fl oz	110
Hi-Spot	8 fl oz	110
Island Lime	8 fl oz	140
Jamaica Cola	8 fl oz	110
Lemon Sour	8 fl oz	100
Peach	8 fl oz	120
Pina Pineapple	8 fl oz	110
Seltzer	8 fl oz	0
Seltzer Cherry	8 fl oz	0
Seltzer Cranberry Lime	8 fl oz	0
Seltzer Grapefruit	8 fl oz	0
Seltzer Lemon Lime	8 fl oz	0

FOOD	PORTION	CALS.
Canada Dry (CONT.)		
Seltzer Mandarin Orange	8 fl oz	0
Seltzer Peach	8 fl oz	0
Seltzer Raspberry	8 fl oz	0
Seltzer Strawberry	8 fl oz	0
Seltzer Tropical	8 fl oz	0
Sunripe Orange	8 fl oz	140
Tahitian Treat	8 fl oz	150
Tonic Water	8 fl oz	100
Tonic Water Twist Of Lime	8 fl oz	100
Vanilla Cream	8 fl oz	120
Vichy Water	8 fl oz	0
Wild Cherry	8 fl oz	110
Clearly 2		
Black Cherry	8 fl oz	2
Key Lime	8 fl oz	2
Clearly Canadian		
Alpine Fruit & Berries	8 fl oz	90
Boysenberry Mist	8 fl oz	2
Country Raspberry	8 fl oz	80
Green Apple	8 fl oz	80
Mountain Blackberry	8 fl oz	100
Orchard Peach Strawberry	8 fl oz	90
Soda	8 fl oz	0
Summer Strawberry	8 fl oz	80
Western Longanberry	8 fl oz	80
Wild Cherry	8 fl oz	90
Coca-Cola		
Cherry	8 fl oz	104
Classic	8 fl oz	97
Classic Caffeine-Free	8 fl oz	97
Coke II	8 fl oz	105
Diet	8 fl oz	1
Diet Cherry	8 fl oz	1
Diet Coke Caffeine-Free	6 oz	tr
Diet Coke Caffeine-free	8 fl oz	1
Cott		
Cola	8 fl oz	110
Ginger Ale	8 fl oz	90
Grape	8 fl oz	130
Orange	8 fl oz	140
Pineapple	8 fl oz	130
Punch	8 fl oz	130
Seltzer	8 fl oz	0

FOOD	PORTION	CALS.
Crush		
Cherry	8 fl oz	140
Grape	8 fl oz	110
Orange	8 fl oz	140
Orange Diet	8 fl oz	0
Pineapple	8 fl oz	140
Strawberry	8 fl oz	130
Tropical Fruit Punch	1 bottle (10 fl oz)	180
Tropical Fruit Punch	1 can (11.5 fl oz)	200
Diet Rite		
Black Cherry Salt/Sodium Free	8 fl oz	2
Cola	8 fl oz	1
Cola Caffeine/Sugar Free	8 fl oz	1
Cola Salt/Sodium Free	8 fl oz	1
Fruit Punch Salt/Sodium Free	8 fl oz	2
Golden Peach Salt/Sodium Free	8 fl oz	2
Key Lime Salt/Sodium Free	8 fl oz	7
Pink Grapefruit Salt/Sodium Free	8 fl oz	2
Red Raspberry Salt/Sodium Free	8 fl oz	3
Tangerine Salt/Sodium Free	8 fl oz	2
White Grape Salt/Sodium Free	8 fl oz	1
Dr Pepper		
Diet	1 oz	tr
Free	1 oz	12
Free Diet	1 oz	tr
Original	1 oz	13
Dr. Nehi		
Soda	8 fl oz	100
Fanta		
Ginger Ale	8 fl oz	86
Grape	8 fl oz	117
Orange	8 fl oz	118
Root Beer	8 fl oz	111
Fresca		
Soda	8 fl oz	3
Health Valley		
Ginger Ale	12 oz	153
Rootbeer Old Fashioned	12 oz	120
Sarsaparilla Rootbeer	12 oz	153
Wild Berry	12 oz	142
Hires		
Cream	8 fl oz	130
Cream Soda Diet	8 fl oz	0
Original Mocha	8 fl oz	100

FOOD	PORTION	CALS.
Hires (CONT.)		
Original Mocha Diet	8 fl oz	5
Root Beer	8 fl oz	130
Root Beer Diet	8 fl oz	0
Kick		
Soda	8 fl oz	120
Like		
Cola	1 oz	13
Cola Sugar Free	1 oz	tr
Lucozade		
Soda	7 oz	136
Manischewitz		
Seltzer No Salt Added No Calories	8 fl oz	0
Mello Yellow		
Diet	8 fl oz	4
Soda	8 fl oz	119
Minute Maid		
Berry	8 fl oz	111
Diet Orange	8 fl oz	2
Fruit Punch	8 fl oz	117
Grape	8 fl oz	121
Grapefruit	8 fl oz	108
Orange	8 fl oz	118
Peach	8 fl oz	110
Pineapple	8 fl oz	109
Raspberry	8 fl oz	111
Soda	8 fl oz	110
Strawberry	8 fl oz	122
Mountain Dew		
Diet	8 fl oz	2
Soda	8 fl oz	118
Mr. PiBB		
Diet	8 fl oz	1
Soda	6 oz	97
Mug		
Cream	8 fl oz	122
Diet Cream	8 fl oz	2
Diet Root Beer	8 fl oz	1
Root Beer	8 fl oz	141
Nehi		
Cream	8 fl oz	120
Fruit Punch	8 fl oz	120
Ginger Ale	8 fl oz	90
Grape	8 fl oz	120

FOOD	PORTION	CALS.
Nehi (CONT.)		
Orange	8 fl oz	130
Peach	8 fl oz	130
Pineapple	8 fl oz	130
Quinine Water	8 fl oz	90
Root Beer	8 fl oz	120
Strawberry	8 fl oz	120
Wild Red	8 fl oz	120
Old Colony		
Grape	8 fl oz	140
Orangina		
Sparkling Citrus	6 fl oz	80
Pepsi		
Caffeine Free	8 fl oz	105
Diet	8 fl oz	1
Diet Caffeine Free	8 fl oz	1
Regular	8 fl oz	105
Ramblin' Root Beer	8 fl oz	120
Razing Razberry		
Cola	8 fl oz	117
Royal Crown		
Caffeine Free Cola	8 fl oz	110
Cherry	8 fl oz	110
Cola	8 fl oz	100
Diet	8 fl oz	1
Diet Caffeine Free	8 fl oz	1
Diet Cranberry Apple Salt/Sodium Free	8 fl oz	2
Diet Cranberry Salt/Sodium Free	8 fl oz	2
Royal Mistic		
'N Juice Black Cherry	12 fl oz	146
'N Juice Peach Vanilla	12 fl oz	146
'N Juice Tangerine Orange	12 fl oz	146
'N Juice Tropical Supreme	12 fl oz	152
'N Juice Wild Berry	12 fl oz	156
Caribbean Fruit Punch	16 fl oz	230
Grape Strawberry	16 fl oz	230
Sparkling Diet With Lime Kiwi	11.1 fl oz	0
Sparkling Diet With Raspberry Boysenberry	11.1 fl oz	0
Sparkling Diet With Royal Peach	11.1 fl oz	0
Sparkling Diet With Wild Cherry	11.1 fl oz	0
Sparkling With Lime Kiwi	11.1 fl oz	112
Sparkling With Mandarin Orange Pineappple	11.1 fl oz	120

FOOD	PORTION	CALS.
Royal Mistic (CONT.)		
Sparkling With Mango Passion	11.1 fl oz	112
Sparkling With Royal Peach	11.1 fl oz	112
Sparkling With Wild Cherry	11.1 fl oz	112
Schweppes		
Bitter Lemon	8 fl oz	110
Club	8 fl oz	0
Club Sodium Free	8 fl oz	0
Diet Ginger Ale Dry Grape	8 fl oz	2
Diet Ginger Ale Raspberry	8 fl oz	0
Ginger Ale	8 fl oz	90
Ginger Ale Dry Grape	8 fl oz	100
Ginger Ale Raspberry	8 fl oz	100
Ginger Beer	8 fl oz	100
Grape	8 fl oz	130
Grapefruit	8 fl oz	110
Lemon Sour	8 fl oz	110
Lemon-Lime	8 fl oz	100
Seltzer Black Berry	8 fl oz	0
Seltzer Lemon	8 fl oz	0
Seltzer Lemon Lime	8 fl oz	0
Seltzer Lime	8 fl oz	0
Seltzer Orange	8 fl oz	0
Seltzer Peaches & Cream	8 fl oz	0
Seltzer Raspberry	8 fl oz	0
Tonic Citrus	8 fl oz	90
Tonic Cranberry	8 fl oz	90
Tonic Raspberry	8 fl oz	90
Tonic Water Diet	8 fl oz	0
Shasta		
Black Cherry	12 oz	162
Cherry Cola	12 oz	140
Citrus Mist	12 oz	170
Club	12 oz	0
Cola	8 oz	98
Cola	12 oz	147
Collins	12 oz	118
Creme	12 oz	154
Diet Birch Beer	12 oz	4
Diet Cola	8 oz	0
Diet Ginger Ale	8 oz	0
Diet Lemon Lime	8 oz	0
Dr. Diablo	12 oz	140
Free Cola	12 oz	151

FOOD	PORTION	CALS.
Shasta (CONT.)		
Fruit Punch	12 oz	173
Ginger Ale	8 oz	80
Ginger Ale	12 oz	120
Grape	12 oz	177
Lemon Lime	12 oz	146
Lemon Lime	8 oz	97
Orange	12 oz	177
Red Berry	12 oz	158
Red Pop	12 oz	158
Root Beer	12 oz	154
Strawberry	12 oz	147
Tonic Water	12 oz	0
Slice		
Diet Lemon Lime	8 fl oz	5
Diet Mandarin	8 fl oz	5
Lemon Lime	8 fl oz	100
Mandarin Orange	8 fl oz	128
Red	8 fl oz	128
Snapple		
Amazin' Grape	8 fl oz	120
Cherry Lime Ricky	8 fl oz	110
Creme D'Vanilla	8 fl oz	130
French Cherry	8 fl oz	120
Kiwi Peach	8 fl oz	120
Kiwi Strawberry	8 fl oz	130
Mango Madness	8 fl oz	130
Passion Supreme	8 fl oz	120
Peach Melba	8 fl oz	120
Raspberry	8 fl oz	120
Seltzer Black Cherry	8 fl oz	0
Seltzer Lemon Lime	8 fl oz	0
Seltzer Original	8 fl oz	0
Seltzer Tangerine	8 fl oz	0
Tru Root Beer	8 fl oz	110
Sprite		
Diet	8 fl oz	3
Soda	8 fl oz	100
Sundrop		
Cherry	8 fl oz	130
Diet	8 fl oz	5
Soda	8 fl oz	140
Sunkist		
Cactus Cooler	8 fl oz	110

FOOD	PORTION	CALS.
Sunkist (CONT.)		
Cherry	8 fl oz	140
Diet Citrus	8 fl oz	0
Diet Orange	8 fl oz	5
Fruit Punch	8 fl oz	130
Orange	8 fl oz	140
Peach	8 fl oz	120
Pineapple	8 fl oz	140
Strawberry	8 fl oz	140
TAB		
Soda	8 fl oz	1
Tropical Chill		
Cola	8 fl oz	117
Diet	8 fl oz	1
Upper 10		
Diet	8 fl oz	3
Diet Salt/Sodium Free	8 fl oz	3
Salt Free	8 fl oz	100
Soda	8 fl oz	100
Welch's		
Sparkling Apple	12 oz	180
Sparkling Grape	12 oz	180
Sparkling Orange	12 oz	180
Sparkling Strawberry	12 oz	180
Wink		
Diet	8 fl oz	5
Soda	8 fl oz	130
Yoo-Hoo		
Original	9 fl oz	150
SOLDIER BEANS		
Bean Cuisine		
Dried	½ cup	115
SOLE		
FRESH		
cooked	1 fillet (4.5 oz)	148
cooked	3 oz	99
lemon raw	3½ oz	85
raw	3½ oz	90
FROZEN		
Gorton's		
Fishmarket Fresh	5 oz	110
Microwave Entree In Lemon Butter	1 pkg	380
Microwave Entree In Wine Sauce	1 pkg	180

FOOD	PORTION	CALS.
Mrs. Paul's		
Light Fillets	1 fillet	240
Van De Kamp's		
Lightly Breaded Fillets	1 (4 oz)	220
Natural Fillets	1 (4 oz)	110
TAKE-OUT		
battered & fried	3.2 oz	211
breaded & fried	3.2 oz	211

SORBET
(*see* ICES AND ICE POPS)

SORGHUM
sorghum	½ cup	325

SOUFFLE
HOME RECIPE

cheese	3.5 oz	253
grand marnier	1 cup	109
lemon chilled	1 cup	176
raspberry chilled	1 cup	173
spinach	1 cup	218

SOUP
CANNED

asparagus cream of as prep w/ milk	1 cup	161
asparagus cream of as prep w/ water	1 cup	87
beef broth ready-to-serve	1 can (14 oz)	27
beef broth ready-to-serve	1 cup	16
beef noodle as prep w/water	1 cup	84
black bean turtle soup	1 cup	218
black bean as prep w/water	1 cup	116
celery cream of as prep w/ milk	1 cup	165
celery cream of as prep w/ water	1 cup	90
celery cream of not prep	1 can (10¾ oz)	219
cheese as prep w/ milk	1 cup	230
cheese as prep w/ water	1 cup	155
cheese not prep	1 can (11 oz)	377
chicken broth as prep w/ water	1 cup	39
chicken cream of as prep w/ milk	1 cup	191
chicken cream of as prep w/ water	1 cup	116
chicken gumbo as prep w/water	1 cup	56
chicken noodle as prep w/ water	1 cup	75
chicken rice as prep w/ water	1 cup	251
clam chowder manhattan as prep w/ water	1 cup	77
clam chowder new england as prep w/ water	1 cup	95

FOOD	PORTION	CALS.
clam chowder new england as prep w/ milk	1 cup	163
consomme w/ gelatin not prep	1 can (10½ oz)	71
consomme w/ gelatin as prep w/ water	1 cup	29
escarole ready-to-serve	1 cup	27
french onion as prep w/ water	1 cup	57
gazpacho ready-to-serve	1 cup	57
minestrone as prep w/water	1 cup	83
mushroom cream of as prep w/ milk	1 cup	203
mushroom cream of as prep w/ water	1 cup	129
oyster stew as prep w/ milk	1 cup	134
oyster stew as prep w/ water	1 cup	59
pepperpot as prep w/ water	1 cup	103
potato cream of as prep w/ milk	1 cup	148
potato cream of as prep w/ water	1 cup	73
scotch broth as prep w/ water	1 cup	80
split pea w/ ham as prep w/ water	1 cup	189
tomato as prep w/ milk	1 cup	160
tomato as prep w/water	1 cup	86
vegetarian vegetable as prep w/ water	1 cup	72
vichyssoise	1 cup	148
American Original		
New England Chowder	4 oz	64
New England Chowder as prep w/ milk	4 oz	145
Campbell		
Asparagus Cream Of as prep	8 oz	80
Bean Homestyle as prep	8 oz	130
Bean With Bacon as prep	8 oz	140
Beef as prep	8 oz	80
Beef Broth as prep	8 oz	16
Beef Noodle Homestyle as prep	8 oz	80
Beef Noodle as prep	8 oz	70
Beefy Mushroom as prep	8 oz	60
Broccoli Cream Of as prep	8 oz	80
Broccoli Cream Of as prep w/ 2% milk	8 oz	140
Celery Cream Of as prep	8 oz	100
Cheddar Cheese as prep	8 oz	110
Chicken Alphabet as prep	8 oz	80
Chicken Noodle-O's as prep	8 oz	70
Chicken Vegetable as prep	8 oz	70
Chicken & Stars as prep	8 oz	60
Chicken 'n Dumplings as prep	8 oz	80
Chicken Barley as prep	8 oz	70
Chicken Broth as prep	8 oz	30
Chicken Broth & Noodles as prep	8 oz	45

FOOD	PORTION	CALS.
Campbell (CONT.)		
Chicken Cream Of as prep	8 oz	110
Chicken Gumbo as prep	8 oz	60
Chicken Mushroom Creamy as prep	8 oz	120
Chicken Noodle Homestyle as prep	8 oz	70
Chicken Noodle as prep	8 oz	60
Chicken With Rice as prep	8 oz	60
Chili Beef as prep	8 oz	140
Chunky Chicken Nuggets w/ Vegetables & Noodles	10¾ oz	190
Clam Chowder Manhattan Style as prep	8 oz	70
Clam Chowder New England as prep	8 oz	80
Clam Chowder New England as prep w/ whole milk	8 oz	150
Consomme as prep	8 oz	25
Curly Noodle With Chicken as prep	8 oz	80
French Onion as prep	8 oz	60
Green Pea as prep	8 oz	160
Healthy Request Bean With Bacon as prep	8 oz	140
Healthy Request Chicken Noodle as prep	8 oz	60
Healthy Request Chicken With Rice as prep	8 oz	60
Healthy Request Cream Of Mushroom as prep	8 oz	60
Healthy Request Cream Of Chicken	8 oz	70
Healthy Request Hearty Chicken Vegetable	8 oz	120
Healthy Request Ready-To-Serve Chicken Broth	8 oz	10
Healthy Request Ready-To-Serve Hearty Minestrone	8 oz	90
Healthy Request Ready-To-Serve Hearty Chicken Noodle	8 oz	80
Healthy Request Ready-To-Serve Hearty Chicken Rice	8 oz	110
Healthy Request Ready-To-Serve Hearty Vegetable	8 oz	110
Healthy Request Ready-To-Serve Hearty Vegetable Beef	8 oz	120
Healthy Request Tomato as prep	8 oz	90
Healthy Request Tomato as prep w/ skim milk	8 oz	130
Healthy Request Vegetable as prep	8 oz	90
Healthy Request Vegetable Beef as prep	8 oz	70
Home Cookin' Bean & Ham	10¾ oz	210

FOOD	PORTION	CALS.
Campbell (CONT.)		
Home Cookin' Beef With Vegetables & Pasta	10¾ oz	140
Home Cookin' Chicken Minestone	10¾ oz	180
Home Cookin' Chicken Gumbo With Sausages	10¾ oz	140
Home Cookin' Chicken Rice	10¾ oz	150
Home Cookin' Chicken With Noodles	10¾ oz	140
Home Cookin' Country Vegetable	10¾ oz	120
Home Cookin' Garden Tomato	10¾ oz	150
Home Cookin' Hearty Lentil	10¾ oz	170
Home Cookin' Minestrone	10¾ oz	140
Home Cookin' Split Pea With Ham	10¾ oz	230
Home Cookin' Vegetable Beef	10¾ oz	140
Minestrone as prep	8 oz	80
Mushroom Cream Of as prep	8 oz	100
Mushroom Golden as prep	8 oz	70
Nacho Cheese as prep	8 oz	110
Nacho Cheese as prep w/ milk	8 oz	180
Noodles & Ground Beef as prep	8 oz	90
Onion Cream Of as prep	8 oz	100
Onion Cream Of as prep w/ whole milk & water	8 oz	140
Oyster Stew as prep	8 oz	70
Oyster Stew as prep w/ whole milk	8 oz	140
Pepper Pot as prep	8 oz	90
Potato Cream Of as prep	8 oz	80
Potato Cream Of as prep w/ whole milk & water	8 oz	120
Ready-To-Serve Chunky Chili Beef	11 oz	290
Ready-To-Serve Chunky Mediterranean Vegetable	9½ oz	170
Ready-To-Serve Chunky Beef	10¾ oz	200
Ready-To-Serve Chunky Beef Stroganoff	10¾ oz	320
Ready-To-Serve Chunky Chicken Corn Chowder	10¾ oz	340
Ready-To-Serve Chunky Chicken Noodle	10¾ oz	200
Ready-To-Serve Chunky Chicken Vegetable	9½ oz	170
Ready-To-Serve Chunky Chicken With Rice	9½ oz	140
Ready-To-Serve Chunky Creamy Chicken Mushroom	10½ oz	270
Ready-To-Serve Chunky Creole Style	10¾ oz	240

FOOD	PORTION	CALS.
Campbell (CONT.)		
Ready-To-Serve Chunky Ham 'n Butter Bean	10¾ oz	280
Ready-To-Serve Chunky Manhattan Style Clam Chowder	10¾ oz	160
Ready-To-Serve Chunky New England Clam Chowder	10¾ oz	290
Ready-To-Serve Chunky Old Fashioned Chicken	10¾ oz	180
Ready-To-Serve Chunky Old Fashioned Vegetable Beef	10¾ oz	190
Ready-To-Serve Chunky Old Fashioned Bean w/ Ham	11 oz	290
Ready-To-Serve Chunky Pepper Steak	10¾ oz	180
Ready-To-Serve Chunky Sirloin Burger	10¾ oz	220
Ready-To-Serve Chunky Split Pea w/ Ham	10¾ oz	230
Ready-To-Serve Chunky Steak & Potato	10¾ oz	200
Ready-To-Serve Chunky Turkey Vegetable	9⅜ oz	150
Ready-To-Serve Low Sodium Chicken Vegetable Beef	10¾ oz	180
Ready-To-Serve Low Sodium Chicken Broth	10½ oz	30
Ready-To-Serve Low Sodium Chicken With Noodles	10¾ oz	170
Ready-To-Serve Low Sodium Mushroom Cream Of	10½ oz	210
Ready-To-Serve Low Sodium Split Pea	10¾ oz	230
Scotch Broth as prep	8 oz	80
Shrimp Cream Of as prep	8 oz	90
Shrimp Cream Of as prep w/ whole milk	8 oz	160
Split Pea With Bacon as prep	8 oz	160
Teddy Bear as prep	8 oz	70
Tomato as prep	8 oz	90
Tomato as prep w/ 2% milk	8 oz	150
Tomato Bisque as prep	8 oz	120
Tomato Homestyle Cream Of as prep	8 oz	110
Tomato Homestyle Cream Of as prep w/ whole milk	8 oz	180
Tomato Rice Old Fashioned as prep	8 oz	110
Tomato Zesty as prep	8 oz	100
Turkey Vegetable as prep	8 oz	70
Turkey Noodle as prep	8 oz	70
Vegetable Homestyle as prep	8 oz	60
Vegetable as prep	8 oz	90

FOOD	PORTION	CALS.
Campbell (CONT.)		
Vegetable Beef as prep	8 oz	70
Vegetable Old Fashioned as prep	8 oz	60
Vegetarian Vegetable as prep	8 oz	80
Won Ton as prep	8 oz	40
College Inn		
Beef Broth	½ can (7 oz)	16
Chicken Broth	½ can (7 oz)	35
Chicken Broth Lower Salt	½ can (7 oz)	20
Gold's		
Borscht	8 oz	100
Borscht Lo-Cal	8 oz	20
Schav	8 oz	25
Gorton's		
New England Clam Chowder as prep w/ whole milk	¼ can	140
Goya		
Black Bean	7.5 oz	160
Hain		
Chicken Broth	8¾ fl oz	70
Chicken Broth No Salt Added	8¾ fl oz	60
Chicken Noodle	9½ fl oz	120
Chicken Noodle No Salt Added	9½ fl oz	120
Creamy Mushroom	9¼ fl oz	110
Italian Vegetable Pasta	9½ fl oz	160
Italian Vegetable Pasta Low Sodium	9½ fl oz	140
Minestrone	9½ fl oz	170
Minestrone No Salt Added	9½ fl oz	160
Mushroom Barley	9½ fl oz	100
New England Clam Chowder	9¼ fl oz	180
Split Pea	9½ fl oz	170
Split Pea No Salt Added	9½ fl oz	170
Turkey Rice	9½ fl oz	100
Turkey Rice No Salt Added	9½ fl oz	120
Vegetable Chicken	9½ fl oz	120
Vegetable Chicken No Salt Added	9½ fl oz	130
Vegetable Broth	9½ fl oz	45
Vegetable Broth Low Sodium	9½ fl oz	40
Vegetable Split Pea	9½ fl oz	170
Vegetable Split Pea No Salt Added	9½ fl oz	170
Vegetarian Lentil	9½ fl oz	160
Vegetarian Lentil No Salt Added	9½ fl oz	160
Vegetarian Vegetable	9½ fl oz	140
Vegetarian Vegetable No Salt Added	9½ fl oz	150

FOOD	PORTION	CALS.
Health Valley		
Beef Broth	7.5 oz	10
Beef Broth No Salt Added	7.5 oz	10
Black Bean	7.5 oz	150
Black Bean No Salt Added	7.5 oz	150
Chicken Broth	7.5 oz	35
Chicken Broth No Salt Added	7.5 oz	35
Chunky Chicken Vegetable	7.5 oz	125
Chunky Five Bean Vegetable	7.5 oz	110
Chunky Five Bean Vegetable No Salt Added	7.5 oz	110
Chunky Vegetable Chicken No Salt Added	7.5 oz	125
Green Split Pea	7.5 oz	180
Green Split Pea No Salt Added	7.5 oz	180
Lentil	7.5 oz	220
Lentil No Salt Added	7.5 oz	220
Manhattan Clam Chowder	7.5 oz	110
Manhattan Clam Chowder No Salt Added	7.5 oz	110
Minestrone	7.5 oz	130
Minestrone No Salt Added	7.5 oz	130
Mushroom Barley	7.5 oz	100
Mushroom Barley No Salt Added	7.5 oz	100
Potato Leek	7.5 oz	130
Potato Leek No Salt Added	7.5 oz	130
Tomato	7.5 oz	130
Tomato No Salt Added	7.5 oz	130
Vegetable	7.5 oz	110
Vegetable No Salt Added	7.5 oz	110
Healthy Choice		
Bean & Ham	1 cup (8.7 oz)	184
Beef & Potato	1 cup (8.5 oz)	119
Chicken Corn Chowder	1 cup (8.8 oz)	176
Chicken Pasta	1 cup (8.6 oz)	118
Chicken With Rice	1 cup (8.4 oz)	108
Chili Beef	1 cup (9.1 oz)	166
Clam Chowder	1 cup (8.8 oz)	123
Country Vegetable	1 cup (8.6 oz)	104
Cream Of Mushroom	1 cup (8.8 oz)	77
Cream Of Chicken With Mushrooms	1 cup (8.9 oz)	127
Cream Of Chicken With Vegetables	1 cup (8.9 oz)	127
Garden Vegetable	1 cup (8.6 oz)	118
Hearty Chicken	1 cup (8.7 oz)	132
Lentil	1 cup (8.7 oz)	146
Minestrone	1 cup (8.6 oz)	112
Old Fashion Chicken Noodle	1 cup (8.8 oz)	137

FOOD	PORTION	CALS.
Healthy Choice (CONT.)		
Split Pea & Ham	1 cup (8.8 oz)	155
Tomato Garden	1 cup (8.6 oz)	106
Turkey With Wild Rice	1 cup (8.4 oz)	92
Vegetable Beef	1 cup (8.8 oz)	130
Hormel		
Bean & Ham	1 cup (7.5 oz)	190
Beef Vegetable	1 cup (7.5 oz)	90
Broccoli Cheese With Ham	1 cup (7.5 oz)	170
Chicken & Rice	1 cup (7.5 oz)	110
Chicken Noodle	1 cup (7.5 oz)	110
New England Clam Chowder	1 cup (7.5 oz)	130
Potato Cheese With Ham	1 cup (7.5 oz)	190
Manischewitz		
Borscht Low Calorie	8 fl oz	20
Borscht With Beets	8 fl oz	80
Schav	1 cup	11
Old El Paso		
Black Bean With Bacon	1 cup (8.6 oz)	160
Chicken Vegetable	1 cup (8.4 oz)	110
Chicken With Rice	1 cup (8.4 oz)	90
Garden Vegetable	1 cup (8.4 oz)	110
Hearty Beef	1 cup (8.4 oz)	120
Hearty Chicken Noodle	1 cup (8.4 oz)	110
Pritikin		
Chicken & Rice	1 cup (8.8 oz)	80
Chicken Broth	1 cup (8.5 oz)	15
Chicken Pasta	1 cup (8.6 oz)	100
Hearty Vegetable	1 cup (8.8 oz)	90
Lentil	1 cup (8.4 oz)	130
Minestrone	1 cup (8.8 oz)	90
Split Pea	1 cup (9.2 oz)	140
Three Bean Chili	½ cup (4.5 oz)	90
Vegetable Broth	1 cup (8.3 oz)	20
Vegetarian Vegetables	1 cup (9 oz)	100
Progresso		
Bean And Ham	1 cup (8.4 oz)	160
Beef	1 can (10.5 fl oz)	180
Beef Barley	1 cup (8.5 oz)	130
Beef Minestrone	1 cup (8.5 oz)	140
Beef Noodle	1 cup (8.5 oz)	140
Beef Vegetable & Rotini	1 cup (8 oz)	120
Broccoli & Shells	1 cup (8.5 oz)	70
Chickarina	1 cup (8.3 oz)	120

FOOD	PORTION	CALS.
Progresso (CONT.)		
Chicken Minestrone	1 cup (8.4 oz)	120
Chicken Vegetables & Penne	1 cup (8.4 oz)	100
Chicken & Wild Rice	1 cup (8.4 oz)	100
Chicken Barley	1 cup (8.5 oz)	110
Chicken Broth	1 cup ((8.2 oz)	20
Chicken Noodle	1 cup (8.4 oz)	80
Chicken Noodle	1 can (10.5 oz)	110
Chicken Rice Vegetable	1 can (10.5 oz)	130
Chicken Rice Vegetable	1 cup (8.4 oz)	110
Clam & Rotini Chowder	1 cup (8.8 oz)	200
Corn Chowder	1 cup (8.6 oz)	180
Cream Of Chicken	1 cup (8.4 oz)	170
Cream Of Mushroom	1 cup (8.4 oz)	140
Creamy Tortellini	1 cup (8.4 oz)	210
Escarole In Chicken Broth	1 cup (8.1 oz)	25
Green Split Pea	1 cup (8.6 oz)	170
Healthy Classics Beef Barley	1 cup (8.5 oz)	140
Healthy Classics Beef Vegetable	1 cup (8.5 oz)	150
Healthy Classics Chicken Noodle	1 cup (8.3 oz)	80
Healthy Classics Chicken Rice With Vegetables	1 cup (8.4 oz)	90
Healthy Classics Cream Of Broccoli	1 cup (8.6 oz)	90
Healthy Classics Garlic & Pasta	1 cup (8.5 oz)	100
Healthy Classics Lentil	1 cup (8.5 oz)	120
Healthy Classics Minestrone	1 cup (8.5 oz)	120
Healthy Classics New England Clam Chowder	1 cup (8.6 oz)	120
Healthy Classics Split Pea	1 cup (8.9 oz)	180
Healthy Classics Tomato Garden Vegetable	1 cup (8.6 oz)	100
Healthy Classics Vegetable	1 cup (8.4 oz)	80
Hearty Black Bean	1 cup (8.5 oz)	170
Hearty Chicken	1 can (10.5 fl oz)	120
Hearty Chicken & Rotini	1 cup (8.4 oz)	90
Hearty Penne In Chicken Broth	1 cup (8.4 oz)	70
Hearty Tomato & Rotini	1 cup (8.4 oz)	90
Hearty Vegetable With Rotini	1 cup (8.4 oz)	110
Homestyle Chicken Vegetable	1 cup (8.4 oz)	100
Lentil	1 can (10.5 fl oz)	170
Lentil	1 cup (8.5 oz)	140
Lentil & Shells	1 cup (8.5 oz)	130
Lentil With Sausage	1 cup (8.5 oz)	170
Macaroni & Bean	1 cup (8.6 oz)	160
Manhattan Clam Chowder	1 cup (8.4 oz)	110

FOOD	PORTION	CALS.
Progresso (CONT.)		
Meatballs & Pasta Pearls	1 cup (8.3 oz)	140
Minestrone	1 can (10.5 fl oz)	170
Minestrone	1 cup (8.4 oz)	130
New England Clam Chowder	1 can (10.5 oz)	220
New England Clam Chowder	1 cup (8.4 oz)	180
Spicy Chicken & Penne	1 cup (8.5 oz)	120
Split Pea With Ham	1 cup (8.5 oz)	160
Tomato	1 cup (8.5 oz)	90
Tomato Tortellini	1 cup (8.4 oz)	120
Tomato Beef & Rotini	1 cup (8.5 oz)	140
Tortellini In Chicken Broth	1 cup (8.3 oz)	80
Vegetable	1 cup (8.4 oz)	90
Zesty Minestrone	1 cup (8.3 oz)	150
Snow's		
Manhattan Clam Chowder as prep w/ water	7.5 fl oz	70
New England Clam Chowder as prep w/ milk	7.5 fl oz	140
New England Corn Chowder as prep w/ milk	7.5 fl oz	150
New England Fish Chowder as prep w/ milk	7.5 fl oz	130
New England Seafood Chowder as prep w/ milk	7.5 fl oz	130
Swanson		
Beef Broth	7¼ oz	18
Chicken Broth	7¼ oz	30
Natural Goodness Clear Chicken Broth	7¼ oz	20
Vegetable Broth	7.25 fl oz	20
Weight Watchers		
Chicken & Rice	1 can (10.5 oz)	110
Chicken Noodle	1 can (10.5 oz)	150
Minestrone	1 can (10.5 oz)	130
Vegetable	1 can (10.5 oz)	130
DRY		
asparagus cream of as prep w/ water	1 cup	59
beef broth	1 pkg (0.2 oz)	14
beef broth as prep w/ water	1 cup	19
beef broth cube	1 cube (3.6 g)	6
beef broth cube as prep w/water	1 cup	8
celery cream of as prep w/ water	1 cup	63
chicken broth	1 pkg (0.2 oz)	16
chicken broth as prep w/water	1 cup	21

FOOD	PORTION	CALS.
chicken broth cube	1 cube (4.8 g)	9
chicken broth cube, as prep w/ water	1 cup	13
chicken cream of as prep w/ water	1 cup	107
chicken noodle as prep w/ water	1 cup	53
french onion not prep	1 pkg (1.4 oz)	115
leek as prep w/ water	1 cup	71
onion as prep w/ water	1 cup	28
tomato as prep w/ water	1 cup	102
4C		
Noodle	8 oz	50
Onion Reduced Salt	8 oz	30
Armour		
Bouillon Cubes Beef	1 (4 g)	5
Bouillon Cubes Chicken	1 (4 g)	5
Arrowhead		
Bean & Barley	¼ cup (1.9 oz)	170
Bean Cuisine		
Bean Bouillabisse	1 cup (7.5 fl oz)	174
Island Black Bean	1 cup (8.6 fl oz)	202
Lots of Lentil	1 cup (7.7 oz)	166
Mesa Maize	1 cup (9.2 fl oz)	179
Rocky Mountain Red Bean	1 cup (8.6 oz)	202
Sante Fe Corn Chowder	1 cup (9.2 oz)	179
Thick As Fog Split Pea	1 cup (8.6 oz)	189
Ultima Pasta E Fagioli	1 cup (8.6 fl oz)	179
White Bean Provencal	1 cup (7.7 fl oz)	166
Campbell		
Bean With Bacon 'n Ham Microwave	7½ oz	230
Chicken Noodle Microwave	7½ oz	100
Chicken Noodle as prep	8 oz	100
Chicken With Rice Microwave	7½ oz	100
Chili Beef Microwave	7½ oz	190
Hearty Noodle as prep	8 oz	90
Noodle as prep	8 oz	110
Onion as prep	8 oz	30
Vegetable as prep	8 oz	40
Vegetable Beef Microwave	7½ oz	100
Campbell's Cup		
Beef Noodle	1 (1.35 oz)	130
Chicken Noodle	1 (1.35 oz)	140
Chicken Noodle w/ White Meat as prep	6 oz	90
Creamy Chicken w/ White Meat as prep	6 oz	90
Hearty Noodles With Vegetables	1 (1.7 oz)	180
Noodle With Chicken Broth as prep	6 oz	90

FOOD	PORTION	CALS.
Casbah		
Black Bean	1 pkg (1.7 oz)	170
Split Pea	1 pkg (2.3 oz)	230
Sweet Corn Chowder	1 pkg (1.2 oz)	125
Vegetarian Chili	1 pkg (1.8 oz)	170
Cup-A-Ramen		
Beef With Vegetables Low Fat as prep	8 oz	220
Beef With Vegetables as prep	8 oz	270
Chicken With Vegetables Low Fat as prep	8 oz	220
Chicken With Vegetables as prep	8 oz	270
Oriental With Vegetables Low Fat as prep	8 oz	220
Oriental With Vegetables as prep	8 oz	270
Shrimp With Vegetables Low Fat as prep	8 oz	230
Shrimp With Vegetables as prep	8 oz	280
Cup-A-Soup		
Chicken Vegetable as prep	1 pkg	90
Chicken Vegetable as prep	1 pkg	50
Chicken Broth as prep	1 pkg	20
Chicken Noodle as prep	1 pkg	50
Cream Of Chicken as prep	1 pkg	70
Cream Of Mushroom as prep	1 pkg	60
Creamy Broccoli & Cheese as prep	1 pkg	70
Green Pea as prep	1 pkg	110
Hearty Chicken Noodle as prep	1 pkg	60
Hearty Chicken Supreme as prep	1 pkg	90
Hearty Harvest Vegetable as prep	1 pkg	90
Ring Noodle as prep	1 pkg	50
Spring Vegetable as prep	1 pkg	50
Tomato as prep	1 pkg	90
Virginia Pea as prep	1 pkg	130
Emes		
Beef Base	1 tsp	18
Chicken Base	1 tsp	18
Fantastic		
Cha-Cha Chili Low Fat	1 pkg	220
George Washington		
Broth & Brown Seasoning	1 serv	6
Broth & Golden Seasoning	1 serv	6
Broth & Onion Seasoning	1 serv	12
Golden Dipt		
Lobster Bisque	¼ pkg	30
Manhattan Clam Chowder	¼ pkg	80
New England Clam Chowder	¼ pkg	24
Seafood Chowder	¼ pkg	70

FOOD	PORTION	CALS.
Golden Dipt (CONT.)		
Shrimp Bisque	¼ pkg	30
Goodman's		
Cup Of Soup Beef	1 pkg (1½ cups)	180
Cup Of Soup Chicken Noodle	1 pkg (1½ cups)	180
Cup Of Soup Vegetable	1 pkg (1½ cups)	180
Matzo Ball & Soup	1 cup	40
Matzo Ball & Soup 50% Less Salt	1 serv	50
Noodleman	1 cup	45
Noodleman Low Sodium	1 cup	50
Onion	1 cup	30
Onion Low Sodium	1 cup	30
Hain		
Cheese & Broccoli	¾ cup	310
Cheese Savory	¾ cup	250
Savory Lentil	¾ cup	130
Savory Minestrone	¾ cup	110
Savory Mushroom	¾ cup	210
Savory Mushroom No Salt Added	¾ cup	250
Savory Onion	¾ cup	50
Savory Onion No Salt Added	¾ cup	50
Savory Potato Leek	¾ cup	260
Savory Split Pea	¾ cup	310
Savory Tomato	¾ cup	220
Savory Vegetable	¾ cup	80
Savory Vegetable No Salt Added	¾ cup	80
Herb-Ox		
Beef Bouillon	1 cube (3.5 g)	10
Beef Instant Bouillon Powder	1 tsp (4 g)	10
Beef Instant Broth & Seasoning Pack	1 pkg (4.5 g)	10
Beef Instant Broth & Seasoning Pack Low Sodium	1 pkg (4 g)	15
Chicken Bouillon	1 cube (4 g)	10
Chicken Instant Bouillon Powder	1 tsp (4 g)	10
Chicken Instant Broth & Seasoning Pack	1 pkg (5 g)	10
Chicken Instant Broth & Seasoning Pack Low Sodium	1 pkg (4 g)	15
Vegetable Bouillon	1 cube (4 g)	10
Hodgson Mill		
13 Bean not prep	1.5 oz	100
Hurst		
15 Bean Soup Beef	1 serv (1.7 oz)	160
15 Bean Soup Cajun	1 serv (1.7 oz)	160
15 Bean Soup Chicken	1 serv (1.7 oz)	160

FOOD	PORTION	CALS.
Hurst (CONT.)		
15 Bean Soup Chili	1 serv (1.7 oz)	160
15 Bean Soup Ham	1 serv (1.7 oz)	160
Spanish-American Black Bean	1 serv (1.3 oz)	120
Ka-Me		
Won Ton Chicken not prep	1 pkg (1.25 oz)	180
Won Ton Pork not prep	1 pkg (1.25 oz)	180
Knorr		
Black Bean Cup-A-Soup as prep	1 pkg	200
Broccoli as prep	8 fl oz	160
Cauliflower as prep	8 fl oz	100
Chef's Series Wild Mushroom as prep	8 fl oz	100
Chick 'N Pasta as prep	8 fl oz	90
Chicken Bouillon as prep	8 fl oz	16
Chicken Flavored Noodle as prep	8 fl oz	100
Chicken Noodle Instant as prep	6 fl oz	25
Fine Herb as prep	8 fl oz	130
Fish Bouillon as prep	8 fl oz	10
French Onion as prep	8 fl oz	50
Hearty Minestrone Cup-A-Soup as prep	1 pkg	150
Lentil Cup-A-Soup as prep	1 pkg	220
Mushroom as prep	8 fl oz	100
Navy Bean Cup-A-Soup as prep	1 pkg	140
Oriental Hot And Sour as prep	8 fl oz	50
Oxtail Hearty Beef as prep	8 fl oz	70
Potato Leek Cup-A-Soup as prep	1 pkg	120
Spinach as prep	8 fl oz	100
Spring Vegetable With Herbs as prep	8 fl oz	30
Tomato Basil as prep	8 fl oz	90
Tortellini In Brodo as prep	8 fl oz	60
Vegetable Cup-A-Soup as prep	1 pkg	100
Vegetable as prep	8 fl oz	35
Vegetarian Vegetable Bouillon as prep	8 fl oz	16
Kojel		
Hearty Potato With Vegetables Instant	1 serv (6 fl oz)	60
Noodle Soup Chicken Flavor Instant	1 serv (6 fl oz)	70
Split Pea Instant	1 serv (6 fl oz)	60
Tomato Instant	1 serv (6 fl oz)	50
Vegetable Chicken Couscous Instant	1 serv (6 fl oz)	80
Lipton		
Recipe Secrets Beefy Mushroom	2 tbsp	35
Recipe Secrets Beefy Onion	1 tbsp	25
Recipe Secrets Golden Herb With Lemon	2 tbsp	35
Recipe Secrets Golden Onion	2 tbsp	60

FOOD	PORTION	CALS.
Lipton (CONT.)		
Recipe Secrets Italian Herb With Tomato	2 tbsp	40
Recipe Secrets Onion	1 tbsp	20
Recipe Secrets Onion Mushroom	2 tbsp	35
Recipe Secrets Savory Herb With Garlic	1 tbsp	35
Recipe Secrets Vegetable	2 tbsp	30
Soup Secrets Chicken Noodle	1 serv	80
Soup Secrets Extra Noodle	1 serv	90
Soup Secrets Giggle Noodle	1 serv	80
Soup Secrets Hearty Chicken Noodle	1 serv	80
Soup Secrets Hearty Noodle With Vegetables	1 serv	70
Soup Secrets Noodle With Chicken Broth	1 serv	60
Soup Secrets Ring-O-Noodle	1 serv	70
Soup Secrets Ruffle Pasta	1 serv	60
Lite Line		
Beef Bouillon Instant Low Sodium	1 tsp	12
Chicken Bouillon Instant Low Sodium	1 tsp	12
Manischewitz		
Minestrone as prep	6 fl oz	50
Split Pea as prep	6 fl oz	45
Vegetable as prep	6 fl oz	50
Maruchan		
Instant Lunch Oriental Noodles Beef	1 pkg (2.25 oz)	290
Instant Lunch Oriental Noodles Chicken	1 pkg (2.25 oz)	290
Instant Lunch Oriental Noodles Chicken Mushroom	1 pkg (2.25 oz)	280
Instant Lunch Oriental Noodles Mushroom	1 pkg (2.25 oz)	290
Instant Lunch Oriental Noodles Pork	1 pkg (2.25 oz)	290
Instant Lunch Oriental Noodles Shrimp	1 pkg (2.25 oz)	290
Instant Lunch Oriental Noodles Toast Onion	1 pkg (2.25 oz)	270
Instant Lunch Oriental Noodles Vegetable Beef	1 pkg (2.25 oz)	290
Instant Wonton Chicken	1 pkg (1.49 oz)	200
Instant Wonton Hot & Sour	1 pkg (1.49 oz)	200
Instant Wonton Oriental	1 pkg (1.49 oz)	190
Instant Wonton Pork	1 pkg (1.49 oz)	200
Instant Wonton Shrimp	1 pkg (1.49 oz)	200
Oriental Noodle Picante Style Beef	1 pkg (2.25 oz)	290
Oriental Noodle Picante Style Chicken	1 pkg (2.25 oz)	290
Oriental Noodle Picante Style Shrimp	1 pkg (2.25 oz)	300
Ramen Beef	½ pkg (1.5 oz)	190
Ramen Chicken	½ pkg (1.5 oz)	190

FOOD	PORTION	CALS.
Maruchan (CONT.)		
Ramen Chicken Mushroom	½ pkg (1.5 oz)	190
Ramen Chili	½ pkg (1.5 oz)	190
Ramen Mushroom	½ pkg (1.5 oz)	190
Ramen Oriental	½ pkg (1.5 oz)	190
Ramen Pork	½ pkg (1.5 oz)	190
Ramen Shrimp	½ pkg (1.5 oz)	190
Wonton Beef	⅓ pkg (0.68 oz)	90
Wonton Chicken	⅓ pkg (0.67 oz)	90
Wonton Pork	⅓ pkg (0.68 oz)	90
Wonton Vegetable	⅓ pkg (0.7 oz)	90
Nile Spice		
Couscous Almondine	1 pkg	200
Couscous Garbanzo	1 pkg	220
Couscous Lentil Curry	1 pkg	200
Couscous Minestrone	1 pkg	180
Couscous Parmesan	1 pkg	200
Homestyle Black Bean	1 pkg	190
Homestyle Chicken Flavored Vegetable	1 pkg	120
Homestyle Lentil	1 pkg	180
Homestyle Minestrone	1 pkg	160
Homestyle Red Beans & Rice	1 pkg	190
Homestyle Split Pea	1 pkg	200
Homestyle Sweet Corn Chowder	1 pkg	120
Italian Tomato	1 pkg	140
Potato Leek	1 pkg	150
Potato Romano	1 pkg	140
Ramen Noodle		
Beef Low Fat as prep	8 oz	160
Beef as prep	8 oz	190
Chicken Low Fat as prep	8 oz	160
Chicken as prep	8 oz	190
Oriental Low Fat as prep	8 oz	150
Oriental as prep	8 oz	190
Pork Low Fat as prep	8 oz	150
Pork as prep	8 oz	200
Ultra Slim-Fast		
Beef Noodle	6 oz	45
Chicken Leek	6 oz	50
Chicken Noodle	6 oz	45
Creamy Broccoli	6 oz	75
Creamy Tomato	6 oz	60
Hearty Vegetable	6 oz	50
Onion	6 oz	45

FOOD	PORTION	CALS.
Ultra Slim-Fast (CONT.)		
Potato Leek	6 oz	80
Weight Watchers		
Instant Beef Broth	1 pkg (0.16 oz)	10
Instant Chicken Broth	1 pkg (0.16 oz)	10
Wyler's		
Beef Bouillon Instant	1 tsp	6
Beef Bouillon Instant Cube	1	6
Chicken Bouillon Instant	1 tsp	8
Chicken Bouillon Instant Cube	1	8
Onion Bouillon Instant	1 tsp	10
Vegetable Bouillon Instant	1 tsp	6
FROZEN		
Jaclyn's		
Barley & Mushroom	7.5 fl oz	90
Split Pea	7.5 fl oz	180
Vegetable	7.5 fl oz	90
Tabatchnick		
Barley Mushroom	1 serv (7.5 oz)	70
Barley Mushroom No Salt Added	1 serv (7.5 oz)	70
Broccoli Cream Of	1 serv (7.5 oz)	90
Cabbage	1 serv (7.5 oz)	60
Chicken With Dumplings	1 serv (7.5 oz)	70
Corn Chowder	1 serv (7.5 oz)	150
Minestrone	1 serv (7.5 oz)	150
New England Potato	1 serv (7.5 oz)	150
New York Chicken	1 serv (7.5 oz)	35
Old Fashion Potato	1 serv (7.5 oz)	70
Pea	1 serv (7.5 oz)	180
Pea No Salt Added	1 serv (7.5 oz)	180
Spinach Cream Of	1 serv (7.5 oz)	90
Vegetable	1 serv (7.5 oz)	110
Vegetable No Salt Added	1 serv (7.5 oz)	110
Wisconsin Cheddar Vegetable	1 serv (7.5 oz)	140
Yankee Bean	1 serv (7.5 oz)	160
SHELF-STABLE		
Lunch Bucket		
Chicken Noodle	1 pkg (7.25 oz)	90
Country Vegetable	1 pkg (7.25 oz)	70
TAKE-OUT		
beef stew soup	1 cup (8.8 oz)	221
black bean turtle soup	1 cup	241
brunswick stew soup	1 cup (8.5 oz)	232
corn & cheese chowder	¾ cup	215

FOOD	PORTION	CALS.
gazpacho	1 cup	46
greek	¾ cup	63
hot & sour	1 serv (14 oz)	173
oxtail	5 oz	64
pasta e fagioli	1 cup (8.8 oz)	194
ratatouille	1 cup (7.5 oz)	266

SOUR CREAM
(see also SOUR CREAM SUBSTITUTES)

FOOD	PORTION	CALS.
sour cream	1 cup	493
sour cream	1 tbsp	26
Breakstone		
Free	2 tbsp (1.1 oz)	35
Half & Half	2 tbsp (1.1 oz)	45
Sour Cream	2 tbsp (1 oz)	60
Cabot		
Light	1 oz	33
Sour Cream	1 oz	60
Friendship		
Light	2 tbsp (1 oz)	35
Sour Cream	2 tbsp (1 oz)	60
Heluva Good Cheese		
Fat-Free	2 tbsp (1.1 oz)	20
Light	2 tbsp (1.1 oz)	40
Sour Cream	2 tbsp (1.1 oz)	60
Hood		
Fat Free	2 tbsp (1 oz)	20
Light	2 tbsp (1 oz)	40
Sour Cream	2 tbsp (1 oz)	60
Knudsen		
Free	2 tbsp (1.1 oz)	35
Hampshire	2 tbsp (1 oz)	60
Light	2 tbsp (1.1 oz)	40
Naturally Yours		
No Fat	2 tbsp (1 fl oz)	15
Sealtest		
Free	2 tbsp (1.1 oz)	35
Light	2 tbsp (1.1 oz)	40
Sour Cream	2 tbsp (1 oz)	60

SOUR CREAM SUBSTITUTES

FOOD	PORTION	CALS.
nondairy	1 cup	479
nondairy	1 oz	59
Pet		
Imitation	1 tbsp	25

FOOD	PORTION	CALS.
Tofutti		
Better Than Sour Cream Sour Supreme	1 oz	50
SOURSOP		
fresh	1	416
fresh cut up	1 cup	150
SOY		
(*see also* ICE CREAM AND FROZEN DESSERTS, MILK SUBSTITUTES, MISO, SOY SAUCE, SOYBEANS, TEMPH AND TOFU)		
lecithin	1 tbsp	104
soy milk	1 cup	79
soya cheese	1.4 oz	128
LaLoma		
Soyagen All Purpose	¼ cup	130
Soyagen Carob	¼ cup	140
Soyagen No Sucrose	¼ cup	130
Worthington		
Soyamel	1 oz	130
SOY SAUCE		
shoyu	1 tbsp	9
soy sauce	1 tbsp	7
tamari	1 tbsp	11
Eden		
Shoyu Organic	1 tbsp (0.5 oz)	15
Shoyu Traditional	1 tbsp (0.5 oz)	15
Tamari Organic Domestic	1 tbsp (0.5 oz)	15
Tamari Organic Imported	1 tbsp (0.5 oz)	15
House Of Tsang		
Dark	1 tbsp (0.6 oz)	10
Ginger Flavored Low Sodium	1 tbsp (0.6 oz)	10
Ginger Flavored	1 tbsp (0.6 oz)	20
Light	1 tbsp (0.6 oz)	5
Low Sodium	1 tbsp (0.6 oz)	5
Mushroom Flavored Low Sodium	1 tbsp (0.6 oz)	10
Ka-Me		
Chinese Dark	1 tbsp (0.5 fl oz)	10
Chinese Light	1 tbsp (0.5 fl oz)	5
Dark	1 tbsp (0.5 fl oz)	10
Japanese	1 tbsp (0.5 fl oz)	5
Light	1 tbsp (0.5 oz)	5
Mild	1 tbsp (0.5 fl oz)	5
Kikkoman		
Lite	1 tbsp	13

FOOD	PORTION	CALS.
Kikkoman (CONT.)		
Soy Sauce	1 tbsp	12
La Choy		
Lite	½ tsp	1
Soy Sauce	½ tsp	2
Trappey		
Chef Magic	1 tbsp (0.5 oz)	23
Tree Of Life		
Shoyu	1 tbsp (0.5 oz)	15
Tamari Reduced Sodium	1 tbsp (0.5 oz)	20
Tamari Wheat Free	1 tbsp (0.5 oz)	15

SOYBEANS

(see also MILK SUBSTITUTES, MISO, SOY, SOY SAUCE, TEMPH, AND TOFU)

dried cooked	1 cup	298
dry-roasted	½ cup	387
green cooked	½ cup	127
roasted	½ cup	405
roasted & toasted	1 oz	129
roasted & toasted	1 cup	490
roasted & toasted salted	1 cup	490
roasted & toasted salted	1 oz	129
sprouts raw	½ cup	43
sprouts steamed	½ cup	38
sprouts stir fried	1 cup	125

SPAGHETTI

(see PASTA, PASTA DINNERS, PASTA SALAD, SPAGHETTI SAUCE)

SPAGHETTI SAUCE

(see also PIZZA, TOMATO)

JARRED		
marinara sauce	1 cup	171
spaghetti sauce	1 cup	272
Classico		
Beef & Pork	4 fl oz	80
Four Cheese	4 fl oz	70
Spicy Red Pepper	4 fl oz	50
Sweet Peppers & Onions	4 fl oz	50
Tomato & Basil	4 fl oz	60
Contadina		
Italian	¼ cup	15
Sauce	¼ cup	20
Thick & Zesty	¼ cup	15
Del Monte		
Traditional	½ cup (4.4 oz)	80

FOOD	PORTION	CALS.
Del Monte (CONT.)		
Traditional No Sugar Added	½ cup (4.4 oz)	60
With Garlic & Onion	½ cup (4.4 oz)	70
With Green Peppers & Mushrooms	½ cup (4.4 oz)	70
With Meat	½ cup (4.4 oz)	40
With Mushrooms	½ cup (4.4 oz)	80
Eden		
Organic	½ cup (4.4 oz)	80
Organic No Salt Added	½ cup (4.4 oz)	80
Enrico's		
Fat Free Organic Basil	½ cup (4 oz)	50
Fat Free Organic Garlic	½ cup (4 oz)	50
Fat Free Organic Hot Pepper	½ cup (4 oz)	50
Fat Free Organic Mushroom	½ cup (4 oz)	60
Fat Free Organic Traditional	½ cup (4 oz)	45
Healthy Choice		
Extra Chunky Garlic & Onion	½ cup (4.4 oz)	43
Extra Chunky Italian Vegetable	½ cup (4.4 oz)	39
Extra Chunky Mushroom	½ cup (4.4 oz)	41
Garlic & Herbs	½ cup (4.4 oz)	47
Super Chunky Mushroom & Sweet Peppers	½ cup (4.4 oz)	44
Super Chunky Tomato, Mushroom & Garlic	½ cup (4.4 oz)	46
Super Chunky Vegetable Primavera	½ cup (4.4 oz)	46
Traditional	½ cup (4.4 oz)	47
With Meat	½ cup (4.4 oz)	47
With Mushrooms	½ cup (4.4 oz)	47
Hunt's		
Chunky	¼ cup (2.2 fl oz)	30
Classic Italian With Parmesan	½ cup (4.4 fl oz)	50
Homestyle Traditional No Sugar Added	½ cup (4.4 fl oz)	60
Traditional	4 oz	70
With Meat	4 oz	70
With Mushrooms	4 oz	70
Mama Rizzo's		
Mushroom Onion	½ cup (4.3 oz)	60
Pepper Mushroom Onion	½ cup (4.3 oz)	60
Pepper Primavera Vegetable	½ cup (4.2 oz)	50
Pepper Tomato Basil Garlic	½ cup (4.7 oz)	60
Primavera Vegetable	½ cup (4.2 oz)	50
Tomato Basil Garlic	½ cup (4.6 oz)	60
Muir Glen		
Organic Cabernet Marinara	½ cup (4.4 oz)	45

FOOD	PORTION	CALS.
Muir Glen (CONT.)		
Organic Chunky Style	½ cup (4.5 oz)	80
Organic Fat Free Tomato Basil	½ cup (4.3 oz)	50
Organic Garlic Onion	½ cup (4.3 oz)	50
Organic Garlic Roasted Garlic	½ cup (4.4 oz)	45
Organic Green Pepper & Mushroom	½ cup (4.5 oz)	70
Organic Italian Herb	½ cup (4.5 oz)	60
Organic Romano Cheese	½ cup (4.5 oz)	90
Organic Sun Dried Tomato	½ cup (4.4 oz)	40
Organic Sweet Pepper Onion	½ cup (4.4 oz)	40
Organic Tomato Basil	½ cup (4.3 oz)	50
Newman's Own		
Marinara	4 oz	70
Marinara With Mushrooms	4 oz	70
Sockarooni	4 oz	70
Prego		
Chunky Sausage & Green Peppers	4 oz	160
Extra Chunky Garden Combination	4 oz	80
Extra Chunky Mushroom & Tomato	4 oz	110
Extra Chunky Mushroom & Green Pepper	4 oz	100
Extra Chunky Mushroom & Onion	4 oz	100
Extra Chunky Mushroom With Extra Spice	4 oz	100
Extra Chunky Tomato & Onion	4 oz	110
Marinara	4 oz	100
Meat Flavored	4 oz	140
Mushroom	4 oz	130
Onion & Garlic	4 oz	110
Regular	4 oz	130
Three Cheese	4 oz	100
Tomato & Basil	4 oz	100
Pritikin		
Chunky Garden	½ cup (4 oz)	50
Marinara	½ cup (4 oz)	60
Original	½ cup (4 oz)	60
Progresso		
Marinara	½ cup (4.3 oz)	90
Meat Flavored	½ cup (4.4 oz)	100
Mushroom	½ cup (4.4 oz)	100
Sauce	½ cup (4.4 oz)	100
Ragu		
Fino Italian Garden Medley	½ cup (4.5 oz)	90
Fino Italian Garlic & Basil	½ cup (4.5 oz)	90
Fino Italian Sliced Mushroom	½ cup (4.5 oz)	90
Fino Italian Tomato & Herb	½ cup (4.5 oz)	90

FOOD	PORTION	CALS.
Ragu (CONT.)		
Fino Italian Zesty Tomato	½ cup (4.5 oz)	90
Gardenstyle Chunky Garden Combination	½ cup (4.5 oz)	120
Gardenstyle Chunky Green & Red Pepper	½ cup (4.5 oz)	120
Gardenstyle Chunky Mushroom & Green Pepper	½ cup (4.5 oz)	120
Gardenstyle Chunky Mushroom & Onion	½ cup (4.5 oz)	120
Gardenstyle Chunky Tomato Garlic & Onion	½ cup (4.5 oz)	120
Gardenstyle Super Mushroom	½ cup (4.5 oz)	120
Gardenstyle Super Vegetable Primavera	½ cup (4.5 oz)	110
Homestyle Mushroom	½ cup (4.5 oz)	120
Homestyle Tomato & Herb	½ cup (4.5 oz)	120
Homestyle With Meat	½ cup (4.5 oz)	130
Light Chunky Mushroom	½ cup (4.4 oz)	50
Light Garden Harvest	½ cup (4.4 oz)	50
Light No Sugar Added	½ cup (4.4 oz)	60
Light Tomato & Herb	½ cup (4.4 oz)	50
Old World Style Marinara	½ cup (4.4 oz)	90
Old World Style Mushrooms	½ cup (4.4 oz)	80
Old World Style Traditional	½ cup (4.4 oz)	80
Old World Style With Meat	½ cup (4.4 oz)	90
Sauce	4 fl oz	80
Thick & Hearty Mushroom	½ cup (4.5 oz)	120
Thick & Hearty Spaghetti Sauce	4 oz	100
Thick & Hearty Tomato & Herb	½ cup (4.5 oz)	120
Thick & Hearty With Meat	1.2 cup (4.5 oz)	130
Tree Of Life		
Pasta Sauce	½ cup (4 oz)	50
Pasta Sauce Calabrese	½ cup (3.9 oz)	60
Pasta Sauce Fat Free Classic	½ cup (3.9 oz)	40
Pasta Sauce Fat Free Mushroom & Basil	½ cup (3.9 oz)	30
Pasta Sauce Fat Free Onion & Garlic	½ cup (3.9 oz)	30
Pasta Sauce Fat Free Sweet Pepper	½ cup (3.9 oz)	30
Pasta Sauce No Salt	½ cup (3.9 oz)	50
Weight Watchers		
Pasta Sauce With Mushrooms	½ cup	60
MIX		
Durkee		
American Style as prep	½ cup	15
Family Style as prep	½ cup	20
Spaghetti Sauce as pre	½ cup	15
With Mushrooms as prep	½ cup	15
Zesty as prep	½ cup	20

FOOD	PORTION	CALS.
French's		
All American as prep	½ cup	20
Italian as prep	½ cup	16
Mushroom as prep	½ cup	20
Thick as prep	½ cup	10
Zesty Pasta as prep	½ cup	20
REFRIGERATED		
Contadina		
Alfredo	½ cup (4.2 fl oz)	400
Four Cheese Sauce With White Wine & Shallots	½ cup (4.2 fl oz)	320
Light Alfredo	½ cup (4.2 fl oz)	190
Light Chunky Tomato	½ cup (4.4 fl oz)	45
Light Garden Vegetable	½ cup (4.4 fl oz)	45
Marinara	½ cup (4.4 fl oz)	80
Pesto With Basil	¼ cup (2 oz)	310
Pesto With Sun Dried Tomatoes	¼ cup (2 oz)	250
Plum Tomato With Basil	½ cup (4.4 fl oz)	70
Spicy Italian Sausage & Bell Pepper	½ cup (4.4 fl oz)	100
Di Giorno		
Alfredo	¼ cup (2.2 oz)	230
Four Cheese	¼ cup (2.2 oz)	200
Light Chunky Tomato With Basil	½ cup (4.5 oz)	70
Light Reduced Fat Alfredo	¼ cup (2.4 oz)	170
Marinara	½ cup (4.5 oz)	100
Olive Oil & Garlic With Grated Cheese	¼ cup (2.1 oz)	370
Pesto	¼ cup (2.2 oz)	320
Plum Tomato & Mushroom	½ cup (4.4 oz)	70
Traditional Meat	½ cup (4.5 oz)	120
TAKE-OUT		
bolognese	5 oz	195

SPANISH FOOD

(see also BEANS, CHIPS, DINNER, PEPPERS, SALSA, SNACKS, SAUCE, TORTILLA)

FOOD	PORTION	CALS.
CANNED		
Chi-Chi's		
Picante Hot	2 tbsp (1 oz)	10
Picante Medium	2 tbsp (1 oz)	10
Picante Mild	2 tbsp (1 oz)	10
Pico De Gallo	2 tbsp (1.2 oz)	10
Derby		
Tamales	2	160
El Molino		
Enchilada Sauce Hot	2 tbsp	16

FOOD	PORTION	CALS.
El Molino (CONT.)		
Green Chili Sauce Mild	2 tbsp	10
Gebhardt		
Enchiladas	2	310
Tamales	2	290
Tamales Jumbo	2	400
Guiltless Gourmet		
Picante Mild	1 oz	6
Queso Mild Cheddar	1 oz	22
Hormel		
Tamales Beef	3 (7.5 oz)	280
Tamales Chicken	3 (7.5 oz)	210
Tamales Hot Spicy Beef	3 (7.5 oz)	280
Tamales Jumbo Beef	2 (6.9 oz)	270
Old El Paso		
Tamales	3 (7.2 oz)	330
Rosarita		
Enchilada Sauce Mild	2.5 oz	25
Picante Chunky Hot	3 tbsp (2 fl oz)	18
Picante Chunky Medium	3 tbsp (2 fl oz)	16
Picante Chunky Mild	3 tbsp (2 oz)	25
Van Camp's		
Tamales	2 (5.1 oz)	210
Wolf Brand		
Tamales	7.5 oz	328
FROZEN		
Amy's Organic		
Enchilada Cheese	1 (4.7 oz)	210
Banquet		
Beef Enchilada	1 pkg (11 oz)	320
Chimichanga Meal	1 pkg (9.5 oz)	470
Enchilada Cheese	1 pkg (11 oz)	350
Enchilada Chicken	1 pkg (11 oz)	360
Family Entree Beef Enchilada w/ Cheese	1 serv (4.67 oz)	130
El Charrito		
Enchiladas 4 Grande Beef	1 pkg (16.5 oz)	890
Healthy Choice		
Beef Burrito Ranchero Medium	1 (5.4 oz)	290
Beef Burrito Ranchero Mild	1 (5.4 oz)	300
Beef Enchilada Rio Grande	1 meal (13.4 oz)	410
Burrito Chicken Con Queso	1 (5.4 oz)	280
Chicken Enchilada Supreme	1 meal (13.4 oz)	390
Enchiladas Suiza Chicken	1 meal (10 oz)	270
Feista Chicken Fajitas	1 meal (7 oz)	260

FOOD	PORTION	CALS.
Jimmy Dean		
Burrito Breakfast Bacon	1 (4 oz)	260
Burrito Breakfast Sausage	1 (4 oz)	250
Le Menu		
Entree LightStyle Enchiladas Chicken	8 oz	280
Lean Cuisine		
Enchanadas Chicken	1 meal (9.9 oz)	220
Enchilada Suiza Chicken	1 meal (9 oz)	290
Life Choice		
Burrito Black Bean	1 meal (13.2 oz)	410
Vegetable Enchilada Sonora	1 meal (14 oz)	420
Lightlife		
Vegetarian Taco	2 oz	51
Old El Paso		
Burrito Bean & Cheese	1 (4.9 oz)	290
Burrito Beef & Bean Hot	1 (5 oz)	320
Burrito Beef & Bean Medium	1 (5 oz)	320
Burrito Beef & Bean Mild	1 (5 oz)	330
Chimichanga Beef	1 (4.5 oz)	370
Chimichanga Chicken	1 (4.5 oz)	350
Patio		
Burrito Bean & Cheese	1 (5 oz)	270
Burrito Chicken	1 (5 oz)	260
Burrito Red Chili	1 (5 oz)	270
Burritos Beef & Bean	1 (5 oz)	280
Burritos Beef & Bean Green Chili	1 (5 oz)	260
Burritos Beef & Bean Red Chili	1 (5 oz)	260
Enchilada Beef Dinner	1 meal (12 oz)	320
Enchilada Cheese Dinner	1 meal (12 oz)	330
Enchilada Chicken	1 pkg (12 oz)	380
Family Entree Beef Enchilada	2 (5.7 oz)	170
Family Entree Enchilada Beef	2 (5.3 oz)	250
Family Entree Enchilada Beef & Cheese	2 (5.3 oz)	250
Family Entree Enchilada Cheese	2 (5.7 oz)	170
Fiesta Dinner	1 meal (12 oz)	340
Mexican Dinner	1 meal (13.25 oz)	440
Salis Con Queso	1 pkg (11 oz)	390
Patio Britos		
Beef & Bean	10 (6 oz)	420
Nacho Beef	10 (6 oz)	410
Nacho Cheese	10 (6 oz)	360
Spicy Chicken	10 (6 oz)	400
Rudy's Farm		
Burrito Beef/Bean	1 (5 oz)	326

FOOD	PORTION	CALS.
Rudy's Farm (CONT.)		
Burrito Hot Beef/Bean	1 (5 oz)	305
Senor Felix's		
Burrito Black Bean	1 (10 oz)	540
Burrito Black Bean Soy	1 (5 oz)	240
Burrito Chicken	1 (10 oz)	520
Burrito Hot Potato	1 (10 oz)	560
Burrito Soy Hot	1 (10 oz)	520
Burritos Charbroiled Chicken	1 + 4 tsp sauce (6.7 oz)	320
Burritos Sonora Style	1 + 4 tsp sauce (6.7 oz)	280
Burritos Yucatan Style	1 + 4 tsp sauce (6.7 oz)	310
Empanadas Chicken	1 (4.7 oz)	340
Empanadas Corn & Rice	1 (4.7 oz)	280
Empanadas Pumpkin & Mushroom	1 (4.7 oz)	260
Empanadas Spinach & Ricotta	1 (4.7 oz)	260
Enchilada Red Pepper	1 (10 oz)	420
Enchilada Soy Verda	1 (10 oz)	430
Enchilada Supreme Soy Cheese	1 (10 oz)	460
Enchilada Verde	1 (5 oz)	423
Tamales Blue Corn & Soy Cheese	2 + 4 tsp sauce (5.7 oz)	240
Tamales Chicken	2 + 4 tsp sauce (5.7 oz)	240
Tamales Gourmet Vegetarian	2 + 4 tsp sauce	240
Taquitos Blue Corn Soy	3 + 4 tsp sauce (5.2 oz)	230
Taquitos Chicken	2 + 4 tsp sauce (5.7 oz)	240
Stouffer's		
Cheese Enchilada	1 pkg (9.75 oz)	370
Chicken Enchilada	1 pkg (10 oz)	370
Swanson		
Enchiladas Beef	13¾ oz	480
Mexican Style Combination	14¼ oz	490
Mexican Style Hungry Man	20¼ oz	820
Today's Tamales		
Cheese & Chili	1 pkg (7 oz)	390
Del Sol	1 pkg (6.5 oz)	310
Original Bean	1 pkg (7 oz)	330
Spicy Taco	1 pkg (7 oz)	310
Tyson		
Fajita Kit Beef	3.84 oz	160
Fajita Kit Chicken	4 oz	80
Weight Watchers		
Chicken Enchilada Suiza	1 pkg (9 oz)	250
Nacho Grande Chicken Enchiladas	1 pkg (9 oz)	290
MIX		
Gebhardt		
Menudo Mix	1 tsp	5

FOOD	PORTION	CALS.
Hain		
Taco Seasoning Mix	1/10 pkg	10
Old El Paso		
Burrito Seasoning Mix	2 tsp (6 g)	20
Dinner Kit Burrito as prep	1	280
Dinner Kit Soft Taco as prep	2	380
Dinner Kit Taco as prep	2	270
Enchilada Sauce Mix	2 tsp (4 g)	10
Taco Mix 40% Less Sodium	2 tsp (6 g)	20
Taco Seasoning Mix	2 tsp (6 g)	20
Ortega		
Taco Meat Seasoning Mix Mild	1 filled taco	90
Quaker		
Masa Harina De Maiz	2 tortillas	137
Masa Trigo	2 tortillas	149
READY-TO-USE		
taco shell baked	1 med (½ oz)	61
taco shell baked w/o salt	1 med (½ oz)	61
Casa Fiesta		
Taco Shells	3.5 oz	480
Chi-Chi's		
Taco Shells White Corned	2 (1 oz)	130
Gebhardt		
Taco Shells	1	50
Old El Paso		
Taco Shells Mini	7 (1.1 oz)	160
Taco Shells Regular	3 (1.1 oz)	170
Taco Shells Super	2 (1.3 oz)	190
Taco Shells White Corn	3 (1.1 oz)	170
Tostaco Shells	1 (0.8 oz)	130
Tostada Shells	3 (1.1 oz)	160
Rosarita		
Taco Shells	1 shell (11 g)	50
Tostada Shells	1 shell (14 g)	60
TAKE-OUT		
burrito w/ apple	1 lg (5.4 oz)	484
burrito w/ apple	1 sm (2.6 oz)	231
burrito w/ beans	2 (7.6 oz)	448
burrito w/ beans & cheese	2 (6.5 oz)	377
burrito w/ beans & chili peppers	2 (7.2 oz)	413
burrito w/ beans & meat	2 (8.1 oz)	508
burrito w/ beans cheese & beef	2 (7.1 oz)	331
burrito w/ beans cheese & chili peppers	2 (11.8 oz)	663
burrito w/ beef	2 (7.7 oz)	523

FOOD	PORTION	CALS.
burrito w/ beef & chili peppers	2 (7.1 oz)	426
burrito w/ beef cheese & chili peppers	2 (10.7 oz)	634
burrito w/ cherry	1 sm (2.6 oz)	231
burrito w/ cherry	1 lg (5.4 oz)	484
chimichanga w/ beef	1 (6.1 oz)	425
chimichanga w/ beef & cheese	1 (6.4 oz)	443
chimichanga w/ beef & red chili peppers	1 (6.7 oz)	424
chimichanga w/ beef cheese & red chili peppers	1 (6.3 oz)	364
enchilada w/ cheese	1 (5.7 oz)	320
enchilada w/ cheese & beef	1 (6.7 oz)	324
enchirito w/ cheese beef & beans	1 (6.8 oz)	344
frijoles w/ cheese	1 cup (5.9 oz)	226
nachos w/ cheese	6 to 8 (4 oz)	345
nachos w/ cheese & jalapeno peppers	6 to 8 (7.2 oz)	607
nachos w/ cheese beans ground beef & peppers	6 to 8 (8.9 oz)	568
nachos w/ cinnamon & sugar	6 to 8 (3.8 oz)	592
taco	1 sm (6 oz)	370
taco salad	1½ cups	279
taco salad w/ chili con carne	1½ cups	288
tostada w/ beans & cheese	1 (5.1 oz)	223
tostada w/ beans beef & cheese	1 (7.9 oz)	334
tostada w/ beef & cheese	1 (5.7 oz)	315
tostada w/ guacamole	2 (9.2 oz)	360

SPARE RIBS
(see PORK)

SPICES
(see individual names, HERBS/SPICES)

SPELT
Arrowhead
Spelt	1 oz	83

SPINACH
CANNED
spinach	½ cup	25

Del Monte
50% Less Salt	½ cup (4 oz)	30
Chopped	½ cup (4 oz)	30
No Salt Added	½ cup (4 oz)	30
Whole Leaf	½ cup (4 oz)	30

Popeye
Chopped	½ cup (4.1 oz)	40

FOOD	PORTION	CALS.
Popeye (CONT.)		
Leaf	½ cup (4.2 oz)	45
Low Sodium	½ cup (4.2 oz)	35
S&W		
Northwest Premium	½ cup	25
Sunshine		
Chopped	½ cup (4.1 oz)	40
FRESH		
cooked	½ cup	21
mustard chopped cooked	½ cup	14
mustard raw chopped	½ cup	17
new zealand chopped cooked	½ cup	11
new zealand raw	½ cup	4
raw chopped	½ cup	6
raw chopped	1 pkg (10 oz)	46
Dole		
Spinach	3 oz	9
Fresh Express		
Spinach	1½ cups (3 oz)	40
FROZEN		
cooked	½ cup	27
Birds Eye		
Chopped	½ cup	20
Creamed	½ cup	90
Leaf	½ cup	20
Budget Gourmet		
Au Gratin	1 pkg (5.5 oz)	160
Fresh Like		
Cut Leaf	3.5 oz	21
Green Giant		
Creamed	½ cup	70
Cut Leaf In Butter Sauce	½ cup	40
Harvest Fresh	½ cup	25
Spinach	½ cup	25
Stouffer's		
Creamed	½ cup (2.25 oz)	150
Souffle	½ cup (4 oz)	150
Tabatchnick		
Creamed	7.5 oz	60
TAKE-OUT		
spanakopita spinach pie	1 cup (6 oz)	196

SPINACH JUICE

juice	3½ oz	7

FOOD	PORTION	CALS.
SPORTS DRINKS		
(see also NUTRITIONAL SUPPLEMENTS)		
Gatorade		
Citrus Cooler	1 cup (8 oz)	50
Fruit Punch	1 cup (8 oz)	50
Grape	1 cup (8 oz)	50
Iced Tea Cooler	1 cup (8 oz)	50
Lemon-Lime	1 cup (8 oz)	50
Lemonade	1 cup (8 oz)	50
Orange	1 cup (8 fl oz)	50
Tropical Fruit	1 cup (8 oz)	50
PowerAde		
Fruit Punch	8 fl oz	72
Grape	8 fl oz	73
Lemon-Lime	8 fl oz	72
Orange	8 fl oz	72
Slice		
All Sport Diet Lemon Lime	8 fl oz	1
All Sport Lemon Lime	8 fl oz	72
All Sport Orange	8 fl oz	74
All Sport Punch	8 fl oz	81
Snapple		
Sport Fruit	1 bottle	80
Sport Lemon	1 bottle	80
Sport Lemon Lime	1 bottle	80
Sport Orange	1 bottle	80
SPOT		
baked	3 oz	134
SQUAB		
breast w/o skin raw	1 (3.5 oz)	135
w/ skin raw	1 squab (6.9 oz)	584
w/o skin raw	1 squab (5.9 oz)	239
SQUASH		
(see also ZUCCHINI)		
CANNED		
crookneck sliced	½ cup	14
Allen		
Yellow	½ cup (4.2 oz)	25
Sunshine		
Yellow	½ cup (4.2 oz)	25
FRESH		
acorn cooked mashed	½ cup	41

FOOD	PORTION	CALS.
acorn cubed baked	½ cup	57
butternut baked	½ cup	41
crookneck raw sliced	½ cup	12
crookneck sliced cooked	½ cup	18
hubbard baked	½ cup	51
hubbard cooked mashed	½ cup	35
scallop raw sliced	½ cup	12
scallop sliced cooked	½ cup	14
spaghetti cooked	½ cup	23
Nature's Pasta		
Spaghetti Squash	1 cup (5.5 oz)	20
FROZEN		
butternut cooked mashed	½ cup	47
crookneck sliced cooked	½ cup	24
Birds Eye		
Winter Cooked	½ cup	45
Southland		
Butternut	4 oz	45
Prepared Squash	3.6 oz	80
SEEDS		
dried	1 oz	154
dried	1 cup	747
roasted	1 oz	148
roasted	1 cup	1184
salted & roasted	1 cup	1184
salted & roasted	1 oz	148
whole roasted	1 oz	127
whole roasted	1 cup	285
whole salted roasted	1 oz	127
whole salted roasted	1 cup	285

SQUID

fried	3 oz	149
raw	3 oz	78

SQUIRREL

roasted	3 oz	147

STAR FRUIT

Sonoma		
Dried	7-9 pieces (1.4 oz)	140

STRAWBERRIES

CANNED		
in heavy syrup	½ cup	117

FOOD	PORTION	CALS.
FRESH		
strawberries	1 cup	45
strawberries	1 pint	97
Dole		
Strawberries	8	50
FROZEN		
sweetened sliced	1 cup	245
sweetened sliced	1 pkg (10 oz)	273
unsweetened	1 cup	52
whole sweetened	1 cup	200
whole sweetened	1 pkg (10 oz)	223
Big Valley		
Strawberries	⅔ cup (4.9 oz)	50
Birds Eye		
Halved In Delicious Syrup	½ cup	120
Halved In Lite Syrup	½ cup	90
Whole In Lite Syrup	½ cup	80

STRAWBERRY JUICE

FOOD	PORTION	CALS.
Juice Works		
Drink	6 oz	100
Kern's		
Nectar	6 fl oz	110
Kool-Aid		
Koolers	1 (8.45 oz)	136
Strawberry	8 oz	98
Libby		
Nectar	1 can (11.5 fl oz)	210
Smucker's		
Juice	8 oz	130
Tang		
Strawberry	8.45 fl oz	121

STUFFING/DRESSING

FOOD	PORTION	CALS.
HOME RECIPE		
bread as prep w/ water & fat	½ cup	251
bread as prep w/ water egg & fat	½ cup	107
MIX		
bread dry as prep	½ cup	178
cornbread as prep	½ cup	179
Arnold		
All Purpose Seasoned	½ oz	50
Corn	½ oz	50
Herb Seasoned	½ oz	50
Sage & Onion	½ oz	50

FOOD	PORTION	CALS.
Betty Crocker		
Chicken	½ cup	180
Traditional Herb	½ cup	180
Brownberry		
Corn	1 oz	103
Herb	1 oz	100
Sage & Onion	1 oz	97
Golden Grain		
Bread Stuffing Chicken	½ cup	180
Bread Stuffing Corn Bread	½ cup	180
Bread Stuffing Herb & Butter	½ cup	180
Bread Stuffing With Wild Rice	½ cup	180
Kellogg's		
Croutettes	1 cup (1.2 oz)	120
Pepperidge Farm		
Corn Bread	1 oz	110
Country Style	1 oz	100
Cube	1 oz	110
Distinctive Apple Raisin	1 oz	110
Distinctive Classic Chicken	1 oz	110
Distinctive Country Garden Herb	1 oz	120
Distinctive Vegetable & Almond	1 oz	110
Distinctive Wild Rice & Mushroom	1 oz	130
Herb Seasoned	1 oz	110
Stove Top		
Beef as prep	½ cup	178
Chicken as prep	½ cup	176
Chicken With Rice as prep	½ cup	182
Cornbread as prep	½ cup	175
Flex Serve Chicken as prep	½ cup	173
Flex Serve Cornbread as prep	½ cup	181
Flex Serve Homestyle Herb as prep	½ cup	173
Long Grain & Wild Rice as prep	½ cup	182
Select Wild Rice & Mushroom	½ cup	172
Wonder		
Seasoned Stuffing	1 cup (0.9 oz)	60
TAKE-OUT		
bread	½ cup (3½ oz)	195
sausage	½ cup	292
STURGEON		
cooked	3 oz	115
raw	3 oz	90
roe raw	3.5 oz	207

FOOD	PORTION	CALS.
smoked	3 oz	147
smoked	1 oz	48
SUCKER		
white baked	3 oz	101
SUGAR		
(*see also* FRUCTOSE, SUGAR SUBSTITUTES, SYRUP)		
brown packed	1 cup (7.7 oz)	828
brown unpacked	1 cup (5.1 oz)	546
maple	1 piece (1 oz)	100
powdered	1 tbsp (0.3 oz)	31
powdered unsifted	1 cup (4.2 oz)	467
white	1 cup (7 oz)	773
white	1 packet (6 g)	25
white	1 tbsp	45
white	1 tsp (4 g)	15
C&H		
White	1 tsp	16
Domino		
White	1 tsp	16
Hain		
Turbinado	1 tbsp	50
Hollywood		
Turbinado	1 tbsp	50
SUGAR SUBSTITUTES		
(*see also* FRUCTOSE)		
Equal		
Packet	1 pkg	4
NatraTaste		
Packet	1 pkg (1 g)	0
S&W		
Liquid Table Sweetener	⅛ tsp	0
Sprinkle Sweet		
Sugar Substitute	1 tsp	2
SugarTwin		
Brown	1 tsp (0.4 g)	2
Packet	1 pkg (0.8 g)	3
Sugar Substitute	1 tsp (0.4 g)	2
Sweet One		
Packet	1 pkg (1 g)	4
Sweet'N Low		
Granulated	1 pkg (1g)	4
*Sweet*10*		
Granular	⅛ tsp	0

FOOD	PORTION	CALS.
Weight Watchers		
Sweetener	1 measure (1 g)	5
SUGAR-APPLE		
fresh	1	146
fresh cut up	1 cup	236
SUNDAE TOPPINGS		
(*see* ICE CREAM TOPPINGS)		
SUNFISH		
pumpkinseed baked	3 oz	97
SUNFLOWER		
dried	1 oz	162
dried	1 cup	821
dry roasted	1 oz	165
dry roasted	1 cup	745
dry roasted salted	1 oz	165
dry roasted salted	1 cup	745
oil roasted	1 cup	830
oil roasted salted	1 cup	830
oil roasted salted	1 oz	175
sunflower butter	1 tbsp	93
sunflower butter w/o salt	1 tbsp	93
toasted	1 oz	176
toasted	1 cup	826
toasted salted	1 oz	176
toasted salted	1 cup	826
Erewhon		
Sunflower Seed Butter	2 tbsp (32 g)	200
Fisher		
Seeds Oil Roasted	1 oz	170
Seeds Salted In Shell shelled	1 oz	160
Seeds Salted In Shell unshelled	1 oz	170
Frito Lay		
Seeds	1 oz	160
Planters		
Kernels	1 pkg (2 oz)	340
Kernels	1 pkg (1.7 oz)	290
Kernels Barbecue	1 pkg (1.7 oz)	290
Kernels Honey Roasted	1 pkg (1.7 oz)	280
Kernels Salted	1 oz	170
Munch'N Go Singles Dry Roasted	1 pkg	120
Nuts Dry Roasted	¼ cup (1.1 oz)	190
Original With Shell Dry Roasted	¾ cup	160

FOOD	PORTION	CALS.
Stone-Buhr		
Seeds Raw	4 tsp (1 oz)	170
SUSHI		
TAKE-OUT		
california roll	1 piece (0.8 oz)	28
kim chi	⅓ cup (5.8 oz)	18
sashimi	1 serving (6 oz)	198
tuna roll	1 piece (0.7 oz)	23
vegetable roll	1 piece (1.2 oz)	27
vinegared ginger	⅓ cup (1.6 oz)	48
wasabi	2 tsp (0.3 oz)	5
yellowtail roll	1 piece (0.6 oz)	25
SWAMP CABBAGE		
chopped cooked	½ cup	10
raw chopped	1 cup	11
SWEET POTATO		
(*see also* YAM)		
CANNED		
in syrup	½ cup	106
pieces	1 cup	183
Princella		
Mashed	⅔ cup (5.1 oz)	120
Royal Prince		
Candied	½ cup (4.9 oz)	210
Halves	3 pieces (5.7 oz)	190
Orange Pineapple	½ cup (4.8 oz)	210
Sugary Sam		
Mashed	⅔ cup (5.1 oz)	120
FRESH		
baked w/ skin	1 (3½ oz)	118
leaves cooked	½ cup	11
mashed	½ cup	172
FROZEN		
cooked	½ cup	88
Mrs. Paul's		
Candied Sweet Potatoes	4 oz	170
Candied Sweets 'N Apples	4 oz	160
TAKE-OUT		
candied	3½ oz	144
SWEETBREADS		
beef braised	3 oz	230
lamb braised	3 oz	199
veal braised	3 oz	218

FOOD	PORTION	CALS.
SWISS CHARD		
cooked	½ cup	18
raw chopped	½ cup	3
SWORDFISH		
cooked	3 oz	132
raw	3 oz	103
SYRUP		
(*see also* ICE CREAM TOPPINGS, PANCAKE/WAFFLE SYRUP)		
corn	2 tbsp	122
corn dark	1 tbsp (0.7 oz)	56
corn dark	1 cup (11.5 oz)	925
corn light	1 cup (11.5 oz)	925
corn light	1 tbsp (0.7 oz)	56
malt	1 tbsp (0.8 oz)	76
malt	1 cup (13 oz)	1222
maple	1 cup (11.1 oz)	824
maple	1 tbsp (0.8 oz)	52
raspberry	3.5 oz	267
rose hip	3.5 oz	33
sorghum	1 cup (11.6 oz)	957
sorghum	1 tbsp (0.7 oz)	61
Eden		
Barley Malt Organic Syrup	1 tbsp (0.7 fl oz)	60
Estee		
Blueberry Lite	¼ cup (2.4 oz)	80
Home Brands		
Maple Rich	1 oz	110
Karo		
Corn Syrup Dark	1 tbsp (21 g)	60
Corn Syrup Dark	1 cup (331 g)	975
Corn Syrup Light	1 tbsp (21 g)	60
Corn Syrup Light	1 cup (331 g)	960
McIlhenny		
Cane	2 tbsp (1.4 oz)	130
Quik		
Strawberry	1⅔ tbsp	100
Red Wing		
Strawberry	2 tbsp (1.4 oz)	110
S&W		
Blueberry Diet	1 tbsp	4
Maple Flavored Diet	1 tbsp	4
Strawberry Diet	1 tbsp	4

FOOD	PORTION	CALS.
Smucker's		
All Flavors Fruit Syrup	2 tbsp	100
Tree Of Life		
Maple	¼ cup (2.1 oz)	200
Rice Syrup	2 tbsp (1 oz)	120
Whistling Wings		
Blueberry	1 oz	45
Raspberry	1 oz	60
TACO		
(*see* SPANISH FOOD)		
TAHINI		
(*see* SESAME)		
TAMARIND		
fresh	1	5
fresh cut up	1 cup	287
TANGERINE		
CANNED		
in light syrup	½ cup	76
juice pack	½ cup	46
FRESH		
sections	1 cup	86
tangerine	1	37
Dole		
Tangerine	2	70
TANGERINE JUICE		
canned sweetened	1 cup	125
fresh	1 cup	106
frzn sweetened as prep	1 cup	110
frzn sweetened not prep	6 oz	344
After The Fall		
Juice	1 can (12 oz)	170
Dole		
Mandarin frzn as prep	8 fl oz	140
Minute Maid		
Frozen	8 fl oz	120
TAPIOCA		
pearl dry	⅓ cup	174
starch	3½ oz	344
General Foods		
Minute Tapioca	1 tbsp	32

FOOD	PORTION	CALS.
TARO		
chips	1 oz	141
chips	10 (0.8 oz)	115
leaves cooked	½ cup	18
raw sliced	½ cup	56
shoots sliced cooked	½ cup	10
sliced cooked	½ cup (2.3 oz)	94
tahitian sliced cooked	½ cup	30
TARRAGON		
ground	1 tsp	5
TEA/HERBAL TEA		
(see also ICE TEA)		
HERBAL		
Bigelow		
Almond Orange	5 fl oz	tr
Apple Orchard	5 fl oz	5
Apple Spice	5 fl oz	tr
Chamomile	5 fl oz	tr
Chamomile Mint	5 fl oz	tr
Cinnamon Orange	5 fl oz	tr
Early Riser	5 fl oz	3
Feeling Free	5 fl oz	1
Fruit & Almond	5 fl oz	1
Hibiscus & Rose Hips	5 fl oz	1
I Love Lemon	5 fl oz	1
Lemon & C	5 fl oz	tr
Looking Good	5 fl oz	1
Mint Blend	5 fl oz	tr
Mint Medley	5 fl oz	1
Orange & C	5 fl oz	tr
Orange & Spice	5 fl oz	1
Peppermint	5 fl oz	tr
Roasted Grains & Carob	5 fl oz	3
Spearmint	5 fl oz	tr
Sweet Dreams	5 fl oz	1
Take-A-Break	5 fl oz	3
Celestial Seasonings		
Almond Sunset	8 fl oz	3
Bengal Spice	8 fl oz	5
Caffeine Free	8 fl oz	2
Chamomile	8 fl oz	2
Cinnamon Apple Spice	8 fl oz	<3
Cinnamon Rose	8 fl oz	<4

FOOD	PORTION	CALS.
Celestial Seasonings (CONT.)		
Country Peach Spice	8 fl oz	3
Cranberry Cove	8 fl oz	2
Emperor's Choice	8 fl oz	4
Ginseng Plus	8 fl oz	3
Grandma's Tummy Mint	8 fl oz	2
Lemon Mist	8 fl oz	3
Lemon Zinger	8 fl oz	4
Mama Bear's Cold Care	8 fl oz	6
Mandarin Orange Spice	8 fl oz	5
Mellow Mint	8 fl oz	2
Mint Magic	8 fl oz	1
Orange Zinger	8 fl oz	6
Peppermint	8 fl oz	2
Peppermint	8 fl oz	2
Raspberry Patch	8 fl oz	4
Red Zinger	8 fl oz	4
Roastaroma	8 fl oz	10
Sleepytime	8 fl oz	4
Spearmint	8 fl oz	5
Strawberry Fields	8 fl oz	4
Sunburst C	8 fl oz	3
Tropical Escape	8 fl oz	1
Wild Forest Blackberry	8 fl oz	2
Lipton		
Tea Bag Almond Pleasure as prep	1 cup	0
Tea Bag Cinnamon Apple as prep	1 cup	0
Tea Bag Cinnamon Spice as prep	1 cup	0
Tea Bag Country Cranberry as prep	1 cup	0
Tea Bag Gentle Orange as prep	1 cup	0
Tea Bag Ginger Twist as prep	1 cup	0
Tea Bag Golden Honey & Lemon as prep	1 cup	0
Tea Bag Lemon Mint Refresher as prep	1 cup	0
Tea Bag Lemon Smoother as prep	1 cup	0
Tea Bag Moonlight Mint as prep	1 cup	0
Tea Bag Mountain Berry	1 cup	0
Tea Bag Orange Refresher as prep	1 cup	0
Tea Bag Peppermint as prep	1 cup	0
Tea Bag Quietly Chamomile as prep	1 cup	0
Tea Bag Wildflower & Honey as prep	1 cup	0
REGULAR		
brewed tea	6 oz	2
instant unsweetened as prep w/ water	8 oz	2

FOOD	PORTION	CALS.
Bigelow		
Chinese Fortune	5 fl oz	1
Cinnamon Stick	5 fl oz	1
Constant Comment	5 fl oz	1
Darjeeling Blend	5 fl oz	1
Earl Gray	5 fl oz	1
English Teatime	5 fl oz	1
Lemon Lift	5 fl oz	1
Orange Pekoe	5 fl oz	1
Peppermint Stick	5 fl oz	1
Plantation Mint	5 fl oz	1
Raspberry Royale	5 fl oz	1
Celestial Seasonings		
Cinnamon Vienna	8 fl oz	2
Earl Grey Extraordinary	8 fl oz	3
English Breakfast Classic	8 fl oz	3
Lemon	8 fl oz	7
Mint	8 fl oz	4
Morning Thunder	8 fl oz	3
Naturally Decaffeinated	8 fl oz	10
Orange Spice	8 fl oz	7
Orange Spice Decaff	8 fl oz	7
Organically Grown	8 fl oz	12
Raspberry	8 fl oz	7
Lipton		
English Blend as prep	1 cup	0
Family Size Bags Decaf as prep	1 qt	0
Family Size Bags as prep	1 qt	0
Instant as prep	1 serv	0
Instant Decaf as prep	1 serv	0
Instant Lemon as prep	1 serv	0
Special Blends Amaretto as prep	1 cup	0
Special Blends Blackberry as prep	1 cup	0
Special Blends Cinnamon as prep	1 cup	0
Special Blends Earl Grey as prep	1 cup	0
Special Blends English Breakfast as prep	1 cup	0
Special Blends Honey & Cinnamon as prep	1 cup	0
Special Blends Honey & Lemon as prep	1 cup	0
Special Blends Honey & Orange as prep	1 cup	0
Special Blends Mint as prep	1 cup	0
Special Blends Orange & Spice as prep	1 cup	0
Special Blends Peach as prep	1 cup	0
Special Blends Raspberry	1 cup	0
Tea Bag Decaf as prep	1	0

FOOD	PORTION	CALS.
Lipton (CONT.)		
Tea Bag Green Tea as prep	1	0
Tea Bag as prep	1	0
Natural Touch		
Kaffree	8 fl oz	0
Nestea		
Tea Bag as prep	6 oz	0
TEFF		
Arrowhead		
Whole Grain	¼ cup (1.6 oz)	160
TEMPEH		
tempeh	½ cup	165
Lightlife		
Garden Vege	4 oz	142
Tempeh	4 oz	182
White Wave		
Burger	1 patty (3 oz)	110
Lemon Broil	1 patty (2 oz)	130
Organic Wild Rice	⅓ block (2.7 oz)	140
Teriyaki Burger	1 patty (3 oz)	110
THYME		
ground	1 tsp	4
Watkins		
Thyme	¼ tsp (0.5 oz)	0
TILEFISH		
cooked	½ fillet (5.3 oz)	220
cooked	3 oz	125
raw	3 oz	81
TOFU		
firm	¼ block (3 oz)	118
firm	½ cup	183
fresh fried	1 piece (½ oz)	35
fuyu salted & fermented	1 block (⅓ oz)	13
koyadofu dried frozen	1 piece (½ oz)	82
okara	½ cup	47
regular	¼ block (4 oz)	88
regular	½ cup	94
Azumaya		
Blue Label	3.5 oz	46
Green Label	3.5 oz	68
Name Age Fried	3.5 oz	144

FOOD	PORTION	CALS.
Azumaya (CONT.)		
Red Label	3.5 oz	68
Casbah		
Gyro as prep w/ tofu	1 patty (2 oz)	105
Jaclyn's		
Grilled In Black Bean Sauce	10.75 oz	270
Grilled In Peanut Sauce	10.75 oz	260
Mori-Nu		
Extra Firm	1 in slice (3 oz)	55
Firm	1 in slice (3 oz)	50
Lite Extra Firm	1 in slice (3 oz)	35
Lite Firm	1 in slice (3 oz)	35
Soft	1 in slice (3 oz)	45
Nasoya		
Extra Firm	⅕ block (3 oz)	90
Firm	⅕ block (3 oz)	80
Silken	⅙ block (3 oz)	50
Soft	⅕ block (3 oz)	60
Spring Creek		
Baked Barbeque	2 oz	88
Baked Cajun	2 oz	87
Baked Teriyaki	2 oz	84
Great Balls Of Tofu!	2 (3 oz)	107
Nigari Firm	4 oz	140
Tofu Salads !Onion Dip	2 oz	46
Tofu Salads !Taco Dip	2 oz	46
Tofu Salads Missing Egg	2 oz	49
Tree Of Life		
Baked	⅕ block (3.2 oz)	150
Firm	⅕ block (3.2 oz)	100
Raw Firm	⅕ block (3.2 oz)	100
Ready Ground Hot & Spicy	⅓ pkg (3 oz)	60
Ready Ground Original	⅓ pkg (3 oz)	60
Ready Ground Savory Garlic	⅓ pkg (3 oz)	60
Reduced Fat	⅕ block (3.2 oz)	90
Savory Baked	⅕ block (3.2 oz)	140
Smoked Hot'N Spicy	½ block (3 oz)	120
Smoked Original	½ block (3 oz)	120
White Wave		
Baked Tofus Teriyaki Oriental Style	¼ block (2 oz)	120
Hard	4 oz	120
International Baked Italian Garlic Herb	¼ pkg (2 oz)	120
International Baked Mexican Jalapeno	¼ pkg (2 oz)	120
International Baked Oriental Teriyaki	¼ pkg (2 oz)	120

FOOD	PORTION	CALS.
White Wave (CONT.)		
International Baked Thai Sesame Peanut	¼ pkg (2 oz)	120
Soft	4 oz	120
YOGURT		
Stir Fruity		
Black Cherry	6 oz	141
Blueberry	6 oz	140
Lemon Chiffon	6 oz	152
Mixed Berry	6 oz	149
Orange	6 oz	143
Peach	6 oz	160
Pina Colada	6 oz	162
Raspberry	6 oz	155
Spiced Apple	6 oz	167
Strawberry	6 oz	140
Tropical Fruit	6 oz	170
TOMATILLO		
fresh	1 (1.2 oz)	11
fresh chopped	½ cup	21
TOMATO		
(*see also* PIZZA, SPAGHETTI SAUCE)		
CANNED		
paste	½ cup	110
puree	1 cup	102
puree w/o salt	1 cup	102
red whole	½ cup	24
sauce	½ cup	37
sauce spanish style	½ cup	40
sauce w/ mushrooms	½ cup	42
sauce w/ onion	½ cup	52
stewed	½ cup	34
w/ green chiles	½ cup	18
wedges in tomato juice	½ cup	34
Claussen		
Kosher	1	9
Contadina		
California Sliced	½ cup	40
Crushed	¼ cup	20
Italian Paste	2 tbsp	40
Italian Style Pear	½ cup	25
Italian Style Stewed	½ cup	40
Mexican Style Stewed	½ cup	40
Pasta Ready Primavera	½ cup	50

FOOD	PORTION	CALS.
Contadina (CONT.)		
Pasta Ready Tomatoes	½ cup	50
Pasta Ready With Crushed Red Pepper	½ cup	60
Pasta Ready With Mushrooms	½ cup	50
Pasta Ready With Olives	½ cup	60
Pasta Ready With Three Cheeses	½ cup	70
Paste	2 tbsp	30
Peeled Whole	½ cup	25
Puree	¼ cup	20
Recipe Ready	½ cup	25
Stewed	½ cup	40
Del Monte		
Paste	2 tbsp (1.2 oz)	30
Peeled Diced	½ cup (4.4 oz)	25
Puree	¼ cup (2.2 oz)	30
Sauce	¼ cup (2.1 oz)	20
Sauce No Salt Added	¼ cup (2.1 oz)	20
Stewed Cajun Style	½ cup (4.4 oz)	35
Stewed Chunky Chili	½ cup (4.5 oz)	30
Stewed Chunky Pasta	½ cup (4.5 oz)	45
Stewed Chunky Pizza	½ cup (4.5 oz)	35
Stewed Chunky Salsa	½ cup (4.5 oz)	35
Stewed Italian Style	½ cup (4.4 oz)	30
Stewed Mexican Style	½ cup (4.4 oz)	35
Stewed Original	½ cup (4.4 oz)	35
Stewed Original No Salt Added	½ cup (4.4 oz)	35
Wedges	½ cup (4.4 oz)	35
Whole Peeled	½ cup (4.4 oz)	25
Eden		
Crushed Organic	¼ cup (2.1 oz)	20
Sauce Lightly Seasoned	¼ cup (2.1 oz)	25
Health Valley		
Sauce	1 cup	70
Sauce Low Sodium	1 cup	70
Hebrew National		
Pickled	⅓ tomato (1 oz)	4
Hunt's		
Choice Cut	½ cup (4.2 oz)	22
Choice Cut Diced Tomatoes & Green Chiles	2 tbsp (0.4 oz)	1
Choice Cut Diced Tomatoes & Italian Herb	½ cup (4.2 oz)	24
Choice Cut Diced Tomatoes & Roasted Garlic	½ cup (4.2 oz)	24
Crushed	½ cup (4.2 oz)	29

FOOD	PORTION	CALS.
Hunt's (CONT.)		
Crushed Angela Mia	½ cup (4.2 oz)	27
Paste	2 tbsp (1.2 oz)	30
Paste Italian	2 tbsp (1.2 oz)	27
Paste No Salt Added	2 tbsp (1.2 oz)	30
Paste With Garlic	2 tbsp (1.2 oz)	28
Pear Shaped	½ cup (4.6 oz)	20
Puree	¼ cup (2.2 oz)	24
Ready Sauce Chunky Chili	¼ cup (2.2 oz)	22
Ready Sauce Chunky Italian	¼ cup (2.2 oz)	26
Ready Sauce Chunky Mexican	¼ cup (2.2 oz)	21
Ready Sauce Chunky Special	¼ cup (2.2 oz)	21
Ready Sauce Chunky Tomato	¼ cup (2.2 oz)	15
Ready Sauce Country Herb	¼ cup (2.2 oz)	33
Ready Sauce Garlic	¼ cup (2.2 oz)	29
Ready Sauce Garlic & Herb	¼ cup (2.2 oz)	26
Ready Sauce Meatloaf Fixins	¼ cup (2.2 oz)	23
Ready Sauce Original	¼ cup (2.2 oz)	30
Sauce	¼ cup (2.2 oz)	16
Sauce Italian	¼ cup (2.2 oz)	32
Sauce No Salt Added	¼ cup (2.2 oz)	16
Sauce With Herb	¼ cup (2.2 oz)	32
Stewed	½ cup (4.2 oz)	33
Stewed Italian	4 oz	40
Tomatoes	½ cup (4.2 oz)	33
Whole	2 (5.2 oz)	22
Muir Glen		
Organic Chunky Sauce	¼ cup (2.3 oz)	20
Organic Crushed With Basil	¼ cup (2.3 oz)	25
Organic Diced	½ cup (4.5 oz)	25
Organic Diced No Salt Added	½ cup (4.5 oz)	25
Organic Ground Peeled	¼ cup (2.3 oz)	10
Organic Italian Style Diced	½ cup (4.4 oz)	25
Organic Paste	2 tbsp (1.2 oz)	30
Organic Puree	¼ cup (2.2 oz)	20
Organic Sauce	¼ cup (2.2 oz)	20
Organic Sauce No Salt Added	¼ cup (2.2 oz)	20
Organic Stewed	½ cup (4.5 oz)	30
Organic Stewed Italian Style	½ cup (4.4 oz)	30
Organic Stewed Mexican Style	½ cup (4.4 oz)	30
Organic Whole Peeled	½ cup (4.6 oz)	30
Old El Paso		
Tomatoes & Jalapenos	¼ cup (2 oz)	15
Tomatoes & Green Chilies	¼ cup (2 oz)	10

FOOD	PORTION	CALS.
Progresso		
Crushed	¼ cup (2.1 oz)	20
Paste	2 tbsp (1.2 oz)	30
Peeled Whole	½ cup (4.2 oz)	25
Peeled w/ Basil	½ cup (4.2 oz)	25
Puree	¼ cup (2.2 oz)	25
Puree Thick Style	¼ cup (2.2 oz)	30
Sauce	¼ cup (2.1 oz)	20
Rosoff's		
Pickled	⅓ tomato (1 oz)	5
S&W		
Aspic Supreme	½ cup	60
Diced In Rich Puree	½ cup	35
Italian Stewed Sliced	½ cup	35
Italian Style w/ Basil	½ cup	25
Paste	6 oz	150
Peeled Ready Cut	½ cup	25
Puree	½ cup	60
Sauce	½ cup	40
Sauce Chunky	½ cup	45
Stewed 50% Salt Reduced	½ cup	35
Stewed Mexican Style	½ cup	40
Stewed Sliced	½ cup	35
Whole Diet	½ cup	25
Whole Peeled	½ cup	25
Schorr's		
Pickled	⅓ tomato (1 oz)	4
Sonoma		
Dried Spice Medley oil drained	1 tbsp (0.5 oz)	50
Pesto	¼ cup (2 oz)	110
Tapenade	1 tbsp (0.7 oz)	70
Tree Of Life		
Sauce	¼ cup (2 oz)	20
DRIED		
sun dried	1 cup	140
sun dried	1 piece	5
sun dried in oil	1 piece (3 g)	6
sun dried in oil	1 cup (4 oz)	235
Sonoma		
Bits	2-3 tsp (5 g)	15
Dried	2-3 halves (5 g)	15
Halves	2-3 halves (5 g)	15
Julienne	7-9 pieces (5 g)	15
Pasta Toss	½ cup (0.7 oz)	70

FOOD	PORTION	CALS.
Sonoma (CONT.)		
Season It	2-3 tsp (5 g)	20
FRESH		
cooked	½ cup	32
green	1	30
red	1 (4½ oz)	26
red chopped	1 cup	35
TAKE-OUT		
stewed	1 cup	80

TOMATO JUICE

beef broth & tomato	5½ oz	61
clam & tomato	1 can (5½ oz)	77
tomato juice	6 oz	32
tomato juice	½ cup	21
Campbell		
Juice	6 oz	40
Del Monte		
Snap-E-Tom	6 fl oz	40
Snap-E-Tom	10 fl oz	60
Snap-E-Tom	8 fl oz	50
Hunt's		
Juice	8 fl oz	22
No Salt Added	8 fl oz	34
Libby		
Juice	6 oz	35
Mott's		
Beefamato	8 fl oz	80
Clamato	8 fl oz	100
Clamato Caesar	8 fl oz	100
Muir Glen		
Organic	8 oz	40
S&W		
California	6 oz	35
Diet	½ cup	35

TONGUE

beef simmered	3 oz	241
lamb braised	3 oz	234
pork braised	3 oz	230

TOPPINGS

(*see* ICE CREAM TOPPINGS)

TORTILLA

(*see also* CHIPS TORTILLA, SPANISH FOOD)

corn	1 (6 in diam)	56

FOOD	PORTION	CALS.
corn w/o salt	1-6 in diam (.9 oz)	56
flour w/o salt	1-8 in diam (1.2 oz)	114
Alvarado St. Bakery		
Burrito Size	1 (2.2 oz)	170
Fajita Size	1 (1.6 oz)	130
El Charrito		
Corn	2	95
Flour	2	170
Mariachi		
Tortilla	1	112
Old El Paso		
Flour	1 (1.4 oz)	150
Soft Taco Tortilla	2 (1.8 oz)	180
Tyson		
Burrito Style Flour	1	170
Burrito Style Hand Stretched Small Flour	1	106
Burrito Style Heat Pressed Large Flour	1	182
Enchilada Style Corn	1	54
Fajito Style Flour	1	89
Soft Taco Flour	1	121
Whole Wheat	1	120
Wonder		
Low Fat Wheat	1 (1.4 oz)	120
Low Fat White	1 (1.4 oz)	110
Zapata		
Tortilla	1 (1.2 oz)	100

TORTILLA CHIPS
(*see* CHIPS)

TREE FERN
chopped cooked	½ cup	28

TRITICALE
dry	½ cup	323
triticale not prep	3.5 oz	329

TROUT
baked	3 oz	162
rainbow cooked	3 oz	129
seatrout baked	3 oz	113
Clear Springs		
Rainbow	3.5 oz	140

TRUFFLES
fresh	3½ oz	25

FOOD	PORTION	CALS.
TUNA		
(*see also* TUNA DISHES)		
CANNED		
light in oil	3 oz	169
light in oil	1 can (6 oz)	399
light in water	3 oz	99
light in water	1 can (5.8 oz)	192
white in oil	3 oz	158
white in oil	1 can (6.2 oz)	331
white in water	1 can (6 oz)	234
white in water	3 oz	116
Bumble Bee		
Chunk Light In Oil	2 oz	160
Chunk Light In Water	2 oz	60
Chunk White In Oil	2 oz	160
Chunk White In Water	2 oz	70
Chunk White In Water Diet	2 oz	60
Solid White In Oil	2 oz	130
Solid White In Water	2 oz	70
Empress		
Chunk Light	2 oz	60
Chunk Light Tongol	2 oz	50
Solid White	2 oz	70
Progresso		
In Olive Oil	¼ cup (2 oz)	160
S&W		
Chunk Light Fancy In Oil	2 oz	140
Chunk Light Fancy In Water	2 oz	60
Fancy White Albacore in Oil	2 oz	160
Tree Of Life		
Tongol In Spring Water	2 oz	60
Tongol In Spring Water No Salt Water	2 oz	70
FRESH		
bluefin cooked	3 oz	157
bluefin raw	3 oz	122
skipjack baked	3 oz	112
yellowfin baked	3 oz	118
TUNA DISHES		
FROZEN		
Chefwich		
Tuna Melt	5 oz	360
Mrs. Paul's		
Microwave Tuna Sandwich	1	200
MIX		
Bumble Bee		
Tuna Mix-ins Classic Italian	⅓ pkg (0.17 oz)	25

FOOD	PORTION	CALS.
Bumble Bee (CONT.)		
Tuna Mix-ins Garden & Herb	⅓ pkg (0.17 oz)	25
Tuna Mix-ins Lemon Herb	⅓ pkg (0.17 oz)	25
Tuna Mix-ins Zesty Tomato	⅓ pkg (0.17 oz)	25
Tuna Helper		
Au Gratin as prep	⅕ pkg (6 oz)	280
Buttery Rice as prep	⅕ pkg (6 oz)	280
Cheesy Noodles as prep	⅕ pkg (7.75 oz)	240
Creamy Mushroom as prep	⅕ pkg (7 oz)	220
Creamy Noodles as prep	⅕ pkg (8 oz)	300
Fettucine Alfredo as prep	⅕ pkg (7 oz)	300
Romanoff as prep	⅕ pkg (8 oz)	290
Tetrazzini as prep	⅕ pkg (6 oz)	240
Tuna Pot Pie as prep	⅙ pkg (5.1 oz)	420
Tuna Salad as prep	⅕ pkg (5.5 oz)	420
READY-TO-USE		
The Spreadables		
Tuna Salad	¼ can	90
Wampler Longacre		
Salad	1 oz	60
TAKE-OUT		
tuna salad	1 cup	383
tuna salad	3 oz	159
tuna salad submarine sandwich w/ lettuce & oil	1	584

TURBOT

european baked	3 oz	104

TURKEY

(*see also* DINNER, HOT DOG, TURKEY DISHES, TURKEY SUBSTITUTES)

CANNED		
w/ broth	½ can (2.5 oz)	116
w/ broth	1 can (5 oz)	231
Armour		
Turkey Loaf	2 oz	110
Hormel		
Chunk	2 oz	70
Chunk Turkey Ham	2 oz	70
Chunk White	2 oz	60
Swanson		
White	2½ oz	80
Underwood		
Chunky Light	2.08 oz	75

FOOD	PORTION	CALS.
FRESH		
back w/ skin roasted	½ back (9 oz)	637
breast w/ skin roasted	4 oz	212
dark meat w/ skin roasted	3.6 oz	230
dark meat w/o skin roasted	1 cup (5 oz)	262
dark meat w/o skin roasted	3 oz	170
ground cooked	3 oz	188
leg w/ skin roasted	2.5 oz	147
leg w/ skin roasted	1 (1.2 lbs)	1133
light meat w/ skin roasted	from ½ turkey (2.3 lbs)	2069
light meat w/ skin roasted	4.7 oz	268
light meat w/o skin roasted	4 oz	183
neck simmered	1 (5.3 oz)	274
skin roasted	1 oz	141
skin roasted	from ½ turkey (9 oz)	1096
w/ skin roasted	8.4 oz	498
w/ skin roasted	½ turkey (4 lbs)	3857
w/ skin neck & giblets roasted	½ turkey (8.8 lbs)	4123
w/o skin roasted	1 cup (5 oz)	238
w/o skin roasted	7.3 oz	354
wing w/ skin roasted	1 (6.5 oz)	426
Butterball		
Ground All White Meat	3 oz	100
Louis Rich		
Ground	3 oz	140
Mr. Turkey		
Ground 85% Fat Free	3.5 oz	210
Ground 91% Fat Free	3.5 oz	170
Perdue		
Breast Tenderloins Cooked	3 oz	110
Breast Boneless Cooked	3 oz	110
Breast Cutlets Thin Sliced Cooked	1 (2.5 oz)	90
Breast Fillets Cooked	3 oz	110
Burger Cooked	1 (3 oz)	170
Cubed Steak Cooked	3 oz	120
Dark Cooked	3 oz	200
Drumsticks Roasted	3 oz	150
Drumsticks Cooked	3 oz	150
Ground Cooked	3 oz	170
Ground Breast Cooked	3 oz	110
Half Breast Cooked	3 oz	170
Thighs Cooked	3 oz	180
Tom Wings Cooked	3 oz	160
White Cooked	3 oz	170

FOOD	PORTION	CALS.
Perdue (CONT.)		
Whole Breast Cooked	3 oz	170
Wings Roasted	1 (3 oz)	180
Wings Drummettes Roasted	1 (3.5 oz)	180
Shady Brook		
Breast Prime Young	3 oz	140
Wings	3 oz	130
Swift-Eckrich		
Ground All White	3 oz	100
Wampler Longacre		
Ground raw	1 oz	60
FROZEN		
roast boneless seasoned light & dark meat roasted	1 pkg (1.7 lbs)	1213
Empire		
Patties	1 (3.1 oz)	200
READY-TO-USE		
bologna	1 oz	57
breast	1 slice (¾ oz)	23
diced light & dark seasoned	½ lb	313
diced light & dark seasoned	1 oz	39
ham thigh meat	2 oz	73
ham thigh meat	1 pkg (8 oz)	291
pastrami	1 pkg (8 oz)	320
pastrami	2 oz	80
patties battered & fried	1 (3.3 oz)	266
patties battered & fried	1 (2.3 oz)	181
patties breaded & fried	1 (3.3 oz)	266
patties breaded & fried	1 (2.3 oz)	181
poultry salad sandwich spread	1 oz	238
poultry salad sandwich spread	1 tbsp	109
prebasted breast w/ skin roasted	1 breast (3.8 lbs)	2175
prebasted breast w/ skin roasted	½ breast (1.9 lbs)	1087
prebasted thigh w/ skin roasted	1 thigh (11 oz)	494
roll light & dark meat	1 oz	42
roll light meat	1 oz	42
salami cooked	1 pkg (8 oz)	446
salami cooked	2 oz	111
turkey loaf breast meat	2 slices (1.5 oz)	47
turkey loaf breast meat	1 pkg (6 oz)	187
turkey sticks battered & fried	1 stick (2.3 oz)	178
turkey sticks breaded & fried	1 stick (2.3 oz)	178
Alpine Lace		
Breast Fat Free	2 oz	50

FOOD	PORTION	CALS.
Carl Buddig		
Honey Turkey	1 oz	40
Turkey	1 oz	50
Turkey Ham	1 oz	40
Empire		
Barbecue Whole	5 oz	250
Bologna	3 slices (1.8 oz)	90
Oven Prepared Breast Slices	3 slices (1.8 oz)	50
Pastrami	3 slices (1.8 oz)	60
Salami	3 slices (1.8 oz)	70
Smoked Breast Slices	3 slices (1.8 oz)	40
Falls		
BBQ	3 oz	140
Gourmet Breast	3 oz	80
Premium Cooked Breast	3 oz	100
Hansel n'Gretel		
Breast Gourmet	1 oz	28
Breast Gourmet Smoked	1 oz	31
Breast Honey	1 oz	28
Breast Lessalt Cooked	1 oz	25
Breast Oven Cooked	1 oz	26
Doubledecker Turkey Corned Beef	1 oz	30
Doubledecker Turkey Ham	1 oz	30
Healthy Choice		
Deli-Thin Honey Roast & Smoked	6 slices (2 oz)	70
Deli-Thin Roasted Breast	6 slices (2 oz)	60
Deli-Thin Smoked Breast	6 slices (2 oz)	60
Deli-Thin Turkey Ham	6 slices (2 oz)	60
Fresh-Trak Honey Roast & Smoked Breast	1 slice (1 oz)	35
Fresh-Trak Oven Roasted Breast	1 slice (1 oz)	35
Honey Roasted & Smoked	1 slice (1 oz)	35
Oven Roasted Breast	1 slice (1 oz)	35
Smoked Breast	1 slice (1 oz)	30
Variety Pack Regular	3 slices (2.2 oz)	70
Hebrew National		
Deli Thin Hickory Smoked	1.8 oz	55
Deli Thin Lemon Garlic	1.8 oz	50
Deli Thin Oven Roasted	1.8 oz	80
Hillshire		
Deli Select Honey Roasted Breast	1 slice	10
Deli Select Oven Roasted Breast	1 slice	10
Deli Select Smoked Breast	1 slice	10
Deli Select Turkey Ham	1 slice	10
Flavor Pack 90-99% Fat Free Honey Roasted Breast	1 slice (0.75 oz)	20

FOOD	PORTION	CALS.
Hillshire (CONT.)		
Flavor Pack 90-99% Fat Free Oven Roasted Breast	1 slice (0.75 oz)	20
Honey Cured Breast	1 oz	35
Lunch 'N Munch Smoked Turkey/ Cheddar	1 pkg (4.5 oz)	350
Lunch 'N Munch Smoked Turkey/ Cheddar/ Brownie	1 pkg (4.5 oz)	400
Lunch 'N Munch Turkey/Cheddar/ Brownie/Hi-C	1 pkg (4.5 oz + 6 fl oz)	500
Smoked Breast	1 oz	35
Hormel		
Light & Lean 97 Breast Sliced	1 slice (1 oz)	30
Light & Lean 97 Breast Smoked	3 oz	80
Light & Lean 97 Cuts	16 pieces (1 oz)	30
Light & Lean 97 Cuts Smoked	16 pieces (1 oz)	30
Louis Rich		
Bologna	1 slice (28 g)	50
Breaded Nuggets	4 (3.2 oz)	260
Breaded Patties	1 (3 oz)	220
Breaded Sticks	3 (3 oz)	230
Carving Board Oven Roasted Breast	2 slices (1.6 oz)	40
Carving Board Oven Roasted Thin Carved Breast	6 slices (2.1 oz)	60
Carving Board Smoked Breast	2 slices (1.6 oz)	40
Chopped Ham	1 slice (1 oz)	46
Cotto Salami	1 slice (28 g)	40
Deli-Thin Smoked Breast	4 slices (1.8 oz)	50
Fat Free Hickory Smoked Breast	1 slice (1 oz)	25
Fat Free Oven Roasted Breast	1 slice (28 g)	25
Ham Round	1 slice (28 g)	34
Ham Square	3 slices (2.2 oz)	70
Hickory Smoked Dinner Slices Breast	1 slice (2.8 oz)	80
Honey Cured Turkey Ham	3 slices (2.2 oz)	70
Honey Roasted Breast	1 slice (1 oz)	30
Honey Roasted Dinner Slices Breast	1 slice (2.8 oz)	80
Oven Roasted Breast	2 oz	60
Oven Roasted Breast	1 slice (1 oz)	30
Oven Roasted Deli-Thin Breast	4 slices (1.8 oz)	50
Oven Roasted Dinner Slices Breast	1 slice (2.8 oz)	70
Pastrami	2 slices (1.6 oz)	45
Salami	1 slice (28 g)	45
Skinless Barbecued Breast	2 oz	60
Skinless Hickory Smoked Breast	2 oz	60
Skinless Honey Roasted Breast	2 oz	60

FOOD	PORTION	CALS.
Louis Rich (CONT.)		
Skinless Oven Roasted Breast	2 oz	50
Smoked Breast	1 slice (1 oz)	25
Smoked White	1 slice (1 oz)	30
Turkey Ham	4 slices (1.8 oz)	60
Mr. Turkey		
Deli Cuts Hardwood Smoked Breast	3 slices	30
Deli Cuts Honey Roasted Breast	3 slices	30
Deli Cuts Oven Roasted Breast	3 slices	30
Deli Cuts Turkey Ham	3 slices	35
Deli Cuts Turkey Pastrami	3 slices	35
Hardwood Smoked Breast	1 slice	30
Hardwood Smoked Turkey Ham	1 slice	35
Honey Cured Turkey Ham	1 slice	30
Oven Roasted Breast	1 slice	30
Smoked Breakfast Turkey Ham	1 oz	30
Turkey Cotto Salami	1 slice	50
Turkey Ham	1 slice	35
Turkey Pastrami	1 slice	30
Oscar Mayer		
Deli-Thin Roast	4 slices (1.8 oz)	50
Deli-Thin Smoked Honey Roasted	4 slices (1.8 oz)	60
Free Oven Roasted Breast	4 slices (1.8 oz)	40
Free Smoked Breast	4 slices (1.8 oz)	40
Healthy Favorites Oven Roasted Breast	4 slices (1.8 oz)	40
Healthy Favorites Smoked Breast	4 slices (1.8 oz)	40
Lunchables Fun Pack Turkey/Pacific Cooler	1 pkg (11.2 oz)	460
Lunchables Fun Pack Turkey/Surger Cooler	1 pkg (11.2 oz)	440
Lunchables Turkey Oven Roasted/Green Onion Cheese	1 pkg (4.5 oz)	380
Lunchables Turkey Smoked/ Ranch & Herb Cheese	1 pkg (4.5 oz)	380
Lunchables Turkey/Cheddar	1 pkg (4.5 oz)	360
Perdue		
Nuggets Dinosaur	3 (3 oz)	200
Sara Lee		
Hardwood Smoked Breast Of Turkey	2 oz	60
Hardwood Smoked Turkey Ham	2 oz	60
Honey Roasted Breast Of Turkey	2 oz	60
Honey Roasted Turkey Ham	2 oz	70
Mesquite Smoked Breast Of Turkey	2 oz	60
Oven Roasted Breast Of Turkey	2 oz	60

FOOD	PORTION	CALS.
Sara Lee (CONT.)		
Peppered Breast Of Turkey	2 oz	50
Seasoned Breast Of Turkey Pastrami	2 oz	60
Tyson		
Breast	1 slice	20
Ham	1 slice	23
Wampler Longacre		
Bologna	1 oz	60
Breast Chops	1 serv (4 oz)	120
Breast Sliced	1 slice (1 oz)	35
Breast Sliced Smoked	1 slice (0.75 oz)	20
Burger	1 (4 oz)	230
Burger	1 (3 oz)	170
Burger Barbecue	1 (4 oz)	240
Chef Select Breast Skinless	1 oz	35
Chef Select Breast Smoked	1 oz	35
Chunk Dark Smoked Cured	1 oz	45
Chunk Ham 12% Water Smoked	1 oz	45
Chunk Ham 20% Water	1 oz	40
Chunk Pastrami	1 oz	35
Cook-In-The-Bag Breast	1 oz	30
Cook-In-The-Bag Breast Mini	1 oz	30
Cook-In-The-Bag Combo Roast	1 oz	35
Cook-In-The-Bag Thigh Roast	1 oz	40
Dark Smoked Cured	1 oz	45
Deli Chef Breast And White Meat No Skin	1 oz	40
Gourmet Breast	1 oz	35
Gourmet Breast Mini	1 oz	35
Gourmet Breast Mini Smoked	1 oz	35
Gourmet Breast Smoked	1 oz	30
Gourmet Brown & Glazed Breast	1 oz	35
Gourmet Brown & Roasted Breast	1 oz	35
Gourmet Honey Cured Breast	1 oz	30
Lean-Lite Breast Skinless	1 oz	35
Lean-Lite Deli Breast	1 oz	35
Lean-Lite Deli Breast Smoked	1 oz	35
Old Fashioned Brown & Roasted Breast	1 oz	35
Pastrami	1 oz	35
Premium Breast Skinless	1 oz	30
Premium Brown & Roasted Breast Skinless	1 oz	16
Roll Combo	1 oz	44
Roll Sliced Breast	1 slice (0.75 oz)	30
Roll White	1 oz	45

FOOD	PORTION	CALS.
Wampler Longacre (CONT.)		
Salami	1 oz	50
Salt Watchers Breast Skinless	1 oz	35
Seasoned Roast	1 oz	40
Sliced Salami	1 slice (0.8 oz)	45
Tenderlings BBQ	1 serv (4 oz)	110
Tenderlings Cajun	1 serv (4 oz)	110
Tenderlings Garlic & Pepper	1 serv (4 oz)	110
Tenderlings Original	1 serv (4 oz)	110
Turkey Ham 12% Water Baked	1 oz	45
Turkey Ham 20% Water Baked	1 oz	40
Unseasoned Roast	1 oz	40
Whole Browned & Roasted	1 oz	60
Weight Watchers		
Deli Thin Smoked Breast	5 slices (⅓ oz)	10
Oven Roasted Breast	2 slices (¾ oz)	25
Oven Roasted Turkey Ham	2 slices (¾ oz)	25
Roasted & Smoked Breast	2 slices (¾ oz)	25

TURKEY DISHES

(*see also* DINNER, TURKEY SUBSTITUTES)

FROZEN		
gravy & turkey	1 cup (8.4 oz)	160
gravy & turkey	1 pkg (5 oz)	95
Hot Pocket		
Stuffed Sandwich Turkey & Ham With Cheese	1 (4.5 oz)	320
Lean Pockets		
Stuffed Sandwich Turkey & Ham With Cheddar	1 (4.5 oz)	260
Stuffed Sandwich Turkey Broccoli & Cheese	1 (4.5 oz)	260
Luigino's		
Gravy Dressing & Turkey	1 pkg (8 oz)	340
Ovenstuffs		
Turkey Turnover	1 (4.75 oz)	350
Weight Watchers		
Honey Dijon Turkey Pretzel Sandwich	1 (4 oz)	230
READY-TO-USE		
Spreadables		
Turkey Salad	¼ can	100
Wampler Longacre		
Meatloaf Italian	1 serv (4 oz)	114
Meatloaf Mexican	1 serv (4 oz)	114

FOOD	PORTION	CALS.
Wampler Longacre (CONT.)		
Meatloaf Original	1 serv (4 oz)	126
Salad	1 oz	60
Salad Turkey Ham	1 oz	50
Teriyaki	1 serv (4 oz)	112
SHELF-STABLE		
Dinty Moore		
American Classics Chicken With Mashed Potatoes	1 bowl (10 oz)	250
American Classics Turkey & Dressing With Gravy	1 bowl (10 oz)	280

TURKEY SUBSTITUTES

Harvest Direct		
TVP Poultry Chunks	3.5 oz	280
TVP Poultry Ground	3.5 oz	280
White Wave		
Meatless Sandwich Slices	2 slices (1.6 oz)	80
Worthington		
Smoked Turkey Slices	4 slices (76 g)	180
Turkee Slices	2 slices (63 g)	130

TURMERIC

ground	1 tsp	8

TURNIPS

CANNED		
greens	½ cup	17
Allen		
Chopped Greens And Diced Turnip	½ cup (4.2 oz)	30
Greens	½ cup (4.2 oz)	25
Luck's		
Turnip Greens w/ Diced Turnips Seasoned w/ Pork	7.5 oz	90
Sunshine		
Chopped Greens And Diced Turnip	½ cup (4.2 oz)	30
Greens	½ cup (4.2 oz)	25
FRESH		
cooked mashed	½ cup (4.2 oz)	47
cubed cooked	½ cup (3 oz)	33
greens chopped cooked	½ cup	15
greens raw chopped	½ cup	7
raw cubed	½ cup (2.4 oz)	25
FROZEN		
greens cooked	½ cup	24

FOOD	PORTION	CALS.
Southland		
Mashed	3.6 oz	90
Rutabaga Yellow Turnips	4 oz	50
TURTLE		
raw	3½ oz	85
TUSK FISH		
raw	3½ oz	79
VANILLA		
Hershey		
Vanilla Milk Chips	¼ cup	240
Virginia Dare		
Vanilla Extract	1 tsp	10
VEAL		
(*see also* DINNER, VEAL DISHES)		
FRESH		
cutlet lean only braised	3 oz	172
cutlet lean only fried	3 oz	156
ground broiled	3 oz	146
loin chop w/ bone lean & fat braised	1 chop (2.8 oz)	227
loin chop w/ bone lean only braised	1 chop (2.4 oz)	155
shoulder w/ bone lean only braised	3 oz	169
sirloin w/ bone lean & fat roasted	3 oz	171
sirloin w/ bone lean only roasted	3 oz	143
VEAL DISHES		
TAKE-OUT		
parmigiana	4.2 oz	279
VEGETABLE JUICE		
vegetable juice cocktail	6 fl oz	34
vegetable juice cocktail	½ cup	22
Mott's		
Vegetable Juice as prep	8 fl oz	60
Muir Glen		
Organic	8 oz	70
Organic Reduced Sodium	8 oz	70
Odwalla		
Vegetable Cocktail	8 fl oz	70
Smucker's		
Vegetable Juice Hearty	8 fl oz	58
Vegetable Juice Hot & Spicy	8 fl oz	58
V8		
No Salt Added	6 fl oz	35

FOOD	PORTION	CALS.
V8 (CONT.)		
Original	6 fl oz	35
Spicy Hot	6 fl oz	35

VEGETABLES MIXED
(*see also individual vegetables,* VEGETABLE JUICE)

CANNED

FOOD	PORTION	CALS.
mixed vegetables	½ cup	39
peas & carrots	½ cup	48
peas & carrots low sodium	½ cup	48
peas & onions	½ cup	30
succotash	½ cup	102
Allen		
Green Beans And Potatoes	½ cup (4.2 oz)	35
Okra & Tomatoes	½ cup (4 oz)	25
Okra Tomatoes & Corn	½ cup (4.1 oz)	30
Chi-Chi's		
Diced Tomatoes & Green Chilies	¼ cup (2.5 oz)	20
Del Monte		
Mixed	½ cup (4.4 oz)	40
Peas And Carrots	½ cup (4.5 oz)	60
Green Giant		
Garden Medley	½ cup	40
Hanover		
Mixed	½ cup	110
Vegetable Salad	½ cup	90
House Of Tsang		
Vegetables & Sauce Cantonese Classic	½ cup (4.2 oz)	70
Vegetables & Sauce Hong Kong Sweet & Sour	½ cup (4.5 oz)	160
Vegetables & Sauce Szechuan Hot & Spicy	½ cup (4.2 oz)	70
Vegetables & Sauce Tokyo Teriyaki	½ cup (4.4 oz)	100
Ka-Me		
Stir Fry	½ cup (4.5 oz)	20
La Choy		
Chop Suey Vegetables	½ cup	10
S&W		
Garden Salad Marinated	½ cup	60
Mixed Vegetables Old Fashion Harvest Time	½ cup	35
Peas & Carrots Water Pack	½ cup	35
Succotash Country Style	½ cup	80
Sweet Peas & Diced Carrots	½ cup	50
Sweet Peas w/ Tiny Pearl Onions	½ cup	60

FOOD	PORTION	CALS.
Seneca		
Peas & Carrots	½ cup	60
Succotash	½ cup	90
Sunshine		
Green Beans And Potatoes	½ cup (4.2 oz)	35
Trappey		
Okra & Tomatoes	½ cup (4 oz)	25
Okra Tomatoes & Corn	½ cup (4.1 oz)	30
FROZEN		
mixed vegetables cooked	½ cup	54
peas & carrots cooked	½ cup	38
peas & onions cooked	½ cup	40
succotash cooked	½ cup	79
Big Valley		
California Blend	¾ cup (3 oz)	25
Italian Blend	¾ cup (3 oz)	30
Oriental Blend	¾ cup (3 oz)	25
Stew Vegetables	⅔ cup (3 oz)	40
Winter Blend	¾ cup (3 oz)	25
Birds Eye		
Broccoli Cauliflower And Carrots With Cheese Sauce	½ pkg	80
Farm Fresh Broccoli And Cauliflower	¾ cup	30
Farm Fresh Broccoli Corn And Red Peppers	⅔ cup	60
Farm Fresh Broccoli Green Beans Pearl Onions and Red Peppers	¾ cup	35
Farm Fresh Broccoli Red Peppers Onions And Mushrooms	¾ cup	30
Farm Fresh Brussels Sprouts Cauliflower And Carrots	¾ cup	40
Farm Fresh Cauliflower Carrots And Snow Peas	⅔ cup	35
In Butter Sauce Broccoli Cauliflower And Carrots	½ cup	40
In Sauce Peas And Pearl Onions With Seasonings	½ cup	70
Internationals Austrian	3.3 oz	70
Internationals Bavarian	3.3 oz	90
Internationals California	3.3 oz	90
Internationals French Country	3.3 oz	70
Internationals Japanese	3.3 oz	60
Internationals New England	3.3 oz	100
Mixed	½ cup	60

FOOD	PORTION	CALS.
Birds Eye (CONT.)		
Peas And Potatoes With Cream Sauce	½ cup	100
Polybag	½ cup	60
Budget Gourmet		
Mandarin Vegetables	1 pkg (5.25 oz)	160
New England Recipe Vegetables	1 pkg (5.5 oz)	230
Spring Vegetables In Cheese Sauce	1 pkg (5 oz)	130
Fresh Like		
California Blend	3.5 oz	31
Chuckwagon Blend	3.5 oz	71
Italian Blend	3.5 oz	33
Midwestern Blend	3.5 oz	42
Mixed	3.5 oz	69
Oriental Blend	3.5 oz	26
Peas & Carrots	3.5 oz	63
Winter Blend	3.5 oz	26
Green Giant		
American Mixtures California	½ cup	25
American Mixtures Heartland	½ cup	25
American Mixtures New England	½ cup	70
American Mixtures San Francisco	½ cup	25
American Mixtures Sante Fe	½ cup	70
American Mixtures Seattle	½ cup	25
Broccoli Cauliflower And Carrots In Cheese Sauce	½ cup	60
Harvest Fresh Mixed Vegetables	½ cup	40
Mixed	½ cup	40
Mixed In Butter Sauce	½ cup	60
One Serve Broccoli Carrots & Rotini In Cheese Sauce	1 pkg	120
One Serve Broccoli Cauliflower And Carrots	1 pkg	25
Valley Combinations Broccoli & Cauliflower	½ cup	60
Hanover		
Broccoli Cut & Cauliflower Cut	½ cup	20
Caribbean Blend	½ cup	20
Garden Medley	½ cup	20
Mixed	½ cup	50
Oriental Blend	½ cup	25
Succotash	½ cup	80
Summer Vegetables	½ cup	35
Vegetables For Soup	½ cup	60

FOOD	PORTION	CALS.
La Choy		
Mixed Fancy	½ cup	12
Ore Ida		
Stew Vegetables	⅔ cup (3 oz)	50
Soglowek		
Golden Vegetarian Nuggets	4 pieces (2.5 oz)	190
Southland		
Peppers & Onions	2 oz	15
Soup Mix Vegetables	3.2 oz	50
Stew Vegetables	4 oz	60
Tree Of Life		
Mixed	½ cup (3 oz)	65
Veg-All		
Country Wisconsin Blend	3.5 oz	52
Scandinavian Blend	3.5 oz	48
Vegetables For Soup (Eight)	3.5 oz	34
Vegetables For Soup (Potatoes)	3.5 oz	53
Vegetables For Stew 4-Way	3.5 oz	51
Vegetables For Stew 5-Way	3.5 oz	54
SHELF-STABLE		
Pantry Express		
Corn Green Beans Carrots Pasta In Tomato Sauce	½ cup	80
Green Beans Potatoes And Mushrooms In A Seasoned Sauce	½ cup	50
Mixed Vegetables	½ cup	35
TAKE-OUT		
caponata	¼ cup	28
curry	1 serving (7.7 oz)	398
pakoras	1 (2 oz)	108
ratatouille	8.8 oz	190
samosa	2 (4 oz)	519
succotash	½ cup	111

VENISON

FOOD	PORTION	CALS.
roasted	3 oz	134
Broken Arrow Ranch		
Antelope Chili Meat	3.5 oz	115
Antelope Ground Venison	3.5 oz	110
Antelope Stew Meat	3.5 oz	110
Nilgai Chili Meat	3.5 oz	115
Nilgai Leg	3.5 oz	100
Nilgai Stew Meat	3.5 oz	110
Venison & Beef Smoked Sausage	6 oz	432

FOOD	PORTION	CALS.
Broken Arrow Ranch (CONT.)		
Venison Meat Chunks	6 oz	175
Venison Salami	6 oz	252
VINEGAR		
cider	1 tbsp	tr
Hain		
Cider	1 tbsp	2
Ka-Me		
Chinese Seasoned	1 tbsp (0.5 fl oz)	5
Rice Wine Chinese	1 tbsp (0.5 fl oz)	5
Rice Wine Japanese	1 tbsp (0.5 oz)	0
Seasoned Rice Japanese	1 tbsp (0.5 fl oz)	10
Nakano		
Rice	1 tbsp	0
Regina		
Red Wine	1 oz	4
Tree Of Life		
Apple Cider Organic	1 tbsp (0.5 oz)	0
Brown Rice	1 tbsp (0.5 oz)	2
White House		
Apple Cider	2 tbsp	2
Red Wine	2 tbsp	4
WAFFLES		
FROZEN		
buttermilk	1, 4 in sq (1.2 oz)	88
plain	1, 4 in sq (1.2 oz)	88
Aunt Jemima		
Blueberry	2 (2.5 oz)	190
Buttermilk	2 (2.5 oz)	170
Cinnamon	2 (2.5 oz)	180
Oatmeal	2 (2.5 oz)	170
Whole Grain	2 (2.5 oz)	170
Belgian Chef		
Belgian	2 (2.5 oz)	140
Downyflake		
Blueberry	2	180
Buttermilk	2	190
Multi-Grain	2	250
Oat Bran	2	260
Regular	2	120
Regular Jumbo	2	170
Rice Bran	2	210
Roman Meal	2	280

FOOD	PORTION	CALS.
Downyflake (CONT.)		
Waffles	2	180
Eggo		
Apple Cinnamon	2 (2.7 oz)	220
Blueberry	2 (2.7 oz)	220
Buttermilk	2 (2.7 oz)	220
Common Sense Oat Bran	2 (2.7 oz)	200
Common Sense Oat Bran With Fruit & Nut	2 (2.9 oz)	220
Homestyle	2 (2.7 oz)	220
Minis Blueberry	12 (3 oz)	240
Minis Cinnamon Toast	12 (3.2 oz)	280
Minis Homestyle	12 (1.8 oz)	240
Nut & Honey	2 (2.7 oz)	240
Nutri-Grain	2 (2.7 oz)	190
Nutri-Grain Multi-Bran	2 (2.7 oz)	180
Nutri-Grain Raisin & Bran	2 (3 oz)	210
Special K	2 (2 oz)	140
Strawberry	2 (2.7 oz)	220
Great Starts		
Belgian Waffles And Sausage	2.85 oz	280
Belgian Waffles Strawberries And Sausage	3.5 oz	210
Waffle With Bacon	2.2 oz	230
Van's		
Belgian 7 Grain	1	80
Belgian Original	1	73
Toaster Apple Cinnamon	1	75
Toaster Honey Almond	1	75
Toaster Multigrain	1	75
Toaster Wheat Free	1	110
Toaster Wheat Free Cinnamon Apple	1	110
Weight Watchers		
Belgian	1 (1.5 oz)	120
HOME RECIPE		
plain	1 (7 in diam)	218
MIX		
plain as prep	1, 7 in diam (2.6 oz)	218

WALNUTS

black dried	1 oz	172
black dried chopped	1 cup	759
english dried	1 oz	182
english dried chopped	1 cup	770
Planters		
Black	1 pkg (2 oz)	340

FOOD	PORTION	CALS.
Planters (CONT.)		
Gold Measure Halves	1 pkg (2 oz)	380
Halves	⅓ cup (1.2 oz)	220
Pieces	¼ cup (1 oz)	190

WATER CHESTNUTS
CANNED

chinese sliced	½ cup	35
Empress		
Sliced	2 oz	14
Whole	2 oz	14
Ka-Me		
Whole In Water	½ cup (4.5 oz)	45
La Choy		
Sliced	¼ cup	18
Whole	4	14
FRESH		
sliced	½ cup	66

WATERCRESS
(*see also* CRESS)

raw chopped	½ cup	2

WATERMELON
FRESH

cut up	1 cup	50
wedge	1/16	152
SEEDS		
dried	1 oz	158
dried	1 cup	602

WAX BEANS
CANNED

Del Monte		
Cut Golden	½ cup (4.3 oz)	20
Owatonna		
Cut	½ cup	20
S&W		
Golden Cut Premium	½ cup	20
Seneca		
Cuts Natural Pack	½ cup	25
Wax Beans	½ cup	25

WHALE

raw	3.5 oz	134

FOOD	PORTION	CALS.

WHEAT
(see also BULGUR, BRAN, CEREAL, COUSCOUS, FLOUR, WHEAT GERM)

sprouted	⅓ cup	71
starch	3½ oz	348
Arrowhead		
Kamut Grain	¼ cup (1.7 oz)	140
Seitan Quick Mix	⅓ cup (1.4 oz)	150
Hodgson Mill		
Vital Wheat Gluten Plus Ascorbic Acid	1 tbsp (0.3 oz)	30
Near East		
Taboule Salad Mix as prep	⅔ cup	120
Wheat Pilaf as prep	1 cup	220
Sonoma		
Wheat Nuts Salted	2 tbsp (0.5 oz)	60
White Wave		
Seitan	½ pkg (4 oz)	140
Seitan Fajita Strips	⅓ cup (1.8 oz)	60
Seitan Marinated Slices	3 slices (1.8 oz)	60

WHEAT GERM

plain toasted	¼ cup	108
plain toasted	1 cup	431
plain untoasted	¼ cup	104
w/ brown sugar & honey toasted	1 cup	426
w/ brown sugar & honey toasted	1 oz	107
Arrowhead		
Wheat Germ	3 tbsp (0.5 oz)	50
Hodgson Mill		
Wheat Germ	2 tbsp (0.5 oz)	55
Kretschmer		
Honey Crunch	¼ cup	105
Original	¼ cup	103
Stone-Buhr		
Untoasted	2 tbsp (0.5 oz)	58

WHEY

acid dry	1 tbsp (3 g)	10
acid fluid	1 cup (8 fl oz)	59
sweet dry	1 tbsp (8 g)	26
sweet fluid	1 cup (8 fl oz)	66
whey cheese	3.5 oz	440

WHIPPED TOPPINGS
(see also CREAM)

cream pressurized	1 cup	154

FOOD	PORTION	CALS.
cream pressurized	1 tbsp	8
nondairy powdered as prep w/ whole milk	1 cup	151
nondairy powdered as prep w/ whole milk	1 tbsp	8
nondairy pressurized	1 tbsp	11
nondairy pressurized	1 cup	184
Cool Whip		
Extra Creamy	1 tbsp	13
Lite	1 tbsp	9
Non Dairy	1 tbsp	11
D-Zerta		
As prep	1 tbsp	7
Dream Whip		
As prep	1 tbsp	9
Estee		
Whipped Topping Sugar Free as prep	2 tbsp	10
Hood		
Instant	2 tbsp	20
Light Instant	2 tbsp	15
Kraft		
Real Cream	2 tbsp (0.4 oz)	20
Whipped Topping	2 tbsp (0.4 oz)	20
La Creme		
Topping	1 tbsp	16
Pet		
Whip	1 tbsp	14
Reddiwip		
Lite	2 tbsp (8 g)	15
Non-Dairy	2 tbsp (8 g)	20
Real Whipped Heavy Cream	2 tbsp (8 g)	30
Real Whipped Light Cream	2 tbsp (8 g)	20

WHITE BEANS

CANNED

white beans	1 cup	306
Goya		
Spanish Style	7.5 oz	130
Progresso		
Cannellini	½ cup (4.6 oz)	100

DRIED

regular cooked	1 cup	249
small cooked	1 cup	253

WHITEFISH

baked	3 oz	146
smoked	3 oz	92
smoked	1 oz	39

FOOD	PORTION	CALS.
WHITING		
cooked	3 oz	98
raw	3 oz	77
WILD RICE		
cooked	½ cup	83
Haddon House		
Extra Fancy	¼ cup (1.6 oz)	170
WINE		
(*see also* CHAMPAGNE, WINE COOLERS)		
madeira	3.5 oz	169
port	3.5 oz	156
red	3½ oz	74
rose	3½ oz	73
sherry	2 oz	84
sweet dessert	2 oz	90
vermouth dry	3½ oz	105
vermouth sweet	3½ oz	167
white	3½ oz	70
Boone's		
Country Kwencher	1 fl oz	24
Delicious Apple	1 fl oz	21
Sangria	1 fl oz	22
Snow Creek Berry	1 fl oz	18
Strawberry Hill	1 fl oz	22
Sun Peak Peach	1 fl oz	18
Wild Island	1 fl oz	18
Carlo Rossi		
Blush	1 fl oz	21
Burgundy	1 fl oz	22
Chablis	1 fl oz	21
Paisano	1 fl oz	23
Red Sangria	1 fl oz	24
Rhine	1 fl oz	21
Vin Rose'	1 fl oz	21
White Grenache	1 fl oz	20
Fairbanks		
Cream Sherry	1 fl oz	42
Port	1 fl oz	44
Sherry	1 fl oz	34
White Port	1 fl oz	44
Gallo		
Blush Chablis	1 fl oz	22
Burgundy	1 fl oz	22

FOOD	PORTION	CALS.
Gallo (CONT.)		
Cabernet Sauvignon	1 fl oz	22
Chablis Blanc	1 fl oz	20
Chardonnay	1 fl oz	23
Classic Burgundy	1 fl oz	21
French Colombard	1 fl oz	21
Hearty Burgundy	1 fl oz	22
Johannisbery Riesling '88	1 fl oz	20
Pink Chablis	1 fl oz	20
Red Rose'	1 fl oz	23
Rhine	1 fl oz	22
Sauvignon Blanc '90	1 fl oz	20
White Grenache '92	1 fl oz	20
White Grenache New Vintage	1 fl oz	20
White Zinfandel '91	1 fl oz	18
White Zinfandel New Vintage	1 fl oz	18
Zinfandel '87	1 fl oz	23
Ka-Me		
Chinese Cooking	2 tbsp (1 fl oz)	20
Sheffield Cellars		
Sherry	1 fl oz	44
Tawny Port	1 fl oz	45
Vermouth Extra Dry	1 fl oz	28
Vermouth Sweet	1 fl oz	43
Very Dry Sherry	1 fl oz	32
WINE COOLERS		
Bartles & Jaymes		
Berry	12 fl oz	210
Margarita	12 fl oz	260
Original	12 fl oz	190
Peach	12 fl oz	210
Pina Colada	12 fl oz	280
Planter's Punch	12 fl oz	230
Strawberry	12 fl oz	210
Strawberry Daquiri	12 fl oz	230
Tropical	12 fl oz	230
WINGED BEANS		
dried cooked	1 cup	252
WOLFFISH		
atlantic baked	3 oz	105
YAM		
(*see also* SWEET POTATO)		
CANNED		
Allen		
Cut	⅔ cup (5.8 oz)	160

FOOD	PORTION	CALS.
Bruce		
Cut	½ cup	139
Mashed	½ cup	130
Vacuum Pack	½ cup	122
Whole	½ cup	139
Princella		
Cut	⅔ cup (5.8 oz)	160
Royal Prince		
Whole	4 pieces (5.9 oz)	200
S&W		
Candied	½ cup	180
Southern Whole In Extra Heavy Syrup	½ cup	139
Sugary Sam		
Cut	⅔ cup (5.8 oz)	160
Trappey		
Whole	4 pieces (5.9 oz)	200
FRESH		
mountain yam hawaii cooked	½ cup	59
yam cubed cooked	½ cup	79

YAMBEAN
| cooked | ¾ cup | 38 |

YARDLONG BEANS
| dried cooked | 1 cup | 202 |

YEAST
baker's compressed	1 cake (0.6 oz)	18
baker's dry	1 pkg (¼ oz)	21
baker's dry	1 tbsp	35
brewer's dry	1 tbsp	25
Fleischmann's		
Active Dry	1 pkg (¼ oz)	20
Fresh Active	1 pkg (0.6 oz)	15
Household Yeast	½ oz	15
RapidRise	1 pkg (¼ oz)	20
Red Star		
Small Flakes	3 tbsp (0.5 oz)	47
Yeast	4 tbsp (0.5 oz)	47
Yeast Flakes	3 tbsp (0.5 oz)	47

YELLOW BEANS
CANNED
| low sodium | ½ cup | 13 |
| yellow beans | ½ cup | 13 |

FOOD	PORTION	CALS.
DRIED		
cooked	1 cup	254
FRESH		
cooked	½ cup	22
raw	½ cup	17
FROZEN		
cooked	½ cup	18
YELLOWEYE BEANS		
CANNED		
B&M		
Baked	½ cup (4.6 oz)	170
DRIED		
Bean Cuisine		
Dried	½ cup	115
YELLOWTAIL		
baked	3 oz	159
YOGURT		
(*see also* YOGURT FROZEN)		
coffee lowfat	8 oz	194
fruit lowfat	4 oz	113
fruit lowfat	8 oz	225
plain	8 oz	139
plain lowfat	8 oz	144
plain no fat	8 oz	127
vanilla lowfat	8 oz	194
Breyers		
1% Fat Black Cherry	8 oz	260
1% Fat Blueberry	8 oz	250
1% Fat Mixed Berry	8 oz	250
1% Fat Peach	8 oz	250
1% Fat Pineapple	8 oz	250
1% Fat Red Raspberry	8 oz	250
1% Fat Strawberry	8 oz	250
1% Fat Strawberry Banana	8 oz	250
1.5% Fat Coffee	8 oz	220
1.5% Fat Plain	8 oz	130
1.5% Fat Vanilla	8 oz	220
Cabot		
All Flavors	8 oz	220
Plain	8 oz	140
Colombo		
Banana Strawberry	8 oz	210

FOOD	PORTION	CALS.
Colombo (CONT.)		
Black Cherry	8 oz	200
Blueberry	8 oz	200
Fat Free Apples 'n Spice	8 oz	190
Fat Free Apricot	8 oz	190
Fat Free Banana Strawberry	8 oz	200
Fat Free Blueberry	8 oz	190
Fat Free Cappuccino	8 oz	180
Fat Free Cherry	8 oz	190
Fat Free Cranberry Strawberry	8 oz	200
Fat Free French Roast	8 oz	180
Fat Free Fruit Cocktail	8 oz	190
Fat Free Lemon	8 oz	170
Fat Free Peach	8 oz	190
Fat Free Plain	8 oz	110
Fat Free Raspberry	8 oz	190
Fat Free Strawberry	8 oz	190
Fat Free Strawberry Pineapple Orange	8 oz	190
Fat Free Vanilla	8 oz	170
French Vanilla	8 oz	180
Light 100 Blueberry	8 oz	100
Light 100 Cherry Vanilla	8 oz	100
Light 100 Coffee & Cream	8 oz	100
Light 100 Creamy Vanilla	8 oz	100
Light 100 Fruit Medley	8 oz	100
Light 100 Juicy Peach	8 oz	100
Light 100 Lemon Creme	8 oz	100
Light 100 Mandarin Orange	8 oz	100
Light 100 Mixed Berries	8 oz	100
Light 100 Raspberry	8 oz	100
Light 100 Strawberry	8 oz	100
Peach Melba	8 oz	200
Plain	8 oz	120
Raspberry	8 oz	200
Strawberry	8 oz	200
Dannon		
Blended Nonfat Blueberry	6 oz	160
Blended Nonfat French Vanilla	6 oz	160
Blended Nonfat Lemon Chiffon	6 oz	150
Blended Nonfat Peach	6 oz	150
Blended Nonfat Raspberry	6 oz	160
Blended Nonfat Strawberry	6 oz	150
Blended Nonfat Strawberry Banana	6 oz	150
Daniamls Lowfat Tropical Punch	4.4 oz	140

FOOD	PORTION	CALS.
Dannon (CONT.)		
Danimals Lowfat Blueberry	4.4 oz	140
Danimals Lowfat Grape Lemonade	4.4 oz	130
Danimals Lowfat Lemon Ice	4.4 oz	130
Danimals Lowfat Orange Banana	4.4 oz	140
Danimals Lowfat Strawberry	4.4 oz	140
Danimals Lowfat Vanilla	4.4 oz	140
Danimals Lowfat Wild Raspberry	4.4 oz	130
Fruit On The Bottom Lowfat Apple Cinnamon	8 oz	240
Fruit On The Bottom Lowfat Blueberry	8 oz	240
Fruit On The Bottom Lowfat Boysenberry	8 oz	240
Fruit On The Bottom Lowfat Cherry	8 oz	240
Fruit On The Bottom Lowfat Mixed Berries	8 oz	240
Fruit On The Bottom Lowfat Orange	8 oz	240
Fruit On The Bottom Lowfat Peach	8 oz	240
Fruit On The Bottom Lowfat Pear	8 oz	240
Fruit On The Bottom Lowfat Raspberry	8 oz	240
Fruit On The Bottom Lowfat Strawberry	8 oz	240
Fruit On The Bottom Lowfat Strawberry Banana	8 oz	240
Light Nonfat Banana Cream Pie	4.4 oz	60
Light Nonfat Cherry Vanilla	1 cup (3.5 oz)	110
Light Nonfat Lemon Chiffon	4.4 oz	60
Light Nonfat Peach	4.4 oz	50
Light Nonfat Strawberry	4.4 oz	50
Light Nonfat Strawberry	1 cup (3.5 oz)	110
Light Nonfat Vanilla	1 cup (3.5 oz)	110
Light 'N Crunchy Nonfat Cappuccino w/ Chocolate	1 pkg	150
Light 'N Crunchy Nonfat Caramel Apple Crunch	1 pkg	150
Light 'N Crunchy Nonfat Raspberry w/ Granola	1 pkg	150
Light 'N Crunchy Nonfat Vanilla w/ Chocolate	1 pkg	150
Light Nonfat Banana Cream Pie	8 oz	100
Light Nonfat Blueberry	8 oz	100
Light Nonfat Creme Caramel	8 oz	100
Light Nonfat Lemon	8 oz	100
Light Nonfat Peach	8 oz	100
Light Nonfat Raspberry	8 oz	100
Light Nonfat Strawberry	8 oz	100
Light Nonfat Strawberry Banana	8 oz	100

FOOD	PORTION	CALS.
Dannon (CONT.)		
Light Nonfat Tropical Fruit	8 oz	100
Light Nonfat Vanilla	8 oz	100
Lowfat Coffee	8 oz	210
Lowfat Coffee	1 cup (8.7 oz)	230
Lowfat Cranberry Raspberry	8 oz	210
Lowfat Lemon	8 oz	210
Lowfat Lemon	1 cup (8.7 oz)	230
Lowfat Plain	1 cup (8.7 oz)	150
Lowfat Plain	8 oz	140
Lowfat Vanilla	8 oz	210
Lowfat Vanilla	1 cup (8.7 oz)	230
Minipack Blended Nonfat Blueberry	4.4 oz	120
Minipack Blended Nonfat Cherry	4.4 oz	110
Minipack Blended Nonfat Peach	4.4 oz	110
Minipack Blended Nonfat Raspberry	4.4 oz	120
Minipack Blended Nonfat Strawberry	4.4 oz	110
Minipack Blended Nonfat Strawberry Banana	4.4 oz	110
Nonfat Plain	1 cup (8.7 oz)	120
Nonfat Plain	8 oz	110
Nonfat Light Cherry Vanilla	8 oz	100
Nonfat Light Strawberry Fruit Cup	8 oz	100
Sprinkl'ins Banana	4.1 oz	140
Sprinkl'ins Cherry Vanilla	4.1 oz	140
Sprinkl'ins Crazy Crunch Cherry w/ Honey Grahams	4.4 oz	170
Sprinkl'ins Crazy Crunch Grape w/ Chocolate Grahams	4.4 oz	160
Sprinkl'ins Crazy Crunch Vanilla w/ Chocolate Grahams	4.4 oz	160
Sprinkl'ins Crazy Crunch Vanilla w/ Honey Grahams	4.4 oz	170
Sprinkl'ins Strawberry	4.1 oz	140
Sprinkl'ins Strawberry Banana	4.1 oz	140
Tropifruta Nonfat Banana	6 oz	150
Tropifruta Nonfat Guava	6 oz	150
Tropifruta Nonfat Mango	6 oz	150
Tropifruta Nonfat Papaya Pineapple	6 oz	150
Tropifruta Nonfat Pina Colada	6 oz	150
Tropifruta Nonfat Strawberry	6 oz	150
Tropifruta Nonfat Strawberry Banana	6 oz	150
Tropifruta Nonfat Strawberry Kiwi	6 oz	150
With Fruit Toppings Banana Creme Strawberry	6 oz	170

FOOD	PORTION	CALS.
Dannon (CONT.)		
With Fruit Toppings Bavarian Creme Raspberry	6 oz	170
With Fruit Toppings Cheesecake Cherry	6 oz	170
With Fruit Toppings Cheesecake Strawberry	6 oz	170
With Fruit Toppings Vanilla Peach & Apricot	6 oz	170
With Fruit Toppings Vanilla Strawberry	6 oz	170
Friendship		
Coffee	8 oz	210
Fruit Crunch Blueberry	6 oz	190
Fruit Crunch Peach	6 oz	190
Fruit Crunch Strawberry	6 oz	190
Fruit Crunch Strawberry Banana	6 oz	190
Plain	8 oz	150
Hood		
Fat Free Blueberry	1 (8 oz)	190
Fat Free Cherry	1 (8 oz)	190
Fat Free Peach	1 (8 oz)	190
Fat Free Plain	1 (8 oz)	130
Fat Free Raspberry	1 (8 oz)	190
Fat Free Strawberry	1 (8 oz)	190
Fat Free Strawberry Banana	1 (8 oz)	190
Fat Free Vanilla	1 (8 oz)	190
Fat Free Swiss Blueberry	1 (8 oz)	210
Fat Free Swiss Lemon	1 (8 oz)	210
Fat Free Swiss Raspberry	1 (8 oz)	210
Fat Free Swiss Strawberry	1 (8 oz)	210
Fat Free Swiss Strawberry Banana	1 (8 oz)	210
Fat Free Swiss Vanilla	1 (8 oz)	210
Knudsen		
1.5% Fat Creamy Lemon	8 oz	220
70 Calories Black Cherry	6 oz	70
70 Calories Blueberry	6 oz	70
70 Calories Lemon	6 oz	70
70 Calories Peach	6 oz	70
70 Calories Pineapple	6 oz	70
70 Calories Red Raspberry	6 oz	70
70 Calories Strawberry	6 oz	70
70 Calories Strawberry Banana	6 oz	70
70 Calories Strawberry Fruit Basket	6 oz	70
70 Calories Vanilla	6 oz	70
Free Lemon	6 oz	160

FOOD	PORTION	CALS.
Knudsen (CONT.)		
Free Mixed Berry	6 oz	170
Free Peach	6 oz	170
Free Red Raspberry	6 oz	170
Free Strawberry	6 oz	170
Free Vanilla	6 oz	170
La Yogurt		
French Style Banana	6 oz	180
French Style Blueberry	6 oz	180
French Style Cherry	6 oz	180
French Style Cherry Vanilla	6 oz	190
French Style Guava	6 oz	180
French Style Key Lime	6 oz	180
French Style Mango	6 oz	180
French Style Mixed Berry	6 oz	180
French Style Nonfat Blueberry	6 oz	70
French Style Nonfat Cherry	6 oz	75
French Style Nonfat Raspberry	6 oz	70
French Style Nonfat Strawberry	6 oz	70
French Style Nonfat Strawberry Banana	6 oz	70
French Style Peach	6 oz	180
French Style Pina Colada	6 oz	180
French Style Raspberry	6 oz	180
French Style Strawberry	6 oz	180
French Style Strawberry Banana	6 oz	180
French Style Strawberry Fruit Cup	6 oz	180
French Style Tropical Orange	6 oz	180
French Style Vanilla	6 oz	170
Latin Style Banana	6 oz	190
Latin Style Guava	6 oz	190
Latin Style Mango	6 oz	190
Latin Style Papaya	6 oz	190
Latin Style Passion Fruit	6 oz	190
Latin Style Strawberry Kiwi	6 oz	180
Light N'Lively		
Free Blueberry	6 oz	190
Free Lemon	6 oz	170
Free Mixed Berry	6 oz	170
Free Peach	6 oz	170
Free Red Raspberry	6 oz	180
Free Strawberry	6 oz	180
Free Strawberry Fruit Cup	6 oz	170
Free Vanilla	6 oz	160
Free 50 Calories Blueberry	4.4 oz	50

FOOD	PORTION	CALS.
Light N'Lively (CONT.)		
Free 50 Calories Peach	4.4 oz	50
Free 50 Calories Red Raspberry	4.4 oz	50
Free 50 Calories Strawberry	4.4 oz	50
Free 50 Calories Strawberry Banana	4.4 oz	50
Free 50 Calories Strawberry Fruit Cup	4.4 oz	50
Free 70 Calories Black Cherry	6 oz	70
Free 70 Calories Blueberry	6 oz	70
Free 70 Calories Lemon	6 oz	70
Free 70 Calories Peach	6 oz	70
Free 70 Calories Red Raspberry	6 oz	70
Free 70 Calories Strawberry	6 oz	70
Free 70 Calories Strawberry Banana	6 oz	70
Free 70 Calories Strawberry Fruit Cup	6 oz	70
Kidpack Banana Berry	4.4 oz	130
Kidpack Berry Blue	4.4 oz	150
Kidpack Cherry	4.4 oz	140
Kidpack Grape	4.4 oz	130
Kidpack Outrageous Orange	4.4 oz	150
Kidpack Tropical Punch	4.4 oz	140
Kidpack Wild Berry	4.4 oz	140
Kidpack Wild Strawberry	4.4 oz	140
Multipack Blueberry	4.4 oz	140
Multipack Peach	4.4 oz	140
Multipack Pineapple	4.4 oz	140
Multipack Red Raspberry	4.4 oz	130
Multipack Strawberry	4.4 oz	140
Multipack Strawberry Banana	4.4 oz	140
Multipack Strawberry Fruit Cup	4.4 oz	140
Lite Line		
Swiss Style Cherry Vanilla	1 cup	240
Swiss Style Peach	1 cup	230
Swiss Style Plain	1 cup	140
Swiss Style Strawberry	1 cup	240
Meadow Gold		
Plain	1 cup	160
Sundae Style Raspberry	1 cup	250
Mountain High		
Blueberry	1 cup	220
Plain	1 cup	200
Weight Watchers		
Ultimate 90 Blueberries 'n Creme	1 cup	90
Ultimate 90 Cappuccino	1 cup	90
Ultimate 90 Cherries Jubilee	1 cup	90

FOOD	PORTION	CALS.
Weight Watchers (CONT.)		
Ultimate 90 Cranberry Raspberry	1 cup	90
Ultimate 90 Lemon Chiffon	1 cup	90
Ultimate 90 Plain	1 cup	90
Ultimate 90 Raspberries 'n Creme	1 cup	90
Ultimate 90 Strawberry	1 cup	90
Ultimate 90 Strawberry Banana	1 cup	90
Ultimate 90 Vanilla	1 cup	90
Utlimate 90 Peach	1 cup	90
Yoplait		
Custard Style Banana	6 oz	190
Custard Style Blueberry	6 oz	190
Custard Style Cherry	6 oz	180
Custard Style Lemon	6 oz	190
Custard Style Mixed Berry	6 oz	180
Custard Style Raspberry	6 oz	190
Custard Style Strawberry	4 oz	130
Custard Style Strawberry	6 oz	190
Custard Style Strawberry Banana	6 oz	190
Custard Style Strawvberry Banana	4 oz	130
Custard Style Vanilla	4 oz	130
Custard Style Vanilla	6 oz	180
Fat Free Blueberry	6 oz	150
Fat Free Cherry	6 oz	150
Fat Free Mixed Berry	6 oz	150
Fat Free Peach	6 oz	150
Fat Free Raspberry	6 oz	150
Fat Free Strawberry	6 oz	150
Fat Free Strawberry Banana	6 oz	150
Light Blueberry	4 oz	60
Light Blueberry	6 oz	80
Light Cherry	6 oz	80
Light Cherry	4 oz	60
Light Peach	4 oz	60
Light Peach	6 oz	80
Light Raspberry	6 oz	80
Light Raspberry	4 oz	60
Light Strawberry	6 oz	80
Light Strawberry	4 oz	60
Light Strawberry Banana	6 oz	80
Light Strawberry Banana	4 oz	60
Nonfat Plain	8 oz	120
Nonfat Vanilla	8 oz	180
Original Apple	6 oz	190

FOOD	PORTION	CALS.
Yoplait (CONT.)		
Original Blueberry	6 oz	190
Original Blueberry	4 oz	120
Original Boysenberry	6 oz	190
Original Cherry	6 oz	190
Original Lemon	6 oz	190
Original Mixed Berry	6 oz	190
Original Orange	6 oz	190
Original Peach	6 oz	190
Original Peach	4 oz	120
Original Pina Colada	6 oz	190
Original Pineapple	6 oz	190
Original Plain	6 oz	130
Original Raspberry	6 oz	190
Original Raspberry	4 oz	120
Original Strawberry	6 oz	190
Original Strawberry	4 oz	120
Original Strawberry Banana	6 oz	190
Original Strawberry Rhubarb	6 oz	190
Original Vanilla	6 oz	180

YOGURT FROZEN
(see also TOFU YOGURT)

FOOD	PORTION	CALS.
chocolate soft serve	½ cup (4 fl oz)	115
vanilla soft serve	½ cup (4 fl oz)	114
Bee-Lite		
Chocolate	4 oz	100
Vanilla	4 oz	110
Ben & Jerry's		
Cherry Garcia	½ cup (3.7 oz)	170
Chocolate Fudge Brownie	½ cup (3.7 oz)	190
Coffee Almond Fudge	½ cup (3.7 oz)	200
English Toffee Crunch	½ cup (3.7 oz)	190
No Fat Cappuccino	½ cup (3.3 oz)	140
Pop Cherry Garcia	1 (3.8 oz)	290
Borden		
Strawberry	½ cup	100
Bresler's		
All Flavors	5 oz	145
All Flavors Lite	5 oz	135
Breyers		
Chocolate	½ cup (2.7 oz)	150
Fight Fat Free Black Cherry Jubilee	1 cup (8 oz)	130
Light Fat Free Apple Pie A La Mode	1 cup (8 oz)	130

FOOD	PORTION	CALS.
Breyers (CONT.)		
Light Fat Free Blueberries n' Cream	1 cup (8 oz)	130
Light Fat Free Cherry Chocolate	1 cup (8 oz)	130
Light Fat Free Classic Strawberry	1 cup (8 oz)	130
Light Fat Free Key Lime Pie	1 cup (8 oz)	130
Light Fat Free Lemon Chiffon	1 cup (8 oz)	130
Light Fat Free Peaches n'Cream	1 cup (8 oz)	130
Light Fat Free Strawberry Cheesecake	1 cup (8 oz)	130
Red Raspberry	½ cup (2.7 oz)	140
Strawberry Banana	½ cup (2.7 oz)	140
Vanilla	½ cup (2.7 oz)	140
Dannon		
Coco-Nut Fudge	½ cup (3 oz)	160
Light Cappuccino	½ cup (2.8 oz)	80
Light Cherry Vanilla Swirl	½ cup (2.8 oz)	90
Light Chocolate	½ cup (2.7 oz)	80
Light Lemon Chiffon	½ cup (2.8 oz)	90
Light Peach Raspberry Melba	½ cup (2.8 oz)	90
Light Strawberry Cheesecake	½ cup (2.8 oz)	90
Light Vanilla	½ cup (2.8 oz)	80
Light Nonfat Cappuccino	8 oz	100
Light'N Crunchy Banana Cream Pie	½ cup (2.8 oz)	110
Light'N Crunchy Mocha Chocolate Chunk	½ cup (2.8 oz)	110
Light'N Crunchy Peanut Chocolate Crunch	½ cup (2.8 oz)	110
Light'N Crunchy Triple Chocolate	½ cup (2.8 oz)	110
Light'N Crunchy Vanilla Blueberry Swirl	½ cup (2.8 oz)	110
Pure Indulgence Cherry Chocolate Cherry	½ cup (3 oz)	150
Pure Indulgence Chunky Chocolate Nut	½ cup (3 oz)	150
Pure Indulgence Cookies'n Cream	½ cup (3 oz)	150
Pure Indulgence Vanilla Raspberry Truffle	½ cup (3 oz)	150
Desserve		
All Flavors	4 oz	70
Dutch Chocolate	4 oz	80
Edy's		
Banana Strawberry	3 oz	80
Blueberry	3 oz	80
Cherry	3 oz	80
Chocolate	3 oz	80
Chocolate Chip	3 oz	100
Citrus Heights	3 oz	80
Cookies'N'Cream	3 oz	100
Marble Fudge	3 oz	100
Perfectly Peach	3 oz	80
Raspberry	3 oz	80

FOOD	PORTION	CALS.
Edy's (CONT.)		
Raspberry Vanilla Swirl	3 oz	80
Strawberry	3 oz	80
Vanilla	3 oz	80
Elan		
Blueberry	4 oz	130
Caramel Almond Praline	4 oz	150
Chocolate	4 oz	130
Chocolate Almond	4 oz	160
Coffee	4 oz	130
Coffee Decaffeinated	4 oz	130
Peach	4 oz	130
Rum Raisin	4 oz	135
Strawberry	4 oz	125
Vanilla	4 oz	130
Fi-Bar		
Chocolate	1	190
Strawberry	1	190
Vanilla	1	190
Friendly's		
Apple Bettie	½ cup (2.6 oz)	140
Fabulous Fudge Swirl	½ cup (2.6 oz)	140
Fudge Berry Swirl	½ cup (2.6 oz)	150
Lowfat Perfectly Peach	½ cup (2.6 oz)	110
Lowfat Purely Chocolate	½ cup (2.6 oz)	120
Lowfat Raspberry Delight	½ cup (2.6 oz)	120
Lowfat Simply Vanilla	½ cup (2.6 oz)	120
Lowfat Strawberry Patch	½ cup (2.6 oz)	110
Mint Chocolate Chip	½ cup (2.6 oz)	130
Strawberry Cheesecake Blast	½ cup (2.6 oz)	140
Toffee Almond Crunch	½ cup (2.6 oz)	160
Good Humor		
Creamsicle Raspberry	1 (2.8 oz)	100
Frista Cup	1 (6.2 oz)	220
Haagen-Dazs		
Banana Nut Blast	½ cup (3.5 oz)	220
Bars Cherry Chocolate Fudge	1 (2.6 oz)	240
Bars Peach	1 (2.5 oz)	90
Bars Pina Colada	1 (2.5 oz)	100
Bars Raspberry & Vanilla	1 (2.5 oz)	90
Bars Strawberry Daiquiri	1 (2.5 oz)	90
Chocolate	½ cup (3.4 oz)	160
Coffee	½ cup (3.4 oz)	160
Fat Free Cherry Vanilla	½ cup (3.3 oz)	140

FOOD	PORTION	CALS.
Haagen-Dazs (CONT.)		
Fat Free Chocolate	½ cup (3.3 oz)	140
Fat Free Coffee	½ cup (3.3 oz)	140
Fat Free Vanilla	½ cup (3.3 oz)	140
Fat Free Vanilla Fudge	½ cup (3.3 oz)	160
Orange Tango	½ cup (3.5 oz)	130
Pina Colada	½ cup (3.4 oz)	130
Raspberry Randevous	½ cup (3.5 oz)	130
Strawberry Cheesecake Craze	½ cup (3.6 oz)	220
Strawberry Duet	½ cup (3.4 oz)	130
Vanilla	½ cup (3.4 oz)	160
Hood		
Bavarian Truffle & Twist	½ cup (2.6 oz)	150
Coffee Toffee Chunk Sundae	½ cup (2.6 oz)	150
Combo Bars	1 (2.2 oz)	90
Cookies & Cream	½ cup (2.6 oz)	140
Grandma's Raisin Oatmeal Cookie Dough	½ cup (2.6 oz)	140
Mixed Berry Swirl	½ cup (2.6 oz)	120
Natural Strawberry	½ cup (2.6 oz)	110
Natural Strawberry Banana	½ cup (2.6 oz)	110
Natural Vanilla	½ cup (2.6 oz)	120
Nonfat Caramel & Brownie Sundae	½ cup (2.6 oz)	120
Nonfat Chocolate Marshmallow	½ cup (2.6 oz)	110
Nonfat Double Raspberry	½ cup (2.6 oz)	120
Nonfat Mocha Fudge	½ cup (2.6 oz)	120
Nonfat Olde Fashioned Vanilla	½ cup (2.6 oz)	110
Nonfat Peach Cobbler A La Mode	½ cup (2.6 oz)	110
Nonfat Strawberry	½ cup (2.6 oz)	100
Nonfat Vanilla Fudge	½ cup (2.6 oz)	120
Raspberry Swirl	½ cup (2.6 oz)	130
Sundae Cups Chocolate & Strawberry	1 (2.2 oz)	110
Vanilla Chocolate Strawberry	½ cup (2.6 oz)	120
Vanilla Swiss Almond Sundae	½ cup (2.6 oz)	150
Just 10		
All Flavors	1 oz	10
Kissed With Honey		
Chocolate	3.5 oz	100
Nonfat Chocolate	3.5 oz	85
Nonfat Vanilla	3.5 oz	85
Vanilla	3.5 oz	100
Meadow Gold		
Strawberry	½ cup	100
Sealtest		
Chocolate	½ cup (2.7 oz)	120

FOOD	PORTION	CALS.
Sealtest (CONT.)		
Mocha Fudge	½ cup (2.6 oz)	130
Vanilla	½ cup (2.6 oz)	120
Tofutti		
Better Than Yogurt Chocolate Fudge	4 fl oz	120
Better Than Yogurt Coffee Mashmallow Swirl	4 fl oz	100
Better Than Yogurt Peach Mango	4 fl oz	100
Better Than Yogurt Strawberry Banana	4 fl oz	100
Better Than Yogurt Vanilla Fudge	4 fl oz	120
Turkey Hill		
Chocolate Cherry Cordial	½ cup (2.6 oz)	130
Chocolate Chip Cookie Dough	½ cup (2.6 oz)	140
Death By Chocolate	½ cup (2.6 oz)	150
Nonfat Chocolate Marshmallow	½ cup (2.4 oz)	130
Nonfat Coffee Cappuccino	½ cup (2.4 oz)	110
Nonfat Mint Cookie 'N Cream	½ cup (2.4 oz)	110
Nonfat Neapolitan	½ cup (2.4 oz)	100
Nonfat Raspberry Chocolate Bliss	½ cup (2.4 oz)	110
Nonfat Southern Lemon Pie	½ cup (2.4 oz)	110
Nonfat Vanilla Fudge	½ cup (2.4 oz)	110
Peach Raspberry	½ cup (2.6 oz)	110
Strawberry	½ cup (2.6 oz)	110
Tin Roof Sundae	½ cup (2.6 oz)	140
Vanilla & Chocolate	½ cup (2.6 oz)	110
Vanilla Bean	½ cup (2.6 oz)	110

ZABAGLIONE
(*see* CUSTARD)

ZUCCHINI

CANNED		
italian style	½ cup	33
Del Monte		
With Italian Tomato Sauce	½ cup (4.2 oz)	30
Progresso		
Italian Style	½ cup (4.2 oz)	40
S&W		
Italian Style	½ cup	45
FRESH		
baby raw	1 (½ oz)	3
raw sliced	½ cup	9
sliced cooked	½ cup	14
FROZEN		
cooked	½ cup	19

FOOD	PORTION	CALS.
Big Valley		
Zucchini	¾ cup (3 oz)	10
Empire		
Breaded	1 (2.9 oz)	100
Southland		
Zucchini Sliced	3.2 oz	15

PART · TWO

RESTAURANT

AND

FAST-FOOD CHAINS

FOOD	PORTION	CALS.

ARBY'S
BEVERAGES

FOOD	PORTION	CALS.
Chocolate Shake	1 (12 oz)	451
Jamocha Shake	1 (12 oz)	384
Vanilla Shake	1 (12 oz)	360

BREAKFAST SELECTIONS

FOOD	PORTION	CALS.
Bacon	2 strips (0.53 oz)	90
Biscuit Plain	1 (2.9 oz)	280
Blueberry Muffin	1 (2.3 oz)	230
Cinnamon Nut Danish	1 (3.5 oz)	360
Croissant Plain	1 (2 oz)	220
Egg Portion	1 serv (1.6 oz)	95
Ham	1 serv (1.5 oz)	45
Sausage	1 (1.3 oz)	163
Swiss	1 serv (0.5 oz)	45
Table Syrup	1 serv (1 oz)	100
Toastix	6 pieces (4.4 oz)	430

DESSERTS

FOOD	PORTION	CALS.
Apple Turnover	1 (3.2 oz)	330
Cheesecake Plain	1 serv (3 oz)	320
Cherry Turnover	1 (3.2 oz)	320
Chocolate Chip Cookie	1 (1 oz)	125
Polar Swirl Butterfinger	1 (11.6 oz)	457
Polar Swirl Heath	1 (11.6 oz)	543
Polar Swirl Oreo	1 (11.6 oz)	329
Polar Swirl Peanut Butter Cup	1 (11.6 oz)	517
Polar Swirl Snickers	1 (11.6 oz)	511

MAIN MENU SELECTIONS

FOOD	PORTION	CALS.
Arby's Sauce	1 serv (0.5 oz)	15
Baked Potato Broccoli'n Cheddar	1 (15.7 oz)	571
Baked Potato Deluxe	1 (15.3 oz)	736
Baked Potato Plain	1 (11.5 oz)	355
Baked Potato w/ Margarine & Sour Cream	1 (14 oz)	578
Barbeque Sauce	1 serv (0.5 oz)	30
Beef Stock Au Jus	1 serv (2 oz)	10
Breaded Chicken Fillet	1 (7.2 oz)	536
Cheddar Cheese Sauce	1 serv (0.75 oz)	35
Cheddar Curly Fried	1 serv (4.25 oz)	333
Chicken Cordon Bleu	1 (8.5 oz)	623
Chicken Finger	2 (3.6 oz)	290
Curly Fries	1 serv (3.5 oz)	300
Fish Fillet Sandwich	1 (7.7 oz)	529
French Fries	1 serv (2.5 oz)	246

FOOD	PORTION	CALS.
Garden Salad	1 (11.9 oz)	61
Grilled Chicken BBQ	1 (7.1 oz)	388
Grilled Chicken Deluxe	1 (8.1 oz)	430
Ham 'n Cheese Sandwich	1 (5.9 oz)	359
Ham'n Cheese Melt	1 (4.9 oz)	329
Honey Mayonnaise Reduced Calorie	1 serv (0.5 oz)	70
Horsey Sauce	1 serv (0.5 oz)	60
Italian Sub	1 (10.1 oz)	675
Italian Sub Sauce	1 serv (0.5 oz)	70
Ketchup	1 serv (0.5 oz)	16
Light Roast Beef Deluxe	1 (6.4 oz)	296
Light Roast Chicken Deluxe	1 (6.8 oz)	276
Light Roast Chicken Salad	1 serv (14.4 oz)	149
Light Roast Turkey Deluxe	1 (6.8 oz)	260
Mayonnaise	1 serv (0.5 oz)	110
Mayonnaise Light Cholesterol Free	1 serv (0.25 oz)	12
Mustard German Style	1 serv (0.16 oz)	5
Parmesan Cheese Sauce	1 serv (0.5 oz)	70
Potato Cakes	2 (3 oz)	204
Roast Beef Arby's Melt w/ Cheddar	1 (5.2 oz)	368
Roast Beef Arby-Q	1 (6.4 oz)	431
Roast Beef Bac'n Cheddar Deluxe	1 (8.1 oz)	539
Roast Beef Beef'n Cheddar	1 (6.7 oz)	487
Roast Beef Gaint	1 (8.1 oz)	555
Roast Beef Junior	1 (4.4 oz)	324
Roast Beef Regular	1 (5.4 oz)	388
Roast Beef Super	1 (8.7 oz)	523
Roast Chicken Club	1 (8.5 oz)	546
Roast Chicken Deluxe	1 (7.6 oz)	433
Roast Chicken Santa Fe	1 (6.4 oz)	436
Side Salad	1 (5 oz)	23
Sub Roll French Dip	1 (6.8 oz)	475
Sub Roll Hot Ham 'n Swiss	1 (9.3 oz)	500
Sub Roll Pilly Beef'n Swiss	1 (10.4 oz)	755
Sub Roll Triple Cheese Melt	1 (8.4 oz)	720
Tartar Sauce	1 serv (1 oz)	140
Turkey Sub	1 (9.8 oz)	550
SALAD DRESSINGS		
Blue Cheese	1 serv (2 oz)	290
Buttermilk Ranch Reduced Calorie	1 serv (2 oz)	50
Honey French	1 serv (2 oz)	280
Italian Reduced Calorie	1 serv (2 oz)	20
Red Ranch	1 serv (0.5 oz)	75
Thousand Island	1 serv (2 oz)	260

FOOD	PORTION	CALS.
SOUPS		
Boston Clam Chowder	1 serv (8 oz)	190
Cream of Broccoli	1 serv (8 oz)	160
Lumberjack Mixed Vegetable	1 serv (8 oz)	90
Old Fashioned Chicken Noodle	1 serv (8 oz)	80
Potato w/ Bacon	1 serv (8 oz)	170
Timberline Chili	1 serv (8 oz)	220
Wisconsin Cheese	1 serv (8 oz)	280
AU BON PAIN		
BAKED GOODS		
Bagel Cinnamon Raisin	1 (4.9 oz)	360
Bagel Onion	1 (5.1 oz)	370
Bagel Plain	1 (4.8 oz)	350
Bagel Poppy Seed	1 (5.1 oz)	380
Baguette Loaf	1 slice (1.8 oz)	140
Braided Roll	1 (1.8 oz)	170
Cheese Loaf	1 slice (1.8 oz)	40
Country Seed Roll	1 (2.6 oz)	220
Croissant Almond	1 (4.3 oz)	560
Croissant Apple	1 (3.4 oz)	260
Croissant Chocolate	1 (3.1 oz)	390
Croissant Cinnamon Raisin	1 (3.7 oz)	380
Croissant Plain	1 (2.1 oz)	270
Croissant Raspberry Cheese	1 (3.5 oz)	380
Croissant Strawberry Cheese	1 (3.5 oz)	370
Croissant Sweet Cheese	1 (3.6 oz)	390
Four Grain Loaf	1 slice (1.8 oz)	130
French Sandwich Roll	1 (1.8 oz)	120
Hearth Roll	1 (2.8 oz)	220
Hearth Sandwich Roll	1 (1.8 oz)	140
Low Fat Muffin Cinnamon Cranapple	1 (4.6 oz)	280
Low Fat Muffin Pineapple	1 (4.2 oz)	280
Low Fat Muffin Triple Berry	1 (4.2 oz)	270
Muffin Blueberry	1 (4.5 oz)	410
Muffin Carrot	1 (5 oz)	480
Muffin Chocolate Chip	1 (4.5 oz)	490
Muffin Corn	1 (4.6 oz)	470
Multigrain Loaf	1 slice (1.8 oz)	130
Parisienne Loaf	1 slice (1.8 oz)	120
Petit Pain Roll	1 (2.5 oz)	200
Rye Loaf	1 slice (1.8 oz)	110
Sandwich Croissant	1 (2.6 oz)	310
Scone Blueberry	1 (4 oz)	430

FOOD	PORTION	CALS.
Scone Cinnamon	1 (4.1 oz)	520
Scone Orange	1 (4.1 oz)	440
Sesame Roll	1 (5.1 oz)	390
BEVERAGES		
Hot Apple Cider	1 lg (20 oz)	350
Hot Apple Cider	1 med (16 oz)	310
Hot Apple Cider	1 sm (10 oz)	190
Hot Raspberry Mocha Blast	1 serv (20 oz)	350
Hot Raspberry Mocha Blast	1 serv (10 oz)	180
Hot Raspberry Mocha Blast	1 serv (16 oz)	300
Iced Caffee Latte	1 sm (9 oz)	130
Iced Caffee Latte	1 med (12 oz)	150
Iced Caffee Latte	1 lg (20.5 oz)	270
Iced Cappuccino	1 sm (9 oz)	110
Iced Cappuccino	1 lg (20.5 oz)	270
Iced Cappuccino	1 med (12 oz)	150
Iced Cocoa	1 lg (20.5 oz)	440
Iced Cocoa	1 med (12 oz)	280
Iced Cocoa	1 sm (9 oz)	200
Iced Mocha Blast	1 sm (9 oz)	180
Iced Mocha Blast	1 med (12 oz)	260
Iced Mocha Blast	1 lg (20.5 oz)	360
Iced Raspberry Mocha Blast	1 serv (16 oz)	210
Iced Raspberry Mocha Blast	1 serv (12 oz)	160
Iced Raspberry Mocha Blast	1 serv (24 oz)	330
Whipped Cream	1 serv (1.2 oz)	160
DESSERTS		
Biscotti	1 (1.5 oz)	200
Biscotti Chocolate	1 (1.7 oz)	240
Cookie Chocolate Chip	1 (2.1 oz)	280
Cookie Oatmeal Raisin	1 (2.1 oz)	250
Cookie Peanut Butter	1 (2.1 oz)	280
Cookie Shortbread	1 (2.4 oz)	390
Danish Raspberry	1 (3.6 oz)	370
Danish Sweet Cheese	1 (3.6 oz)	420
Pecan Roll	1 (6.8 oz)	900
SALAD DRESSINGS		
Bleu Cheese	3 oz	410
Buttermilk Ranch	3 oz	310
Ceasar	3 oz	380
Fat Free Tomato Basil	3 oz	70
Greek	3 oz	440
Honey Mustard	3 oz	380
Lemon Basil Vinaigrette	3 oz	330

FOOD	PORTION	CALS.
Lite Italian	3 oz	230
Mandarin Orange	3 oz	380
Sesame French	3 oz	370
SALADS AND SALAD BARS		
Antipasto	1 serv (12.9 oz)	410
Caesar	1 serv (8.9 oz)	270
Chicken Caesar	1 serv (11.4 oz)	360
Chicken Tarragon	1 serv (16 oz)	470
Garden	1 lg (10.6 oz)	160
Garden	1 sm (7.5 oz)	100
Greek	1 serv (10.5 oz)	300
Oriental Chicken	1 serv (14.2 oz)	230
Tuna	1 serv (15 oz)	490
SANDWICHES AND FILLINGS		
Brie	½ serv (1.5 oz)	140
Cheddar Cheese	½ serv (1.5 oz)	170
Chicken Cracked Pepper	1 serv (3.9 oz)	140
Chicken Tarragon	1 serv (4 oz)	240
Country Ham	1 serv (3.7 oz)	150
Grilled Chicken	1 serv (3.9 oz)	140
Herb Cheese	½ serv (1.5 oz)	150
Hot Croissant Ham & Cheese	1 (4.2 oz)	380
Hot Croissant Spinach & Cheese	1 (3.6 oz)	270
Hot Croissant Turkey & Cheddar	1 (4.2 oz)	390
Lite Cream Cheese	1 serv (1.9 oz)	110
Provolone	½ serv (1.5 oz)	150
Roast Beef	1 serv (3.7 oz)	140
Swiss	½ serv (1.5 oz)	160
Tuna Salad	1 serv (4.5 oz)	360
Turkey Breast	1 serv (3.7 oz)	120
SOUPS		
Beef Barley	1 serv (12 oz)	112
Beef Barley	1 serv (8 oz)	75
Beef Barley	1 serv (16 oz)	150
Beef Stew	1 serv (16 oz)	280
Beef Stew	1 serv (8 oz)	140
Beef Stew	1 serv (12 oz)	210
Broccoli & Cheddar	1 serv (16 oz)	520
Broccoli & Cheddar	1 serv (12 oz)	390
Broccoli & Cheddar	1 serv (8 oz)	260
Chicken & Sausage Gumbo	1 serv (12 oz)	230
Chicken & Sausage Gumbo	1 serv (16 oz)	310
Chicken & Sausage Gumbo	1 serv (8 oz)	160
Chicken Noodle	1 serv (8 oz)	80

FOOD	PORTION	CALS.
Chicken Noodle	1 serv (12 oz)	120
Chicken Noodle	1 serv (16 oz)	170
Chicken Wild Rice	1 serv (12 oz)	130
Chicken Wild Rice	1 serv (16 oz)	180
Chicken Wild Rice	1 serv (8 oz)	90
Chili	1 serv (16 oz)	460
Chili	1 serv (8 oz)	230
Chili	1 serv (12 oz)	340
Clam Chowder	1 serv (16 oz)	540
Clam Chowder	1 serv (8 oz)	270
Clam Chowder	1 serv (12 oz)	400
Corn Chowder	1 serv (8 oz)	260
Corn Chowder	1 serv (12 oz)	390
Corn Chowder	1 serv (16 oz)	530
Cream Of Broccoli	1 serv (12 oz)	330
Cream Of Broccoli	1 serv (8 oz)	220
Cream Of Broccoli	1 serv (16 oz)	440
Cream Of Chicken With Wild Rice	1 serv (16 oz)	330
Cream Of Chicken With Wild Rice	1 serv (12 oz)	250
Cream Of Chicken With Wild Rice	1 serv (8 oz)	160
Garden Vegetable	1 serv (1 cup)	29
Garden Vegetable	1 serv (16 oz)	58
Garden Vegetable	1 serv (12 oz)	45
Seafood Gumbo	1 serv (12 oz)	190
Seafood Gumbo	1 serv (8 oz)	130
Seafood Gumbo	1 serv (16 oz)	260
Split Pea	1 serv (16 oz)	352
Split Pea	1 serv (12 oz)	265
Split Pea	1 serv (8 oz)	176
Tomato Florentine	1 serv (16 oz)	122
Tomato Florentine	1 serv (12 oz)	90
Tomato Florentine	1 serv (8 oz)	61
Tomato Tortellini	1 serv (8 oz)	60
Tomato Tortellini	1 serv (12 oz)	90
Tomato Tortellini	1 serv (16 oz)	110
Vegetable Stew	1 serv (8 oz)	60
Vegetable Stew	1 serv (12 oz)	100
Vegetable Stew	1 serv (16 oz)	130
Vegetarean Chili	1 serv (12 oz)	210
Vegetarean Chili	1 serv (8 oz)	139
Vegetarean Chili	1 serv (16 oz)	278
Vegetarian Lentil	1 serv (8 oz)	130
Vegetarian Lentil	1 serv (12 oz)	200
Vegetarian Lentil	1 serv (16 oz)	270

FOOD	PORTION	CALS.
BASKIN-ROBBINS		
Sugar Cone	1	60
Waffle Cone	1	140
FROZEN YOGURT		
Cafe Mocha	½ cup (4 fl oz)	70
Chocolate Nonfat	½ cup	110
Chocolate Vanilla	½ cup	110
Dutch Chocolate Chip Bar	1	260
Pralines Vanilla Bar	1	250
Strawberry Low-Fat	½ cup (4 fl oz)	120
Strawberry Nonfat	½ cup	110
Wild Cherry	½ cup (4 fl oz)	70
ICE CREAM		
Almond Butter Crunch Light	½ cup	130
Butter Pecan	½ cup	160
Butterfinger	½ cup	170
Caramel Banana Fat Free	½ cup	100
Cherry Cordial Sugar Free	½ cup	100
Chewy Babyruth	½ cup	190
Chilly Burgers Vanilla	1	240
Chocolate	½ cup	150
Chocolate Almond	½ cup	170
Chocolate Chip	½ cup	150
Chocolate Chip Sugar Free	½ cup	100
Chocolate Fudge	½ cup	170
Chocolate Mousse Royale	½ cup	180
Chocolate Raspberry Truffle	½ cup	180
Chocolate Vanilla Fat Free	½ cup	100
Chocolate Wonder Fat Free	½ cup	120
Chunky Banana Sugar Free	½ cup	80
Coconut Caramel Nut Light	½ cup	130
Cookies N Cream	½ cup	160
Double Raspberry Light	½ cup	120
Espresso N Cream Light	½ cup	120
French Vanilla	½ cup	170
Fudge Brownie	½ cup	180
Gold Medal Ribbon	½ cup	150
Jamoca Almond Fudge	½ cup	150
Jamoca Swirl Fat Free	½ cup	100
Jamoca Swiss Almond Sugar Free	½ cup	90
Just Peachy Fat Free	½ cup	100
Kahula N Cream	½ cup	160
Mint Chocolate Chip	½ cup	150

FOOD	PORTION	CALS.
Peanut Butter Chocolate	½ cup	190
Pineapple Cheesecake Fat Free	½ cup	110
Pineapple Coconut Sugar Free	½ cup	90
Pistachio Almond	½ cup	160
Praline Dream Light	½ cup	130
Pralines N Cream	½ cup	160
Reeses Peanut Butter Cup	½ cup	170
Rocky Road	½ cup	170
Strawberry Sugar Free	½ cup	80
Thin Mint Chip Sugar Free	½ cup	90
Tiny Toon Adventures Toonwiches Chocolate	1	330
Tiny Toon Adventures Toonwiches Vanilla	1	340
Tiny Toon Adventures Bar Mint Chocolate Chip	1	230
Tiny Toon Adventures Bar Vanilla	1	210
Vanilla	½ cup	140
Vanilla Fudge Light	½ cup	110
Very Berry Strawberry	½ cup	120
World Class Chocolate	½ cup	160
ICES AND ICE POPS		
Daiquiri Ice	1 scoop	140
Rainbow Sherbet	1 scoop	160
Sorbet Strawberry	½ cup (4 fl oz)	100
BEN & JERRY'S		
Sugar Cone	1	48
FROZEN YOGURT		
Cherry Garcia	½ cup (2.7 oz)	140
Chocolate Chip Cookie Dough	½ cup (2.7 oz)	180
Chocolate Fudge Brownie	½ cup (2.7 oz)	160
Coffee Almond Fudge	½ cup (2.7 oz)	180
English Toffee Crunch	½ cup (2.7 oz)	180
No Fat Cappuccino	½ cup (2.7 oz)	120
No Fat Chocolate	½ cup (2.7 oz)	120
No Fat Peach Melba	½ cup (2.7 oz)	110
No Fat Raspberry	½ cup (2.7 oz)	120
No Fat Strawberry	½ cup (2.7 oz)	120
No Fat Vanilla	½ cup (2.7 oz)	120
Strawberry Cheesecake	½ cup (2.7 oz)	140
Vanilla Fudge	½ cup (2.7 oz)	140
ICE CREAM		
Apple Pie	½ cup (2.7 oz)	200
Aztec Harvests Coffee	½ cup (2.7 oz)	180
Banana Walnut	½ cup (2.7 oz)	240

FOOD	PORTION	CALS.
Butter Pecan	½ cup (2.7 oz)	250
Cappuccino Chocolate Chunk	½ cup (2.7 oz)	220
Cherry Garcia	½ cup (2.7 oz)	200
Cherry Vanilla	½ cup (2.7 oz)	180
Chocolate Amaretto	½ cup (2.7 oz)	180
Chocolate Chip Cookie Dough	½ cup (2.7 oz)	230
Chocolate Fudge Brownie	½ cup (2.7 oz)	200
Chocolate Orange Fudge	½ cup (2.7 oz)	190
Chocolate Peanut Butter Cookie Dough	½ cup (2.7 oz)	240
Chocolate Raspberry Swirl	½ cup (2.7 oz)	190
Chubby Hubby	½ cup (2.7 oz)	260
Chunky Monkey	½ cup (2.7 oz)	240
Cinnamon	½ cup (2.7 oz)	180
Coconut Almond Fudge Chip	½ cup (2.7 oz)	260
Coffee Toffee Crunch	½ cup (2.7 oz)	240
Deep Dark Chocolate	½ cup (2.7 oz)	200
Double Chocolate Fudge Swirl	½ cup (2.7 oz)	210
Egg Nog	½ cup (2.7 oz)	190
English Toffee Crunch	½ cup (2.7 oz)	240
Maple Walnut	½ cup (2.7 oz)	240
Mint Chocolate Chunk	½ cup (2.7 oz)	220
Mint Chocolate Cookie	½ cup (2.7 oz)	220
Mint Fudge Swirl	½ cup (2.7 oz)	200
Mocha Fudge	½ cup (2.7 oz)	200
New York Super Fudge Chunk	½ cup (2.7 oz)	240
Peach	½ cup (2.7 oz)	170
Peanut Butter Cup	½ cup (2.7 oz)	260
Pistachio Pistachio	½ cup (2.7 oz)	220
Praline Pecan	½ cup (2.7 oz)	250
Rain Forest Crunch	½ cup (2.7 oz)	240
Reverse Chocolate Chunk	½ cup (2.7 oz)	230
Rum Raisin	½ cup (2.7 oz)	200
Strawberry	½ cup (2.7 oz)	170
Sweet Cream Cookie	½ cup (2.7 oz)	220
Vanilla	½ cup (2.7 oz)	190
Vanilla Bean	½ cup (2.7 oz)	190
Vanilla Caramel Fudge	½ cup (2.7 oz)	180
Vanilla Chocolate Chunk	½ cup (2.7 oz)	220
Vanilla Fudge Brownie	½ cup (2.7 oz)	200
Wavy Gravy	½ cup (2.7 oz)	260
White Russian	½ cup (2.7 oz)	190
ICES		
Lemon Daiquiri	½ cup (2.7 oz)	120
Mandarin	½ cup (2.7 oz)	130

FOOD	PORTION	CALS.
Marguerita Lime	½ cup (2.7 oz)	120
Pina Colada Sorbet	½ cup (2.7 oz)	120
Raspberry	½ cup (2.7 oz)	120
BIG BOY		
ICE CREAM		
Frozen Yogurt	1 serv	72
Frozen Yogurt Shake	1 serv	184
No-No Frozen Dessert	1 serv	75
MAIN MENU SELECTIONS		
Baked Cod Dinner	1 serv	392
Baked Cod Dijon Dinner	1 serv	455
Baked Potato	1	163
Bran Muffin	1	367
Breast of Chicken Dinner	1 serv	358
Breast of Chicken w/ Mozzarella Dinner	1 serv	379
Breast of Chicken w/ Mozzarella Sandwich	1	390
Broiled Cod Dijon Dinner	1 serv	455
Broiled Cod Dinner	1 serv	392
Cajun Chicken Dinner	1 serv	358
Cajun Cod Dinner	1 serv	392
Carrots	1 serv	35
Chicken Breast Salad w/ Dijon And Pita Bread	1 serv	377
Corn	1 serv	90
Dijon Sauce	1 serv	63
Dinner Salad	1	19
Green Beans	1 serv	28
Mixed Vegetables	1 serv	27
Peas	1 serv	77
Promise Margarine	1 pat (5 g)	35
Rice	1 serv	114
Roll	1	139
Spaghetti Marinara Dinner	1 serv	450
Stir Fry Vegetable	1 serv	408
Stir Fry Dinner Chicken 'n Vegetable	1 serv	562
Turkey Pita	1	224
Vegetable Pita	1	144
SALAD DRESSINGS		
Buttermilk	1 serv	36
SOUPS		
Cabbage	1 cup	37
Cabbage	1 bowl	43
BOJANGLES		
BAKED SELECTIONS		
Biscuit	1 (2.4 oz)	239

FOOD	PORTION	CALS.
Cajun Roast Multi-Grain Roll	1	100
Cinnamon Twist	1 (3.5 oz)	431
MAIN MENU SELECTIONS		
Biscuit Sandwich Bacon	1 (2.6 oz)	294
Biscuit Sandwich Bacon & Cheese	1 (3 oz)	422
Biscuit Sandwich Bacon & Egg	1 (4.2 oz)	386
Biscuit Sandwich Bacon, Egg & Cheese	1 (4.6 oz)	428
Biscuit Sandwich Chicken Filet	1 (3.6 oz)	399
Biscuit Sandwich Chicken Filet & Cheese	1 (6 oz)	441
Biscuit Sandwich Chicken Filet & Egg	1 (7.2 oz)	491
Biscuit Sandwich Chicken Filet, Egg & Cheese	1 (7.6 oz)	533
Biscuit Sandwich Country Ham	1 (3.6 oz)	314
Biscuit Sandwich Country Ham & Cheese	1 (4 oz)	356
Biscuit Sandwich Country Ham & Egg	1 (5.2 oz)	406
Biscuit Sandwich Country Ham, Egg & Cheese	1 (5.6 oz)	448
Biscuit Sandwich Egg	1 (3.9 oz)	331
Biscuit Sandwich Egg & Cheese	1 (4.3 oz)	373
Biscuit Sandwich Sausage	1 (4.3 oz)	448
Biscuit Sandwich Sausage & Cheese	1 (4.7 oz)	490
Biscuit Sandwich Sausage & Egg	1 (5.9 oz)	540
Biscuit Sandwich Sausage, Egg & Cheese	1 (6.3 oz)	582
Biscuit Sandwich Steak	1 (5.1 oz)	488
Biscuit Sandwich Steak & Cheese	1 (5.5 oz)	530
Biscuit Sandwich Steak & Egg	1 (6.7 oz)	580
Biscuit Sandwich Steak, Egg & Cheese	1 (7.1 oz)	622
Bo*Biscuit Canadian Bacon, Egg & Cheese	1 (5.2 oz)	417
Botato Rounds	1 serv (3.1 oz)	285
Buffalo Bites	1 serv	260
Cajun Pintos	1 serv (2.5 oz)	124
Cajun Roast Breast	1 serv	156
Cajun Roast Green Beans	1 serv	28
Cajun Roast Leg	1 serv	80
Cajun Roast Thigh	1 serv	170
Cajun Roast Wing	1 serv	100
Cole Slaw	1 serv (3.6 oz)	105
Dirty Rice	1 serv (2.9 oz)	167
Mashed Potatoes & Gravy	1 serv (3.6 oz)	165
Sandwich Cajun Filet	1 serv (6.7 oz)	550
Sandwich Grilled Filet	1 serv (5.8 oz)	429
Sandwich Grilled Filet Deluxe	1 serv (6.2 oz)	502
Sandwich Grilled Filet w/o Mayonnaise	1 serv (5.2 oz)	329
Seasoned Fries	1 serv (4 oz)	252

FOOD	PORTION	CALS.
Skinfree Southern Breast	1 serv (4.2 oz)	271
Skinfree Southern Leg	1 serv (1.9 oz)	128
Skinfree Southern Thigh	1 serv (3.4 oz)	264
Spiced Cajun Breast	1 serv (4.8 oz)	385
Spiced Cajun Leg	1 serv (3.2 oz)	245
Spiced Cajun Thigh	1 serv (3.7 oz)	335

BOSTON MARKET
DESSERTS

FOOD	PORTION	CALS.
Brownie	1 (3.3 oz)	450
Cookie Chocolate Chip	1 (2.8 oz)	340
Cookie Oatmeal Raisin	1 (2.8 oz)	320

MAIN MENU SELECTIONS

FOOD	PORTION	CALS.
½ Chicken w/ Skin	1 serv (10 oz)	630
¼ Dark Meat Chicken w/ Skin	1 serv (4.6 oz)	330
¼ Dark Meat Chicken w/o Skin	1 serv (3.6 oz)	210
¼ White Meat Chicken w/ Skin	1 serv (5.4 oz)	330
¼ White Meat Chicken w/o Skin Or Wing	1 serv (3.6 oz)	160
BBQ Baked Beans	¾ cup (7.1 oz)	330
Buttered Corn	¾ cup (5.1 oz)	190
Butternut Squash	¾ cup (6.8 oz)	160
Caesar Salad Entree	1 serv (10 oz)	520
Caesar Salad w/o Dressing	1 serv (8 oz)	225
Caesar Side Salad	1 (4 oz)	210
Chicken Caesar Salad	1 serv (13 oz)	670
Chicken Gravy	1 serv (1 oz)	15
Chicken Salad Sandwich	1 (10.7 oz)	680
Chicken Sandwich w/ Cheese & Sauce	1 serv (12.4 oz)	760
Chicken Sandwich w/o Cheese & Sauce	1 (10 oz)	430
Chunky Chicken Salad	3.4 cup (5.5 oz)	390
Cole Slaw	¾ cup (6.5 oz)	280
Corn Bread	1 (2.4 oz)	200
Cranberry Relish	¾ cup (7.9 oz)	370
Creamed Spinach	¾ cup (6.4 oz)	300
Fruit Salad	¾ cup (5.5 oz)	70
Ham & Turkey Club w/ Cheese & Sauce	1 (13.3 oz)	890
Ham & Turkey Club w/o Cheese & Sauce	1 (9.3 oz)	430
Ham Sandwich w/ Cheese & Sauce	1 (11.8 oz)	760
Ham Sandwich w/o Cheese & Sauce	1 (9.3 oz)	450
Ham w/ Cinnamon Apples	1 serv (8 oz)	350
Homestyle Mashed Potatoes & Gravy	¾ cup (6.6 oz)	200
Hot Cinnamon Apples	¾ cup (6.4 oz)	250
Macaroni & Cheese	¾ cup (6.7 oz)	280
Mashed Potatoes	⅔ cup (5.6 oz)	180

FOOD	PORTION	CALS.
Meat Loaf Sandwich w/ Cheese	1 (13.8 oz)	860
Meat Loaf Sandwich w/o Cheese	1 (12.3 oz)	690
Mediterranean Pasta Salad	¾ cup (4.5 oz)	170
New Potatoes	¾ cup (4.6 oz)	140
Original Chicken Pot Pie	1 serv (14.9 oz)	750
Rice Pilaf	⅔ cup (5.1 oz)	180
Rotisserie Turkey Breast Skinless	1 serv (5 oz)	170
Steamed Vegetables	⅔ cup (3.7 oz)	35
Stuffing	¾ cup (6.1 oz)	310
Tortellini Salad	¾ cup (5.6 oz)	380
Turkey Sandwich w/ Cheese & Sauce	1 (11.8 oz)	710
Turkey Sandwich w/o Cheese & Sauce	1 (9.3 oz)	400
Zucchini Marinara	¾ cup (6.6 oz)	80
SOUPS		
Chicken	¾ cup (6.8 oz)	80
Chicken Tortilla	1 cup (8.4 oz)	220

BROWN'S CHICKEN

Breadsticks w/ Garlic Butter	1 serv (12 oz)	1593
Breast	3 oz	284
Coleslaw	3 oz	131
Corn Fritters	3 oz	415
Corn On Cob	3 oz	126
Fettucini Alfredo	1 serv (12 oz)	1507
French Fries	3 oz	503
Gizzard	3 oz	387
Leg	3 oz	287
Liver	3 oz	341
Mostaccioli w/ Meat	1 serv (12 oz)	835
Mostaccioli w/o Meat	1 serv (12 oz)	792
Mushrooms	3 oz	289
Potato Salad	3 oz	94
Ravioli w/ Meat	1 serv (12 oz)	865
Ravioli w/o Meat	1 serv (12 oz)	822
Shrimp	3 oz	277
Thigh	3 oz	355
Wing	3 oz	385

BURGER KING
BEVERAGES

Shake Chocolate	1 med (10 oz)	310
Shake Chocolate Syrup Added	1 med (12 oz)	460
Shake Strawberry Syrup Added	1 med (12 oz)	430
Shake Vanilla	1 med (10 oz)	310

FOOD	PORTION	CALS.
BREAKFAST SELECTIONS		
AM Express Grape Jelly	1 serv (0.4 oz)	30
AM Express Strawberry Jam	1 serv (0.4 oz)	30
AM Express Dip	1 serv (1 oz)	80
Croissan'wich Bacon, Egg & Cheese	1 (4.1 oz)	350
Croissan'wich Ham, Egg & Cheese	1 (5.1 oz)	351
Croissan'wich Sausage, Egg & Cheese	1 (5.6 oz)	530
French Toast Sticks	1 serv (4.9 oz)	500
Hash Browns	1 serv (2.5 oz)	220
Land O'Lakes Whipped Classic Blend	1 serv (0.4 oz)	65
MAIN MENU SELECTIONS		
American Cheese	1 slice (0.9 oz)	90
BK Big Fish Sandwich	1 (8.9 oz)	720
BK Broiler Chicken Sandwich	1 (8.7 oz)	540
Bacon Bits	1 serv (3 g)	15
Broiled Chicken Salad w/o Dressing	1 serv (10.6 oz)	200
Bull's Eye Barbecue Sauce	1 serv (0.5 oz)	20
Cheeseburger	1 (5 oz)	380
Chicken Sandwich	1 (8 oz)	700
Chicken Tenders	6 pieces (3.1 oz)	250
Croutons	1 serv (0.2 oz)	30
Dipping Sauce Barbecue	1 serv (1 oz)	35
Dipping Sauce Honey	1 serv (1 oz)	90
Dipping Sauce Ranch	1 serv (1 oz)	170
Dipping Sauce Sweet & Sour	1 serv (1 oz)	45
Double Cheeseburger	1 (7.5 oz)	600
Double Cheeseburger w/ Bacon	1 (7.8 oz)	540
Double Whopper	1 (12.3 oz)	870
Dutch Apple Pie	1 serv (4 oz)	310
French Fries	1 med (4.1 oz)	400
Garden Salad w/o Dressing	1 (7.5 oz)	90
Hamburger	1 (4.5 oz)	330
Ketchup	1 serv (0.5 oz)	15
Lettuce	1 leaf (0.7 oz)	0
Mayonnaise	1 serv (1 oz)	210
Mustard	1 serv (3 g)	0
Onion	1 serv (0.5 oz)	5
Onion Rings	1 serv (4.4 oz)	310
Pickles	1 serv (0.5 oz)	0
Side Salad w/o Dressing	1 (4.7 oz)	50
Tartar Sauce	1 serv (1 oz)	180
Tomato	1 serv (1 oz)	6
Whopper	1 (9.5 oz)	640
Whopper Double w/ Cheese	1 (13.2 oz)	960

FOOD	PORTION	CALS.
Whopper Jr.	1 (5.9 oz)	420
Whopper Jr. w/ Cheese	1 (6.3 oz)	460
Whopper w/ Cheese	1 (10.3 oz)	730
SALAD DRESSINGS		
Bleu Cheese	1 serv (1 oz)	160
French	1 serv (1 oz)	140
Light Italian Reduced Calorie	1 serv (1 oz)	15
Ranch	1 serv (1 oz)	180
Thousand Island	1 serv (1 oz)	140

CAPTAIN D'S

FOOD	PORTION	CALS.
DESSERTS		
Carrot Cake	1 piece (4 oz)	**434**
Cheesecake	1 piece (4 oz)	**420**
Chocolate Cake	1 piece (4 oz)	303
Lemon Pie	1 piece (4 oz)	351
Pecan Pie	1 piece (4 oz)	458
MAIN MENU SELECTIONS		
Baked Potato	1	278
Breadstick	1	113
Broiled Chicken Lunch	1 serv	503
Broiled Chicken Platter	1 serv	802
Broiled Chicken Sandwich	1 (8.2 oz)	451
Broiled Fish Lunch	1 serv	435
Broiled Fish Platter	1 serv	734
Broiled Shrimp Lunch	1 serv	421
Broiled Shrimp Platter	1 serv	720
Cheese	1 slice (1 oz)	54
Cob Corn	1 serv (9.5 oz)	251
Cocktail Sauce	1 lg serv (1 fl oz)	34
Cocktail Sauce	1 serv (1 fl oz)	137
Cole Slaw	1 pt (16 oz)	633
Cole Slaw	1 serv (4 oz)	158
Crackers	4 (0.5 oz)	50
Cracklins	1 serv (1 oz)	218
Dinner Salad w/o Dressing	1 (2.5 oz)	27
French Fried Potatoes	1 serv (3.5 oz)	302
Fried Okra	1 serv (4 oz)	300
Green Beans Seasoned	1 serv (4 oz)	46
Hushpuppies	6 (6.7 oz)	756
Hushpuppy	1 (1.1 oz)	126
Imitation Sour Cream	1 serv	29
Margarine	1 serv	102
Non-Dairy Creamer	1 serv	14

FOOD	PORTION	CALS.
Rice	1 serv (4 oz)	124
Stuffed Crab	1 serving	91
Sugar	1 pkg	18
Sweet & Sour Sauce	1 serv (1.8 fl oz)	52
Sweet & Sour Sauce	1 lg serv (4 fl oz)	206
Tartar Sauce	1 serv (1 fl oz)	75
Tartar Sauce	1 lg serv (4 fl oz)	298
Vegetable Medley	1 serv	36
White Beans	1 serv (4 oz)	126
SALAD DRESSINGS		
Blue Cheese	1 pkg (1 fl oz)	105
French	1 pkg (1 fl oz)	111
Light Italian	1 serv	16
Ranch	1 pkg (1 fl oz)	92

CARL'S JR.

FOOD	PORTION	CALS.
BAKED SELECTIONS		
Cheese Danish	1 (4.1 oz)	400
Cheesecake Strawberry Swirl	1 serv (3.5 oz)	300
Chocolate Cake	1 serv (3 oz)	300
Chocolate Chip Cookie	1 (2.5 oz)	370
Cinnamon Roll	1 (4.2 oz)	420
Muffin Blueberry	1 (4.2 oz)	340
Muffin Bran	1 (4.7 oz)	370
BEVERAGES		
Shake Chocolate	1 sm (13.5 oz)	390
Shake Strawberry	1 sm (13.5 oz)	400
Shake Vanilla	1 sm (13.5 fl oz)	330
BREAKFAST SELECTIONS		
Bacon	2 strips (0.3 oz)	40
Breakfast Burrito	1 (5.3 oz)	430
Breakfast Quesadilla Cheese	1 (5.2 oz)	300
English Muffin w/ Margarine	1 (2.6 oz)	230
French Toast Dips w/o Syrup	1 serv (3.7 oz)	410
Grape Jelly	1 serv (0.5 oz)	35
Hash Brown Nuggets	1 serv (3.3 oz)	270
Sausage	1 patty (1.8 oz)	200
Scrambed Eggs	1 serv (3.5 oz)	160
Strawberry Jam	1 serv (0.5 oz)	35
Sunrise Sandwich	1 (4.6 oz)	370
Table Syrup	1 serv (1 oz)	90
MAIN MENU SELECTIONS		
American Cheese	1 slice (0.5 oz)	60
BBQ Chicken Sandwich	1 (6.7 oz)	310

FOOD	PORTION	CALS.
BBQ Sauce	1 serv (1.1 oz)	50
Big Burger	1 (6.8 oz)	470
Breadstick	1 (0.3 oz)	35
Carl's Catch Fish Sandwich	1 (7.5 oz)	560
Chicken Club Sandwich	1 (8.8 oz)	550
Chicken Stars	6 pieces (3 oz)	230
CrissCut Fries	1 lg (5.7 oz)	550
Croutons	1 serv (7 g)	35
Double Western Bacon Cheeseburger	1 (11.5 oz)	970
Famous Big Star Hamburger	1 (8.6 oz)	610
French Fries	1 reg (4.4 oz)	370
Great Stuff Potato Bacon & Cheese	1 (14.2 oz)	630
Great Stuff Potato Broccoli & Cheese	1 (14.2 oz)	530
Great Stuff Potato Plain	1 (9.4 oz)	290
Great Stuff Potato Sour Cream & Chive	1 (10.9 oz)	430
Hamburger	1 (3.1 oz)	200
Honey Sauce	1 serv (1 oz)	90
Hot & Crispy Sandwich	1 (5 oz)	400
Mustard Sauce	1 serv (1 oz)	45
Onion Rings	1 serv (5.3 oz)	520
Salsa	1 serv (0.9 oz)	10
Sante Fe Chicken Sandwich	1 (7.9 oz)	530
Super Star Hamburger	1 (11.2 oz)	820
Sweet N'Sour Sauce	1 serv (1 oz)	50
Swiss Cheese	1 slice (0.5 oz)	45
Western Bacon Cheeseburger	1 (8.1 oz)	870
Zucchini	1 serv (5.9 oz)	380
SALAD DRESSINGS		
1000 Island	2 fl oz	250
Blue Cheese	2 fl oz	310
French Fat Free	2 fl oz	70
House	2 fl oz	220
Italian Fat Free	2 fl oz	15
SALADS AND SALAD BARS		
Salad-To-Go Charbroiled Chicken	1 serv (12 oz)	260
Salad-To-Go Garden	1 (4.8 oz)	50

CARVEL

FOOD	PORTION	CALS.
FROZEN YOGURT		
Vanilla No Sugar Added	4 fl oz	100
ICE CREAM		
Brown Bonnet Cone	1	380
Chipsters	1	380
Chocolate	4 fl oz	180

FOOD	PORTION	CALS.
Chocolate No Fat	4 fl oz	90
Flying Saucers	1	240
Ice Cream Cupcakes	1	210
Vanilla	4 fl oz	190
Vanilla No Fat	4 fl oz	120
SHERBET		
Assorted Flavors	4 oz	150

CHICK-FIL-A
DESSERTS

Cheesecake	1 slice (3.1 oz)	270
Cheesecake w/ Blueberry Topping	1 slice (4.1 oz)	290
Cheesecake w/ Strawberry Topping	1 slice (4.1 oz)	290
Fudge Nut Brownie	1 (2.6 oz)	350
Icedream Cone	1 sm (4.5 oz)	140
Icedream Cup	1 sm (7.5 oz)	350
Lemon Pie	1 slice (3.5 oz)	280

MAIN MENU SELECTIONS

Carrot & Raisin Salad	1 sm (2.7 oz)	150
Chargrilled Chicken Club Sandwich w/o Dressing	1 (8.2 oz)	390
Chargrilled Chicken Deluxe Sandwich	1 (7.4 oz)	290
Chargrilled Chicken Garden Salad	1 serving (14 oz)	170
Chargrilled Chicken Sandwich	1 (5.3 oz)	280
Chargrilled Chicken w/o Bun or Pickles	1 piece (2.8 oz)	130
Chick-n-Q Sandwich	1 (6.1 oz)	370
Chick-n-Strips	4 (4.2 oz)	230
Chick-n-Strips Salad	1 serv (15.9 oz)	290
Chicken Sandwich	1 (5.9 oz)	290
Chicken Deluxe Sandich	1 (8 oz)	300
Chicken Salad Plate	1 serv (16.5 oz)	290
Chicken Salad Sandwich On Whole Wheat	1 (5.9 oz)	320
Chicken w/o Bun or Pickles	1 piece (3.7 oz)	160
Cole Slaw	1 sm (2.8 oz)	130
Grilled 'n Lites	2 skewers (2.7 oz)	100
Hearty Breast of Chicken Soup	1 cup (7.6 oz)	110
Nuggets	8 (3.9 oz)	290
Tossed Salad	1 serv (4.6 oz)	70
Waffle Potato Fries	1 sm (3 oz)	290
Waffle Potato Fries w/o Salt	1 sm (3 oz)	290

CHILI'S
DESSERTS

Diet By Chocolate Cake	1 serv	370
Diet By Chocolate Cake w/ Yogurt	1 serv	465

FOOD	PORTION	CALS.
Diet By Chocolate Cake w/ Yogurt & Fudge Topping	1 serv	534
MAIN MENU SELECTIONS		
Guiltless Grill Chicken Fijitas	1 serv	726
Guiltless Grill Chicken Platter	1 serv	563
Guiltless Grill Chicken Salad w/ Dressing	1 serv	254
Guiltless Grill Chicken Sandwich	1	527
Guiltless Grill Veggie Pasta	1 serv	590
Guiltless Grill Veggie Pasta w/ Chicken	1 serv	696

CHURCH'S CHICKEN

FOOD	PORTION	CALS.
Apple Pie	1 serv (3.1 oz)	280
Biscuit	1 (2.1 oz)	250
Breast	1 serv (2.8 oz)	200
Cajun Rice	1 serv (3.1 oz)	130
Cole Slaw	1 serv (3 oz)	92
Corn On The Cob	1 serv (5.7 oz)	139
French Fries	1 serv (2.7 oz)	210
Leg	1 serv (2 oz)	140
Okra	1 serv (2.8 oz)	210
Potatoes & Gravy	1 serv (3.7 oz)	90
Tender Strip	1 (1.1 oz)	80
Thigh	1 serv (2.8 oz)	230
Wing	1 serv (3.1 oz)	250

COLOMBO FROZEN YOGURT

FOOD	PORTION	CALS.
Alpine Strawberry Nonfat	4 fl oz	100
Banana Strawberry Nonfat	4 fl oz	50
Brazlian Banana Nonfat	4 fl oz	100
Butter Pecan Nonfat	4 fl oz	100
Cappuccino Nonfat	4 fl oz	100
Cherry Amaretto Nonfat	4 fl oz	50
Cherry Vanilla Nonfat	4 fl oz	100
Chocolate Nonfat	4 fl oz	50
Coconut Cooler Nonfat	4 fl oz	100
Cool Berry Blue Nonfat	4 fl oz	100
Country Pumpkin Nonfat	4 fl oz	100
Double Dutch Chocolate Nonfat	4 fl oz	100
Egg Nog Nonfat	4 fl oz	100
French Vanilla Lowfat	4 fl oz	110
French Vanilla Nonfat	4 fl oz	100
Georgia Peach Nonfat	4 fl oz	100
German Fudge Chocolate Nonfat	4 fl oz	100
Hawaiian Pineapple Nonfat	4 fl oz	100
Hazelnut Amaretto Nonfat	4 fl oz	100

FOOD	PORTION	CALS.
Honey Almond Nonfat	4 fl oz	100
Irish Cream Nonfat	4 fl oz	100
New York Cheesecake Nonfat	4 fl oz	100
Old World Chocolate Lowfat	4 fl oz	110
Orange Bavarian Creme Nonfat	4 fl oz	100
Peanut Butter Lowfat	4 fl oz	110
Pecan Praline Nonfat	4 fl oz	100
Pina Colada Nonfat	4 fl oz	100
Raspberry Nonfat	4 fl oz	50
Rockin' Raspberry Nonfat	4 fl oz	100
Simply Vanilla Lowfat	4 fl oz	110
Simply Vanilla Nonfat	4 fl oz	100
Strawberry Nonfat	4 fl oz	50
Tropical Tango Nonfat	4 fl oz	100
Vanilla Nonfat	4 fl oz	50
White Chocolate Almond Nonfat	4 fl oz	100
Wild Strawberry Lowfat	4 fl oz	110

D'ANGELO SANDWICH SHOPS
SALADS AND SALAD BARS

FOOD	PORTION	CALS.
D'Lite Chicken	1 serv	345
D'Lite Roast Beef	1 serv	355
D'Lite Tuna	1 serv	295
D'Lite Turkey	1 serv	355

SANDWICHES

FOOD	PORTION	CALS.
D'Lite Pocket Classic Vegetable	1	340
D'Lite Pocket Crunchy Vegetable	1	350
D'Lite Pocket Ginger Stir Fry Chicken	1	400
D'Lite Pocket Roast Beef	1	330
D'Lite Pocket Spicy Steak	1	425
D'Lite Pocket Steak	1	390
D'Lite Pocket Stuffed Turkey	1	510
D'Lite Pocket Turkey	1	350
D'Lite Small Sub Crunchy Vegetable	1	385
D'Lite Small Sub Roast Beef	1	365
D'Lite Small Sub Stuffed Turkey	1	545
D'Lite Small Sub Turkey	1	365

DAIRY QUEEN
FOOD SELECTIONS

FOOD	PORTION	CALS.
Cheese Dog	1 (4 oz)	290
Chicken Breast Fillet Sandwich	1 (6.7 oz)	430
Chicken Breast Fillet Sandwich w/ Cheese	1 (7.2 oz)	480
Chicken Strip Basket w/ BBQ Sauce	1 serv (10.2 oz)	810
Chicken Strip Basket w/ Gravy	1 serv (13.1 oz)	860

FOOD	PORTION	CALS.
Chili 'n' Cheese Dog	1 (5 oz)	330
Chili Dog	1 (4.5 oz)	280
DQ Homestyle Bacon Double Cheeseburger	1 (8.9 oz)	610
DQ Homestyle Cheeseburger	1 (5.3 oz)	340
DQ Homestyle Deluxe Double Cheeseburger	1 (8.5 oz)	540
DQ Homestyle Deluxe Double Hamburger	1 (7.4 oz)	440
DQ Homestyle Double Cheeseburger	1 (7.7 oz)	540
DQ Homestyle Hamburger	1 (4.8 oz)	290
DQ Homestyle Ultimate Burger	1 (9.4 oz)	670
Fish Fillet Sandwich	1 (6 oz)	370
Fish Fillet Sandwich w/ Cheese	1 (6.5 oz)	420
French Fries	1 reg (3.5 oz)	300
French Fries	1 sm (2.5 oz)	210
French Fries	1 lg (4.5 oz)	390
Grilled Chicken Breast Fillet Sandwich	1 (6.5 oz)	310
Hot Dog	1 (3.5 oz)	240
Onion Rings	1 serv (3 oz)	240
ICE CREAM		
Banana Split	1 (12.9 oz)	510
Blizzard Butterfinger	1 reg (16 oz)	750
Blizzard Butterfinger	1 sm (12 oz)	520
Blizzard Chocolate Sandwich Cookie	1 sm (12 oz)	520
Blizzard Chocolate Sandwich Cookie	1 reg (16 oz)	640
Blizzard Chocolate Chip Cookie Dough	1 reg (16 oz)	950
Blizzard Chocolate Chip Cookie Dough	1 sm (12 oz)	660
Blizzard Heath	1 sm (12 oz)	560
Blizzard Heath	1 reg (16 oz)	820
Blizzard Reese's Peanut Butter Cup	1 sm (12 oz)	590
Blizzard Reese's Peanut Butter Cup	1 reg (16 oz)	790
Blizzard Strawberry	1 reg (16 oz)	570
Blizzard Strawberry	1 sm (12 oz)	400
Breeze Heath	1 reg (16 oz)	710
Breeze Heath	1 sm (12 oz)	470
Breeze Strawberry	1 reg (16 oz)	460
Breeze Strawberry	1 sm (12 oz)	320
Buster Bar	1 (5.2 oz)	450
Cone Chocolate	1 reg (7.5 oz)	360
Cone Chocolate	1 sm (5 oz)	240
Cone Vanilla	1 sm (5 oz)	230
Cone Vanilla	1 lg (8.9 oz)	410
Cone Vanilla	1 reg (7.5 oz)	350
Cone Yogurt	1 reg (7.5 oz)	280
Cone Dipped	1 reg (8.2 oz)	510
Cone Dipped	1 sm (5.5 oz)	340

FOOD	PORTION	CALS.
Cup Of Yogurt	1 reg (6.9 oz)	230
DQ Bar Caramel Nut	1 (2.8 oz)	260
DQ Bar Fudge	1 (2.3 oz)	50
DQ Bar Vanilla Orange	1 (2.3 oz)	60
DQ Heart Cake	1/10 of cake (4.8 oz)	270
DQ Lemon Freez'r	1/2 cup (3.2 oz)	80
DQ Log Cake Undecorated	1/8 of cake (4.7 oz)	280
DQ Nonfat Frozen Yogurt	1/2 cup (3 oz)	100
DQ Round Cake 10 in	1/12 of cake (6.6 oz)	360
DQ Round Cake 8 in	1/8 of cake (6.2 oz)	340
DQ Sandwich	1 (2.1 oz)	150
DQ Sheet Cake Undecorated	1/20 of cake (6 oz)	350
DQ Soft Serve Chocolate	1/2 cup (3.3 oz)	150
DQ Soft Serve Vanilla	1/2 cup (3.3 oz)	140
DQ Treatzza Pizza Heath	1/8 of pie (2.3 oz)	180
DQ Treatzza Pizza M&M	1/8 of pie (2.4 oz)	190
DQ Treatzza Pizza Peanut Butter Fudge	1/8 of pie (2.5 oz)	220
DQ Treatzza Pizza Strawberry Banana	1/8 of pie (2.7 oz)	180
Dilly Bar Chocolate	1 (3 oz)	210
Dilly Bar Chocolate Mint	1 (2.7 oz)	190
Dilly Bar Toffee w/ Heath Pieces	1 (2.8 oz)	210
Fudge Nut Bar	1 (5 oz)	410
Malt Chocolate	1 sm (14.7 oz)	650
Malt Chocolate	1 reg (19.9 oz)	880
Misty Cooler Strawberry	1 (11.9 oz)	190
Misty Slush	1 reg (20.9 oz)	290
Misty Slush	1 sm (15.9 oz)	220
Peanut Buster Parfait	1 (10.7 oz)	730
Queen's Choice Big Scoop Chocolate	1 (4 oz)	250
Queen's Choice Big Scoop Vanilla	1 (4 oz)	250
Shake Chocolate	1 sm (13.9 oz)	560
Shake Chocolate	1 reg (18.9 oz)	770
Starkiss	1 (3 oz)	80
Strawberry Shortcake	1 (8.5 oz)	430
Sundae Chocolate	1 sm (6 oz)	290
Sundae Chocolate	1 reg (7.5 oz)	410
Yogurt Sundae Strawberry	1 reg (7.9 oz)	300

DELTACO

BEVERAGES

FOOD	PORTION	CALS.
M&M's Toppers	1 serv	256
Oreos Toppers	1 serv	257
Shake Chocolate	1 sm	549
Shake Chocolate	1 med	755

FOOD	PORTION	CALS.
Shake Orange	1 sm	609
Shake Orange	1 med	837
Shake Strawberry	1 sm	486
Shake Strawberry	1 med	668
Shake Vanilla	1 sm	514
Shake Vanilla	1 med	707
Snickers Toppers	1 serv	254
BREAKFAST SELECTIONS		
Burrito Beef And Egg	1	529
Burrito Breakfast	1	256
Burrito Egg And Cheese	1	443
Burrito Egg and Bean	1	470
Burrito Steak And Egg	1	500
CHILDREN'S MENU SELECTIONS		
Kid's Meal Hamburger	1 meal	617
Kid's Meal Taco	1 meal	532
MAIN MENU SELECTIONS		
American Cheese	1 slice	53
Beans And Cheese	1	122
Burrito Chicken	1	264
Burrito Combination	1	413
Burrito Del Beef	1	440
Burrito Deluxe Chicken	1	549
Burrito Deluxe Combo	1	453
Burrito Deluxe Del Beef	1	479
Burrito Green	1	229
Burrito Green Regular	1	330
Burrito Macho Beef	1	893
Burrito Macho Combo	1	774
Burrito Red	1	235
Burrito Red Regular	1	342
Burrito Spicy Chicken	1	392
Burrito The Works	1	448
Cheeseburger	1	284
Chicken Salad	1	254
Chicken Salad Deluxe	1	716
Del Burger	1	385
Del Cheeseburger	1	439
Double Del Cheeseburger	1	618
French Fries	1 sm	242
French Fries	1 reg	404
French Fries	1 lg	566
Fries Chili Cheese	1 serv	562
Fries Deluxe Chili Cheese	1 serv	600

FOOD	PORTION	CALS.
Fries Nacho	1 serv	669
Guacamole	1 oz	60
Hamburger	1	231
Hot Sauce	1 pkg	2
Nacho Cheese Sauce	1 side order	100
Nachos	1 serv	390
Nachos Macho	1	1089
Quesadilla	1	257
Quesadilla Chicken	1	544
Quesadilla Regular	1	483
Quesadilla Spicy Jack	1	254
Quesadilla Spicy Jack Chicken	1	537
Quesadilla Spicy Jack Regular	1	476
Salsa	2 oz	14
Salsa Dressing	1 oz	33
Soft Taco	1	146
Soft Taco Chicken	1	197
Soft Taco Deluxe Double Beef	1	211
Soft Taco Double Beef	1	178
Sour Cream	1 oz	60
Taco	1	140
Taco Chicken	1	186
Taco Deluxe Double Beef	1	205
Taco Double Beef	1	172
Taco Salad	1	235
Taco Salad Deluxe	1	741
Tostada	1	140

DENNY'S
BREAKFAST SELECTIONS

Applesauce	1 serv (2 oz)	40
Bacon	4 strips	145
Bagel	1	230
Banana	1	105
Banana Strawberry Medley	1 serv	95
Belgian Waffle	1	320
Biscuit Plain	1	215
Biscuit w/ Sausage Gravy	1 serv	465
Blueberry Topping	1 serv (3 oz)	110
Cantaloup	¼	100
Chicken Fried Steak & Eggs w/o Bread	1 serv	650
Cinnamon Roll	1	670
Cream Cheese	1 oz	100
Egg	1	120

FOOD	PORTION	CALS.
English Muffin	1	150
French Toast	1 serv	325
Grand Slam	1 serv	860
Grapefruit	½	40
Grapes	1 serv	50
Grits	1 serv	160
Ham	1 serv	170
Hashed Browns	1 serv	210
Honeydew	¼	125
Moon Over My Hammy	1 serv	980
Muffin Blueberry	1	310
Omelette Chili Cheese	1 serv	445
Omelette Denver	1 serv	735
Omelette Ham'n Cheddar	1 serv	490
Omelette Mexican	1 serv	550
Omelette Senior	1 serv	650
Omelette Ultimate	1 serv	745
Omelette Vegetable	1 serv	585
Pancakes Buttermilk	3	410
Sausage	4 links	225
Senior Grand Slam	1 serv	535
Senior Omelette	1 serv	640
Senior Starter	1 serv	550
Slams All-American w/o Bread	1 serv	980
Slams French	1 serv	915
Slams Harvest	1 serv	1055
Slams International	1 serv	975
Slams Scram w/o Bread	1 serv	1080
Slams Southern	1 serv	895
Steak & Eggs w/o Bread	1 serv	800
Strawberry Topping	1 serv (3 oz)	80
Syrup	1 serv (2 oz)	160
Toast w/o Butter	2 pieces	140
Whipped Butter	1 tbsp	65
Whipped Topping	1 serv (2 oz)	23
DESSERTS		
Apple Pie	1 serv	520
Apple Pie w/ Equal	1 serv	460
Banana Split	1 serv	850
Blueberry Cream Cheese Pie	1 serv	700
Cherry Cream Cheese Pie	1 serv	685
Cherry Pie	1 serv	635
Cherry Pie w/ Equal	1 serv	510
Chocolate Cake	1 serv	370

FOOD	PORTION	CALS.
Coconut Cream Pie	1 serv	480
Double Dip Sundae	1 serv	545
French Silk Pie Cheese	1 serv	510
Hot Fudge Sundae	1 serv	495
Hot Fudge Cake Sundae	1 serv	730
Ice Cream Scoop	1 serv	135
Ice Cream Shake	1 serv	525
Key Lime Pie	1 serv	590
MAIN MENU SELECTIONS		
Buffalo Wings w/o Dressing	1 serv	350
Burger Bacon Swiss	1	745
Burger Patty Melt	1	780
Chicken Fried Steak	1 serv	465
Chicken Strips	1 serv	580
Chicken Strips w/o Dressing	1 serv	580
Chili Fries	1 serv	585
Club Sandwich	1	485
Coleslaw	1 serv	105
Denny Burger	1	485
French Fries	1 serv	285
Fried Chicken	1 serv	460
Grilled Breast Of Chicken	1 serv (4 oz)	125
Grilled Breast Of Chicken	1 serv (6 oz)	190
Grilled Catfish	1 serv	475
Grilled Rainbow Trout	1 serv	490
Liver w/ Bacon & Onions	1 serv	585
Mozzarella Sticks	4	350
Nachos Supreme	1 serv	770
Prime Rib	1 serv (8 oz)	570
Quesadilla	1 serv	460
Quesadilla Chicken	1 serv	580
Roast Beef w/ Bread, Gravy, Potatoes	1 serv	600
Roast Turkey w/ Stuffing & Gravy	1 serv	490
Sandwich Bacon, Lettuce & Tomato	1	490
Sandwich Chicken Melt	1 serv	700
Sandwich French Dip	1 serv	575
Sandwich Grilled Cheese	1	715
Sandwich Grilled Chicken	1	665
Sandwich Mega Melt	1 serv	945
Sandwich Prime Time	1 serv	930
Sandwich Roast Beef Deluxe	1 serv	850
Sandwich Super Bird	1	585
Sandwich Tuna Melt Supreme	1	805
Sandwich Veggie Cheese Melt	1	565

FOOD	PORTION	CALS.
Senior Chicken Fried Steak	1 serv	425
Senior Fried Chicken	1 serv	480
Senior Grilled Catfish Dinner w/o Vegetable	1 serv	450
Senior Grilled Cheese Sandwich	1 serv	360
Senior Grilled Chicken Dinner w/o Vegetable	1 serv	245
Senior Liver w/ Bacon & Onions	1 serv	435
Senior Roast Beef Dinnner w/o Vegetable	1 serv	280
Senior Roast Turkey & Stuffing w/o Vegetable	1 serv	440
Senior Sirloin Tips w/o Vegebable	1 serv	220
Senior Spaghetti w/ Meatballs	1 serv	580
Senior Tuna Salad Sandwich	1	260
Senior Turkey Sandwich	1	340
Spaghetti w/ Meatballs	1 serv	1000
Spaghetti w/ Sauce	1 serv	605
Stir Fry Chicken w/ Vegetables & Rice Pilaf	1 serv	435
Works Burger	1	950
SALAD DRESSINGS		
Bleu Cheese	1 oz	120
Creamy Italian	1 oz	100
French	1 oz	100
French Reduced Calorie	1 oz	70
Honey Mustard	1 oz	100
Italian Reduced Calorie	1 oz	16
Ranch	1 oz	110
Thousand Island	1 oz	120
SALADS AND SALAD BARS		
Caesar	1 serv	325
California Grilled Chicken	1 serv	290
Chef's	1 serv	370
Crispy Chicken Salad	1 serv	905
Crispy Chicken Salad w/o Tortilla Shell	1 serv	465
Garden Salad	1 serv	115
Grilled Chicken Caesar	1 serv	655
Taco Salad	1 serv	905
Taco Salad w/o Tortilla Shell	1 serv	470
SOUPS		
Cheese	1 serv	315
Chicken Noodle	1 serv	60
Chili With Beans	1 serv	160
Clam Chowder	1 serv	220
Cream Of Broccoli	1 serv	200
Cream of Potato	1 serv	230
Vegetable Beef	1 serv	80

FOOD	PORTION	CALS.
DOMINO'S PIZZA		
12 INCH		
Deep Dish Cheese	2 slices (7.2 oz)	560
Deep Dish Ham	2 slices (7.7 oz)	577
Deep Dish Italian Sausage & Mushroom	2 slices (8.3 oz)	618
Deep Dish Pepperoni	2 slices (7.6 oz)	622
Deep Dish Veggie	2 slices (8.3 oz)	576
Deep Dish X-Tra Cheese & Pepperoni	2 slices (8.2 oz)	671
Hand-Tossed Cheese	2 slices (5.2 oz)	344
Hand-Tossed Ham	2 slices (5.6 oz)	362
Hand-Tossed Italian Sausage & Mushroom	2 slices (6.2 oz)	402
Hand-Tossed Pepperoni	2 slices (5.6 oz)	406
Hand-Tossed Veggie	2 slices (6.2 oz)	360
Hand-Tossed X-Tra Cheese & Pepperoni	2 slices (6.2 oz)	455
Thin Crust Cheese	⅓ pie (4.9 oz)	364
Thin Crust Ham	⅓ pie (5.6 oz)	388
Thin Crust Italian Sausage & Mushroom	⅓ pie (6.3 oz)	442
Thin Crust Pepperoni	⅓ pie (5.5 oz)	447
Thin Crust Veggie	⅓ pie (6.3 oz)	386
Thin Crust X-Tra Cheese & Pepperoni	⅓ pie (6.2 oz)	512
DUNKIN' DONUTS		
BAKED GOODS		
Bagel Cinnamon Raisin	1 (3 oz)	220
Bagel Onion	1 (3 oz)	200
Bagel Plain	1 (3 oz)	200
Bismark	1 (2.8 oz)	310
Bow Tie	1 (2.5 oz)	250
Brownie Blondie w/ Chocolate Chips	1 (2.4 oz)	300
Brownie Fudge	1 (2.4 oz)	290
Brownie Peanut Butter Blondie	1 (2.4 oz)	330
Cake Donut Blueberry	1 (2.4 oz)	230
Cake Donut Blueberry Crumb	1 (2.6 oz)	260
Cake Donut Butternut	1 (2.6 oz)	340
Cake Donut Chocolate	1 (2.1 oz)	210
Cake Donut Chocolate Coconut	1 (2.4 oz)	250
Cake Donut Chocolate Glazed	1 (2.5 oz)	250
Cake Donut Cinnamon	1 (2.3 oz)	300
Cake Donut Coconut	1 (2.5 oz)	320
Cake Donut Double Chocolate	1 (2.6 oz)	260
Cake Donut Old Fashioned	1 (2.1 oz)	280
Cake Donut Peanut	1 (2.6 oz)	340
Cake Donut Powdered	1 (2.4 oz)	310
Cake Donut Sugared	1 (2.4 oz)	310

FOOD	PORTION	CALS.
Cake Donut Toasted Coconut	1 (2.5 oz)	320
Cake Donut Whole Wheat Glazed	1 (2.7 oz)	230
Coffee Roll	1 (2.6 oz)	280
Coffee Roll Chocolate Frosted	1 (2.7 oz)	290
Coffee Roll Cinnamon Raisin	1 (3.1 oz)	330
Coffee Roll Maple Frosted	1 (2.7 oz)	300
Coffee Roll Vanilla Frosted	1 (2.7 oz)	300
Cookie Chocolate Chocolate Chunk	1 (1.5 oz)	200
Cookie Chocolate Chunk	1 (1.5 oz)	200
Cookie Chocolate Chunk w/ Nut	1 (1.5 oz)	200
Cookie Chocolate White Chocolate Chunk	1 (1.5 oz)	200
Cookie Oatmeal Raisin Pecan	1 (1.5 oz)	190
Cookie Peanut Butter Chocolate Chunk w/ Nuts	1 (1.5 oz)	210
Cookie Peanut Butter Chocolate Chunk w/ Peanuts	1 (1.5 oz)	210
Cream Cheese Plain	1 serv (1 oz)	100
Croissant Almond	1 (2.7 oz)	360
Croissant Cheese	1 (2.5 oz)	240
Croissant Chocolate	1 (2.5 oz)	370
Croissant Plain	1 (2.1 oz)	270
Crullers/Sticks Dunkin' Donut	1 (2.1 oz)	240
Crullers/Sticks Glazed	1 (3 oz)	340
Crullers/Sticks Glazed Chocolate	1 (3.2 oz)	410
Crullers/Sticks Jelly	1 (3.2 oz)	330
Crullers/Sticks Plain	1 (2.1 oz)	260
Crullers/Sticks Powdered	1 (2.3 oz)	290
Crullers/Sticks Sugar	1 (2.2 oz)	270
Eclair	1 (3.2 oz)	290
English Muffin	1 (2 oz)	130
French Roll	1 (2.1 oz)	140
Fritter Apple	1 (3.3 oz)	300
Fritter Glazed	1 (2.7 oz)	290
Muffin Banana Nut	1 (3.3 oz)	340
Muffin Blueberry	1 (3.3 oz)	310
Muffin Cherry	1 (3.3 oz)	330
Muffin Chocolate Chip	1 (3.3 oz)	400
Muffin Corn	1 (3.3 oz)	350
Muffin Cranberry Orange Nut	1 (3.5 oz)	310
Muffin Honey Raisin Bran	1 (3.3 oz)	330
Muffin Lemon Poppy Seed	1 (3.3 oz)	360
Muffin Oat Bran	1 (3.2 oz)	290
Muffin Lowfat Apple n' Spice	1 (3.3 oz)	220
Muffin Lowfat Banana	1 (3.3 oz)	240

FOOD	PORTION	CALS.
Muffin Lowfat Blueberry	1 (3.3 oz)	230
Muffin Lowfat Bran	1 (3.3 oz)	260
Muffin Lowfat Cherry	1 (3.3 oz)	230
Muffin Lowfat Corn	1 (3.3 oz)	250
Muffin Lowfat Cranberry Orange	1 (3.3 oz)	230
Munchkins Butternut	3 (2 oz)	230
Munchkins Chocolate Glazed	3 (2 oz)	180
Munchkins Cinnamon	4 (2 oz)	240
Munchkins Coconut	3 (1.7 oz)	200
Munchkins Glazed Cake	3 (2.1 oz)	220
Munchkins Glazed Raised	4 (2.1 oz)	210
Munchkins Jelly	3 (1.9 oz)	170
Munchkins Lemon	3 (2 oz)	160
Munchkins Plain	4 (1.8 oz)	200
Munchkins Powdered Sugar	4 (2 oz)	240
Munchkins Sugar Raised	6 (1.9 oz)	210
Munchkins Toasted Coconut	3 (1.8 oz)	210
Tart Apple	1 (3.4 oz)	310
Tart Blueberry	1 (3.4 oz)	300
Tart Lemon	1 (3.4 oz)	280
Tart Raspberry	1 (3.4 oz)	310
Tart Strawberry	1 (3.4 oz)	310
Turnover Apple	1 (3.8 oz)	350
Turnover Blueberry	1 (3.8 oz)	370
Turnover Lemon	1 (3.8 oz)	350
Turnover Raspberry	1 (3.8 oz)	380
Turnover Strawberry	1 (3.8 oz)	380
Yeast Donut Apple Crumb	1 (2.6 oz)	250
Yeast Donut Apple n' Spice	1 (2.5 oz)	230
Yeast Donut Bavarian Kreme	1 (2.5 oz)	250
Yeast Donut Black Raspberry	1 (2.4 oz)	240
Yeast Donut Boston Kreme	1 (2.8 oz)	270
Yeast Donut Chocalate Kreme Filled	1 (2.6 oz)	320
Yeast Donut Chocolate Frosted	1 (2.1 oz)	210
Yeast Donut Glazed	1 (1.6 oz)	160
Yeast Donut Jelly Filled	1 (2.4 oz)	240
Yeast Donut Lemon	1 (2.5 oz)	240
Yeast Donut Maple Frosted	1 (2.1 oz)	210
Yeast Donut Marble Frosted	1 (2.1 oz)	210
Yeast Donut Strawberry	1 (2.4 oz)	240
Yeast Donut Strawberry Frosted	1 (2.1 oz)	220
Yeast Donut Sugar Raised	1 (1.6 oz)	170
Yeast Donut Vanilla Frosted	1 (2.1 oz)	220

FOOD	PORTION	CALS.
BREAKFAST SELECTIONS		
Croissant Sandwich Egg & Cheese	1 (5 oz)	430
Croissant Sandwich Egg, Bacon & Cheese	1 (5.4 oz)	500
Croissant Sandwich Egg, Ham & Cheese	1 (6 oz)	530
Croissant Sandwich Egg, Sausage & Cheese	1 (6.9 oz)	630
COFFEE		
Cream	1 serv (1 oz)	60
Dark Roast	1 serv (10 oz)	5
Decaf	1 serv (10 oz)	0
French Vanilla	1 serv (10 oz)	5
Hazelnut	1 serv (10 oz)	5
Regular	1 serv (10 oz)	5
LUNCH SELECTIONS		
Croissant Sandwich Broccoli & Cheese	1 (6.1 oz)	370
Croissant Sandwich Chicken Salad	1 (7.6 oz)	540
Croissant Sandwich Ham & Cheese	1 (6.7 oz)	710
Croissant Sandwich Roast Beef & Cheese	1 (6 oz)	490
Croissant Sandwich Seafood Salad	1 (7.6 oz)	480
Croissant Sandwich Tuna Salad	1 (7.5 oz)	540
SOUPS		
Beef Barley	1 serv (8 oz)	90
Beef Noodle	1 serv (8 oz)	90
Chicken Noodle	1 serv (8 oz)	80
Chili	1 serv (8 oz)	170
Chili Con Carne w/ Beans	1 serv (8 oz)	300
Cream Of Broccoli	1 serv (8 oz)	200
Cream Of Potato	1 serv (8 oz)	190
Harvest Vegetable	1 serv (8 oz)	80
Manhattan Clam Chowder	1 serv (8 oz)	70
Minestrone	1 serv (8 oz)	100
New England Clam Chowder	1 serv (8 oz)	200
Split Pea w/ Ham	1 serv (8 oz)	190

EL POLLO LOCO

FOOD	PORTION	CALS.
DESSERTS		
Cheesecake	1 serv (3.5 oz)	310
Churro	1 serv (1.25 oz)	130
MAIN MENU SELECTIONS		
Beans	1 serv (4 oz)	100
Burrito Bean, Rice & Cheese	1 (9 oz)	530
Burrito Chicken	1 (7 oz)	310
Burrito Classic Chicken	1 (9.5 oz)	560
Burrito Gilled Steak	1 (11 oz)	740
Burrito Loco Grande Chicken	1 (13 oz)	680

FOOD	PORTION	CALS.
Burrito Spicy Hot Chicken	1 (10 oz)	570
Burrito Steak	1 (6 oz)	450
Burrito Vegetarian	1 (6 oz)	340
Burrito Whole Wheat Chicken	1 (10.5 oz)	510
Cheddar Cheese	1 serv (1 oz)	90
Chicken Breast	1 piece (3 oz)	160
Chicken Leg	1 piece (1.75 oz)	90
Chicken Thigh	1 piece (2 oz)	180
Chicken Wing	1 (1.5 oz)	110
Coleslaw	1 serv (3 oz)	100
Corn	1 serv (3 oz)	110
Fajita Meal Chicken	1 (17.5 oz)	780
Fajita Meal Steak	1 (17.5 oz)	1040
Guacamole	1 serv (1 oz)	60
Potato Salad	1 serv (4 oz)	180
Rice	1 serv (2 oz)	110
Salsa	1 serv (2 oz)	10
Sour Cream	1 serv (1 oz)	50
Taco Chicken	1 (5 oz)	180
Taco Steak	1 (4.5 oz)	250
Tortilla Corn	1 (1 oz)	60
Tortilla Flour	1 (1 oz)	90
SALAD DRESSINGS		
Blue Cheese	1 serv (1 oz)	80
Deluxe French	1 serv (1 oz)	60
Honey Dijon Mustard	1 serv (1 oz)	50
Italian Reduced Calorie	1 serv (1 oz)	25
Ranch	1 serv (1 oz)	75
Thousand Island	1 serv (1 oz)	110
SALADS AND SALAD BARS		
Chicken Salad	1 (12 oz)	160
Side Salad	1 (9 oz)	50

FRIENDLY'S
FROZEN YOGURT

Apple Bettie	½ cup (2.6 oz)	140
Chocolate Fudge Brownie	½ cup (2.6 oz)	160
Fabulous Fudge Swirl	½ cup (2.6 oz)	140
Fudge Berry Swirl	½ cup (2.6 oz)	150
Lowfat Perfectly Peach	½ cup (2.6 oz)	110
Lowfat Purely Chocolate	½ cup (2.6 oz)	120
Lowfat Raspberry Delight	½ cup (2.6 oz)	120
Lowfat Simply Vanilla	½ cup (2.6 oz)	120
Lowfat Strawberry Patch	½ cup (2.6 oz)	110

FOOD	PORTION	CALS.
Mint Chocolate Chip	½ cup (2.6 oz)	130
Strawberry Cheesecake Blast	½ cup (2.6 oz)	140
Toffee Almond Crunch	½ cup (2.6 oz)	160
ICE CREAM		
Black Raspberry	½ cup	150
Chocolate Almond Chip	½ cup	170
Forbidden Chocolate	½ cup	150
Fudge Nut Brownie	½ cup	200
Heath English Toffee	½ cup (2.7 oz)	190
Purely Pictachio	½ cup	160
Vanilla	½ cup	150
Vienna Mocha Chunk	½ cup	180

FRULLATI CAFE

FOOD	PORTION	CALS.
BAKED GOODS		
Muffin Banana Nut	1 (4 oz)	394
Muffin Cranberry Orange	1 (4 oz)	357
Muffin Fat Free Apple Streusel	1 (4 oz)	260
Muffin Fat Free Chocolate	1 (4 oz)	260
Muffin Fat Free Very Berry	1 (4 oz)	260
Muffin Sugar Free Blueberry	1 (4 oz)	308
Muffin Wild Blueberry	1 (4 oz)	344
BEVERAGES		
Apple Juice	1 serv (12 oz)	131
Carrot Juice	1 serv (12 oz)	111
Celery Juice	1 serv (12 oz)	22
Lemondae	1 serv	209
Lemondae Apple	1 serv	245
Lemondae Cherry	1 serv	237
Lemondae Orange	1 serv	270
Lemondae Strawberry	1 serv	234
Orange Banana Juice	1 serv (12 oz)	150
Orange Juice	1 serv (12 oz)	126
Smoothie A La Frullati	1 lg	426
Smoothie A La Frullati	1 sm	275
Smoothie Affinity	1 sm	226
Smoothie Affinity	1 lg	378
Smoothie Fiesta	1 lg	257
Smoothie Fiesta	1 sm	234
Smoothie Peach Banana	1 lg	289
Smoothie Peach Banana	1 sm	266
Smoothie Pina Colada	1 sm	236
Smoothie Pina Colada	1 lg	387
Smoothie Strawberry Banana	1 lg	188

FOOD	PORTION	CALS.
Smoothie Strawberry Banana	1 sm	165
Smoothie Strawberry Blueberry	1 sm	90
Smoothie Strawberry Blueberry	1 lg	113
Smoothie Strawberry Fruit	1 sm	79
Smoothie Strawberry Fruit	1 lg	101
Smoothie Strawberry Watermelon	1 lg	123
Smoothie Strawberry Watermelon	1 sm	100
DESSERTS		
Frozen Yogurt	1 lg	263
Frozen Yogurt	1 reg	205
Frozen Yogurt	1 sm	146
Yogurt Smoothie Cappuccino	1 serv	472
Yogurt Smoothie Chocolate Fudge	1 serv	555
Yogurt Smoothie Fiesta	1 serv	432
Yogurt Smoothie Oreo Cookie	1 serv	566
Yogurt Smoothie Peach	1 serv	486
Yogurt Smoothie Peach Banana	1 serv	519
Yogurt Smoothie Peanut Butter	1 serv	630
Yogurt Smoothie Pina Colada	1 serv	519
Yogurt Smoothie Strawberry Banana	1 serv	514
Yogurt Smoothie Strawberry Fruit	1 serv	487
Yogurt Smoothie Strawberry Vanilla	1 serv	462
Yogurt Smoothie Strawberry Watermelon	1 serv	503
SALADS AND SALAD BARS		
Fruit Salad	1 lg	148
Fruit Salad	1 sm	99
Garden Salad	1 sm	56
Garden Salad w/ Italian Fat Free Dressing	1 lg	72
Pasta Salad	1 sm	179
Pasta Salad	1 lg	256
SANDWICHES		
Chicken On Croissant	1	481
Chicken On Honey Wheat	1	297
Chicken On Jewish Rye	1	261
Chicken On Pita	1	281
Chicken On White	1	291
Ham & Cheese On Croissant	1	797
Ham & Cheese On Honey Wheat	1	613
Ham & Cheese On Jewish Rye	1	577
Ham & Cheese On Pita	1	597
Ham & Cheese On White	1	607
Roast Beef On Croissant	1	631
Roast Beef On Honey Wheat	1	348
Roast Beef On Jewish Rye	1	312

FOOD	PORTION	CALS.
Roast Beef On Pita	1	332
Roast Beef On White	1	342
Tuna On Croissant	1	480
Tuna On Honey Wheat	1	295
Tuna On Jewish Rye	1	259
Tuna On Pita	1	280
Tuna On White	1	289
Turkey On Croissant	1	566
Turkey On Honey Wheat	1	342
Turkey On Jewish Rye	1	306
Turkey On Pita	1	326
Turkey On White	1	338
Veggie On Croissant	1	510
Veggie On Honey Wheat	1	227
Veggie On Jewish Rye	1	191
Veggie On Pita	1	211
Veggie On White	1	221

GODFATHER'S PIZZA

Golden Crust Cheese	1/10 lg (3.5 oz)	261
Golden Crust Cheese	1/8 med (3.1 oz)	229
Golden Crust Cheese	1/6 sm (3 oz)	213
Golden Crust Combo	1/6 sm (4.5 oz)	273
Golden Crust Combo	1/8 med (4.5 oz)	283
Golden Crust Combo	1/10 lg (5.1 oz)	322
Original Crust Cheese	1/6 sm (3.5 oz)	239
Original Crust Cheese	1/10 lg (4 oz)	271
Original Crust Cheese	1/8 med (3.5 oz)	242
Original Crust Cheese	1/4 mini (2 oz)	138
Original Crust Combo	1/10 lg (5.5 oz)	332
Original Crust Combo	1/6 sm (5 oz)	299
Original Crust Combo	1/4 mini (2.8 oz)	164
Original Crust Combo	1/8 med (5.2 oz)	318

GODIVA

Almond Butter Dome	3 pieces (1.5 oz)	240
Bouchee Au Chocolat	1 piece (1.5 oz)	210
Bouchee Ivory Raspberry	1 pieces (1 oz)	160
Gold Ballotin	3 pieces (1.5 oz)	210
Truffle Amaretto Di Saronno	2 pieces (1.5 oz)	210
Truffle Deluxe Liqueur	2 pieces (1.5 oz)	210

H.SALT SEAFOOD

Chicken	3 oz	108
Cod	3 oz	62

FOOD	PORTION	CALS.
Hamburger	3 oz	228
Pork Loin	3 oz	254
Sirloin Steak	3 oz	239

HAAGEN-DAZS

FROZEN YOGURT

FOOD	PORTION	CALS.
Brownie Nut Blast	½ cup (3.5 oz)	215
Chocolate	½ cup (3.4 oz)	160
Coffee	½ cup (3.4 oz)	161
Orange Tango	½ cup (3.5 oz)	132
Pina Colada	½ cup (3.4 oz)	139
Raspberry Randezvous	½ cup (3.5 oz)	132
Soft Serve Coffee	½ cup (3.3 oz)	145
Soft Serve Nonfat Chocolate	½ cup (3.3 oz)	116
Soft Serve Nonfat Chocolate Mousse	½ cup (3.3 oz)	86
Soft Serve Nonfat Vanilla	½ cup (3.3 oz)	114
Soft Serve Nonfat Vanilla Mousse	½ cup (3.3 oz)	78
Strawberry Cheesecake Craze	½ cup (3.6 oz)	213
Strawberry Duet	½ cup (3.4 oz)	135
Vanilla	½ cup (3.4 oz)	162
Vanilla Almond Crunch	½ cup (3.4 oz)	198

ICE CREAM

FOOD	PORTION	CALS.
Bar Chocolate	1 (2.7 oz)	247
Bar Coffee	1 (2.7 oz)	249
Bar Vanilla	1 (2.7 oz)	251
Belgian Chocolate Chocolate	½ cup (3.6 oz)	315
Brownies A La Mode	½ cup (3.5 oz)	284
Butter Pecan	½ cup (3.7 oz)	304
Cappuccino Commotion	½ cup (3.6 oz)	305
Caramel Cone Explosion	½ cup (3.6 oz)	298
Chocolate	½ cup (3.7 oz)	249
Chocolate Chocolate Chip	½ cup (3.7 oz)	282
Chocolate Chocolate Mint	½ cup (3.6 oz)	285
Coffee	½ cup (3.7 oz)	251
Coffee Chip	½ cup (3.6 oz)	285
Cookie Dough Dynamo	½ cup (3.6 oz)	298
Cookies & Cream	½ cup (3.6 oz)	264
Deep Chocolate Peanut Butter	½ cup (3.7 oz)	339
Macadamia Brittle	½ cup (3.7 oz)	282
Macadamia Nut	½ cup (3.6 oz)	309
Midnight Cookies & Cream	½ cup (3.6 oz)	285
Peanut Butter Burst	½ cup (2.6 oz)	314
Pralines & Cream	½ cup (3.6 oz)	278
Rum Raisin	½ cup (3.7 oz)	256

FOOD	PORTION	CALS.
Strawberry	½ cup (3.7 oz)	242
Strawberry Cheesecake Craze	½ cup (3.7 oz)	273
Swiss Chocolate Almond	½ cup (3.6 oz)	288
Triple Brownie Overload	½ cup (3.5 oz)	296
Vanilla	½ cup (3.7 oz)	252
Vanilla Chip	½ cup (3.6 oz)	266
Vanilla Fudge	½ cup (3.7 oz)	268
Vanilla Swiss Almond	½ cup (3.7 oz)	288
SORBET		
Mango	½ cup (4 oz)	107
Raspberry	½ cup (4 oz)	110
Soft Serve Lemonade	½ cup (3.3 oz)	113
Soft Serve Mango	½ cup (3.3 oz)	107
Soft Serve Raspberry	½ cup (3.3 oz)	106
Strawberry	½ cup (4 oz)	118
Zesty Lemon	½ cup (4 oz)	111
HARDEE'S		
BEVERAGES		
Orange Juice	1 serv (11 oz)	140
Shake Chocolate	1 (12.2 oz)	370
Shake Peach	1 (12.1 oz)	390
Shake Strawberry	1 (12.7 oz)	420
Shake Vanilla	1 (12.2 oz)	349
BREAKFAST SELECTIONS		
Bacon & Egg Biscuit	1 (4.4 oz)	490
Bacon, Egg & Cheese Biscuit	1 (4.8 oz)	530
Big Country Breakfast Bacon	1 (7.6 oz)	740
Big Country Breakfast Sausage	1 (9.6 oz)	930
Biscuit 'N' Gravy	1 (7.8 oz)	510
Cinnamon 'N' Raisin Biscuit	1 (2.8 oz)	370
Country Ham Biscuit	1 (3.8 oz)	430
Frisco Breakfast Sandwich Ham	1 (6.5 oz)	460
Ham Biscuit	1 (4 oz)	400
Ham, Egg & Cheese Biscuit	1 (5.6 oz)	500
Hash Rounds	1 serv (2.8 oz)	230
Rise 'N' Shine Biscuit	1 (2.9 oz)	390
Sausage & Egg Biscuit	1 (5.2 oz)	560
Sausage Biscuit	1 (4.1 oz)	510
Three Pancakes	1 serv (4.8 oz)	280
Three Pancakes w/ 1 Sausage Pattie	1 serv (6.2 oz)	430
Three Pancakes w/ 2 Bacon Strips	1 serv (5.3 oz)	350
Ultimate Omelet Biscuit	1 (4.9 oz)	530
ICE CREAM		
Cool Twist Sundae Hot Fudge	1 (5.5 oz)	290

FOOD	PORTION	CALS.
Cool Twist Sundae Strawberry	1 (5.8 oz)	210
Cool Twist Cone Chocolate	1 (4.1 oz)	180
Cool Twist Cone Vanilla	1 (4.1 oz)	170
Cool Twist Cone Vanilla/ Chocolate	1 (4.1 oz)	180
MAIN MENU SELECTIONS		
Bacon Cheeseburger	1 (7.9 oz)	600
Big Cookie	1 (2.0 oz)	280
Big Deluxe Burger	1 (8.5 oz)	530
Cheeseburger	1 (4.2 oz)	300
Chicken Breast	1 piece (5.2 oz)	370
Chicken Fillet	1 (7.5 oz)	470
Chicken Leg	1 piece (2.4 oz)	170
Chicken Thigh	1 piece (4.2 oz)	330
Chicken Wing	1 piece (2.3 oz)	200
Cole Slaw	1 serv (4 oz)	240
Fisherman's Fillet	1 (7.6 oz)	500
French Fries	1 med (5.0 oz)	350
French Fries	1 sm (3.4 oz)	240
French Fries	1 lg (6.1 oz)	430
Frisco Burger	1 (8.5 oz)	760
Gravy	1 serv (1.5 fl oz)	20
Hamburger	1 (3.6 oz)	260
Hot Ham 'N' Cheese	1 (5.7 oz)	350
Marinated Chicked Grill	1 (7.1 oz)	202
Mashed Potatoes	1 serv (4 oz)	70
Mushroom 'N' Swiss Burger	1 (7.1 oz)	520
Quarter-Pound Cheeseburger	1 (6.5 oz)	490
Regular Roast Beef	1 (4.4 oz)	270
SALAD DRESSINGS		
French Fat Free	1 serv (2 oz)	70
Ranch	1 serv (2 oz)	290
Thousand Island	1 serv (2 oz)	250
SALADS AND SALAD BARS		
Garden Salad	1 (10.2 oz)	210
Grilled Chicken Salad	1 (11.5 oz)	150
Side Salad	1 (4.6 oz)	25
IHOP		
Pancake Buckwheat	1 (2.5 oz)	134
Pancake Buttermilk	1 (2 oz)	108
Pancake Country Griddle	1 (2.25 oz)	134
Pancake Egg	1 (2 oz)	102
Pancake Harvest Grain 'N Nut	1 (2.25 oz)	160
Waffle	1 (4 oz)	305

FOOD	PORTION	CALS.
Waffle Belgian	1 (6 oz)	408
Waffle Belgian Harvest Grain 'N Nut	1 (6 oz)	445

JACK IN THE BOX
BEVERAGES
2% Milk	1 serv (8 fl oz)	120
Coca-Cola Classic	1 sm (16 fl oz)	190
Coffee	1 cup (8 fl oz)	5
Diet Coke	1 sm (16 fl oz)	0
Dr Pepper	1 sm (16 fl oz)	190
Iced Tea	1 sm (16 fl oz)	0
Milk Shake Chocolate	1 reg (11 fl oz)	390
Milk Shake Strawberry	1 reg (10 fl oz)	330
Milk Shake Vanilla	1 reg (10 fl oz)	350
Orange Juice	1 serv (6 fl oz)	80
Ramblin' Root Beer	1 sm (16 fl oz)	240
Sprite	1 sm (16 fl oz)	190

BREAKFAST SELECTIONS
Breakfast Jack	1 (4.2 oz)	300
Country Crock Spread	1 pat (5 g)	25
Grape Jelly	1 serv (0.5 oz)	40
Hash Browns	1 serv (2 oz)	100
Pancake Platter	1 serv (5.6 oz)	400
Pancake Syrup	1 serv (1.5 fl oz)	120
Sausage Croissant	1 (6.4 oz)	670
Scrambled Egg Pocket	1 (6.4 oz)	430
Sourdough Breakfast Sandwich	1 (5.2 oz)	380
Supreme Croissant	1 (6 oz)	570
Ultimate Breakfast Sandwich	1 (8.5 oz)	620

DESSERTS
Cheesecake	1 serv (3.5 oz)	310
Chocolate Chip Cookie Dough Cheesecake	1 serv (3.6 oz)	360
Hot Apple Turnover	1 (3.9 oz)	350

MAIN MENU SELECTIONS
¼ lb. Burger	1 (6 oz)	510
American Cheese	1 slice (0.4 oz)	45
Bacon & Cheddar Potato Wedges	1 serv (9.3 oz)	800
Bacon Bacon Cheeseburger	1 (8.5 oz)	710
Barbeque Dipping Sauce	1 serv (1 fl oz)	45
Cheeseburger	1 (3.9 oz)	320
Chicken Caesar Sandwich	1 (8.3 oz)	520
Chicken Fajita Pita	1 (6.9 oz)	280
Chicken Sandwich	1 (5.6 oz)	400
Chicken Strips Breaded	4 pieces (3.9 oz)	290

FOOD	PORTION	CALS.
Chicken Strips Breaded	6 pieces (6.2 oz)	450
Chicken Supreme	1 (8.6 oz)	620
Chinese Hot Sauce	1 pkg (5 g)	10
Double Cheeseburger	1 (5.3 oz)	450
Egg Rolls	5 pieces (10 oz)	750
Egg Rolls	3 pieces (5.8 oz)	440
Fish Supreme	1 (8.6 oz)	590
French Fries	1 reg (6.7 oz)	350
French Fries	1 sm (2.4 oz)	220
Grilled Chicken Fillet	1 (7.4 oz)	430
Grilled Sourdough Burger	1 (7.8 oz)	670
Guacamole	1 serv (0.9 oz)	50
Hamburger	1 (3.4 oz)	280
Hot Sauce	1 pkg (0.5 fl oz)	5
Jumbo Fries	1 serv (4.3 oz)	400
Jumbo Jack	1 (8 oz)	560
Jumbo Jack With Cheese	1 (8.5 oz)	650
Ketchup	1 pkg (0.3 oz)	10
Mayonnaise	1 pkg (0.7 oz)	150
Monterey Roast Beef Sandwich	1 (8.4 oz)	540
Mustard	1 pkg (6 g)	5
Onion Rings	1 serv (3.6 oz)	380
Salsa	1 serv (1 fl oz)	10
Seasoned Curly Fries	1 serv (3.8 oz)	360
Sour Cream	1 serv (1 oz)	60
Soy Sauce	1 serv (0.3 oz)	5
Spicy Crispy Chicken Sandwich	1 (7.9 oz)	560
Stuffed Jalapenos	7 pieces (4.8 oz)	420
Stuffed Jalapenos	10 pieces (6.8 oz)	600
Super Scoop French Fries	1 serv (6.5 oz)	590
Super Taco	1 (4.4 oz)	280
Sweet & Sour Dipping Sauce	1 serv (1 fl oz)	40
Swiss-Style Cheese	1 slice (0.4 oz)	40
Taco	1 (2.7 oz)	190
Tartar Dipping Sauce	1 pkg (1 oz)	150
Teriyaki Bowl Chicken	1 serv (15.4 oz)	580
The Colassus Burger	1 (10.1 oz)	1100
The Outlaw Burger	1 (8.2 oz)	720
The Really Big Chicken Sandwich	1 (12.5 oz)	900
Ultimate Cheeseburger	1 (9.8 oz)	1030
SALAD DRESSINGS		
Blue Cheese	1 serv (2 fl oz)	210
Buttermilk House	1 serv (2 fl oz)	290
Buttermilk House Dipping Sauce	1 serv (0.9 fl oz)	130

FOOD	PORTION	CALS.
Italian Low Calorie	1 serv (2 fl oz)	25
Thousand Island	1 serv (2 fl oz)	250
SALADS AND SALAD BARS		
Croutons	1 serv (0.4 oz)	50
Garden Chicken Salad	1 serv (8.9 oz)	200
Side Salad	1 (3.4 oz)	70

KFC

BAKED SELECTIONS

Biscuit	1 (2.0 oz)	200
Cornbread	1 (2 oz)	228

MAIN MENU SELECTIONS

BBQ Baked Beans	1 serv (3.9 oz)	132
Chicken Pot Pie	1 (13.4 oz)	700
Cole Slaw	1 serv (3.2 oz)	114
Colonel's Chicken Sandwich	1 (5.9 oz)	482
Colonel's Rotisserie Gold Quarter Breast & Wing	1 serv (6.2 oz)	335
Colonel's Rotisserie Gold Quarter Breast & Wing Skin Removed	1 serv (4.1 oz)	199
Colonel's Rotisserie Gold Quarter Thigh & Leg	1 serv (5.1 oz)	333
Colonel's Rotisserie Gold Quarter Thigh & Leg Skin Removed	1 serv (4.1 oz)	217
Corn On The Cob	1 ear (5.3 oz)	222
Crispy Strips	4 (4 oz)	323
Extra Tasty Crispy Breast	1 (5.9 oz)	470
Extra Tasty Crispy Drumstick	1 (2.4 oz)	190
Extra Tasty Crispy Thigh	1 (4.2 oz)	370
Extra Tasty Crispy Whole Wing	1 (1.9 oz)	200
Garden Rice	1 serv (3.8 oz)	75
Green Beans	1 serv (3.6 oz)	36
Hot & Spicy Breast	1 (6.5 oz)	530
Hot & Spicy Drumstick	1 (2.3 oz)	190
Hot & Spicy Thigh	1 (3.8 oz)	370
Hot & Spicy Whole Wing	1 (1.9 oz)	210
Hot Wings	6 (4.8 oz)	471
Kentucky Nuggets	6 (3.4 oz)	284
Macaroni & Cheese	1 serv (4 oz)	162
Mashed Potatoes With Gravy	1 serv (4.2 oz)	109
Mean Greens	1 serv (3.9 oz)	52
Original Chicken Sandwich	1 (7.2 oz)	497
Original Recipe Breast	1 (4.8 oz)	360
Original Recipe Drumstick	1 (1.8 oz)	130

FOOD	PORTION	CALS.
Original Recipe Thigh	1 (3.3 oz)	260
Original Recipe Whole Wing	1 (1.7 oz)	150
Potato Salad	1 serv (4.4 oz)	180
Potato Wedges	1 serv (3.3 oz)	192
Red Beans & Rice	1 serv (3.9 oz)	114
Value BBQ Chicken Sandwich	1 (5.3 oz)	296

KENNY ROGERS ROASTERS
MAIN MENU SELECTIONS

FOOD	PORTION	CALS.
½ Chicken w/ Skin	1 serv (9.06 oz)	515
½ Chicken w/o Skin & Wing	1 serv (7.03 oz)	313
¼ Chicken Dark Meat w/ Skin	1 serv (4.35 oz)	271
¼ Chicken Dark Meat w/o Skin & Wing	1 serv (3.29 oz)	169
¼ Chicken White Meat w/ Skin	1 serv (4.71 oz)	244
¼ Chicken White Meat w/o Skin & Wing	1 serv (3.74 oz)	144
Baked Sweet Potato	1 (9 oz)	263
Chicken Caesar Salad	1 serv (9.4 oz)	285
Cinnamon Apples	1 serv (5.27 oz)	199
Cole Slaw	1 serv (5.05 oz)	225
Corn Muffin	1 (2 oz)	175
Corn On The Cob	1 (2.25 oz)	68
Corn Stuffing	1 serv (7.1 oz)	326
Creamy Parmesan Spinach	1 serv (5.3 oz)	119
Garlic Parsley Potatoes	1 serv (6.5 oz)	259
Honey Baked Beans	1 serv (6.6 oz)	148
Italian Green Beans	1 serv (6.1 oz)	116
Macaroni & Cheese	1 serv (5.51 oz)	197
Pasta Salad	1 serv (5 oz)	236
Pita BBQ Chicken	1 (7.33 oz)	401
Pita Chicken Caesar	1 (9.2 oz)	606
Pita Roasted Chicken	1 (10.8 oz)	685
Pot Pie Chicken	1 (12 oz)	708
Potato Salad	1 serv (7.01 oz)	390
Real Mashed Potatoes	1 serv (8 oz)	295
Rice Pilaf	1 serv (5 oz)	173
Roasted Chicken Salad	1 serv (16.9 oz)	292
Sandwich Turkey	1 (9.2 oz)	385
Side Salad	1 serv (4.73 oz)	23
Sour Cream & Dill Pasta Salad	1 serv (5 oz)	233
Steamed Vegetables	1 serv (4.25 oz)	48
Sweet Corn Niblets	1 serv (5 oz)	112
Tomato Cucumber Salad	1 serv (6 oz)	123
Turkey Sliced Breast	1 serv (4.5 oz)	158
Zucchini & Squash Santa Fe	1 serv (5 oz)	70

FOOD	PORTION	CALS.
SALAD DRESSINGS		
Blue Cheese	1 serv (2.47 oz)	370
Buttermilk Ranch	1 serv (2.47 oz)	430
Caesar	1 serv (2.47 oz)	340
Honey French	1 serv (2.47 oz)	350
Honey Mustard	1 serv (2.47 oz)	320
Italian Fat Free	1 serv (2.47 oz)	35
Thousand Island	1 serv (2.47 oz)	330
SOUPS		
Chicken Noodle	1 bowl (10 oz)	91
Chicken Noodle	1 cup (6 oz)	55

KRYSTAL

FOOD	PORTION	CALS.
BEVERAGES		
Chocolate Shake	1 (16 fl oz)	275
BREAKFAST SELECTIONS		
Biscuit	1 (2.5 oz)	244
Biscuit Bacon	1 (2.9 oz)	306
Biscuit Bacon, Egg & Cheese	1 (4.7 oz)	421
Biscuit Country Ham	1 (3.7 oz)	334
Biscuit Egg	1 (4 oz)	327
Biscuit Gravy	1 (7.5 oz)	419
Biscuit Sausage	1 (4.1 oz)	437
Sunriser	1 (3.8 oz)	259
DESSERTS		
Apple Pie	1 serv (4.5 oz)	300
Donut Plain	1 (1.3 oz)	150
Donut w/ Chocolate Icing	1 (1.8 oz)	212
Donut w/ Vanilla Icing	1 (1.8 oz)	198
Lemon Meringue Pie	1 serving (4 oz)	340
Pecan Pie	1 serv (4 oz)	450
MAIN MENU SELECTIONS		
Bacon Cheeseburger	1 (7.4 oz)	521
Big K	1 (8 oz)	540
Burger Plus	1 (6.5 oz)	415
Burger Plus w/ Cheese	1 (7.1 oz)	473
Cheese Krystal	1 (2.5 oz)	187
Chili	1 lg (12 oz)	327
Chili	1 reg (8 oz)	218
Chili Cheese Pup	1 (2.7 oz)	211
Chili Pup	1 (2.5 oz)	182
Corn Pup	1 (2.3 oz)	214
Crispy Crunchy Chicken Sandwich	1 (5.75 oz)	467
Double Cheese Krystal	1 (4.5 oz)	337

FOOD	PORTION	CALS.
Double Krystal	1 (4 oz)	277
Fries	1 lg (5.3 oz)	463
Fries	1 reg (4.1 oz)	358
Fries	1 sm (3 oz)	262
Krys Kross Fries	1 serv (4.3 oz)	486
Krys Kross Fries Chili Cheese	1 serv (6.8 oz)	625
Krys Kross Fries w/ Cheese	1 serv (5.3 oz)	515
Krystal	1 (2.2 oz)	158
Plain Pup	1 (1.9 oz)	160

LITTLE CAESARS
MAIN MENU SELECTIONS

Crazy Bread	1 piece (1.4 oz)	106
Crazy Sauce	1 serv (6 oz)	170
Deli-Style Sandwich Ham & Cheese	1 (11.6 oz)	728
Deli-Style Sandwich Italian	1 (11.9 oz)	740
Deli-Style Sandwich Veggie	1 (11.9 oz)	647
Hot Oven-Baked Sandwich Cheeser	1 (12.1 oz)	822
Hot Oven-Baked Sandwich Meatsa	1 (15 oz)	1036
Hot Oven-Baked Sandwich Pepperoni	1 (11.2 oz)	899
Hot Oven-Baked Sandwich Supreme	1 (13.1 oz)	894
Hot Oven-Baked Sandwich Veggie	1 (13.7 oz)	669

PIZZA

Baby Pan!Pan!	1 serv (8.4 oz)	616
Pan!Pan! Cheese	1 med slice (2.9 oz)	181
Pan!Pan! Pepperoni	1 med slice (3 oz)	199
Pizza!Pizza! Cheese	1 med slice (3.2 oz)	201
Pizza!Pizza! Pepperoni	1 med slice (3.3 oz)	220

SALAD DRESSINGS

1000 Island	1 serv (1.5 oz)	183
Blue Cheese	1 serv (1.5 oz)	160
Caesar	1 serv (1.5 oz)	255
French	1 serv (1.5 oz)	166
Greek	1 serv (1.5 oz)	268
Italian	1 serv (1.5 oz)	200
Italian Fat Free	1 serv (1.5 oz)	15
Ranch	1 serv (1.5 oz)	221

SALADS AND SALAD BARS

Antipasto Salad	1 serv (8.4 oz)	176
Caesar Salad	1 serv (5 oz)	140
Greek Salad	1 serv (10.3 oz)	168
Tossed Salad	1 serv (8.5 oz)	116

LONG JOHN SILVER'S
BEVERAGES

Diet Coke	1 serv (8 oz)	1

FOOD	PORTION	CALS.
DESSERTS		
Apple Crumb Cheesecake	1 serv (3.5 oz)	300
Chocolate Cream Pie	1 serv (2.6 oz)	280
Double Lemon Pie	1 serv (3.4 oz)	350
Key Lime Cream Cheese Pie	1 serv (3 oz)	310
Pineapple Cream Cheesecake	1 serv (3.2 oz)	310
MAIN MENU SELECTIONS		
Baked Potato	1 (8 oz)	210
Battered Chicken	1 piece (2 oz)	120
Battered Clams	1 serv (3 oz)	300
Battered Fish	1 piece (2.9 oz)	170
Battered Shrimp	1 piece (0.4 oz)	35
Cheese Sticks	1 serv (1.6 oz)	160
Coleslaw	1 serv (3.4 oz)	140
Corn Cobbette	1 piece (3.3 oz)	140
Corn Cobbette w/o Butter	1 (3.1 oz)	80
Flavorbaked Chicken	1 piece (3.5 oz)	150
Flavorbaked Chicken (1 piece) Rice Baked Potato Green Beans	1 serv	448
Flavorbaked Chicken (1 piece) Rice Side Salad	1 serv	275
Flavorbaked Chicken & Fish Rice Baked Potato Green Beans	1 serv	538
Flavorbaked Fish	1 piece (3.1 oz)	120
Flavorbaked Fish (2 pieces) Rice Baked Potato Green Bean	1 serv	518
Flavorbaked Fish (2 pieces) Rice Side Salad	1 serv	345
Fries	1 serv (3 oz)	250
Green Beans	1 serv (3.5 oz)	30
Honey Mustard Sauce	1 serv (0.4 fl oz)	20
Hushpuppy	1 (0.8 oz)	60
Ketchup	1 serv (.32 oz)	10
Lettuce	1 serv (0.5 oz)	8
Margarine	1 serv (0.2 oz)	35
Mayonnaise	1 serv (0.5 oz)	100
Montery Jack Cheese	1 serv (0.5 oz)	50
Popcorn Chicken	1 serv (3.3 oz)	250
Popcorn Fish	1 serv (3.6 oz)	290
Popcorn Shrimp	1 serv (3.3 oz)	280
Rice Pilaf	1 serv (3 oz)	140
Sandwich Batter Dipped Fish No Sauce	1 (5.4 oz)	320
Sandwich Flavorbaked Chicken	1 (5.8 oz)	290
Sandwich Flavorbaked Fish	1 (6 oz)	320
Sandwich Ultimate Fish	1 (6.4 oz)	430

FOOD	PORTION	CALS.
Sandwich Bun	1 (1.7 oz)	130
Shrimp Sauce	1 serv (0.4 oz)	15
Sour Cream	1 serv (1 oz)	60
Sweet'N'Sour Sauce	1 serv (0.4 fl oz)	20
Tartar Sauce	1 serv (0.4 fl oz)	35
Tomato	1 serv (0.7 oz)	6
SALAD DRESSINGS		
Fat-Free French	1 serv (1.5 oz)	50
Fat-Free Ranch	1 serv (1.5 fl oz)	50
Italian	1 serv (1 oz)	130
Malt Vinegar	1 serv (0.3 fl oz)	0
Ranch Dressing	1 serv (1 fl oz)	170
Thousand Island	1 serv (1 oz)	110
SALADS AND SALAD BARS		
Ocean Chef Salad	1 serv (8.1 oz)	100
Side Salad	1 (4.3 oz)	25

LYONS RESTAURANTS
MAIN MENU SELECTIONS

Light & Healthy Halibut Brochette	1 serv	502
Light & Healthy Lime & Cilantro Chicken	1 serv	511

MACHEEZMO MOUSE
CHILDREN'S MENU SELECTIONS

El Bento Kid	1 serv (7 oz)	235
Quesadilla Kid Cheese	1 serv (5 oz)	360
Quesadilla Kid Chicken	1 serv (7 oz)	430
Taco Kid Cheese	1 serv (6 oz)	285
Taco Kid Chicken	1 (8 oz)	355
MAIN MENU SELECTIONS		
Beans	1 oz	35
Bento Stick	1 oz	30
Boss Sauce	1 oz	30
Broccoli	1 oz	4
Burrito Chicken	1 (13 oz)	580
Burrito Combo	1 (14 oz)	630
Burrito Vegetarian	1 (14 oz)	655
Cheese	1 oz	81
Chicken	1 oz	35
Chili	1 oz	43
Chips	1 oz	140
Cilantro	1 oz	8
Dinner Rice, Beans, Broccoli	1 serv (10 oz)	328
Dinner Rice, Beans, Salad	1 serv (12 oz)	344
El Bento	1 serv (16 oz)	600

FOOD	PORTION	CALS.
El Bento Deluxe	1 serv (20 oz)	740
Enchilada Chicken	1 (12 oz)	533
Enchilada Chili	1 (12 oz)	549
Enchilada Veggie	1 (14 oz)	623
Enchilada Sauce	1 oz	6
Fresh Greens	1 oz	2
Green Sauce	1 oz	5
Guacamole	1 oz	100
Marinated Veggies	1 oz	10
Mexican Cheese	1 oz	100
Mustard Dressing	1 oz	25
Power Salad Chicken	1 serv (16 oz)	275
Power Salad Veggie	1 serv (13 oz)	200
Rice	1 oz	45
Salad Chicken	1 serv (15 oz)	430
Salad Veggie Taco	1 serv (16 oz)	655
Salsa	1 oz	4
Snack Famouse #5	1 serv (14 oz)	585
Snack Nacho Grande	1 serv (9 oz)	841
Snack Quesadilla Cheese	1 serv (6 oz)	377
Snack Quesadilla Chicken	1 serv (10 oz)	450
Snack Tacos Chicken	1 serv (6 oz)	290
Snack Tacos Chili	1 serv (6 oz)	314
Snack Tacos Veggie	1 serv (6 oz)	290
Sour Cream	1 oz	23
Tortilla Corn	3 (1 oz)	60
Tortilla Flour	1 oz	80
Tortilla Wheat	1 oz	80
Veggie Deluxe	1 serv (18 oz)	665
Yogurt Nonfat	1 oz	20

MANHATTAN BAGEL

Blueberry	1 (4 oz)	260
Cheddar Cheese	1 (4 oz)	270
Chocolate Chip	1 (4 oz)	290
Cinnamon Raisin	1 (4 oz)	280
Egg	1 (4 oz)	270
Everything	1 (4 oz)	290
Garlic	1 (4 oz)	270
Marble	1 (4 oz)	260
Oat Bran Raisin Walnut	1 (4 oz)	270
Onion	1 (4 oz)	270
Plain	1 (4 oz)	260
Poppy	1 (4 oz)	300

FOOD	PORTION	CALS.
Pumpernickel	1 (4 oz)	250
Rye	1 (4 oz)	260
Salt	1 (4 oz)	260
Sesame	1 (4 oz)	310
Spinach	1 (4 oz)	270
Whole Wheat	1 (4 oz)	260

MAX & IRMA'S
MAIN MENU SELECTIONS

FOOD	PORTION	CALS.
Cocktail Sauce	1 oz	33
Fruit Smoothie	1 serv (10 oz)	114
Garden Burger	1 serv (14 oz)	467
Gourmet Garden Burger	1 serv (154 oz)	484
Grilled Zucchini & Mushroom Pasta	1 serv (15 oz)	448
Grilled Zucchini & Mushroom Pasta With Chicken	1 serv (18 oz)	621
Peel & Eat Shrimp	1 serv (6 oz)	166
Ranch Mayonnaise Low Fat	1 serv (1 oz)	22

MCDONALD'S
BAKED SELECTIONS

FOOD	PORTION	CALS.
Apple Pie Baked	1 (2.7 oz)	260
Danish Apple	1 (3.7 oz)	360
Danish Cheese	1 (3.7 oz)	410
Danish Cinnamon Raisin	1 (3.7 oz)	430
Danish Raspberry	1 (3.7 oz)	400
Fat Free Muffin Apple Bran	1 (2.5 oz)	170

BEVERAGES

FOOD	PORTION	CALS.
Apple Juice	1 serv (6 oz)	80
Coca-Cola Classic	1 sm (16 oz)	150
Cocoa-Cola Classic	1 child serv (12 oz)	110
Cocoa-Cola Classic	1 med (21 oz)	210
Cocoa-Cola Classic	1 lg (32 oz)	310
Diet Coke	1 sm (16 oz)	1
Diet Coke	1 lg (32 oz)	0
Diet Coke	1 child serv (12 oz)	0
Diet Coke	1 med (21 oz)	0
Hi-C Orange	1 sm (16 oz)	160
Hi-C Orange	1 child serv (12 oz)	120
Hi-C Orange	1 med (21 oz)	240
Hi-C Orange	1 lg (32 oz)	350
Milk 1%	1 serv (8 oz)	100
Orange Juice	1 serv (6 oz)	80
Shake Chocolate	1 sm (14.5 oz)	340
Shake Strawberry	1 sm (14.5 oz)	340

FOOD	PORTION	CALS.
Shake Vanilla	1 sm (14.5 oz)	340
Sprite	1 sm (16 fl oz)	150
Sprite	1 med (21 oz)	210
Sprite	1 child serv (12 oz)	110
Sprite	1 lg (32 oz)	310
BREAKFAST SELECTIONS		
Bacon Egg & Cheese Biscuit	1 (5.3 oz)	450
Biscuit	1 (2.7 oz)	260
Cheerios	1 pkg (0.7 oz)	70
Egg McMuffin	1 (4.8 oz)	290
English Muffin	1 (1.9 oz)	140
Hash Browns	1 serv (1.9 oz)	130
Hotcakes Plain	1 serv (5.3 oz)	310
Hotcakes w/ Margarine & Syrup	2 serv (7.8 oz)	580
Sausage	1 (1.5 oz)	170
Sausage Biscuit	1 (4.2 oz)	430
Sausage Biscuit w/ Egg	1 (6 oz)	520
Sausage McMuffin	1 (3.9 oz)	360
Sausage McMuffin w/ Egg	1 (5.7 oz)	440
Scrambled Eggs	2 (3.6 oz)	170
Wheaties	1 pkg (0.8 oz)	80
DESSERTS		
McDonaldland Cookies	1 pkg (2 oz)	260
Nuts For Sundaes	1 serv (7 g)	40
Sundae Hot Fudge	1 (6.3 oz)	290
Yogurt Cone Lowfat Vanilla	1 (3.2 oz)	120
Yogurt Sundae Lowfat Hot Caramel	1 (6.4 oz)	310
Yogurt Sundae Lowfat Strawberry	1 (6.2 oz)	240
MAIN MENU SELECTIONS		
Arch Deluxe	1 (8.7 oz)	570
Barbeque Sauce	1 pkg (1 oz)	45
Big Mac	1 (7.6 oz)	530
Cheeseburger	1 (4.2 oz)	320
Chicken McNuggets	6 pieces (3.8 oz)	300
Chicken McNuggets	4 pieces (2.6 oz)	200
Chicken McNuggets	9 pieces (5.8 oz)	450
Filet-O-Fish	1 (5 oz)	360
French Fries	1 sm (2.4 oz)	210
French Fries	1 lg (5.2 oz)	450
French Fries	1 super (6.2 oz)	540
Hamburger	1 (3.7 oz)	270
Honey Mustard	1 pkg (0.5 oz)	50
Hot Mustard	1 pkg (1 oz)	60
McChicken Sandwich	1 (6.7 oz)	510

FOOD	PORTION	CALS.
McGilled Chicken Classic	1 (6.6 oz)	260
McNuggets Sauce Honey	1 pkg (0.5 oz)	45
Quarter Pounder	1 (6 oz)	420
Quarter Pounder w/ Cheese	1 (7 oz)	530
Sweet 'N Sour Sauce	1 pkg (1 oz)	50
SALAD DRESSINGS		
1000 Island	1 pkg (2.2 oz)	190
Bleu Cheese	1 pkg (2.1 oz)	190
Lite Vinaigrette	1 pkg (2.2 oz)	50
Ranch	1 pkg (2.1 oz)	230
Red French Reduced Calorie	1 pkg (2.4 oz)	160
SALADS AND SALAD BARS		
Bacon Bits	1 pkg (3 g)	15
Chef Salad	1 serv (11 oz)	210
Croutons	1 pkg (0.4 oz)	50
Fajita Chicken Salad	1 serv (10 oz)	160
Garden Salad	1 serv (8.2 oz)	80
Side Salad	1 serv (4.9 oz)	45

MORRISON'S

FOOD	PORTION	CALS.
DESSERTS		
Boston Cream Cake	1 slice	218
MAIN MENU SELECTIONS		
Baked Potato	1	220
Broccoli	1 serv (4 oz)	37
Cabbage	1 serv (4 oz)	36
Cantaloupe Compote	1 serv (4 oz)	130
Cauliflower	1 serv (4 oz)	68
Chicken Stew & Dumplings	1 serv (7 oz)	362
Chicken Teriyaki	1 serv (5.5 oz)	232
French Bread	1 slice	207
Grilled Chicken Pecan Salad	1 serv (6 oz)	298
Lima Beans	1 serv (4 oz)	170
Okra & Tomatoes	1 serv (5 oz)	40
Pinto Beans	1 serv (4 oz)	105
Plain Jello	1 serv (3 oz)	131
Rutabagas	1 serv (4 oz)	33
Sliced Tomato	4 slices	40
Soft Roll	1 (2 oz)	170
Strawberries Peaches & Bananas	1 serv (6 oz)	203
Turnip Greens	1 serv (4 oz)	30
Watermelon	1 serv (6 oz)	102
Yellow Squash	1 serv (4 oz)	22
SALADS AND SALAD BARS		
Garden Salad	1 serv (2.5 oz)	75
Tossed Salad	1 serv (3 oz)	30

FOOD	PORTION	CALS.
MY FAVORITE MUFFIN		
Basic Muffin	⅓ muffin	220
Double Chocolate	⅓ muffin	190
Fat Free Bavarian	⅓ muffin	100
Fat Free Bavarian Chocolate	⅓ muffin	130
NATHAN'S		
BEVERAGES		
Lemonade	32 fl oz	378
Lemonade	16 fl oz	189
Lemonade	22 fl oz	260
MAIN MENU SELECTIONS		
Breaded Chicken Sandwich	1 (7.2 oz)	510
Charbroiled Chicken Sandwich	1 (4.5 oz)	288
Cheese Steak Sandwich	1 (6.1 oz)	485
Chicken 2 Pieces	1 serv (7.1 oz)	693
Chicken 4 Pieces	1 serv (14.2 oz)	1382
Chicken Platter 2 Pieces	1 serv (14.8 oz)	1096
Chicken Platter 4 Pieces	1 serv (21.9 oz)	1788
Chicken Salad	1 serv (12.7 oz)	154
Double Burger	1 (7.3 oz)	671
Filet of Fish Platter	1 serv (22 oz)	1455
Filet of Fish Sandwich	1 (5.2 oz)	403
Frank Nuggets	15 pieces (6.9 oz)	764
Frank Nuggets	11 pieces (5.1 oz)	563
Frank Nuggets	7 pieces (3.2 oz)	357
Frankfurter	1 (3.2 oz)	310
French Fries	1 serv (8.6 oz)	514
Fried Clam Platter	1 serv (13.1 oz)	1024
Fried Clam Sandwich	1 (5.4 oz)	620
Fried Shrimp	1 serv (4.4 oz)	348
Fried Shrimp Platter	1 serv (12.6 oz)	796
Hamburger	1 (4.7 oz)	434
Knish	1 (5.9 oz)	318
Pastrami Sandwich	1 (4.1 oz)	325
Sauteed Onions	1 serv (3.5 oz)	39
Super Burger	1 (7.6 oz)	533
Turkey Sandwich	1 (4.9 oz)	270
SALADS AND SALAD BARS		
Garden Salad	1 serv (10.9 oz)	193
OLIVE GARDEN		
Baked Lasagna	1 lunch serv	330
Breadstick	1	70
Breadstick w/o margarine	1	30

FOOD	PORTION	CALS.
Breadstick w/o margarine & garlic salt	1	30
Eggplant Parmigiana	1 lunch serv	220
Fettuccine Alfredo	1 lunch serv	790
Garden Fare Dinner Capellini Pomodoro	1 serv (16.6 oz)	420
Garden Fare Dinner Capellini Primavera	1 serv (18.1 oz)	380
Garden Fare Dinner Chicken Giardino	1 serv (18.6 oz)	480
Garden Fare Dinner Grilled Herb Chicken w/ Peppers	1 serv (17.5 oz)	470
Garden Fare Dinner Shrimp Primavera	1 serv (17.5 oz)	420
Garden Fare Dinner Spaghetti w/ Marinara Sauce	1 serv (16.2 oz)	500
Garden Fare Dinner Spaghetti w/ Sicilian Sauce	1 serv (15.9 oz)	530
Garden Fare Dinner Venetian Grilled Chicken	1 serv (9.5 oz)	360
Garden Fare Lunch Capellini Pamodoro	1 serv (10.2 oz)	290
Garden Fare Lunch Capellini Primavera	1 serv (12.1 oz)	270
Garden Fare Lunch Shrimp Primavera	1 serv (11.6 oz)	320
Garden Fare Lunch Spaghetti w/ Marinara Sauce	1 serv (11.2 oz)	350
Garden Fare Lunch Spaghetti w/ Sicilian Sauce	1 serv (11.2 oz)	370
Garden Salad	1 serving	230
Minestrone Soup	1 serv (6 oz)	80
Pasta e Fagioli	6 fl oz	140
Raspberry Sorbetto	1 serv (6 oz)	170
Salad Dressing	1 tbsp	60
Veal Marsala	1 dinner serv	330
Veal Parmigiana	1 dinner serv	590
Veal Piccata	1 dinner serv	230

PICCADILLY CAFETERIA
BAKED SELECTIONS

Corn Sticks	1 (2 oz)	165
French Bread	1 slice	132
Garlic Bread	1 serv (15.8 oz)	1154
Mexican Corn Bread	1 piece	220
Roll	1 (2 oz)	130
Roll Whole Wheat	1 (1.7 oz)	117
Texas Toast	1 serv (15.5 oz)	1088

BEVERAGES

Iced Tea	1 serv (6.5 oz)	2
Punch	1 serv (9 oz)	133

DESSERTS

Apple Pie	1 slice (7.2 oz)	439

FOOD	PORTION	CALS.
Cantaloupe	1 serv (9 oz)	89
Cantaloupe	1 serv (5.5 oz)	55
Chocolate Cream Pie	1 slice (7.5 oz)	512
Custard	1 cup (5.4 oz)	183
Custard Pie	1 slice (6.2 oz)	412
Dole Whip Topping	1 serv (3 oz)	68
Fresh Fruit Plate	1 serv (21.1 oz)	389
Gelatin	1 serv (4.75 oz)	128
Honeydew Melon	1 serv (5.5 oz)	55
Honeydew Melon	1 serv (9 oz)	89
Lemon Chiffon Pie	1 slice (6.3 oz)	481
Pound Cake	1 slice (3.8 oz)	371
Watermelon	1 serv (11 oz)	100
MAIN MENU SELECTIONS		
Au Jus	1 serv (3 oz)	5
Baby Lima Beans	1 serv (4.5 oz)	151
Baked Potato	1	218
Baked Potato w/ Topping	1	350
Beef Chopped Steak Fried	1 serv (4 oz)	311
Beef Leg Roast	1 serv (4 oz)	311
Beef Liver Fried	1 serv (4.5 oz)	430
Beef Tips Braised	1 serv (10 oz)	470
Black-eyed Peas w/ Pork Jowls	1 serv (4 oz)	108
Broccoli Buttered	1 serv (4 oz)	77
Broccoli & Rice Au Gratin	½ cup	184
Carrots Young Buttered	½ cup	90
Cauliflower Buttered	1 serv	80
Chicken Baked w/o Skin	¼ chicken	352
Chicken Teriyaki	1 serv (4 oz)	445
Chicken Teriyaki Polynesian	1 serv (4 oz)	537
Corn	1 serv (4.5 oz)	128
Cornbread Stuffing	1 serv (4.5 oz)	164
Crackers	4 (0.4 oz)	51
Cranberry Sauce	1 serv (1.5 oz)	64
Eggplant Escalloped	½ cup	180
Fish Baked	1 serv (7 oz)	195
Green Beans	1 serv (4.5 oz)	77
Ham Baked	1 serv (4 oz)	224
Macaroni & Cheese	½ cup	317
Mashed Potatoes	1 serv (4.8 oz)	120
Meatballs Baked & Spaghetti	1 serv (11.5 oz)	108
New Potatoes Boiled	½ cup	148
Okra Smothered	1 serv (4 oz)	121
Onion Sauce	1 serv (4 oz)	152

FOOD	PORTION	CALS.
Rice	½ cup	99
Rice Polynesian	1 serv (4 oz)	140
Spaghetti Baked	1 serv (9.5 oz)	256
Squash Baked Italian	1 serv (4.75 oz)	73
Squash Mixed Yellow & Zucchini	1 serv (4 oz)	72
Squash Yellow Baked French Style	⅓ cup	86
Turkey Breast	1 serv (3 oz)	99
Vegetables Unseasoned	1 serv (5 oz)	29
SALADS AND SALAD BARS		
Broccoli Salad	1 serv (4 oz)	202
Cabbage Combination Salad	1 serv (4.5 oz)	50
Carrot & Raisin Salad	1 serv (4.5 oz)	321
Cole Slaw w/ Cream	1 serv (4 oz)	182
Cucumber & Celery Salad	1 serv (4 oz)	82
Fruit Salad	1 serv (6 oz)	59
Neptune Salad	1 serv	361
Spinach Tossed Salad	1 serv (4 oz)	88
Spring Salad Bowl	1 serv (4 oz)	22
SOUPS		
Gumbo Chicken	1 serv (8 oz)	92
Gumbo Seafood	1 serv (8 oz)	98
Vegetable	1 serv (8 oz)	49
PIZZA HUT		
Beef Medium Hand Tossed	1 slice (4.2 oz)	260
Beef Medium Pan	1 slice (4.2 oz)	286
Beef Medium Thin 'N Crispy	1 slice (3.5 oz)	229
Bigfoot Cheese	1 slice (2.7 oz)	186
Bigfoot Pepperoni	1 slice (2.8 oz)	205
Bigfoot Pepperoni Mushroom Italian Sausage	1 slice (3.2 oz)	214
Cheese Medium Hand Tossed	1 slice (3.8 oz)	235
Cheese Medium Pan	1 slice (3.8 oz)	261
Cheese Medium Thin 'N Crispy	1 slice (3 oz)	205
Ham Medium Hand Tossed	1 slice (3.7 oz)	213
Ham Medium Pan	1 slice (3.7 oz)	239
Ham Medium Thin 'N Crispy	1 slice (3 oz)	184
Italian Sausage Medium Hand Tossed	1 slice (4.1 oz)	267
Italian Sausage Medium Pan	1 slice (4.1 oz)	293
Italian Sausage Medium Thin 'N Crispy	1 slice (3.3 oz)	236
Meat Lover's Medium Hand Tossed	1 slice (4.6 oz)	314
Meat Lover's Medium Pan	1 slice (4.6 oz)	340
Meat Lover's Medium Thin 'N Crispy	1 slice (3.9 oz)	288
Pepperoni Lover's Medium Hand Tossed	1 slice (4.3 oz)	306

FOOD	PORTION	CALS.
Pepperoni Lover's Medium Pan	1 slice (4.3 oz)	332
Pepperoni Lover's Medium Thin N'Crispy	1 slice (3.7 oz)	289
Pepperoni Medium Hand Tossed	1 slice (3.6 oz)	238
Pepperoni Medium Pan	1 slice (3.6 oz)	265
Pepperoni Medium Thin 'N Crispy	1 slice (2.9 oz)	215
Personal Pan Pepperoni	1 pie (9 oz)	637
Personal Pan Supreme	1 pie (11.5 oz0	722
Pork Topping Medium Hand Tossed	1 slice (4.2 oz)	268
Pork Topping Medium Pan	1 slice (4.2 oz)	294
Pork Topping Medium Thin 'N Crispy	1 slice (3.5 oz)	237
Super Supreme Medium Hand Tossed	1 slice (5 oz)	296
Super Supreme Medium Pan	1 slice (5 oz)	323
Super Supreme Medium Thin 'N Crispy	1 slice (4.3 oz)	270
Supreme Medium Hand Tossed	1 slice (4.8 oz)	284
Supreme Medium Pan	1 slice (4.8 oz)	311
Supreme Medium Thin 'N Crispy	1 slice (4.1 oz)	257
Veggie Lover's Medium Hand Tossed	1 slice (4.7 oz)	216
Veggie Lover's Medium Pan	1 slice (4.7 oz)	243
Veggie Lover's Medium Thin 'N Crispy	1 slice	186

POLLO TROPICAL
(see TROPIGRILL)

PONDEROSA
BEVERAGES

Chocolate Milk	8 oz	208
Lemonade	6 oz	68
ICE CREAM		
Ice Milk Chocolate	3.5 oz	152
Ice Milk Vanilla	3.5 oz	150
Topping Caramel	1 oz	100
Topping Chocolate	1 oz	89
Topping Strawberry	1 oz	71
Topping Whippped	1 oz	80
MAIN MENU SELECTIONS		
BBQ Sauce	1 tbsp	25
Bake 'R Broil Fish	1 serv (5.2 oz)	230
Baked Potato	1 (7.2 oz)	145
Beans Baked	1 serv (4 oz)	170
Beans Green	1 serv (3.5 oz)	20
Breaded Cauliflower	1 serv (4 oz)	115
Breaded Okra	1 serv (4 oz)	124
Breaded Onion Rings	1 serv (4 oz)	213
Breaded Zucchini	1 serv (4 oz)	102
Carrots	1 serv (3.5 oz)	31

FOOD	PORTION	CALS.
Cheese Herb Garlic Spread	1 tbsp	100
Cheese Sauce	2 oz	52
Chicken Breast	1 serv (5.5 oz)	90
Chicken Wings	2	213
Chopped Steak	5.3 oz	296
Chopped Steak	4 oz	225
Corn	1 serv (3.5 oz)	90
Fish Fried	1 serv (3.2 oz)	190
Fish Nuggets	1	31
French Fries	1 serv (3 oz)	120
Gravy Brown	2 oz	25
Gravy Turkey	2 oz	25
Halibut Broiled	1 serv (6 oz)	170
Hot Dog	1	144
Italian Breadsticks	1	100
Kansas City Strip	5 oz	138
Macaroni And Cheese	4 oz	67
Margarine Liquid	1 tbsp	100
Mashed Potatoes	1 serv (4 oz)	62
Meatballs	1	58
Mini Shrimp	6	47
New York Strip Choice	10 oz	314
New York Strip Choice	8 oz	384
Pasta Shells Plain	2 oz	78
Peas	1 serv (3.5 oz)	67
Porterhouse	13 oz	441
Porterhouse Choice	16 oz	640
Potato Wedges	1 serv (3.5 oz)	130
Ribeye	5 oz	219
Ribeye Choice	6 oz	281
Rice Pilaf	1 serv (4 oz)	160
Roll Dinner	1	184
Roll Sourdough	1	110
Roughy Broiled	1 serv (5 oz)	139
Salmon Broiled	1 serv (6 oz)	192
Sandwich Steak	4 oz	408
Scrod Baked	1 serv (7 oz)	120
Shrimp Fried	7 pieces	231
Sirloin Choice	7 oz	241
Sirloin Tips Choice	5 oz	473
Spaghetti Plain	2 oz	78
Spaghetti Sauce	4 oz	110
Steak Kabobs Meat Only	3 oz	153
Stuffing	4 oz	230

FOOD	PORTION	CALS.
Sweet/Sour Sauce	1 oz	37
Swordfish Broiled	1 serv (6 oz)	271
T-Bone	8 oz	176
T-Bone Choice	10 oz	444
Teriyaki Steak	5 oz	174
Tortilla Chips	1 oz	150
Trout Broiled	1 serv (5 oz)	228
Winter Mix	1 serv (3.5 oz)	25
SALAD DRESSINGS		
Blue Cheese	1 oz	130
Cole Slaw	1 oz	150
Creamy Italian	1 oz	103
Cucumber Reduced Calorie	1 oz	69
Italian Reduced Calorie	1 oz	31
Parmesan Pepper	1 oz	150
Ranch	1 oz	147
Salad Oil	1 tbsp	120
Sour Cream	1 tbsp	26
Sweet-N-Tangy	1 oz	122
Thousand Island	1 oz	113
SALADS AND SALAD BARS		
Alfalfa Sprouts	1 oz	10
Apple	1	80
Apples Canned	4 oz	90
Applesauce	4 oz	80
Banana	1	87
Banana Chips	0.2 oz	25
Banana Pudding	1 oz	52
Bean Sprouts	1 oz	10
Beets Diced	4 oz	55
Breadsticks Sesame	2	35
Broccoli	1 oz	9
Cabbage Green	1 oz	9
Cabbage Red	1 oz	1
Cantaloupe	1 wedge	13
Carrots	1 oz	12
Cauliflower	1 oz	8
Celery	1 oz	4
Cheese Imitation Shredded	1 oz	90
Cheese Spread	1 oz	98
Cherry Peppers	2 pieces	7
Chicken Salad	3.5 oz	212
Chow Mein Noodles	0.2 oz	25
Cocktail Sauce	1 oz	34

FOOD	PORTION	CALS.
Coconut Shredded	0.2 oz	25
Cottage Cheese	4 oz	120
Croutons	1 oz	115
Cucumber	1 oz	4
Eggs Diced	2 oz	94
Fruit Cocktail	4 oz	97
Garbanzo Beans	1 oz	102
Gelatin Plain	4 oz	71
Granola	0.2 oz	24
Grapes	10	34
Green Onion	1	7
Green Pepper	1 oz	6
Ham Diced	2 oz	120
Honeydew	1 wedge	24
Lemon	1 wedge	3
Lettuce	1 oz	5
Macaroni Salad	3.5 oz	335
Margarine Whipped	1 tbsp	34
Meal Mates Sesame Crackers	2	45
Melba Snacks	2	18
Mousse Chocolate	1 oz	78
Mousse Strawberry	1 oz	74
Mushrooms	1 oz	8
Olives Black	1	4
Olives Green	1	3
Onions Red & Yellow	1 oz	11
Orange	1	45
Pasta Salad	3.5 oz	269
Peaches Canned	4 oz	70
Peanuts Chopped	0.2 oz	30
Pears Canned	4 oz	98
Pickles Dill Spears	0.14 oz	tr
Pickles Sweet Chips	0.14 oz	4
Pineapple Tidbits	4 oz	95
Pineapple Fresh	1 wedge	11
Potato Salad	3.5 oz	126
Radishes	1 oz	4
Ritz	2	40
Saltine Crackers	2	25
Spiced Apple Rings	4 oz	100
Spinach	1 oz	7
Strawberries	2 oz	14
Strawberry Glaze	1 oz	37
Sunflower Seeds	0.2 oz	31

FOOD	PORTION	CALS.
Tartar Sauce	1 oz	85
Tomatoes	1 oz	6
Turkey Ham Salad	3.5 oz	186
Turkey Julienne	1 oz	29
Vanilla Wafer	2	35
Watermelon	1 wedge	111
Yogurt Fruit	4 oz	115
Yogurt Vanilla	4 oz	110
Zucchini	1 oz	5

POPEYES

FOOD	PORTION	CALS.
Apple Pie	1 serv (3.1 oz)	290
Biscuit	1 serv (2.3 oz)	250
Breast Mild	1 (3.7 oz)	270
Breast Spicy	1 (3.7 oz)	270
Cajun Rice	1 serv (3.9 oz)	150
Cole Slaw	1 serv (4 oz)	149
Corn On The Cob	1 serv (5.2 oz)	127
French Fries	1 serv (3 oz)	240
Leg Mild	1 (1.7 oz)	120
Leg Spicy	1 (1.7 oz)	120
Nuggets	1 serv (4.2 oz)	410
Nuggets Mild Tender	1 (1.2 oz)	110
Nuggets Spicy Tender	1 (1.2 oz)	110
Onion Rings	1 serv (3.1 oz)	310
Potatoes & Gravy	1 serv (3.8 oz)	100
Red Beans & Rice	1 serv (5.9 oz)	270
Shrimp	1 serv (2.8 oz)	250
Thigh Mild	1 (3.1 oz)	300
Thigh Spicy	1 (3.1 oz)	300
Wing Mild	1 (1.6 oz)	160
Wing Spicy	1 (1.6 oz)	160

PUDGIE'S FAMOUS CHICKEN

FOOD	PORTION	CALS.
Fried Chicken	3.5 oz	233

QUINCY'S

BAKED SELECTIONS

FOOD	PORTION	CALS.
Banana Nut	1 serv (2 oz)	165
Biscuit	1 (2.5 oz)	270
Cornbread	1 serv (2 oz)	140
Yeast Roll	1 (1.5 oz)	160

BREAKFAST SELECTIONS

FOOD	PORTION	CALS.
Bacon	1 serv (0.25 oz)	35
Corned Beef Hash	1 serv (4.5 oz)	210

FOOD	PORTION	CALS.
Country Ham	1 serv (1.5 oz)	90
Escalloped Apples	1 serv (3.5 oz)	120
Oatmeal	1 serv	175
Pancakes	1 (1.5 oz)	95
Sausage Gravy	1 serv (4 oz)	70
Sausage Links	1 (2 oz)	225
Sausage Patties	1 (2 oz)	230
Scrambled Eggs	1 serv (2 oz)	95
Steak Fingers	1 serv (3.5 oz)	360
Syrup	1 oz	75
DESSERTS		
Banana Pudding	1 serv (5 oz)	240
Brownie Pudding Cake	1 serv (4 oz)	310
Chocolate Chip Cookies	1 (0.5 oz)	60
Cobbler Apple	1 serv (6 oz)	255
Cobbler Cherry	1 serv (6 oz)	410
Cobbler Peach	1 serv (6 oz)	305
Frozen Yogurt	1 serv (4 oz)	135
Hot Toppings Caramel	1 serv (1 oz)	105
Hot Toppings Fudge	1 serv (1 oz)	105
Hot Toppings Pineapple	1 serv (1 oz)	70
Sugar Cookie	1 (0.5 oz)	60
MAIN MENU SELECTIONS		
Baked Potato	1 (12 oz)	370
Beef Chopped Steak	1 serv (5.75 oz)	470
Beef Filet	1 (5.5 oz)	330
Blackeyed Peas	1 serv (4 oz)	75
Broccoli & Rice Casserole	1 serv (4 oz)	100
Broccoli w/ Cheese Sauce	1 serv (12 oz)	250
Cabbage Steamed	1 serv (4 oz)	85
Candied Yams	1 serv (4 oz)	250
Carrots Steamed	1 serv (4 oz)	85
Corn On The Cob	1 serv (6 oz)	140
Corn Whole Kernel	1 serv (4 oz)	110
Country Style Steak	1 serv (5 oz)	380
Country Style Steak Sandwich	1 serv (9 oz)	520
Green Beans	1 serv (4 oz)	25
Green Peas	1 serv (4 oz)	60
Grilled Chicken Large	1 serv (9.5 oz)	250
Grilled Chicken Regular	4.75 oz	125
Grilled Chicken Sandwich	1 serv (8.5 oz)	305
Grilled Trout	6 oz	300
Hashrounds	1 serv (2.75 oz)	230
Homestyle Chicken Filet	1 serv (6 oz)	410

FOOD	PORTION	CALS.
Macaroni & Cheese	1 serv (4 oz)	165
Mashed Potatoes	1 serv (4 oz)	70
Mushrooms	1 serv (3 oz)	115
New Potatoes	1 serv (4 oz)	190
Pinto Beans	1 serv (4 oz)	70
Prime Rib	1 serv (8 oz)	570
Prime Rib	1 serv (16 oz)	1145
Quarter Pound Hamburger	1 serv (7.5 oz)	410
Refried Beans	1 serv (4 oz)	140
Ribeye	9.5 oz	870
Ribeye	1 serv (7.25 oz)	670
Rice Pilaf	1 serv (3.5 oz)	105
Sirloin Large	7.75 oz	850
Sirloin Petite	4 oz	450
Sirloin Regular	5.75 oz	650
Sirloin Strip	1 serv (9.5 oz)	595
Sirloin Tips	1 serv (4 oz)	240
Squash	1 serv (4 oz)	110
Stir Fry Beef	1 serv (16 oz)	950
Stir Fry Chicken	1 serv (15.75 oz)	780
T-Bone	14 oz	1610
Turnip Greens	1 serv (4 oz)	75
Vegetable Medley	1 serv (4 oz)	35
SALAD DRESSINGS		
Blue Cheese	1 serv (1 oz)	155
French	1 serv (1 oz)	125
Honey Mustard	1 serv (1 oz)	100
Italian	1 serv (1 oz)	134
Light 1000 Island	1 serv (1 oz)	65
Light Creamy Italian	1 serv (1 oz)	65
Light French	1 serv (1 oz)	85
Light Italian	1 serv (1 oz)	20
Parmesan Peppercorn	1 serv (1 oz)	150
Ranch	1 serv (1 oz)	110
SOUPS		
Chili With Beans	1 serv (6 oz)	235
Clam Chowder	1 serv (6 oz)	180
Cream Of Broccoli	1 serv (6 oz)	170
Vegetable Beef	1 serv (6 oz)	90

RAX

BEVERAGES		
Chocolate Shake	1 (11 fl oz)	445
DESSERTS		
Chocolate Chip Cookie	1 (2 oz)	262

FOOD	PORTION	CALS.
MAIN MENU SELECTIONS		
Bacon	1 slice (0.1 oz)	14
Baked Potato	1 (10 oz)	264
Baked Potato w/ 1 Tbsp Margarine	1 (10.5 oz)	364
Barbecue Sauce	1 pkg (0.4 oz)	11
Beef Bacon 'N Cheddar	1 (6.7 oz)	523
Cheddar Cheese Sauce	1 fl oz	29
Country Fried Chicken Breast Sandwich	1 (7.4 oz)	618
Deluxe Roast Beef	1 (7.9 oz)	498
French Fries	1 serv (3.25 oz)	282
Grilled Chicken Breast Sandwich	1 (6.9 oz)	402
Grilled Chicken Garden Salad w/ French Dressing	1 serv (12.7 oz)	477
Grilled Chicken Garden Salad w/ Lite Italian Dressing	1 serv (12.7 oz)	264
Mushroom Sauce	1 fl oz	16
Philly Melt	1 (8.2 oz)	396
Regular Rax	1 (4.7 oz)	262
Swiss Slice	1 slice (0.4 oz)	42
SALAD DRESSINGS		
French	2 fl oz	275
Lite Italian	2 fl oz	63
SALADS AND SALAD BARS		
Gourmet Garden Salad w/ French Dressing	1 serv (10.7 oz)	409
Gourmet Garden Salad w/ Lite Italian Dressing	1 serv (10.7 oz)	305
Gourmet Garden Salad w/o Dressing	1 serv (8.7 oz)	134
Grilled Chicken Garden Salad w/o Dressing	1 serv (10.7 oz)	202

RED LOBSTER

FOOD	PORTION	CALS.
CHILDREN'S MENU SELECTIONS		
Cheeseburger	1 serv	1040
Fried Chicken Fingers	1 serv	680
Fried Shrimp	1 serv	650
Grilled Chicken Teneders	1 serv	580
Hamburger	1 serv	920
Popcorn Shrimp	1 serv	650
Popcorn Shrimp & Cheesesticks	1 serv	750
Spaghetti & Cheesesticks	1 serv	830
DESSERTS		
Carrot Cake	1 serv (6.5 oz)	730
Cheesecake	1 serv (5.5 oz)	530
Fudge Overboard	1 serv	620
Ice Cream	1 serv (4.5 oz)	140

FOOD	PORTION	CALS.
Key Lime Pie	1 serv (5 oz)	450
Raspberry Cobbler	1 serv (3 oz)	530
Sensational 7	1 serv	790
MAIN MENU SELECTIONS		
Admiral's Feast	1 serv	1060
Appetizer Calamari	1 serv	350
Appetizer Chicken Fingers	1 serv	390
Appetizer Chilled Shrimp In The Shell	1 serv (6 oz)	110
Appetizer Crab & Shrimp Cakes	1 serv	480
Appetizer Crab Add-On	1 serv	60
Appetizer Fresh Fried Mushrooms	1 serv	790
Appetizer Lobster Quesadilla	1 serv	760
Appetizer Lobster Stuffed Mushroom	1 serv	400
Appetizer Mozzarella Cheesesticks	1 serv	730
Appetizer Parmesan Zucchini	1 serv	620
Appetizer Shrimp Cocktail	1 serv	50
Appetizer Stuffed Mushrooms	1 serv	420
Applesauce	1 serv (4 oz)	90
Atlantic Cod	1 serv (8 oz)	200
Atlantic Cod	1 lunch serv (5 oz)	110
Atlantic Salmon	1 lunch serv (5 oz)	200
Atlantic Salmon	1 serv (8 oz)	340
Baked Atlantic Cod	1 serv	220
Baked Atlantic Haddock	1 serv	220
Baked Flounder	1 lunch serv	190
Baked Potato	1 (8 oz)	130
Broccoli	1 serv (3 oz)	25
Broiled Fisherman's Platter	1 serv	600
Broiled Seafarer's Platter	1 serv	450
Caesar Salad w/ Dressing	1 serv	240
Catfish	1 serv (8 oz)	220
Catfish	1 lunch serv (5 oz)	130
Catfish Santa Fe	1 serv	340
Catfish Sante Fe	1 lunch serv	180
Chicken Fingers	1 lunch serv	390
Chicken Fresco	1 serv	1320
Chicken Fresco	1 lunch serv	660
Clam Strips	1 lunch serv	360
Clam Strips	1 serv	720
Cocktail Sauce	1 oz	30
Cole Slaw	1 serv (4 oz)	190
Crab Alfredo	1 serv	1170
Crab Alfredo	1 lunch serv	590
Fish & Shrimp Combo	1 serv	730

FOOD	PORTION	CALS.
Fish Nuggets	1 lunch serv	320
Fish Seasoning Add On For Blackened Dinner	1 serv	70
Fish Seasoning Add On For Blackened Lunch	1 serv	50
Fish Seasoning Add On For Broiled Dinner	1 serv	45
Fish Seasoning Add On For Broiled Lunch	1 serv	35
Fish Seasoning Add On For Grilled Dinner	1 serv	35
Fish Seasoning Add On For Grilled Lunch	1 serv	25
Fish Seasoning Add On For Lemon Pepper Dinner	1 serv	35
Fish Seasoning Add On For Lemon Pepper Lunch	1 serv	30
Fish Seasoning Add On For Sante Fe Style Dinner	1 serv	60
Fish Seasoning Add On For Sante Fe Style Lunch	1 serv	40
Flounder	1 lunch serv (5 oz)	130
Flounder	1 serv (8 oz)	220
French Fries	1 serv (4 oz)	350
Fried Flounder	1 lunch serv	230
Fried Shrimp	12 lg	500
Fried Shrimp	1 lunch serv	270
Garden Salad w/o Dressing	1 serv	50
Garlic Cheese Biscuit	1	140
Grilled Cheeseburger	1	580
Grilled Chicken Breasts	1 serv	230
Grilled Chicken Salad w/o Dressing	1 serv	320
Grouper	1 serv (8 oz)	220
Grouper	1 lunch serv (5 oz)	130
Haddock	1 serv (8 oz)	210
Haddock	1 lunch serv (5 oz)	120
Halibut	1 lunch serv (5 oz)	150
Halibut	1 serv (8 oz)	260
King Salmon	1 lunch serv (5 oz)	250
King Salmon	1 serv (8 oz)	420
Lake Trout	1 serv (8 oz)	340
Lake Trout	1 lunch serv (5 oz)	200
Lemon Pepper Grilled Mahi Mahi	1 serv	240
Lobster Shrimp & Scallop Scampi	1 lunch serv	430
Lobster Shrimp & Scallop Scampi	1 serv	870
Mahi Mahi	1 lunch serv (5 oz)	130
Mahi Mahi	1 serv (8 oz)	220
Maine Lobster Steamed	1 serv (1.25 lb)	160
Maine Lobster Stuffed	1 serv (2 lb)	430
Marinara Sauce	1 serv	50

FOOD	PORTION	CALS.
Melted Butter	1 oz	200
Neptune's Feast	1 serv	1210
New York Strip Steak	1 serv	560
Perch	1 serv (8 oz)	220
Perch	1 lunch serv (5 oz)	130
Pollack	1 lunch serv (5 oz)	120
Pollock	1 serv (8 oz)	120
Popcorn Shrimp	1 serv	580
Popcorn Shrimp	1 lunch serv	380
Red Rockfish	1 serv (8 oz)	230
Red Rockfish	1 lunch serv (5 oz)	130
Red Snapper	1 serv (8 oz)	240
Red Snapper	1 lunch serv (5 oz)	140
Rice Pilaf	1 serv (4 oz)	180
Roasted Vegetables	1 serv (6 oz)	120
Roasted Vegetables	1 lunch serv (4 oz)	80
Sailor's Platter	1 lunch serv	250
Sandwich Blackened Catfish	1	340
Sandwich Broiled Fish	1	300
Sandwich Cajun Grilled Chicken	1	370
Sandwich Classic Fish	1	520
Sandwich Grilled Chicken	1	290
Sassy Sauce	1 oz	80
Seafood Broil	1 lunch serv	310
Shrimp & Chicken	1 serv	340
Shrimp Caesar Salad w/o Dressing	1 serv	240
Shrimp Carbonara	1 lunch serv	650
Shrimp Carbonara	1 serv	1290
Shrimp Combo	1 serv	380
Shrimp Feast	1 serv	470
Shrimp Milano	1 serv	1190
Shrimp Milano	1 lunch serv	590
Shrimp Scampi	1 lunch serv	110
Smothered Chicken	1 serv	530
Snow Crab Legs	1 serv	110
Sockeye Salmon	1 lunch serv (5 oz)	240
Sockeye Salmon	1 serv (8 oz)	410
Sole	1 serv (8 oz)	220
Sole	1 lunch serv (5 oz)	130
Soup Bread Salad w/o Dressing	1 lunch serv	430
Steak & Fried Shrimp	1 serv	780
Steak & Rock Lobster Tail	1 serv	570
Swordfish	1 serv (8 oz)	290
Swordfish	1 lunch serv (5 oz)	170

FOOD	PORTION	CALS.
Tartar Sauce	1 oz	160
Teriyaki Grilled Chicken Breast	1 serv	240
Twice Baked Potato	1	430
Walleye	1 serv (8 oz)	210
Walleye	1 lunch serv (5 oz)	120
Yellow Lake Perch	1 serv (8 oz)	220
Yellow Lake Perch	1 lunch serv (5 oz)	130
SALAD DRESSINGS		
Blue Cheese	1 serv	170
Buttermilk Ranch	1 serv	110
Caesar	1 serv	170
Dijon Honey Mustard	1 serv	140
Fat Free Ranch	1 serv	50
Lite Red Wine Vinaigrette	1 serv	50
SOUPS		
Bayou Style Gumbo	1 serv (6 oz)	120
Broccoli Cheese	1 serv	160
Clam Chowder	1 serv (6 oz)	130

ROY ROGERS

BEVERAGES		
Orange Juice	11 fl oz	140
BREAKFAST SELECTIONS		
3 Pancakes	1 serv (4.8 oz)	280
3 Pancakes w/ 1 Sausage	1 serv (6.2 oz)	430
3 Pancakes w/ 2 Bacon	1 serv (5.3 oz)	350
Bagel Cinnamon Raisin	1 (4 oz)	300
Bagel Plain	1 (4 oz)	300
Big Country Platters w/ Bacon	1 serv (7.6 oz)	740
Big Country Platters w/ Ham	1 serv (9.4 oz)	710
Big Country Platters w/ Sausage	1 serv (9.6 oz)	920
Biscuit	1 (2.9 oz)	390
Biscuit Bacon	1 (3.1 oz)	420
Biscuit Bacon & Egg	1 (4.2 oz)	470
Biscuit Cinnamon 'N' Raisin	1 (2.8 oz)	370
Biscuit Ham & Cheese	1 (4.5 oz)	450
Biscuit Ham & Egg	1 (5.1 oz)	460
Biscuit Ham, Egg & Cheese	1 (5.6 oz)	500
Biscuit Sausage	1 (4.1 oz)	510
Biscuit Sausage & Egg	1 (5.2 oz)	560
Hashrounds	1 serv (2.8 oz)	230
Sourdough Ham, Egg & Cheese	1 (6.8 oz)	480
DESSERTS		
Strawberry Shortcake	1 serv (6.6 oz)	480

FOOD	PORTION	CALS.
ICE CREAM		
Ice Cream Cone	1 (4.1 oz)	180
Sundae Hot Fudge	1 (6 oz)	320
Sundae Strawberry	1 (5.5 oz)	260
MAIN MENU SELECTIONS		
¼ Cheeseburger	1 (6 oz)	510
¼ Hamburger	1 (5.5 oz)	460
¼ Roaster Dark Meat	7.4 oz	490
¼ Roaster Dark Meat w/ Skin Off	4 oz	190
¼ Roaster White Meat	8.6 oz	500
¼ Roaster White Meat w/ Skin Off	4.7 oz	190
Bacon Cheeseburger	1 (5.9 oz)	520
Baked Beans	1 serv (5 oz)	160
Baked Potato	1 (3.9 oz)	130
Baked Potato w/ Margarine	1 (4.4 oz)	240
Baked Potato w/ Margarine & Sour Cream	1 (5.4 oz)	300
Cheeseburger	1 (4.2 oz)	300
Chicken Fillet Sandwich	1 (8.3 oz)	500
Cole Slaw	1 serv (5 oz)	295
Cornbread	1 serv (2.7 oz)	310
Fisherman's Fillet	1 (6.5 oz)	490
Fried Chicken Breast	1 (5.2 oz)	370
Fried Chicken Leg	1 (2.4 oz)	170
Fried Chicken Thigh	1 (4.2 oz)	330
Fried Chicken Wing	1 (2.3 oz)	200
Fry	1 reg (5 oz)	350
Fry	1 lg (6.1 oz)	430
Gravy	1 serv (1.5 fl oz)	20
Grilled Chicken Sandwich	1 (8.3 oz)	340
Hamburger	1 (3.8 oz)	260
Mashed Potatoes	1 serv (5 oz)	92
Nuggets	6 (4 oz)	290
Nuggets	9 (6.2 oz)	460
Pizza	1 serv (4.75 oz)	282
Roast Beef Sandwich	1 (5.7 oz)	260
Sourdough Grilled Chicken	1 (10.1 oz)	500
SALADS AND SALAD BARS		
Garden Salad	1 (9.3 oz)	190
Grilled Chicken Salad	1 serv (9.8 oz)	120
Side Salad	1 (4.9 oz)	20

SCHLOTZSKY'S DELI

PIZZA		
Chicken & Pesto	1	634

FOOD	PORTION	CALS.
Onion & Mushroom	1	577
Smoked Turkey & Jalapeno	1	589
Vegetarian	1	555
SALAD AND SALAD BARS		
Chicken Chef	1 serv	192
Turkey Club	1 serv	233
SANDWICHES		
Chicken Breast	1 sm	514
Dijon Chicken Breast	1 sm	469
Smoked Turkey	1 sm	510
The Original	1 sm	598
SOUPS		
Creole Vegetable	1 serv (8 fl oz)	120
Red Bean	1 serv (8 fl oz)	110
Shrimp & Okra	1 serv (8 fl oz)	100
Spicy Chicken	1 serv (8 fl oz)	120

SHAKEY'S

MAIN MENU SELECTIONS

FOOD	PORTION	CALS.
3 Piece Fried Chicken And Potatoes	1 serv	947
5 Piece Fried Chicken And Potatoes	1 serv	1700
Hot Ham And Cheese	1	550
Potatoes	15 pieces	950
Spaghetti With Meat Sauce And Garlic Bread	1 serv	940
Super Hot Hero	1	810
PIZZA		
Homestyle Crust Cheese	1 slice	303
Homestyle Crust Onion, Green Pepper, Black Olives, Mushrooms	1 slice	320
Homestyle Crust Pepperoni	1 slice	343
Homestyle Crust Sausage, Mushroom	1 slice	343
Homestyle Crust Sausage, Pepperoni	1 slice	374
Homestyle Crust Shakey's Special	1 slice	384
Thick Crust Cheese	1 slice	170
Thick Crust Green Pepper, Black Olives, Mushrooms	1 slice	162
Thick Crust Pepperoni	1 slice	185
Thick Crust Sausage, Mushrooms	1 slice	179
Thick Crust Sausage, Pepperoni	1 slice	177
Thick Crust Shakey's Special	1 slice	208
Thin Crust Cheese	1 slice	133
Thin Crust Onion, Green Pepper, Black Olives, Mushrooms	1 slice	125
Thin Crust Pepperoni	1 slice	148

FOOD	PORTION	CALS.
Thin Crust Sausage, Mushroom	1 slice	141
Thin Crust Sausage, Pepperoni	1 slice	166
Thin Crust Shakey's Special	1 slice	171

SHONEY'S
BREAKFAST SELECTIONS

FOOD	PORTION	CALS.
100% Natural	½ cup	244
Ambrosia Salad	¼ cup	75
Apple		81
Apple Butter	1 tbsp	37
Apple Grape Surprise	¼ cup	19
Apple Ring	1	15
Apple sliced	1 slice	13
Bacon	1 strip	36
Beef Stick	1	43
Biscuit	1	170
Blueberries	¼ cup	21
Blueberry Muffin	1	107
Bread Pudding	1 sq	305
Breakfast Ham	1 slice	26
Brunch Cake Apple	1 sq	160
Brunch Cake Banana	1 sq	152
Brunch Cake Carrot	1 sq	150
Brunch Cake Pineapple	1 sq	147
Brunch Cake Sour Cream	1 sq	160
Buttered Toast	2 slices	163
Cantaloupe Sliced	1 slice	8
Cantaloupe diced	½ cup	28
Captain Crunch Berry	½ cup	73
Cheese Sauce	1 ladle	26
Chicken Pieces	1 piece	40
Chocolate Pudding	¼ cup	81
Cinnamon Honey Bun	1	344
Cottage Cheese	1 tbsp	12
Cottage Fries	¼ cup	62
Country Gravy	¼ cup	82
Croissant	1	260
Donut Mini Cinnamon	1 (14 g)	56
DoughNugget	1	157
Egg Fried	1	159
Egg Scrambled	¼ cup	95
English Muffin w/ margarine	1	140
Fluff	¼ cup	16
French Toast	1 slice	69

FOOD	PORTION	CALS.
Fruit Delight	¼ cup	54
Fruit Topping All Flavors	1 tbsp	24
Glaced Fruit	¼ cup	51
Golden Pound Cake	1 slice	134
Grape Jelly	1 tbsp	60
Grapefruit Canned	¼ cup	24
Grapes	25	57
Grits	¼ cup	57
Hashbrowns	¼ cup	43
Home Fries	¼ cup	53
Honey Bun	1	265
Honeydew Sliced	1 slice	13
Jelly Packet	1	40
Jr. Bun Chocolate	1	141
Jr. Bun Honey	1	141
Jr. Bun Maple	1	141
Kiwi Sliced	1 slice	11
Marble Cake w/ Icing	1 slice	136
Mixed Fruit	¼ cup	37
Mushroom Topping	1 oz	25
Oleo Whipped	1 tbsp	70
Omelette Topping	1 spoonful	23
Orange	1 med	65
Orange Sections	1 section	7
Oriental Salad	¼ cup	79
Pancake	1	41
Pear	1	98
Pineapple Bits	1 tbsp	9
Pineapple Fresh Sliced	1 slice	10
Pistachio Pineapple Salad	¼ cup	98
Prunes	1 tbsp	19
Raisin Bran	½ cup	87
Raisin English Muffin w/ Margarine	1	158
Sausage Link	1	91
Sausage Patty	1	136
Sausage Rice	¼ cup	110
Shortcake	1	60
Sirloin Steak Charbroiled	6 oz	357
Smoked Sausage	1	103
Snow Salad	¼ cup	72
Strawberries	5	23
Syrup Light	1 ladle	60
Syrup Low-Cal	2.2 oz	98
Tangerine	1	37

FOOD	PORTION	CALS.
Trix	½ cup	54
Waldorf Salad	¼ cup	81
Watermelon Sliced	1 slice	9
Whipped Topping	1 scoop	10
CHILDREN'S MENU SELECTIONS		
Jr. Burger All-American	1 serv	234
Kid's Chicken Dinner (fried)	1 serv	244
Kid's Fish N' Chips (includes fries)	1 serv	337
Kid's Fried Shrimp	1 serv	194
Kid's Spaghetti	1 serv	247
DESSERTS		
Apple Pie A La Mode	1 slice	492
Carrot Cake	1 slice	500
Strawberry Pie	1 slice	332
Walnut Brownie A La Mode	1	576
ICE CREAM		
Hot Fudge Cake	1 slice	522
Hot Fudge Sundae	1	451
Strawberry Sundae	1	380
MAIN MENU SELECTIONS		
All-American Burger	1	501
BBQ Sauce	1 souffle cup	41
Bacon Burger	1	591
Baked Fish	1 serv	170
Baked Fish Light	1 serv	170
Baked Ham Sandwich	1	290
Baked Potato	10 oz	264
Beef Patty Light	1 serv	289
Charbroiled Chicken	1 serv	239
Charbroiled Chicken Sandwich	1	451
Chicken Fillet Sandwich	1	464
Chicken Tenders	1 serv	388
Cocktail Sauce	1 souffle cup	36
Country Fried Sandwich	1	588
Country Fried Steak	1 serv	449
Fish N' Chips (includes fries)	1 serv	639
Fish N' Shrimp	1 serv	487
Fish Sandwich	1	323
French Fries	3 oz	189
French Fries	4 oz	252
Fried Fish Light	1 serv	297
Grecian Bread	1 slice	80
Grilled Bacon & Cheese Sandwich	1	440
Grilled Cheese Sandwich	1	302

FOOD	PORTION	CALS.
Half O'Pound	1 serv	435
Ham Club On Whole Wheat	1	642
Hawaiian Chicken	1 serv	262
Italian Feast	1 serv	500
Lasagna	1 serv	297
Liver N' Onions	1 serv	411
Mushroom Swiss Burger	1	616
Old-Fashioned Burger	1	470
Onion Rings	1	52
Patty Melt	1	640
Philly Steak Sandwich	1	673
Reuben Sandwich	1	596
Ribeye	6 oz	605
Rice	3.5 oz	137
Sauteed Mushrooms	3 oz	75
Sauteed Onions	2.5 oz	37
Seafood Platter	1 serv	566
Shoney Burger	1	498
Shrimp Bite-Size	1 serv	387
Shrimp Broiled	1 serv	93
Shrimp Sampler	1 serv	412
Shrimper's Feast	1 serv	383
Shrimper's Feast Large	1 serv	575
Sirloin	6 oz	357
Slim Jim Sandwich	1	484
Spaghetti	1 serv	496
Steak N' Shrimp (charbroiled shrimp)	1 serv	361
Steak N' Shrimp (fried shrimp)	1 serv	507
Sweet N' Sour Sauce	1 souffle cup	58
Tartar Sauce	1 souffle cup	84
Turkey Club On Whole Wheat	1	635
SALAD DRESSINGS		
Biscayne Lo-Cal	2 tbsp	62
Blue Cheese	2 tbsp	113
Creamy Italian	2 tbsp	135
French	2 tbsp	124
Golden Italian	2 tbsp	141
Honey Mustard	2 tbsp	165
Ranch	2 tbsp	95
Rue French	2 tbsp	122
Thousand Island	2 tbsp	130
W.W. Italian	2 tbsp	10
SALADS AND SALAD BARS		
Ambrosia Salad	¼ cup	75

FOOD	PORTION	CALS.
Apple Grape Surprise	¼ cup	19
Apple Ring	1	15
Bacon Bits	1 spoonful	15
Beet Onion Salad	¼ cup	25
Broccoli	¼ cup	4
Broccoli Cauliflower Carrot Salad	¼ cup	53
Broccoli Cauliflower Ranch	¼ cup	65
Broccoli & Cauliflower	¼ cup	98
Carrot	¼ cup	10
Carrot Apple Salad	¼ cup	99
Cauliflower	¼ cup	8
Celery	1 tbsp	5
Cheese Shredded	1 tbsp	21
Chocolate Pudding	¼ cup	81
Chow Mein Noodles	1 spoonful	13
Cole Slaw	¼ cup	69
Cottage Cheese	1 tbsp	12
Croutons	1 spoonful	13
Cucumber	1 tbsp	1
Cucumber Lite	¼ cup	12
Don's Pasta	¼ cup	82
Egg Diced	1 tbsp	15
Fruit Delight	¼ cup	54
Fruit Topping All Flavors	¼ cup	64
Glaced Fruit	¼ cup	51
Granola	1 spoonful	25
Grapefruit	¼ cup	24
Green Pepper	1 tbsp	1
Italian Vegetable	¼ cup	11
Jello	¼ cup	40
Jello Fluff	¼ cup	16
Kidney Bean Salad	¼ cup	55
Lettuce	1.8 oz	7
Macaroni Salad	¼ cup	207
Margarine Whipped	1 tsp	23
Melba Toast	2	20
Mixed Fruit Salad	¼ cup	37
Mixed Squash	¼ cup	49
Mushrooms	1 tbsp	1
Oil	1 tsp	45
Olives Black	2	10
Olives Green	2	8
Onion Sliced	1 tbsp	1
Oriental Salad	¼ cup	79

FOOD	PORTION	CALS.
Pea Salad	¼ cup	73
Pepperoni	1 tbsp	30
Pickle Chips	1 slice	5
Pickle Spear	1 spear	2
Pineapple Bits	1 tbsp	9
Pistachio Pineapple Salad	¼ cup	98
Prunes	1 tbsp	19
Radish	1 tbsp	1
Raisins	1 spoonful	26
Rotelli Pasta	¼ cup	78
Seign Salad	¼ cup	72
Snow Delight	¼ cup	72
Spaghetti Salad	¼ cup	81
Spinach	¼ cup	1
Spring Pasta	¼ cup	38
Summer Salad	¼ cup	114
Sunflower Seeds	1 spoonful	40
Three Bean Salad	¼ cup	96
Trail Mix	1 spoonful	30
Turkey Ham	1 tbsp	12
Waldorf	¼ cup	81
Wheat Bread	1 slice	71
SOUPS		
Bean	6 fl oz	63
Beef Cabbage	6 fl oz	86
Broccoli Cauliflower	6 fl oz	124
Cheddar Chowder	6 fl oz	91
Cheese Florentine Ham	6 fl oz	110
Chicken Gumbo	6 fl oz	60
Chicken Noodle	6 fl oz	62
Chicken Rice	6 fl oz	72
Clam Chowder	6 fl oz	94
Corn Chowder	6 fl oz	148
Cream Of Broccoli	6 fl oz	75
Cream Of Chicken	6 fl oz	136
Cream Of Chicken Vegetable	6 fl oz	79
Onion	6 fl oz	29
Potato	6 fl oz	102
Tomato Florentine	6 fl oz	63
Tomato Vegetable	6 fl oz	46
Vegetable Beef	6 fl oz	82

SIZZLER

DESSERTS

Chocolate & Vanilla Soft Serve	4 oz	136

FOOD	PORTION	CALS.
Chocolate Syrup	1 oz	90
Strawberry Topping	1 oz	70
Whipped Topping	1 tbsp	12
HOT BUFFET		
Broccoli Cheese Soup	1 serv (4 oz)	139
Chicken Noodle Soup	1 serv (4 oz)	31
Chicken Wings	1 oz	73
Clam Chowder	1 serv (4 oz)	118
Fettucine	2 oz	80
Focaccia Bread	2 pieces	108
Marinara Sauce	1 oz	13
Meatballs	4	157
Minestrone Soup	1 serv (4 oz)	36
Nacho Cheese Soup	1 serv (4 oz)	120
Potato Skins	2 oz	160
Refried Beans	¼ cup	62
Saltine Crackers	2	25
Spaghetti	2 oz	80
Taco Filling	2 oz	103
Taco Shells	1	50
Vegetable Sirloin Soup	1 serv (4 oz)	60
MAIN MENU SELECTIONS		
Buttery Dipping Sauce	1 serv (1.5 oz)	330
Cheese Toast	1 piece	273
Cocktail Sauce	1 serv (1.5 oz)	40
Dakota Ranch Steak	1 (6 oz)	316
Dakota Ranch Steak	1 (8 oz)	421
Dakota Ranch Steak	1 (9.5 oz)	500
French Fries	1 serv (4 oz)	358
Hamburger	1	626
Hibachi Chicken Breast w/ Pineapple	5 oz	193
Hibachi Sauce	1 serv (1.5 oz)	57
Lemon Herb Chicken Breast	5 oz	140
Malibu Chicken Patty	1	310
Malibu Sauce	1 serv (1.5 oz)	283
Margarine Whipped	1½ tbsp	105
Potato Baked Plain	1 (4 oz)	105
Rice Pilaf	1 serv (6 oz)	256
Salmon	8 oz	110
Sante Fe Chicken Breast	5 oz	150
Shrimp Broiled	5 oz	150
Shrimp Fried	4 pieces	223
Shrimp Mini	4 oz	152
Shrimp Scampi	5 oz	143

FOOD	PORTION	CALS.
Sour Dressing	2 tbsp	60
Swordfish	8 oz	315
Tartar Sauce	1 serv (1.5 oz)	170
SALAD DRESSINGS		
Blue Cheese	1 oz	111
Honey Mustard	1 oz	160
Italian Lite	1 oz	14
Japanese Rice Vinegar Fat Free	1 oz	10
Parmesan Italian	1 oz	100
Ranch	1 oz	120
Ranch Reduced Calorie	1 oz	90
Thousand Island	1 oz	143
SALADS AND SALAD BARS		
Alfafa Sprouts	¼ cup	2
Avocado	½	153
Bean Sprouts	¼ cup	8
Beets	¼ cup	13
Bell Peppers	2 oz	8
Broccoli	½ cup	12
Cabbage Red	¼ cup	5
Cantoupe	½ cup	28
Carrot & Raisin Salad	2 oz	130
Carrots	¼ cup	12
Chinese Chicken Salad	2 oz	54
Chives	1 oz	62
Cottage Cheese	2 oz	51
Cucumber	2 oz	7
Eggs	1 oz	44
Garbanzo Beans	¼ cup	63
Grapes	½ cup	29
Guacamole	1 oz	42
Honeydew Melon	½ cup	30
Iceberg Lettuce	1 cup	7
Jicama	2 oz	13
Kidney Beans	¼ cup	52
Kiwifruit	2 oz	35
Mediterranean Minted Fruit Salad	2 oz	29
Mexican Fiesta Salad	2 oz	54
Mushrooms	¼ cup	4
Old Fashioned Potato Salad	2 oz	84
Onions Red	2 tbsp	8
Peaches	¼ cup	34
Peas	¼ cup	31
Pineapple	½ cup	38

FOOD	PORTION	CALS.
Real Bacon Bits	1 tbsp	27
Red Herb Potato Salad	2 oz	121
Romaine Lettuce	1 cup	9
Salsa	1 oz	7
Seafood Louis Pasta Salad	2 oz	64
Seafood Salad	2 oz	56
Spicy Jicama Salad	2 oz	16
Spinach	½ cup	6
Strawberries	½ cup	22
Teriyaki Beef Salad	2 oz	49
Tomatoes Cherry	¼ cup	12
Tuna Pasta Salad	2 oz	133
Turkey Ham	1 oz	62
Watermelon	½ cup	26
Zucchini	¼ cup	5

SKIPPER'S

BEVERAGES

Root Beer Float	1 (12 oz)	302

DESSERTS

Jell-O	1 serv (2.75 oz)	55

MAIN MENU SELECTIONS

Baked Fish With Margarine & Seas	1 serv (4.4 oz)	147
Baked Potato	1 (6 oz)	145
Captain's Cut	1 piece (2.6 oz)	160
Cocktail Sauce	1 tbsp	20
Coleslaw	1 serv (5 oz)	289
Corn Muffin	1 (2 oz)	91
English Style Fish	1 piece (2.4 oz)	187
French Fries	1 serv (3.5 oz)	239
Green Salad (no dressing)	1 serv (4 oz)	24
Ketchup	1 tbsp	17
Margarine	1 serv (0.5 oz)	50
Shrimp Fried Cajun	1 serv (4 oz)	342
Shrimp Fried Jumbo	1 piece (.65 oz)	51
Shrimp Fried Original	1 serv (4 oz)	266
Tartar Original	1 tbsp	65

SOUPS

Clam Chowder	1 pint (12 fl oz)	200
Clam Chowder	1 cup (6 fl oz)	100

SONIC DRIVE-IN

#1 Hamburger	1 (6.6 oz)	409
#2 Hamburger	1 (6.6 oz)	323
B-L-T Sandwich	1 (6.1 oz)	327

FOOD	PORTION	CALS.
Bacon Cheeseburger	1 (7.2 oz)	548
Chicken Sandwich Breaded	1 (7.4 oz)	455
Chili Pie	1 (3.7 oz)	327
Corn Dog	1 (3 oz)	280
Extra-Long Cheese Coney	1 (8.9 oz)	635
Fish Sandwich	1 (6.1 oz)	277
French Fries	1 lg (6.7 oz)	315
French Fries	1 reg (5 oz)	233
French Fries w/ Cheese	1 lg (7.7 oz)	219
Grilled Cheese Sandwich	1 (2.8 oz)	288
Grilled Chicken Sandwich w/o Dressing	1 (6.4 oz)	215
Hickory Burger	1 (5.1 oz)	314
Jalapeno Burger Double Meat & Cheese	1 (9.1 oz)	638
Mini Burger	1 (3.5 oz)	246
Onion Rings	1 reg (3.5 oz)	404
Onion Rings	1 lg (5 oz)	577
Regular Cheese Coney	1 (5 oz)	358
Regular Cheese Coney w/ Onions	1 (5.3 oz)	361
Regular Hot Dog	1 (3.5 oz)	258
Steak Sandwich Breaded	1 (3.9 oz)	631
Super Sonic Burger w/ Mustard Double Meat & Cheese	1 (10.1 oz)	644
Super Sonic Burger w/ Mayo Double Meat & Cheese	1 (10.1 oz)	730
Tater Tots	1 serv (3 oz)	150
Tater Tots w/ Cheese	1 serv (3.6 oz)	220

STARBUCKS

FOOD	PORTION	CALS.
Americano Grande	1 serv	10
Americano Short	1 serv	5
Americano Tall	1 serv	5
Cappuccino Grande Lowfat Milk	1 serv	110
Cappuccino Grande Nonfat Milk	1 serv	80
Cappuccino Grande Whole Milk	1 serv	140
Cappuccino Short Lowfat Milk	1 serv	60
Cappuccino Short Nonfat Milk	1 serv	40
Cappuccino Short Whole Milk	1 serv	70
Cappuccino Tall Lowfat Milk	1 serv	80
Cappuccino Tall Nonfat Milk	1 serv	60
Cappuccino Tall Whole Milk	1 serv	110
Cocoa w/ Whipping Cream Grande Lowfat Milk	1 serv	350
Cocoa w/ Whipping Cream Grande Nonfat Milk	1 serv	310

FOOD	PORTION	CALS.
Cocoa w/ Whipping Cream Grande Whole Milk	1 serv	400
Cocoa w/ Whipping Cream Short Lowfat Milk	1 serv	180
Cocoa w/ Whipping Cream Short Nonfat Milk	1 serv	160
Cocoa w/ Whipping Cream Short Whole Milk	1 serv	210
Cocoa w/ Whipping Cream Tall Lowfat Milk	1 serv	270
Cocoa w/ Whipping Cream Tall Nonfat Milk	1 serv	230
Cocoa w/ Whipping Cream Tall Whole Milk	1 serv	300
Drip Coffee Grande	1 serv	10
Drip Coffee Short	1 serv	5
Drip Coffee Tall	1 serv	10
Espresso Doppio	1 serv	5
Espresso Macchiato Doppio Lowfat Milk	1 serv	15
Espresso Macchiato Doppio Nonfat Milk	1 serv	15
Espresso Macchiato Doppio Whole Milk	1 serv	15
Espresso Macchiato Solo Lowfat Milk	1 serv	10
Espresso Macchiato Solo Nonfat Milk	1 serv	10
Espresso Macchiato Solo Whole Milk	1 serv	15
Espresso Solo	1 serv	5
Latte Grande Lowfat Milk	1 serv	170
Latte Grande Nonfat Milk	1 serv	130
Latte Grande Whole Milk	1 serv	220
Latte Short Lowfat Milk	1 serv	80
Latte Short Nonfat Milk	1 serv	60
Latte Short Whole Milk	1 serv	100
Latte Tall Lowfat Milk	1 serv	140
Latte Tall Nonfat Milk	1 serv	110
Latte Tall Whole Milk	1 serv	180
Latte Iced Grande Lowfat Milk	1 serv	170
Latte Iced Grande Nonfat Milk	1 serv	130
Latte Iced Grande Whole Milk	1 serv	210
Latte Iced Short Lowfat Milk	1 serv	90
Latte Iced Short Nonfat Milk	1 serv	70
Latte Iced Short Whole Milk	1 serv	120
Latte Iced Tall Lowfat Milk	1 serv	120
Latte Iced Tall Nonfat Milk	1 serv	90
Latte Iced Tall Whole Milk	1 serv	150
Mocha w/ Whipping Cream Grande Lowfat Milk	1 serv	350
Mocha w/ Whipping Cream Grande Nonfat Milk	1 serv	310
Mocha w/ Whipping Cream Grande Whole Milk	1 serv	390
Mocha w/ Whipping Cream Short Lowfat Milk	1 serv	170

FOOD	PORTION	CALS.
Mocha w/ Whipping Cream Short Nonfat Milk	1 serv	150
Mocha w/ Whipping Cream Short Whole Milk	1 serv	180
Mocha w/ Whipping Cream Tall Lowfat Milk	1 serv	260
Mocha w/ Whipping Cream Tall Nonfat Milk	1 serv	230
Mocha w/ Whipping Cream Tall Whole Milk	1 serv	290
Mocha w/o Whipping Cream Grande Lowfat Milk	1 serv	230
Mocha w/o Whipping Cream Grande Nonfat Milk	1 serv	190
Mocha w/o Whipping Cream Grande Whole Milk	1 serv	260
Mocha w/o Whipping Cream Short Lowfat Milk	1 serv	120
Mocha w/o Whipping Cream Short Nonfat Milk	1 serv	100
Mocha w/o Whipping Cream Short Whole Milk	1 serv	150
Mocha w/o Whipping Cream Tall Lowfat Milk	1 serv	170
Mocha w/o Whipping Cream Tall Nonfat Milk	1 serv	140
Mocha w/o Whipping Cream Tall Whole Milk	1 serv	190
Mocha Syrup Grande	1 serv (2 oz)	80
Mocha Syrup Short	1 serv (1 oz)	40
Mocha Syrup Tall	1 serv (1.5 oz)	60
Steamed Lowfat Milk Grande	1 serv	180
Steamed Lowfat Milk Short	1 serv	90
Steamed Lowfat Milk Tall	1 serv	140
Steamed Nonfat Milk Grande	1 serv	130
Steamed Nonfat Milk Short	1 serv	60
Steamed Nonfat Milk Tall	1 serv	100
Steamed Whole Milk Grande	1 serv	230
Steamed Whole Milk Short	1 serv	110
Steamed Whole Milk Tall	1 serv	180
Whipping Cream Grande	1 serv (1.1 oz)	110
Whipping Cream Short	1 serv (0.7 oz)	70
Whipping Cream Tall	1 serv (0.8 oz)	80

STUFF'N TURKEY

FOOD	PORTION	CALS.
Chef's Salad	1 serv	288
Grilled Turkey Breast	1 serv	244
Homemade Turkey Salad	1 serv	651
Real Fresh Roasted Turkey Breast	1 serv	384
Rotisserie Turkey Breast	1 serv	251
Thanksgiving Dinner On A Sandwich	1 serv	605

FOOD	PORTION	CALS.
Turkey Powerhouse	1 serv	482
Turkey Barbecue	1 serv	478

SUBWAY
COOKIES
Chocolate Chip	1 (1.3 oz)	161
Chocolate Chip M&M	1 (1.3 oz)	162
Chocolate Chip Walnut	1 (1.3 oz)	165
Chocolate Chunk	1 (1.3 oz)	160
Double Chocolate Brazil Nut	1 (1.3 oz)	200
Oatmeal Raisin	1 (1.3 oz)	147
Peanut Butter	1 (1.3 oz)	169
Sugar	1 (1.3 oz)	178
Toffee Crunch	1 (1.3 oz)	153
White Chocolate Chip	1 (1.3 oz)	166
White Chocolate Macadamia Nut	1 (1.3 oz)	174

SALAD DRESSINGS
Creamy Italian	1 tbsp	65
Fat Free French	1 tbsp	15
Fat Free Italian	1 tbsp	5
Fat Free Ranch	1 tbsp	12
French	1 tbsp	65
Ranch	1 tbsp	87
Thousand Island	1 tbsp	65

SALADS AND SALAD BARS
Bread Bowl	1 serv	290
Roasted Chicken Breast Fillet	1 serv	143
Subway Club	1 serv	123
Subway Seafood & Crab	1 serv	238
Subway Seafood & Crab w/ Light Mayonnaise	1 serv	155
Tuna	1 serv	345
Tuna w/ Light Mayonnaise	1 serv	194
Turkey Breast	1 serv	99
Veggie Delight	1 serv	45

SUBS AND SANDWICHES
6-Inch Cold Classic Italian B.M.T.	1	434
6-Inch Cold Cold Cut Trio	1	347
6-Inch Cold Ham	1	273
6-Inch Cold Roast Beef	1	299
6-Inch Cold Subway Club	1	300
6-Inch Cold Subway Seafood & Crab	1	415
6-Inch Cold Subway Seafood & Crab w/ Light Mayonniase	1	333

FOOD	PORTION	CALS.
6-Inch Cold Tuna	1	522
6-Inch Cold Tuna w/ Light Mayonnaise	1	372
6-Inch Cold Turkey Breast	1	276
6-Inch Cold Turkey Breast & Ham	1	275
6-Inch Cold Veggie Delight	1	223
6-Inch Hot Meatball	1	411
6-Inch Hot Roasted Chicken Breast Fillet	1	321
6-Inch Hot Steak & Cheese	1	363
6-Inch Hot Subway Melt	1	361
Bacon	2 strips	45
Cheese	2 triangles	41
Jumbo Deli Bologna	1	446
Jumbo Deli Ham	1	259
Jumbo Deli Roast Beef	1	335
Jumbo Deli Subway Seafood & Crab	1	472
Jumbo Deli Subway Seafood & Crab w/ Light Mayonnaise	1	348
Jumbo Deli Tuna w/ Light Mayonnaise	1	406
Jumbo Deli Tuna w/ Light Mayonnaise	1	632
Jumbo Deli Turkey Breast	1	290
Junior Deli Bologna	1	270
Junior Deli Ham	1	218
Junior Deli Roast Beef	1	232
Junior Deli Subway Seafood & Crab	1	279
Junior Deli Subway Seafood & Crab w/ Light Mayonnaise	1	238
Junior Deli Tuna	1	332
Junior Deli Tuna w/ Light Mayonnaise	1	257
Junior Deli Turkey Breast	1	218
Light Mayonnaise	1 tsp	18
Mayonnaise	1 tsp	37
Mustard	2 tsp	8
Olive Oil Blend	1 tsp	45
Vinegar	1 tsp	1

T.J. CINNAMONS

FOOD	PORTION	CALS.
Doughnuts Cake	2	454
Doughnuts Raised	2	352
Mini-Cinn Plain	1	75
Mini-Cinn With Icing	1	80
Original Gourmet Cinnamon Roll Plain	1	630
Original Gourmet Cinnamon Roll With Icing	1	686
Petite Cinnamon Roll Plain	1	185
Petite Cinnamon Roll With Icing	1	202

FOOD	PORTION	CALS.
Sticky Bun Cinnamon Pecan	1	607
Sticky Bun Petite Cinnamon Pecan	1	255
Triple Chocolate Classic Roll Plain	1	412
Triple Chocolate Classic Roll With Icing	1	462

TCBY

FOOD	PORTION	CALS.
Nonfat All Flavors	1 reg (8.2 fl oz)	226
Nonfat All Flavors	1 kiddie (3.2 fl oz)	88
Nonfat All Flavors	1 lg (10.5 fl oz)	289
Nonfat All Flavors	1 giant (31.6 fl oz)	869
Nonfat All Flavors	1 sm (5.9 fl oz)	162
Nonfat All Flavors	1 super (15.2 fl oz)	418
Regular All Flavors	1 lg (10.5 fl oz)	341
Regular All Flavors	1 giant (31.6 fl oz)	1027
Regular All Flavors	1 sm (5.9 fl oz)	192
Regular All Flavors	1 kiddie (3.2 fl oz)	104
Regular All Flavors	1 super (15.2 fl oz)	494
Sugar Free All Flavors	1 sm (5.9 fl oz)	118
Sugar Free All Flavors	1 lg (10.5 fl oz)	210
Sugar Free All Flavors	1 reg (8.2 fl oz)	164
Sugar Free All Flavors	1 super (15.2 fl oz)	304
Sugar Free All Flavors	1 kiddie (3.2 fl oz)	64
Sugar Free All Flavors	1 giant (31.6 fl oz)	632

TGI FRIDAY'S

FOOD	PORTION	CALS.
Chili Yogurt	1 serv	30
Corn Salsa	1 serv	175
Fresh Vegetable Medley w/ Potato	1 serv	470
Fresh Vegetable Medley w/ Rice	1 serv	407
Friday's Gardenburger	1	445
Garden Dagwood Sandwich	1 serv	375
Pacific Coast Chicken	1 serv	415
Pacific Coast Tuna	1 serv	410
Pea Salsa	1 serv (6.4 oz)	175
Plum Sauce	1 serv	105
Salad & Baked Potato	1 serv	250
Turkey Burger	1 (9.8 oz)	410

TACO BELL

FOOD	PORTION	CALS.
Bean Burrito	1 (6.9 oz)	390
Burrito Supreme	1 (8.7 oz)	440
Burrito Beef	1	431
Burrito Combo	1	407
Chilito	1	383
Cinnamon Twists	1 serv	171

FOOD	PORTION	CALS.
Green Sauce	1 oz	4
Guacamole	0.6 oz	34
Jalapeno Peppers	3.5 oz	20
Light 7-Layer Burrito	1 (9.7 oz)	440
Light Bean Burrito	1 (6.9 oz)	330
Light Burrito Supreme	1 (8.7 oz)	350
Light Chicken Burrito	1 (6 oz)	290
Light Chicken Burrito Supreme	1 (8.7 oz)	410
Light Soft Taco	1 (3.5 oz)	180
Light Soft Taco Chicken	1 (4.2 oz)	180
Light Soft Taco Supreme	1 (4.5 oz)	200
Light Taco	1 (2.7 oz)	140
Light Taco Salad w/ Chips	1 (18.8 oz)	680
Light Taco Salad w/o Chips	1 (16.2 oz)	330
Light Taco Supreme	1 (5.6 oz)	160
MexiMelt Beef	1	266
MexiMelt Chicken	1	257
Mexican Pizza	1	575
Nacho Cheese Sauce	2 oz	103
Nachos	1 serv	346
Nachos Bellgrande	1	649
Pico De Gallo	1 oz	6
Pintos 'N Cheese	1	190
Ranch Dressing	2.5 oz	236
Red Sauce	1 oz	10
Salsa	0.3 oz	18
Soft Taco	1 (3.5 oz)	220
Soft Taco Supreme	1 (4.5 oz)	270
Sour Cream	0.66 oz	46
Taco	1 (2.7 oz)	180
Taco Salad	1 (18.8 oz)	860
Taco Salad w/o Shell	1	484
Taco Sauce	1 pkg	2
Taco Sauce Hot	1 pkg	3
Taco Supreme	1	230
Tostada	1	243

TACO JOHN'S
CHILDREN'S MENU SELECTIONS

Kid's Meal Softshell Taco	1 serv (8.5 oz)	623
Kid's Meal Taco Burger	1 serv (8.75 oz)	668
Kids's Meal Crispy Taco	1 serv (8 oz)	575

DESSERTS

Choco Taco	1 serv (3.5 oz)	320

FOOD	PORTION	CALS.
Churro	1 serv (1.5 oz)	147
Flauta Apple	1 serv (2 oz)	84
Flauta Cherry	1 serv (2 oz)	143
Flauta Cream Cheese	1 serv (2 oz)	181
MAIN MENU SELECTIONS		
Bean Burrito	1 (6 oz)	294
Beans Refried	1 serv (9.25 oz)	301
Beef Burrito	1 (5.25 oz)	309
Chicken Fajita Burrito	1 (6.25)	294
Chicken Fajita Salad w/o Bowl	1 serv (11 oz)	254
Chicken Fajita Salad w/o Dressing	1 serv (12.25 oz)	561
Chicken Fajita Softshell	1 (4 oz)	149
Chili Texas Style w/ 2 Saltines	1 serv (9.25 oz)	297
Chimichanga Platter	1 serv (18.5 oz)	922
Combination Burrito	1 (6 oz)	378
Crispy Tacos	1 serv (3 oz)	178
Double Enchilada Platter	1 serv (18.5 oz)	901
Mexi Rolls w/ Guacamole	1 serv (9.75 oz)	839
Mexi Rolls w/ Nacho Cheese	1 serv (9.75 oz)	813
Mexi Rolls w/ Salsa	1 serv (9.75 oz)	754
Mexi Rolls w/ Sour Cream	1 serv (9.75)	854
Mexican Pizza	1 (9.75 oz)	636
Mexican Rice	1 serv (8 oz)	567
Nacho Cheese	1 serv (2 oz)	80
Nachos	1 serv (3.5 oz)	294
Potato Oles	1 serv (5.55 oz)	442
Potato Oles w/ Nacho Cheese	1 serv (7.55 oz)	523
Salad Dressing House	1 serv (2 oz)	114
Sampler Platter	1 serv (25 oz)	1276
Sierra Chicken Fillet Sandwich	1 (8.5 oz)	500
Smothered Burrito Platter	1 serv (19 oz)	972
Softshell Taco	1 (4 oz)	165
Sour Cream	1 oz	60
Super Burrito	1 (8.5 oz)	424
Super Nachos	1 serv (13 oz)	848
Taco Bravo	1 (6 oz)	332
Taco Burger	1 (5 oz)	275
Taco Salad w/o Bowl	1 (11 oz)	276
Taco Salad w/o Dressing	1 (10.5 oz)	469

TACOTIME

Beef	1 serv (2.5 oz)	115
Burrito Casita	1 (12 oz)	602
Burrito Casita w/o Sour Cream Dressing	1 (11 oz)	537

FOOD	PORTION	CALS.
Burrito Crisp Bean	1 (5.25 oz)	391
Burrito Crisp Meat	1 (5.25 oz)	393
Burrito Soft Bean	1 (9 oz)	547
Burrito Soft Bean w/o Cheese	1 (8.25 oz)	462
Burrito Soft Combo	1 (9 oz)	550
Burrito Soft Combo w/o Cheese	1 (8.25 oz)	465
Burrito Soft Meat	1 (9 oz)	552
Burrito Soft Meat w/o Cheese	1 (8.25 oz)	467
Burrito Veggie	1 (11.25 oz)	535
Burrito Veggie w/o Sour Cream	1 (10.75 oz)	502
Burrito Veggie w/o Sour Cream & Cheese	1 (10.25 oz)	477
Casa Sauce	1 serv (1 oz)	40
Cheese	1 serv (0.75 oz)	85
Chicken	1 serv (3 oz)	135
Chips	1 serv (2 oz)	239
Crustos	1 serv (3.5 oz)	373
Empanada Cherry	1 (4 oz)	250
Guacamole	1 serv (1 oz)	50
Hot Sauce	1 serv (1 oz)	10
Lettuce	1 serv (0.5 oz)	2
Mexi-Fries	1 reg (4 oz)	266
Mexi-Fries	1 lg (8 oz)	532
Mexican Brown Rice	1 serv (4 oz)	160
Mexican Dressing No Fat	1 serv (2 oz)	20
Olives	1 serv (0.50 oz)	16
Ranchero Salsa	1 serv (2 oz)	18
Refritos	1 serv (7 oz)	378
Refritos w/o Cheese	1 serv (6.25 oz)	293
Sauce	1 serv (1 oz)	14
Side Salad w/o Dressing	1 serv (3.75 oz)	106
Side Salad w/o Dressing & Cheese	1 serv (3.25 oz)	51
Soft Flour Taco	1 (6.5 oz)	416
Soft Flour Taco w/o Cheese	1 (5.75 oz)	331
Soft Taco Chicken	1 (6.5 oz)	390
Soft Taco Chicken w/o Cheese	1 (6 oz)	335
Sour Cream	1 serv (1 oz)	65
Sour Cream Dressing	1 serv (1.5 oz)	135
Taco	1 (4 oz)	218
Taco Cheese Burger	1 (8.25 oz)	589
Taco Cheese Burger w/o Thousand Island Dresssing	1 (7.25 oz)	482
Taco Cheese Burger w/o Thousand Island Dresssing & Cheese	1 (6.5 oz)	397
Taco Shell 6 in	1 (0.5 oz)	78

FOOD	PORTION	CALS.
Taco Salad	1 serv (9.25 oz)	447
Taco Salad Chicken	1 serv (11 oz)	571
Taco Salad Chicken w/o Sour Cream Dressing	1 serv (9.5 oz)	436
Taco Salad Chicken w/o Sour Cream Dressing & Cheese	1 serv (9 oz)	381
Taco Salad w/o Sour Cream Dressing	1 serv (7.75 oz)	347
Taco Salad w/o Sour Cream Dressing & Cheese	1 serv (7 oz)	262
Thousand Island Dressing	1 serv (1 oz)	107
Tomato	1 serv (0.50 oz)	3
Tortilla 6 in	1 (1 oz)	50
Tortilla Flour 10 in	1 (2.25 oz)	199
Tortilla Flour 8 in	1 (1.25 oz)	107
Tortilla Fried Flour 10 in	1 (2.5 oz)	209
Tortilla Fried Flour 8 in	1 (1.5 oz)	170
Tortilla Wheat 11 in	1 (3.5 oz)	175
Tostada Meat	1 serv (7.5 oz)	409
Tostada Meat w/o Cheese	1 serv (6.75 oz)	324
Tostada Delight Meat	1 (9.75 oz)	560
Tostada Delight Meat w/o Sour Cream	1 (8.75 oz)	495
Tostada Delight Meat w/o Sour Cream & Cheese	1 (8 oz)	410
Veggie Salad w/o Dressing	1 serv (8.5 oz)	357
Veggie Salad w/o Dressing & Cheese	1 serv (8 oz)	302

TROPIGRILL

(Restaurants in this chain may also be called Pollo Tropical. Menu items are the same for both.)

Banana Tropical	1 serv (7.55 oz)	498
Black Beans (combo meal portion)	1 serv (4.78 oz)	153
Black Beans (side)	1 serv (8.39 oz)	269
Boiled Yuca	1 serv (12 oz)	334
Boneless Breast	1 serv (3.14 oz)	140
Cheese Potatoes	1 serv (7.42 oz)	177
Chicken ¼ Dark Meat	1 serv (4.52 oz)	298
Chicken ¼ Dark Meat w/o Skin	1 serv (3.42 oz)	170
Chicken ¼ White Meat	1 serv (5.09 oz)	295
Chicken ¼ White Meat w/o Skin	1 serv (3.82 oz)	167
Chicken Caesar Sandwich	1 (6.4 oz)	457
Chicken Sandwich	1 (7.92 oz)	442
Congri	1 serv (7.08 oz)	439
Vegetable Kabob	1 (3.07 oz)	106
White Rice	1 serv (6.82 oz)	341

FOOD	PORTION	CALS.
Yellow Rice	1 serv (7 oz)	294
Yucatan Fries	1 serv (5.3 oz)	440

UNO RESTAURANT
DeepDish Pizza	1 serving	770

VILLAGE INN
French Toast Cinnamon Raisin	1 serv	809
Fruit & Nut Pancakes Low Cholesterol	1 serv	936
Omelette Chcken & Cheese	1 serv	721
Omelette Fresh Veggie	1 serv	704
Omelette Mushroom & Cheese	1 serv	680
Turkey & Vegetable Scrambled Sensation	1 serv	726

WENDY'S
CHILDREN'S MENU SELECTIONS

Kid's Meal Cheeseburger	1 (4.3 oz)	320
Kid's Meal Hamburger	1 (3.9 oz)	270

DESSERTS

Chocolate Chip Cookie	1 (2 oz)	270
Frosty Dairy Dessert	1 sm (12 oz)	340
Frosty Dairy Dessert	1 lg (20 fl oz)	570
Frosty Dairy Dessert	1 med (16 fl oz)	460

MAIN MENU SELECTIONS

¼ lb Hamburger Patty	1 (2.6 oz)	200
2 Oz Hamburger Patty	1 (1.3 oz)	100
American Cheese	1 slice (0.6 oz)	70
American Cheese Jr.	1 slice (0.4 oz)	45
Bacon	1 strip (0.2 oz)	30
Baked Potato Bacon & Cheese	1 (13.3 oz)	540
Baked Potato Broccoli & Cheese	1 (14.4 oz)	470
Baked Potato Cheese	1 (13.4 oz)	570
Baked Potato Chili & Cheese	1 (15.4 oz)	620
Baked Potato Plain	1 (10 oz)	310
Baked Potato Sour Cream & Chives	1 (11 oz)	380
Big Bacon Classic	1 (10.1 oz)	610
Breaded Chicken Fillet	1 (3.5 oz)	230
Breaded Chicken Sandwich	1 (7.3 oz)	440
Cheddar Cheese Shredded	2 tbsp (0.6 oz)	70
Chicken Club Sandwich	1 (7.7 oz)	500
Chicken Nuggets	6 pieces (3.3 oz)	280
Chili	1 sm (8 oz)	210
Chili	1 lg (12 oz)	310
French Fries	1 med (4.6 oz)	380
French Fries	1 Biggie (5.6 oz)	460

FOOD	PORTION	CALS.
French Fries	1 sm (3.2 oz)	260
Grilled Chicken Fillet	1 (2.5 oz)	100
Grilled Chicken Sandwich	1 (6.2 oz)	290
Honey Mustard Reduced Calorie	1 tsp (0.2 oz)	25
Jr. Bacon Cheeseburger	1 (6 oz)	410
Jr. Cheeseburger	1 (4.5 oz)	320
Jr. Cheeseburger Deluxe	1 (6.3 oz)	360
Jr. Hamburger	1 (4.1 oz)	270
Kaiser Bun	1 (2.4 oz)	190
Ketchup	1 tsp (0.2 oz)	10
Lettuce	1 leaf (0.5 oz)	0
Mayonnaise	1½ tsp (0.3 oz)	30
Mustard	½ tsp (0.2 oz)	5
Nuggets Sauce Barbeque	1 pkg (1 oz)	50
Nuggets Sauce Honey	1 pkg (0.5 oz)	45
Nuggets Sauce Sweet & Sour	1 pkg (1 oz)	45
Nuggets Sauce Sweet Mustard	1 pkg (1 oz)	50
Onion	4 rings (0.5 oz)	0
Pickles	4 slices (0.4 oz)	0
Plain Single	1 (4.7 oz)	360
Saltines	2 (0.2 oz)	25
Sandwich Bun	1 (2 oz)	160
Single With Everything	1 (7.7 oz)	420
Sour Cream	1 pkt (1 oz)	60
Whipped Margarine	1 pkg (0.5 oz)	60
SALAD DRESSINGS		
Blue Cheese	2 tbsp (1 oz)	170
French	2 tbsp (1 oz)	120
French Fat Free	2 tbsp (1 fl oz)	30
French Sweet Red	2 tbsp (1 oz)	130
Hidden Valley Ranch	2 tbsp (1 oz)	90
Hidden Valley Ranch Reduced Fat Reduced Calorie	2 tbsp (1 oz)	60
Italian Caesar	2 tbsp (1 fl oz)	150
Italian Caesar	2 tbsp (1 oz)	150
Italian Reduced Fat Reduced Calorie	2 tbsp (1 oz)	40
Salad Oil	1 tbsp (0.5 fl oz)	130
Thousand Island	2 tbsp (1 oz)	130
Wine Vinegar	1 tbsp (0.5 fl oz)	0
SALADS AND SALAD BARS		
Applesauce	2 tbsp (1.4 oz)	30
Bacon Bits	2 tbsp (0.5 oz)	45
Bananas & Strawberry Glaze	¼ cup (1.6 oz)	30
Broccoli	¼ cup (0.5 oz)	0

FOOD	PORTION	CALS.
Cantaloupe	1 piece (1.6 oz)	15
Carrots	¼ cup (0.6 oz)	5
Cauliflower	¼ cup (0.6 g)	0
Ceasar Side Salad	1 (3.1 oz)	110
Cheese Shredded Imitation	2 tbsp (0.6 oz)	50
Chicken Salad	2 tbsp (1.2 oz)	70
Chow Mein Noodles	¼ cup (0.2 oz)	35
Cole Slaw	2 tbsp (1.3 oz)	45
Cottage Cheese	2 tbsp (1.1 oz)	30
Croutons	2 tbsp (0.2 oz)	30
Cucumbers	2 slices (0.5 oz)	0
Deluxe Garden Salad	1 (9.5 oz)	110
Eggs Hard Cooked	2 tbsp (0.9 oz)	40
Green Peas	2 tbsp (0.7 oz)	15
Green Peppers	2 pieces (0.3 oz)	0
Grilled Chicken Salad	1 (11.9 oz)	200
Honeydew Melon Sliced	1 piece (1.8 oz)	20
Lettuce Iceberg/Romaine	1 cup (2.6 oz)	10
Mushrooms	¼ cup (0.5 oz)	0
Orange Sliced	2 slices (1.1 oz)	15
Parmesan Cheese Grated	2 tbsp (0.5 oz)	70
Pasta Salad	2 tbsp (1.2 oz)	35
Peaches Sliced	1 piece (1 oz)	15
Pepperoni Sliced	6 slices (0.2 oz)	30
Pineapple Chunks	4 pieces (1.1 oz)	20
Potato Salad	2 tbsp (1.3 oz)	80
Pudding Chocolate	¼ cup (1.8 oz)	70
Pudding Vanilla	¼ cup (1.8 oz)	70
Red Onions	3 rings (0.5 oz)	0
Seafood Salad	¼ cup (1.3 oz)	70
Sesame Breadstick	1 (0.1 oz)	15
Side Salad	1 (5.4 oz)	60
Soft Breadstick	1 (1.5 oz)	130
Strawberries	1 (0.9 oz)	10
Sunflower Seeds & Raisins	2 tbsp (0.5 oz)	80
Taco Salad	1 (17.9 oz)	590
Tomatoes Wedged	1 piece (0.9 oz)	5
Turkey Ham Diced	2 tbsp (0.8 oz)	50
Watermelon Wedged	1 piece (2.2 oz)	20

WHATABURGER
BAKED SELECTIONS

FOOD	PORTION	CALS.
Apple Turnover	1	215
Blueberry Muffin	1	239

FOOD	PORTION	CALS.
Buttermilk Biscuit	1	280
Cookie Chocolate Chunk	1	247
Cookie Macadamia Nut	1	269
Cookie Oatmeal Raisin	1	222
Cookie Peanut Butter	1	262
Pecan Danish	1	270
BEVERAGES		
Shake Chocolate	1 (12 fl oz)	364
Shake Strawberry	1 (12 fl oz)	352
Shake Vanilla	1 (12 fl oz)	325
BREAKFAST SELECTIONS		
Biscuit With Bacon	1	359
Biscuit With Egg And Cheese	1	434
Biscuit With Egg, Cheese And Bacon	1	511
Biscuit With Egg, Cheese And Sausage	1	601
Biscuit With Gravy	1	479
Biscuit With Sausage	1	446
Breakfast Platter With Bacon	1 serv	695
Breakfast Platter With Sausage	1 serv	785
Breakfast On A Bun	1	455
Breakfast On A Bun Bacon	1	365
Butter	1 pkg	36
Egg Omelette Sandwich	1	288
Grape Jelly	1 pkg	38
Hash Brown	1	150
Honey	1 pkg	27
Margarine	1 pkg	25
Pancake Syrup	1 pkg	169
Pancakes	3	259
Pancakes w/ Sausage	1 serv	426
Srambled Eggs	2 eggs	189
Strawberry Jam	1 pkg	37
MAIN MENU SELECTIONS		
Bacon	1 slice	38
Baked Potato	1	310
Baked Potato w/ Broccoli Cheese Topping	1	453
Baked Potato w/ Chesse Topping	1	510
Baked Potato w/ Mushroom Topping	1	360
Cheese Large	1 serv	89
Cheese Small	1 serv	46
Chicken Sandwich Grilled	1	442
Chicken Sandwich Grilled w/o Dressing	1	385
Club Crackers	1 pkg	31
Croutons	1 serv	29

FOOD	PORTION	CALS.
Fajita Taco Beef	1	326
Fajita Taco Chicken	1	272
French Fries	1 junior	221
French Fries	1 reg	332
French Fries	1 lg	442
Garden Salad w/o dressing	1	56
Grilled Chicken Salad	1 serv	150
Jalapeno Pepper	1	3
Justaburger	1	276
Onion Rings	1 reg	329
Onion Rings	1 lg	493
Picante Sauce	1 pkg	5
Sour Cream	1 serv (2 oz)	121
Steak Sandwich	1	387
Taquito Bacon	1 serv	335
Taquito Potato	1 serv	446
Taquito Sausage	1 serv	443
Turkey Sandwich Grilled	1	439
Whataburger	1	598
Whataburger Double Meat	1	823
Whataburger Jr.	1	300
Whatacatch	1	475
Whatachick'n Deluxe	1	573
Whatachick'n Sandwich	1	501
SALAD DRESSINGS		
French	1 pkg	249
Ranch	1 pkg	364
Thousand Island	1 pkg	280
Vinaigrette Lite	1 pkg	36

WHITE CASTLE

Bun Only	1	74
Cheese Only	0.3 oz	31
Cheeseburger	2 (3.6 oz)	310
Fish w/o Tarter Sandwich	1	155
French Fries	1 reg	301
Grilled Chicken Sandwich	2 (4 oz)	250
Grilled Chicken Sandwich w/ Sauce	2 (4.8 oz)	290
Hamburger	2 (3.2 oz)	270
Onion Rings	1 reg	245
Sausage Sandwich	1	196
Sausage & Egg Sandwich	1	322

WINCHELL'S DONUTS

Apple Fritter	1 (4.25 oz)	580

FOOD	PORTION	CALS.
Cinnamon Crumb	1 (2 oz)	240
Cinnamon Roll	1 (3 oz)	360
Glazed Jelly	1 (3 oz)	300
Glazed Round	1 (1.75 oz)	210
Glazed Twist	1 (1.75 oz)	210
Iced Chocolate Bar	1 (2 oz)	220
Iced Chocolate Cake	1 (2 oz)	230
Iced Chocolate Devil's Food	1 (2 oz)	240
Iced Chocolate French	1 (1.89 oz)	220
Iced Chocolate Raised	1 (1.75 oz)	210
Plain	1 (1.58 oz)	200
Plain Donut Hole	1 (0.4 oz)	50

ZUZU

FOOD	PORTION	CALS.
Bean & Cheese Burrito Platter	1 serv	475
Beans	1 cup	210
Cheese Enchilada Platter	1 serv	395
Chicken Burrito Platter	1 serv	580
Chicken Taco Platter	1 serv	440
Chicken Taco w/o Mexican Cream	1	125
Frozen Yogurt	1 serv	200
Green Salad w/o Dressing or Avocado	1	20
Grilled Chicken Salad w/o Dressing	1 serv	305
Rice	1 cup	150
Salsa Roja Epazote	¼ cup	8
Tortilla Corn	1	35
Tortilla Flour	1	60

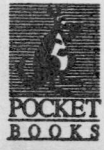